HANDBOOK OF

Drug
Therapy
in
Psychiatry

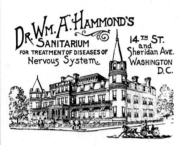
Advertisement from *Harper's New Monthly Magazine*, 1892, from the author's collection.

HANDBOOK OF

Drug Therapy in Psychiatry

THIRD EDITION

Jerrold G. Bernstein, MD

Assistant Clinical Professor
Department of Psychiatry
Harvard Medical School
and
Assistant Psychiatrist
Massachusetts General Hospital
and
Visiting Scientist
Department of Brain and Cognitive Sciences
Clinical Research Center
Massachusetts Institute of Technology

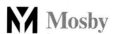 Mosby

St. Louis Baltimore Boston Carlsbad Chicago Naples New York Philadelphia Portland
London Madrid Mexico City Singapore Sydney Tokyo Toronto Wiesbaden

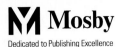

Dedicated to Publishing Excellence

A Times Mirror
Company

Editor: Laura DeYoung
Editorial Assistant: Alicia E. Moten
Project Manager: John Rogers
Designer: Renée Duenow
Manufacturing Supervisor: Linda Ierardi

THIRD EDITION
Copyright © 1995 by Mosby–Year Book, Inc.

Previous editions copyrighted 1988, 1983

Printed in the United States of America
Composition by Graphic World, Inc.
Printing/binding by R.R. Donnelley & Sons Company

Mosby–Year Book, Inc.
11830 Westline Industrial Drive
St. Louis, Missouri 63146

Library of Congress Cataloging in Publication Data

Bernstein, Jerrold G., 1941–
    Handbook of drug therapy in psychiatry / Jerrold G. Bernstein. — 3rd ed.
      p.   cm.
    Includes bibliographical references and index.
    ISBN 0-8016-8101-4
    1. Psychopharmacology—Handbooks, manuals, etc. 2. Psychotropic drugs—
Handbooks, manuals, etc.   3. Mental illness—Chemotherapy—Complications—
Handbooks, manuals, etc. I. Title.
    [DNLM: 1. Mental Disorders—drug therapy. 2. Psychotropic Drugs—
therapeutic use. WM 402 B531h 1995]
    RC483.B47   1995
    616.89′18—dc20   —dc20
    DNLM/DLC
    for Library of Congress   95-17730
                                        CIP

95 96 97 98 99 / 9 8 7 6 5 4 3 2 1

He who learns in order to teach
is granted the means to learn and to teach;
but he who learns in order to practice,
is granted the means to learn and to teach,
to observe and to practice.

Rabbi Ishmael
Ethics of the Fathers
(Mishna: *Pirke Avos*)

To my wife, Arlene,
who has provided continuing support and encouragement.
To our daughter, Janet and her husband, Daniel
and the next generation, Moshe Yechiel.
To our son, David,
for his continuing good advice and computer expertise.
And in memory of my parents.

About the Author

Jerrold G. Bernstein, MD, is *Assistant Clinical Professor of Psychiatry at Harvard Medical School* and Assistant Psychiatrist at the Massachusetts General Hospital. He is a Visiting Scientist in the Department of Brain and Cognitive Sciences, Clinical Research Center at Massachusetts Institute of Technology.

Dr. Bernstein, who has done both laboratory and clinical research, is the author of numerous research and clinical articles and books, including the first 2 editions of the *Handbook of Drug Therapy in Psychiatry,* which was published in 1983 and 1988 by PSG Publishing Company, Inc, Littleton, Mass. Dr. Bernstein is the editor of *Clinical Psychopharmacology,* published in two editions, 1978 and 1984, by PSG Publishing Company, Inc.

Dr. Bernstein has lectured and presented courses and symposia on drug therapy of psychiatric illnesses throughout the United States. He is a member of many professional and scientific societies, including the American Psychiatric Association, American College of Physicians, American Psychosomatic Society, and the Society of Biological Psychiatry. Dr. Bernstein was, for 11 years, Associate Medical Director of a psychiatric hospital and currently divides his time between research, teaching, and the clinical practice of psychopharmacology.

Foreword to the First Edition

N ew knowledge has increased so rapidly that psychopharmacology has become a group of scientific disciplines attempting to test the efficacy of various drugs in clinical trials and understand their mode of action on various neuropharmacologic and neuroendocrine systems. In parallel with these scientific advances, clinical psychopharmacologic practice has deeply influenced not only psychiatry but also other branches of medicine, particularly neurology, internal medicine and primary care.

In writing this volume, Dr. Jerrold Bernstein set three goals for himself: first, to summarize in practical terms, the current knowledge about the use of drugs in the treatment of patients with mental disorders; second, to relate clinical practice to scientific knowledge as to the modes of action of these drugs; and third, to incorporate his own extensive personal experience in research and in the care of psychiatric patients.

He has achieved his goals admirably. This volume is a comprehensive, readable guide for psychiatrists, medical students, psychiatric residents and nonpsychiatric physicians, particularly those in primary care and internal medicine. In addition, patients and their families may find this volume useful, particularly because of its systematic and understanding attention to the dilemmas and difficulties that patients and their families experience. The author responds to the need for psychiatrists and other physicians to carefully explain the nature of the patient's disorder, the goals to be achieved by the drugs and the likely pattern of improvement, as well as possible adverse effects.

This volume by a well-trained researcher and experienced clinician will go a long way toward bridging the gap between theory and practice in the clinical care of the mentally ill.

Gerald J. Klerman, MD
Harrington Professor of Psychiatry
Harvard Medical School
Director, Stanley Cobb
Psychiatric Research Laboratories
Massachusetts General Hospital
1983

ix

Foreword to the Second Edition

W ho among the many outstanding psychiatric clinicians of 40 years ago could have guessed or speculated that the synapse would become the focus of their therapeutic interventions? In fact, at that time few pharmaceutical agents were available to psychiatrists except for barbiturates and stimulants.

Among its many virtues, *The Handbook of Drug Therapy in Psychiatry* serves the purpose of bringing those who have slipped behind in psychopharmacology up to speed. The clear prose and lucid explanations in this book afford easy access to the present state of knowledge in this field. For the practicing psychiatrist who does not need a refresher course in the basics, this book will serve as an excellent reference in the general theory and practice of drug therapy in psychiatry.

Thomas P. Hackett, MD
Eben S. Draper Professor of Psychiatry
Harvard Medical School
Chief of Psychiatry
Massachusetts General Hospital
1988

Preface

The purpose of this handbook is to present a comprehensive discussion of the application of pharmacologic agents in the treatment of psychiatric patients and the complications that may arise from this form of therapy. This book has been designed to provide information on some of the biological aspects of psychiatric illnesses and mechanisms of action of psychotropic medications. In the past four decades, psychopharmacology has advanced from a small splinter within psychiatry to giant timbers, which are being used to construct new knowledge that can be applied to alleviate human suffering. Psychopharmacology draws heavily on information from neuroscience and is simultaneously contributing to the growth of this new scientific discipline.

Since the publication of the first edition of this book, many new and important psychotropic drugs have become available. Indeed, availability of selective serotonin reuptake inhibitors including fluoxetine, paroxetine and particularly sertraline has revolutionized the treatment of depression, obsessive compulsive disorder and panic disorder. Atypical neuroleptics, including clozapine and particularly risperidone may ultimately have a similar impact on the treatment and prophylaxis of psychotic disorders; simultaneous antagonism of dopamine receptors and 5-HT_2 serotonin sites may account for greater efficacy against negative schizophrenic symptoms and lesser extrapyramidal side effects, although the former drug has many potentially serious adverse effects, while risperidone lacks major adverse effects and appears free of the risk of leucopenia and agranulocytosis.

Laboratory and clinical research has further clarified the mechanisms of action of psychotropic drugs and provided new clinical approaches to optimize their therapeutic efficacy and reduce the risk of adverse drug reactions. Extensive investigations and clinical studies have demonstrated the potential utility of a variety of nonpsychotropic medications in the treatment of psychiatric illnesses. Research has also provided additional evidence for the biochemical etiologies of a variety of psychiatric conditions and has demonstrated the likelihood of genetic, biochemical, and therapeutic relationships between a number of psychiatric disorders formerly seen as separate and distinct entities.

The first edition of this book was written shortly after the introduction of the third edition of the *Diagnostic and Statistical Manual of Mental Disorders* (DSM-III) while the second edition followed the introduction of DSM-III-R. The current edition follows the recent publication of the newest diagnostic criteria, as presented in DSM-IV, from which I have quoted criteria, with permission of the American Psychiatric Association. It is my hope that with the advent of DSM-IV a better understanding of the nomenclature and criteria of different psychiatric disorders can facilitate advances in psychopharmacologic research and practice. In the new edition of this handbook, I have attempted to discuss many topics not covered in the previous editions and present more detailed discussions of many areas of psychopharmacology based on newer research and more extensive clinical experience of myself and others.

Many controversies exist regarding the biological etiology of psychopathology as well as the mechanisms of action of various psychotropic drugs. Considerable research in the past two decades has helped to further support genetic and biochemical factors in the etiology of a wide range of psychiatric conditions, and has further clarified many aspects of the therapeutic action and adverse effects of both psychotropic and nonpsychotropic drugs. I have tried to avoid confusing the reader with controversial issues regarding mechanisms of action and varying techniques in the administration of psychotropic medication by perhaps oversimplifying the issue and presenting the most practical available information on a given question. Perhaps the risk of oversimplifying is that the reader may disagree with some of my statements, for which I apologize, but I hope that what is gained from this approach will be a discussion that is understandable to the majority of readers.

With the help of computer-generated bibliographic information, I have read and reviewed a vast number of research and clinical publications and tried to select those references which not only help to document some of the points that I have made, but which may also be useful to the reader in furthering his own knowledge. I have also relied heavily on my clinical experience in the treatment of psychiatric patients in hospital and outpatient settings to provide information and advice that may be of practical value to the reader. Although research investigations are important in establishing knowledge, the clinical experience of others has taught me a great deal and I hope that my own clinical experience will help others.

My goal in writing this volume is to provide a textbook covering the general field of psychopharmacology that will be of interest to psychiatrists, nonpsychiatric physicians, and other mental health professionals as well as those being trained in medicine and mental health. In writing the first edition of this book, it was my feeling that what was needed was a volume that would present a broad base of information, which could be readily translated into the day-to-day practice of psychiatry. I have been gratified to receive many telephone calls and letters and to meet personally many people throughout the United States who have read the previous editions and found them helpful in their own practices. It is my sincere hope that this new edition will likewise be seen as a useful textbook and guide in the clinical practice of psychopharmacology.

My bias, for which I offer no apology, is that psychiatry must be seen as a branch of medicine, based on an organic understanding of the nervous system, the dysfunctions which affect it, and the drugs which will modify those dysfunctions. I urge all who will follow a career in psychiatry to obtain a firm grounding in scientific medicine, neurochemistry, and pharmacology. This is not to say that psychological concepts and psychotherapy are without value, but rather to acknowledge that with increasing understanding, more of the disorders that we treat will eventually be seen in the broader context of medical illnesses.

Regardless of how well we understand the etiology of psychiatric illnesses and how effective our medications may be, patient compliance remains an important limiting factor in the efficacy of pharmacologic intervention. The relationship between the patient and physician is the most critical determinant of therapeutic compliance. Interpersonal and psychotherapeutic skills can do much to enhance this relationship and facilitate effective pharmacotherapy. Though much has been written recently about noncompliance and the patient's right to refuse treatment, these are clearly not new problems. Ben Sira wrote in the second century BCE: "The L-rd has created medicines out of the earth, and a sensible man will not refuse them."

Jerrold G. Bernstein, MD
Newton Centre, Massachusetts

Acknowledgments

This book has been written as a guide to practicing clinicians. My formal training in internal medicine, clinical pharmacology, and psychiatry have all contributed immeasurably to make this task possible. I have tried to weave basic scientific information from biochemistry, pharmacology, clinical studies, and experience together in an attempt to synthesize these diverse but interrelated areas of knowledge. I have learned much from my teachers, sometimes more from my students, and usually, most from my patients. I have enjoyed the opportunity to work with medical students since my own graduation from medical school. In the past 20 years, I have been privileged to learn much from the residents that I have taught at the Massachusetts General Hospital. Shortly after the publication of the first edition of this handbook, I became affiliated with the Massachusetts Institute of Technology, where I have enjoyed continuing and exciting interchanges with scientific colleagues and with physicians, who have come there to study basic science and conduct clinical investigations. Throughout my years as a physician and psychiatrist, I have had the opportunity to evaluate and treat many patients with challenging illnesses. The opportunity to try novel approaches and to occasionally observe unexpected drug side effects has helped me to gain a better appreciation for the value and vicissitudes of psychopharmacologic intervention.

I am grateful to the many scientists and clinicians who have helped to shape my training and career. I am indebted to Dr. Edward J. Walaszek and the late Professor Bruno Minz for my early training in pharmacology at the University of Kansas. The late Drs. Louis Weinstein and Samuel Proger were of inestimable help during my internship and residency in internal medicine at New England Medical Center. Dr. David Rall of the National Institutes of Health provided rigorous scientific training. The late Dr. Aldo A. Luisada of Chicago and Dr. Roman W. DeSanctis of the Massachusetts General Hospital contributed immeasurably to my understanding of cardiovascular disease. Dr. Jan Koch-Weser formerly of the Massachusetts General Hospital not only contributed to my knowledge of clinical pharmacology and research methodology, but taught me to think clearly and express myself in writing. Dr. Jack H. Mendelson, under whom I received my training in psychiatry, continually encouraged me and stimulated my interest in the biological basis of mental illness.

My knowledge of psychopharmacology has been enriched by the warm friendship and colleagal relationship which I shared for many years with the late Dr. Gerald L. Klerman, who has contributed immeasurably to the field of

xvii

clinical psychopharmacology. Dr. Jonathan Cole has always been available to me as a source of ideas and encouragement in trying to define new psychopharmacologic approaches. My close association with Dr. Richard J. Wurtman, Director of the Clinical Research Center at Massachusetts Institute of Technology, has strengthened my knowledge of the scientific underpinnings of clinical psychopharmacology and provided continuing encouragement to explore potential novel therapeutic approaches.

The friendship and support of Dr. Thomas P. Hackett has been very meaningful and important to me since we first worked together more than twenty-five years ago. I feel honored that one of the last things which Dr. Hackett wrote was the foreword to the second edition, completed just weeks before his death.

When I first began working in this field, the literature was small and could be searched with ease during a day at the library. Tremendous advances have been made in the past four decades and the literature has expanded exponentially. Since any good textbook can at best serve to whet the reader's appetite for the field, a selection of important and current references must be provided not only to support the statements made, but to direct the reader to sources of additional data and information. I thank David Bernstein, who conducted extensive computer-assisted searches of databases so that the reader will have access to current and relevant references.

Contents

HANDBOOK OF

Drug
Therapy
in
Psychiatry

CHAPTER 1

Receptors, Drugs, and Neurotransmitters

OVERVIEW

1. Clinical use of psychotropic drugs requires an understanding of the interactions with neurotransmitters and their receptor sites.
2. Dopamine receptor density is increased in the brain in schizophrenia.
3. Antipsychotic drugs block dopamine receptors; new agents also antagonize $5HT_2$ receptors.
4. Depression appears to result from deficiencies of transmitters such as dopamine, norepinephrine, and serotonin or alteration of their receptors.
5. Antidepressants increase dopamine, norepinephrine, and serotonin activity in brain and downregulate receptors.
6. Deficient acetylcholine neurotransmission correlates with cognitive and memory impairment associated with aging and many psychotropic drugs.
7. Amino acids and other dietary precursors enhance brain neurotransmitter synthesis and may have therapeutic benefits in depression and cognitive disorders.
8. Abnormalities in brain norepinephrine, serotonin, and γ-aminobutyric acid neurotransmission may be the basis of anxiety disorders, and alterations in these systems may be the mechanism by which drugs alleviate anxiety.

Historically, psychiatry had its roots in the medical specialty of neurology. Psychiatry moved away from this brain-based discipline and more into the realm of social science and psychology. During the latter half of the twentieth century, psychiatry has gradually evolved back toward a brain-based medical specialty. Accidental discoveries of the behavioral and cognitive effects of drugs such as chlorpromazine, reserpine, and the monoamine oxidase inhibitors have contributed much to a scientific understanding of the relationships between brain function, psychiatric illness, and modern therapy. The applications of physical and chemical techniques in basic biology have given rise to a whole new realm of neuroscience. Positron emission tomography (PET) and single photon emission tomography (SPECT) have allowed us to examine brain physiology and neurotransmission in living human subjects.[1] Through the PET scan, increased density of dopamine receptors has been observed in nontreated schizophrenic patients.[2] Both techniques have revealed changes in acetylcholine receptors in patients with Alzheimer's disease and are being employed to examine neurochemical changes and the response to pharmacologic interventions in affective disorders.[1] As a result of the application of neuroscience techniques and studies of the response to pharmacologic intervention, it is becoming increasingly difficult to ignore the role of brain physiology and chemistry in psychiatric illness and treatment. A half century ago, it would have seemed like science fiction to think that the administration of a tablet or injection could abolish hallucinations or delusions or alleviate a profoundly incapacitating depression. Today, some of the psychodynamic concepts previously used to explain schizophrenia, depression, and panic disorder are beginning to sound fictional.

This chapter reviews concepts of the interaction of chemical substances with receptor sites present in the nervous system of living organisms. Rather than focus on the complexities of organic, physical, and biological chemistry, this topic is discussed in a simplified manner so that it can be readily understood and applied to the practice of pharmacotherapy in the psychiatric patient. This discussion addresses those neurotransmitters which are best known and have relevance to current knowledge and psychotropic drug action, although numerous other neurotransmitters and receptors remain to be understood and fit into the puzzle. Such understanding will eventually relate neuroscience to clinical practice. Since the focus of this volume is the treatment of the psychiatric patient, this chapter deals with the interaction of neurotransmitters, drugs, and receptor sites and the impact of this interaction on human behavior and mood.

NEUROPHYSIOLOGY AND NEUROTRANSMISSION

The human brain is composed of several billion neurons. Each neuron consists of a cell body with multiple short fibers, termed dendrites, which receive information from other neurons. Each neuron also has extending from the cell body a fiber known as an axon, which may be either short or long. The axon transmits information from the cell body to other neurons. Electrical impulses arising in the cell body travel through the axon to a specialized terminal known as the synapse. At the synaptic ending neurotransmitter substances are released which diffuse across the synaptic cleft and thereby transmit information to the dendrite of the next neuron.[3,4] Since the fibers of the multitude of neurons within the brain do not make physical connection with one another, electrical impulses generated within one neuron cannot jump the gap to the next neuron. Communication between them is dependent on the release of specialized chemical substances termed neurotransmitters. The ability of vast numbers of nerve fibers to transmit information between the billions of neurons within the brain involves a large number of neurotransmitter substances and their specialized sites of action, known as receptors. This complex neuronal circuitry and the specialized action of a variety of neurotransmitters regulate information

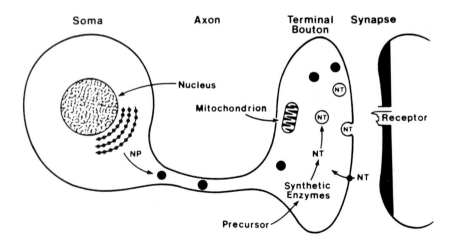

Fig. 1-1 Schematic representation of the neuron. The figure presents the main structural components of the neuron (not shown in scale) emphasizing those aspects involved in chemical neurotransmission. NP, Neuropeptide; NT, neurotransmitter. (*From Coyle JT (section ed): Neuroscience; In Tasman A, Goldfinger SM (eds):* APA annual review of psychiatry; *Washington DC, American Psychiatric Press, 1991, vol 10, pp 397-528.*)

handling, memory, mood, and behavior.[3] Structural and functional areas of the brain appear to be at least partially differentiated by their relative concentrations of chemically distinct neurotransmitters. The complexity of the electrochemical processes necessary for normal brain function makes the possibility of dysfunction readily understandable. As the electrical impulse travels down the axon, it causes the release of transmitters at the axon terminal. The transmitter substance then alters permeability of the dendritic membrane of the next neuron, resulting in either depolarization or hyperpolarization of the dendrites of the next neuron.[3] Once the transmitter has performed its function, it must be removed to terminate its action. It is understandable that the failure to terminate the action of a released neurotransmitter would be likely to prolong, inhibit, or exaggerate its action.[4] Likewise, the production and release of excess neurotransmitter or excessive sensitivity of the receptor site to the action of the neurotransmitter would produce an exaggerated effect at the cellular level, which may be seen as a clinical abnormality. On the other hand, deficient synthesis or release of neurotransmitter molecules, or decreased sensitivity of the receptor site, also would be likely to produce a physiologic abnormality which, again, could be manifested clinically in abnormalities of thought processes, mood, or behavior.[4]

Electron microscopic examination of neuronal junctions reveals that the width of the synaptic cleft separating the presynaptic membrane of the axon terminal from the postsynaptic membrane of the dendrite is approximately 100 to 500 nm.[4] Within the presynaptic terminal are numerous small synaptic vesicles. It is in these vesicles that neurotransmitter substances are stored prior to their release. Once the electrical impulse has triggered the release of the neurotransmitter from the vesicles, the transmitter diffuses across the synaptic cleft, stimulates the postsynaptic receptors, and is released from those receptors back into the synaptic cleft.[3,4] In the case of acetylcholine, one of the more ubiquitous neurotransmitters, there is rapid hydrolysis through the action of the enzyme acetylcholinesterase.[5] In the case of norepinephrine, another prominent CNS transmitter, a portion of the released substance is repackaged into synaptic vesicles within the presynaptic nerve terminal. The remainder of the norepinephrine is then metabolically degraded through the action of the enzyme monoamine oxidase (MAO). That portion of the released norepinephrine which has been repackaged into synaptic vesicles is not vulnerable to MAO-catalyzed inactivation, and it may be released again in response to an electrical impulse traveling down the axon in the fashion previously described.[3,6]

CLINICAL ASPECTS OF NEUROTRANSMITTERS

Having discussed in simplified form some aspects of neurotransmitter function, and before considering receptor sites and the actions of transmitters and drugs on them, some clinical aspects should be considered.[7] Neurotransmitter substances are formed endogenously within the CNS as well as within the autonomic nervous system. These substances are synthesized by the action of enzymes on simpler chemical molecules absorbed into the circulation as a result of the metabolism of food. Neurotransmitter chemicals are complex charged molecules. Although the brain receives voluminous blood flow, the passage of substances from the circulation into the brain is selective. This selectivity is the result of what has been termed the blood-brain barrier.[3] For a circulating chemical to reach neuronal elements within the brain, it must pass through not only the dense capillary wall but also through a fatty barrier called the glial sheath. This sheath is made up of glial feet which are extensions of nearby astrocyte cells.[3] The structure and function of the blood-brain barrier is potentially protective, preventing certain substances from entering the brain, and is potentially disadvantageous, limiting access to the brain of certain chemical substances that we might wish to administer for therapeutic purposes. Due to the nature of this barrier and the molecular structure of neurotransmitter substances, we are unable to increase brain concentration of these substances by administering them directly to the patient.[2,3]

The administration of neurotransmitter precursors will allow these substances to reach the brain and increase synthesis of certain neurotransmitters.[8] Oral administration of choline, a dietary precursor of acetylcholine formation, can increase brain concentrations of this neurotransmitter.[9] Oral administration of tyrosine,[10] the precursor of norepinephrine, and of tryptophan,[11,12] the precursor of serotonin, will increase brain concentrations of these neurotransmitters and may have therapeutic value in depression, which may result from a deficit of these neurotransmitters.[13] The best known clinical use of a neurotransmitter precursor is the therapeutic use of levodopa in Parkinson's disease.[14]

The termination of action of neurotransmitters through their metabolic breakdown has previously been mentioned. If the metabolic breakdown of certain neurotransmitters can be reduced or inhibited, the concentration and most likely the physiologic action of the neurotransmitter would be enhanced. Physostigmine inhibits cholinesterase, the enzyme responsible for terminating the action of acetylcholine.[5] Cholinergic activity can be enhanced by the administration of physostigmine since decreased breakdown of acetylcholine leads to increased cholinergic activity. Physostigmine has been used for a number of years in the evaluation and treatment of patients suffering from toxic deliria induced by the administration of excessive doses of anticholinergic drugs.[15,16] The MAO inhibitors were the first effective antidepressant drugs. They also provided neuropharmacologists with an opportunity to understand some of the connections between neurotransmitters and mood.[4] By inhibiting enzymatic breakdown of norepinephrine and other centrally occurring monoamine neurotransmitters, MAO inhibitor antidepressants, such as phenelzine, allow for increased brain concentration of neurotransmitters whose actions may be deficient in depressed patients. Tricyclic antidepressants (TCAs) inhibit nerve reuptake of both norepinephrine and serotonin; serotonin-selective reuptake inhibitors (SSRIs) inhibit only serotonin reuptake mechanisms, while bupropion inhibits dopamine and possibly norepinephrine reuptake, thus increasing availability of these neurotransmitters and alleviating neurotransmitter deficits which appear to underlie a variety of psychiatric illnesses.[4] Thus a variety of techniques aimed at either enhancing neurotransmitter synthesis or inhibiting inactivation have found their way into the practice of clinical psychiatry and have provided tools for understanding nervous system function.[4,8,15]

RECEPTORS, TRANSMITTERS, AND DRUGS

Having considered the formation and release of neurotransmitter substances as a result of the propagation of electrical impulses down the axon into the axon terminal, and their diffusion across the synaptic cleft to their site of action at the postsynaptic membrane, it is important now to consider the receptor site. A variety of complex protein molecules are present within the membrane structure of each of the multitude of specialized cells that make up the human body.[2-4] The variety of specialized receptor sites within the body is enormous, yet on the surface of any individual cell there may be only a few thousand receptor sites.[3] Any given cell may have one specific type of receptor or a variety of receptors. In recent years we have begun to learn more about the specific nature of receptors, although the theoretical concept originated about a century ago.[3,4]

Postsynaptic membranes contain specialized membrane-bound protein molecules that act as receptors. These specialized molecules respond selectively to endogenously released chemical transmitter substances including neurotransmitters and a variety of hormones.[3,4] The selectivity of receptor sites appears to be based on their individual physicochemical properties which make them uniquely responsive to particular molecular configurations.[4] If endogenously released chemical substances act through combination with selective receptor sites, then one may question the relevance of this to the actions of newly developed therapeutic agents. In general, exogenously administered drugs act within the body by affecting a receptor site whose presence is presumably for the purpose of responding to an endogenous substance of physicochemical properties resembling those of the drug.[5,6] Thus we have synthetically produced pharmaceutical products whose structural similarity is close enough to endogenously occurring substances that the drug product may mimic the naturally occurring substance. For example, the amphetamines are spoken of as sympathomimetic drugs because their action mimics the response to sympathetic nervous system stimulation. Indeed, they are chemically similar to norepinephrine, the naturally occurring transmitter active within the sympathetic nervous system.[6] Arecoline, a potent cholinergic compound, is called parasympathomimetic or cholinomimetic because its action mimics stimulation of the parasympathetic nervous system, presumably as a result of its ability to combine with and stimulate acetylcholine-sensitive receptor sites.[5,17]

Drugs and endogenous substances (agonists) combine with specific receptors and produce specific responses. The combination of a drug or agonist with the receptor site is dependent on the specific molecular structure of the agonist and the availability of properly matched characteristics of the receptor. This interaction gives rise to the concept of structure-activity relationship.[18] In order for a drug to combine with the receptor, it must bear a structural similarity to the naturally occurring agonist for that receptor. This bonding is dependent on specific chemical and physical characteristics of the agonist, the drug, and the receptor.[4,18] As we learn more about receptors, it becomes apparent that many subtypes of receptors for a specific agonist may occur. These subtypes of receptors are characterized by responsiveness to a variety of agonist and antagonist (receptor-blocking) compounds. It has been known for several decades that two types of cholinergic receptors exist, the nicotinic receptor and the muscarinic receptor. In the last few years, three subtypes of muscarinic receptors, M_1, M_2, and M_3, have been described and characterized.[19] For many years, we have been aware of the existence of alpha- and beta-adrenergic receptors; more recently, $alpha_1$-, $alpha_2$-, $beta_1$- and $beta_2$-receptors have been identified and characterized.[20] Likewise, recent work has identified multiple types of serotonin receptors, including 5-HT_1, 5-HT_2, and 5-HT_3.[21] Three functionally different types of dopamine receptors, D_1, D_2, and D_3, have also been identified.[4,21]

The muscarinic cholinergic receptor has been most extensively studied. This receptor appears to be composed of three or more subunits, each with a molecular weight of 40,000, which carry binding sites for cholinergic agonists and antagonists.[4,5] The interaction of agonist compounds with the receptor results in changes in sodium flux through the membrane as a result of change in state of a specific ionophore or ion-conductance modulator. Evidence suggests that this ionophore is a protein distinct from the receptor, with a molecular weight of 43,000, and that the receptor and ionophore are strongly associated with the cell membrane.[18,19] Those chemical substances which stimulate a receptor site and produce a physiologic effect similar to that produced by the action of the naturally occurring transmitter on that site are spoken of as agonists.[5] Chemical compounds whose molecular structure allows them to combine with receptor sites without stimulating the site or producing an agonist effect are known as antagonists.[4] An antagonist may be thought of as a receptor-blocking drug. The action of such compounds at receptor sites occupies the receptor and makes it unavailable to respond to endogenously released transmitter substances or exogenously administered agonist compounds.

Haloperidol exerts its antipsychotic action as a result of its ability to combine with and block dopamine receptor sites; thus it is a dopamine receptor antagonist.[22] Chlorpromazine is a relatively weak dopamine receptor antagonist which also blocks alpha-adrenergic receptors.[7] The ability of this compound to block alpha-adrenergic receptor sites in the peripheral vasculature accounts for its considerable ability to lower blood pressure.[7] Propranolol is a beta-adrenergic antagonist, which will decrease myocardial work, heart rate, and blood pressure[6] by blocking these receptor sites. Some drugs exert mixed agonist-antagonist

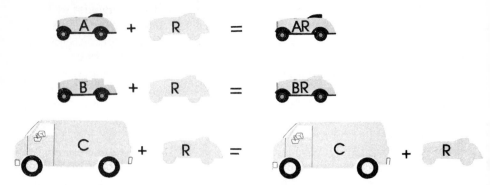

Fig. 1-2 Interaction of agonists (A) and antagonists (B) with receptors (R). A may be an endogenous agonist or an administered drug which conforms structurally and combines with the receptor (R) producing a response (AR) (eg, dopamine stimulates dopamine receptors). B is a drug that is similar but not identical to the naturally occurring agonist (A) and will thus combine with and occupy the receptor (R), blocking it (BR) and preventing the endogenous agonist from acting on the receptor to produce a response (eg, haloperidol blocks dopamine receptors preventing their stimulation by endogenous dopamine). C is an endogenous or exogenous compound that is structurally different from the receptor's agonist (A) and will therefore not combine with the receptor; thus C acts neither as an agonist nor as an antagonist (eg, the polypeptide, substance P, will not stimulate or block dopamine receptors but will act on specific substance P receptors).

activity and thereby may initially stimulate a receptor site and then block its further stimulation by other compounds, whether they be endogenously released or exogenously administered.[3,4]

CHEMICAL TRANSMITTERS IN BRAIN FUNCTION

Most psychiatrists have at least a passing acquaintance with the neurotransmitter role of acetylcholine, norepinephrine, dopamine, and serotonin, since the actions of many psychotropic drugs are linked to these transmitters.[3,4] It must be emphasized, however, that these transmitters, which we have come to accept as the most important ones, act at only a minority of the nerve terminals within the CNS.[3] Neuropeptides and a variety of amino acid–derived substances appear to have an even larger role in central neurotransmission.[4]

In some areas of the brain, γ-aminobutyric acid (GABA) serves a neurotransmitter function.[23] This compound may account for transmission in 25% to 40% of brain synapses.[4] GABA has the ability to inhibit firing of some neurons, and appears to function as the major inhibitory neurotransmitter.[23] The amino acid glycine appears to serve a similar inhibitory transmitter function in a large number of spinal cord and brainstem synapses.[3] Glutamic acid and aspartic acid, present in large concentration within the brain, appear

Box 1-1 A humorous view of the binding of ligands to receptors showing the role of structure specificity and of receptor antagonists

The Structurally Specific, Stereospecific, Saturable Binding of Pepperoni to Pizza

The binding of pepperoni (P) to pizza (Pizza) is well known (Doonesbury, 1982). In a recent study we have undertaken to elucidate the characteristics and mechanism of this binding. The following is a summary of the results of that study.

We have successfully demonstrated that the binding of the ligand P to Pizza is structurally specific, in that prior exposure of Pizza to various concentrations of kolbase, bratwurst or kosher salami will reduce, or in the extreme case prevent, the subsequent binding of P. This clearly demonstrates the structural specificity of the binding.

The suspected stereospecificity of the binding was confirmed when it was found that P would not bind to the underside of the Pizza. The specific receptor is presumed to be mozzarella (MMM) cheese because it had to be present for binding to occur. The binding characteristics of P to Pizza and to MMM were found to be very similar. Thus, while not absolutely certain, it does appear that it is the cheese that binds. The affinity of P for MMM was quantitatively related to the number of MMM strands appearing when separation of P from MMM was attempted. P was

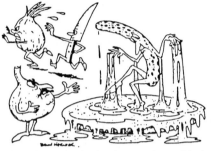

also shown, quite inadvertently, to bind (but not well) to napkins and trousers.

The binding of P to Pizza was found to be saturable, reaching satiation as an asymptomatic hyburpola. Onions and garlic both exerted alliosteric effects. Garlic's effect was potently expressed whereas onion's effect was dicey.

The structurally specific, stereospecific, saturable binding of P to Pizza is readily antagonized by a variety of agents, including olive oil (in excess) and anchovies. Of these, the anchovies appear to compete with P for binding sites while olive oil's antagonism is insurmountable.

The competitive antagonisms by anchovies and kosher salami each show quite different kinetics leading to the suggestion that there may be at least two different receptors for P. We have chosen to call these receptors P_1 and Poo-Poo.

Finally, it must be reported that, the above results notwithstanding, P's binding to Pizza is probably not of great functional significance and P may exert at best only a modulatory effect.

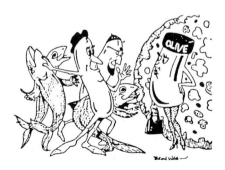

PAUL S. GUTH
Department of Pharmacology,
Tulane University,
New Orleans, LA 70112, U.S.A.

Reproduced from *Trends in Pharmacological Sciences (TIPS)*, December 1982, page 467, by permission of the author and the publisher, Elsevier Publications, Cambridge UK.

to act as excitatory neurotransmitters.[3] The widespread distribution of these amino acids throughout the brain and other body tissues has made it more difficult to study their role in neural function compared with those neurotransmitters whose distribution is somewhat more discrete.[3] A variety of peptide substances, derived from several amino acid molecules linked together, act as hormones and neurotransmitters in the brain and throughout the body.[4] Opiatelike peptides known as enkephalins bind to specific sites within the CNS and are known to mediate pain perception. Opiate receptors are sensitive not only to these endogenously produced compounds but also to exogenously administered narcotic analgesics. A larger molecule made up of methionine-enkephalin, linked to 26 other amino acids, is known as beta-endorphin. It is present in a high concentration within the pituitary and may serve a neurotransmitter function.[4,24] Another polypeptide, substance P, appears to have a role as a neurotransmitter mediating pain sensation.[25] This substance, along with GABA, may function as a naturally occurring tranquilizer, although much investigative work is still needed to clarify this role. Since each specific neuron within the brain utilizes primarily a single type of neurotransmitter compound, we have come to classify neurons not only on the basis of their physical structure and location but also on the basis of which neurotransmitter they release.

NEUROTRANSMISSION IN SPECIFIC NERVE TRACTS

There are two major norepinephrine tracts within the brain. The ventral pathway has cell bodies in several locations of the brainstem and axons that extend into the medial forebrain bundle and terminate at synapses, mainly in the hypothalamus and limbic system. This tract has terminals within the pleasure centers of the lateral hypothalamus, and appears to have a functional role in affective behaviors, including euphoria and depression.[4] The other major norepinephrine tract, the dorsal pathway, has cell bodies that are discretely localized to the locus ceruleus within the brainstem. Its axons also ascend in the medial forebrain bundle dorsal to those of the ventral pathway.[4] Terminals of the dorsal pathway are primarily localized in the cerebral cortex and hippocampus. Some axons from the locus ceruleus descend to form synapses with Purkinje cells within the cerebellum. Some cells of the locus ceruleus give off axons that branch ascending fibers to the cerebral cortex, as well as the cerebellum. Thus a single neuron may influence widespread areas of the brain. There is evidence that the dorsal norepinephrine pathway to the cerebral cortex may be associated with the control of alertness.[4]

There are a number of discrete dopaminergic tracts. The most prominent one has cell bodies in the substantia nigra and axons that terminate in the caudate nucleus and putamen, two structures of the corpus striatum which function to coordinate motor activity.[4] In Parkinson's disease there is deterioration of this pathway, giving rise to tremor and motor disorders that characterize this condition. Administration of the dopamine precursor, levodopa, helps to restore the neurotransmitter that is depleted and thus alleviates some of the symptoms of Parkinson's disease.[26] Other dopamine pathways have cell bodies close to the substantia nigra just dorsal to the interpeduncular nucleus, with terminals in the nucleus accumbens and olfactory tubercle which are components of the limbic system.[4] Furthermore, dopaminergic neurons within the cerebral cortex appear to have a role in emotional behavior. The ability of antipsychotic drugs to control symptoms of psychosis is directly related to blockade of these dopamine receptor sites.[27] Dopaminergic cells in the arcuate nucleus of the hypothalamus, with terminals in the median eminence, probably regulate the release of hypothalamic hormones, which then act on the pituitary gland to regulate the release of pituitary hormones.[27] Dopamine inhibits the release of prolactin from the pituitary gland. Dopamine-blocking antipsychotic drugs thus elevate plasma levels of the hormone prolactin, potentially giving rise to the side effects of abnormal milk secretion and amenorrhea when these therapeutic agents are administered to women.[4,27]

There are at least three subtypes of dopamine-sensitive receptors in the brain.[27,28] The dopamine receptor just described, the one thought to be most important to the action of neuroleptic drugs, is known as D_2.[27,28] The D_1 receptors are found on intrinsic striatal neurons; they are involved in parathormone release and stimulate adenylate cyclase. These receptors are less sensitive to neuroleptic drugs than are D_2 receptors. D_3 receptors are likewise relatively insensitive to neuroleptics; they are involved apparently in autoregulation of dopamine neurons and are found on intrinsic striatal neurons as well as nigrostriatal terminals. The D_2 receptors are found on intrinsic striatal neurons and on corticostriate afferents, as well as in the pituitary gland. D_2 sites are not associated with increased adenylate cyclase, but are highly sensitive to neuroleptics and are the receptors generally referred to in the action of psychoactive drugs on behavior.[28]

Cell bodies of the serotonin-containing neurons are localized in a series of nuclei of the lower midbrain and upper pons known as the raphe nuclei. It appears that most cells within these nuclei are serotonergic.[4] Axons of these cells ascend primarily in the medial forebrain bundle and give off terminals in all regions of the brain, although mostly within the hypothalamus. Destruction of the raphe nuclei in experimental animals produces agitation and insomnia.[4] Administration of the serotonin precursors, L-tryptophan or 5-hydroxytryptophan, will correct serotonin depletion and induce sleep in experimental animals.[29] The serotonin precursor, L-tryptophan, has been employed clinically in normal subjects and patients with insomnia to induce sleep.[30] Stimulation of the raphe nuclei in experimental animals likewise induces sleep.[29]

NEUROCHEMICAL BASES OF MENTAL DISORDERS

Over the years, a variety of attempts have been made to find chemical abnormalities in the blood and urine of individuals suffering from mental disorders. One limitation of studies of the biochemical mechanisms of mental disorders has been the fact that neurotransmitters present within the brain are also present in other body tissues. Thus measurements of chemical substances in body fluids reflect not only what is happening in the CNS but within other tissues as well. In the early years of this research, a variety of abnormalities were proposed to explain schizophrenia, affective disorders, and other disturbances of mental function. Actively psychotic schizophrenic patients have a very low incidence of allergic disorders and are relatively insensitive to the injection of test doses of histamine, due to the presence of increased serum concentrations of the metabolizing enzyme histaminase.[31] Over the years, various studies found apparent abnormalities in blood or urine concentrations of neurotransmitters and their metabolites; however, it was never possible to definitively attach a specific neurochemical defect to a specific psychiatric illness and be certain that the chemical defect reflected changes within the brain, rather than in the periphery.

Early experiments attempting to unravel the biochemistry of psychosis revealed that administration of the amino acids tryptophan or methionine could produce an exacerbation of psychotic symptoms in schizophrenic patients who are clinically in remission.[31] Other studies found that MAO inhibitor drugs could exacerbate symptoms in asymptomatic schizophrenic patients, presumably as a result of inhibition of catecholamine neurotransmitter metabolism.[31] The interaction of hallucinogenic drugs with serotonergic neurons may explain the ability of these compounds to provoke psychotic symptoms in normal subjects.[31]

Since data from studies of body fluids of patients have not been fully reliable and since, unlike other organs, we cannot remove a sample of brain tissue for analysis, our attempts to correlate brain chemistry with disease states depend on indirect documentation. An important source of data regarding chemical mechanisms of mental disorders involves the study of behavioral and cognitive responses to the administration of various drugs, neurotransmitter precursors, and enzyme inhibitors.

Recently developed radioisotope techniques of neuroscience have begun to be applied to the study of a wide range of psychiatric disorders. Utilizing these techniques, we are able to study electrophysiologic, metabolic, and neurochemical phenomena within the brains of living patients. The techniques include measurement of regional cerebral blood flow (rCBF), computerized EEG and evoked potential mapping, single photon emission computed tomography (SPECT), positron emission tomography (PET), and magnetic resonance imaging (MRI).[1] PET and SPECT are of particular interest because they allow us to study neurotransmitter receptors within the living brain, relatively noninvasively.[1] Studies utilizing these techniques have begun to reveal neurotransmitter receptor abnormalities in patients with a variety of psychiatric disorders. Unfortunately, the high cost and technical details of these approaches limit their current use to the research setting. It is hoped that in the future these techniques may be applied productively in the diagnosis of various psychiatric conditions, and perhaps also in monitoring responses to pharmacologic intervention.

Postmortem studies of brain tissue have revealed larger numbers of dopamine D_2 receptors in the basal ganglia of schizophrenic patients than are present in patients without a prior history of neurologic or psychiatric disease.[2] It has been suggested that the increased numbers of D_2 receptors found were related to prior treatment with neuroleptic drugs, rather than to the illness itself.[2] Studies employing PET have demonstrated significantly increased D_2 receptor density in the caudate nucleus of 15 schizophrenic patients in comparison with 11 normal volunteers.[2] Of the 15 patients studied, 10 had never received neuroleptic medication. The finding that D_2 receptors are substantially increased in schizophrenic patients who have never received neuroleptic drugs suggests that the abnormality is directly related to the disease process itself. Alternatively, the increased D_2 receptor number may reflect presynaptic factors such as increased endogenous dopamine concentration. Either condition, however, supports the concept that the dopamine receptor abnormality seen in schizophrenia is not simply the result of prior pharmacotherapy.[2]

PET and SPECT have demonstrated metabolic changes within the frontal lobes of affectively ill patients. Studies have found a decrease in glucose metabolic rate in patients with bipolar affective disorder and an increase in glucose metabolic rate in patients with unipolar affective disorder.[1,32] One study found higher metabolic rates in the frontal cortex of depressed patients treated with amoxapine and lower metabolic rates in imipramine-treated patients. Both these antidepressants elevated the glucose metabolic rate in the occipital cortex.[32] This study suggested that the differential effects of these two antidepressants observed by the PET technique were indicative of rapid downregulation of serotonin $5HT_2$ receptors by amoxapine and the absence of this effect with imipramine.[32]

Several lines of evidence indicate that patients with Alzheimer's disease have impaired cholinergic transmission within the brain. Patients with this disorder exhibit increased sensitivity to anticholinergic drugs and appear to have an impairment in their ability to synthesize acetylcholine. Quinuclidinyl benzoate (QNB) is a compound which binds with high affinity to the muscarinic cholinergic receptor. Utilizing iodine 123–labeled QNB and the technique of SPECT, impairment in muscarinic receptor binding function was found in a patient with Alzheimer's disease.[33] It is likely that the application of brain-imaging techniques will help to further elucidate the neurochemical abnormalities in Alzheimer's disease and a wide range of other neurologic and psychiatric disorders.

PSYCHOTIC ILLNESS

Although the currently available neuroleptics are rather widely divergent in their chemical structure, they have one unifying characteristic in common—namely, their ability to antagonize or block dopamine receptor sites. Their clinical potency closely parallels their affinity for these receptor sites.[22] Inhibition of dopamine receptors accelerates the firing rate of dopamine neurons, increasing dopamine metabolites. Chronic blockade of dopamine receptors by prolonged administration of antipsychotic drugs produces supersensitivity at receptor sites and increased numbers of dopamine receptors.[4] These changes appear to correlate with the primary adverse effects of antipsychotic drugs, namely, the possibility of producing tardive dyskinesia. Dopamine receptors can be measured by monitoring the binding to neuronal membranes of radioactive derivatives of neuroleptic drugs. To determine whether a drug blocks dopamine receptors, one ascertains if it will reduce the amount of radioactive neuroleptic bound to these sites. The relative potency of neuroleptics in blocking dopamine receptors measured in this way parallels their clinical potency, as previously mentioned.[22] Only drugs with neuroleptic activity antagonize dopamine receptors within the dose range used clinically. As will be discussed in chapter 4, the atypical agent clozapine and the newer antipsychotic risperidone antagonize serotonin 5-HT$_2$ receptors as well as D$_2$ receptors, which may explain their lesser likelihood of producing extrapyramidal side effects and tardive dyskinesia.

In contrast to this specificity of action, the potency of neuroleptics as antagonists of nondopamine neurotransmitter receptor sites does not correlate with antipsychotic potency.[34,35] The findings correlating dopamine receptor blockade with clinical potency of antipsychotic drugs suggests that an abnormality in dopamine release or action may underlie schizophrenic illness.[36] Amphetamines, when administered in large doses, produce a psychotic state that is clinically indistinguishable from paranoid schizophrenia.[36] Furthermore, when administered to schizophrenic patients, even low doses of amphetamines may exacerbate psychotic symptoms. The symptoms precipitated by amphetamine administration in schizophrenic patients vary from individual to individual and correlate well with the pattern of symptoms previously seen in the particular patients under study.[4] The structural similarity of the amphetamines to norepinephrine and dopamine suggests that these compounds may facilitate the action of the catecholamine neurotransmitters within the brain.[6,36] Amphetamines trigger the release of norepinephrine and dopamine from nerve endings into the synaptic cleft.[6] Although the final answer is not available on the mechanism of schizophrenic illness, the ability of agents which stimulate dopamine action to exacerbate psychosis, and the salutary effects of dopamine-blocking drugs on psychotic symptoms, strongly suggest that dopamine has a pivotal etiologic role in this form of psychotic illness.

It must be borne in mind that schizophrenia runs in families and that strong evidence supports a genetic factor in the etiology of this psychotic illness. Although the risk of developing schizophrenia is about 1% in the general population, 10% of siblings of schizophrenics are likely to develop the illness and 14% of children of affected patients are likely to develop schizophrenia.[31] If both parents suffer from schizophrenia, it is likely that about half their children will become schizophrenic,[4] although one may argue that environmental factors play a role in this predisposition. Studies of identical twins reared apart from each other and from their biologic parents have attempted to correct for environmental influence, thus focusing on the factors of genetic predisposition. Studies by Kety et al. of biologic and adoptive relatives of adopted children who later developed schizophrenia or schizophrenia-like disorders were compared for the presence of psychiatric disturbance.[37] As a control, biologic and adoptive relatives of nonschizophrenic adoptees were also evaluated. There was a much higher incidence of definite severe schizophrenia in the biologic relatives of schizophrenic adoptees than among those of control adoptees.[37] In contrast, schizophrenia-like disorders, such as schizoid personality, had about the same frequency in the two groups of relatives. This suggests that definite schizophrenia has a genetic basis which is lacking in the other disorders.

When the initial Copenhagen study was extended to the entire country of Denmark, a total of 74 schizophrenic adoptees and more than 1000 relatives were evaluated. In addition to corroborating the results of the initial study, the second investigation identified subtypes in the relatives with greater certainty.[37] Biologic relatives of adoptees with definite schizophrenia had a high incidence of chronic but not of acute schizophrenia. Strikingly, biologic relatives of acute schizophrenics showed very little evidence of schizophrenia-related disorders. Thus we have further evidence that chronic schizophrenia has a genetic determinant not shared by acute schizophrenic illness.[37] Although psychologic and environmental factors cannot be excluded in the genesis of schizophrenic illness, the evidence overwhelmingly supports the occurrence of a genetic predisposition to the development of a biochemical neurotransmitter defect in the etiology of this condition.[4,31]

AFFECTIVE ILLNESS

In affective illness there is strong evidence for a genetic predisposition. In a summary of twin studies of affective illness, the overall concordance rate for bipolar illness in monozygotic twins was 72%, while the corresponding figure for dizygotic twins was only 14%.[38] In unipolar affective illness the concordance rate for monozygotic twins was 40%, while for dizygotic twins there was a concordance of only 11%. Numerous studies have suggested that the incidence of bipolar illness is much higher among relatives of bipolar patients than among relatives of unipolar patients.[4,38] A high frequency of hypomanic personality traits, even in the absence of clear affective illness, has been noted in family members of patients suffering from bipolar affective illness. Depressive personality traits are common in family members of patients suffering from bipolar affective illness and from unipolar depression.[39] Alcoholism, which also appears to have a genetic predisposition, tends to be more common in the families of patients with major affective illness than in the population as a whole.[4] Although the etiologic role of life stresses in the precipitation of affective illness may be important, the genetic contribution appears to be of greater significance in those patients who begin to experience depression earlier in their life and in those individuals who have multiple recurrent affective episodes, whether they be depressive or manic episodes.[4] As in the case of schizophrenic illness, a genetic predisposition appears to give rise to a biochemical neurotransmitter defect that eventually, on one or more occasions, becomes manifested in the life of the individual by affective symptoms. As in the case of schizophrenic illness, direct measurements of abnormal chemical factors within the brain cannot be made. Likewise, data from studies of biological fluids have provided only limited etiologic information.

Clinical and biochemical responses to administered drugs have provided most of the useful information supporting a biochemical etiology in affective illness. Serotonin and norepinephrine have both been implicated in the etiology of affective illness; both are localized in the limbic system and hypothalamus, brain areas that are known to be involved in the regulation of emotions.[4] Two serendipitous observations made about 40 years ago have given rise to much of our current appreciation of neurochemical correlates in mood disorders. Reserpine, widely used in the treatment of hypertension, frequently produced severe depressive illness and suicidal behavior, even in individuals with no prior history of affective disease.[31] This drug weakens binding sites for dopamine, norepinephrine, and serotonin within the synaptic vesicles, causing these transmitters to gradually leak out into the synapse and become metabolically degraded.[31] The other important finding was the observation of hypomanic and manic behavior in tuberculous patients being treated with iproniazid. This compound was known to inhibit the enzyme monoamine oxidase, thus impairing the ability of the brain to metabolize monoamine neurotransmitters such as norepinephrine and serotonin.[7] Reserpine depletion of these neurotransmitters was associated with the production of severe depressive states, while iproniazid-induced enhancement of the brain concentration of these neurotransmitters was able to elevate mood or induce mania.[31]

Another accidental finding, which occurred much later, was the observation that the antihypertensive drug alpha-methyldopa, which is known to interfere with the synthesis and release of norepinephrine, was capable of inducing severe depression.[40] In the search for safer and more effective antipsychotic drugs, the chlorpromazine derivative imipramine was administered experimentally to patients. Although this compound unfortunately lacked antipsychotic efficacy, an incidental observation revealed its ability to improve mood in depressed individuals.[31] Imipramine and related tricyclic antidepressants inhibit nerve reuptake mechanisms, the primary mode of inactivation of serotonin and norepinephrine.[4,31] Thus we have additional evidence correlating a decrement or increment in neurotransmitter activity with changes in mood state.

It would appear from these observations that any intervention decreasing central monoamine transmitter function would induce depression and that interventions enhancing central monoamine neurotransmission would exert an antidepressant effect. Electrically induced seizures in rats increase turnover of brain norepinephrine and appear to produce a net increase in both brain level and synthesis of this neurotransmitter.[41] Numerous studies have revealed decreased urinary excretion of MHPG (3-methoxy-4-hydroxyphenylglycol) in some depressed patients.[42] Urinary levels of MHPG have been observed to increase following a series of electroconvulsive therapy (ECT) treatments, suggesting a correlation between increased norepinephrine turnover and improvement in mood.[4,41] Those individuals who have low pretreatment MHPG are thought to represent depressive disorders whose mechanism involves decreased norepinephrine activity. Another group of depressed patients, whose urinary and MHPG excretion is normal, may show abnormally low CSF levels of the serotonin metabolite 5-hydroxyindolacetic acid (5-HIAA).[42] CSF levels of 5-HIAA increase toward normal following ECT in many patient studies.[41] Thus the metabolic changes in both serotonin and norepinephrine that have been associated with ECT help to explain the mechanism of action of this effective therapeutic agent, and also lend further evidence for a biochemical understanding of depression. Among the tricyclic, SSRI, and heterocyclic antidepressant drugs, various compounds appear to exert selective action with respect to enhancing central serotonergic or noradrenergic (norepinephrine) activity.[31,32,42] This selective biochemical action may correlate with some selectivity of the therapeutic action of these compounds.

Manic behavior appears to have both clinical and neurochemical abnormalities that are essentially opposite those seen in depression.[4] Those drugs that improve depressive symptoms may trigger or worsen mania.[31] Drugs that may provoke depression, such as reserpine and neuroleptics, have an antimanic action.[31] Since acetylcholine appears to act in opposition to the catecholamine neurotransmitters, it would seem that cholinergic stimulation should decrease manic symptoms. The administration of anticholinergic drugs may worsen manic symptoms. The experimental administration of physostigmine (a cholinesterase inhibitor), arecoline (a direct cholinergic stimulant), or choline (an acetylcholine precursor) has been shown to exert antimanic activity. This activity correlates with the ability of each of these compounds to increase central cholinergic function.[8,31,43] The neurochemical action of lithium remains quite intriguing, because this compound is capable of controlling and preventing mania; it also has the ability to improve and protect against recurrent episodes of depression. Information now becoming available suggests that lithium interacts with serotonergic, catecholaminergic, and cholinergic sites within the brain. Furthermore, lithium appears to have a regulatory function in effecting the passage of sodium and perhaps other ions across cell membranes.[44]

ANXIETY

The central biochemical correlates of anxiety are less well understood than are the neurochemical correlates of schizophrenia and affective illness. Specific benzodiazepine receptor sites have been identified within brain tissue.[45] Indeed, the role of GABA and substance P has been mentioned earlier in the context of their possible function as naturally occurring tranquilizers. The benzodiazepine receptor is functionally and perhaps structurally coupled to a receptor for GABA, the major inhibitory neurotransmitter.[4,45] Buspirone, which is structurally different from the benzodiazepines, appears to exert an antianxiety effect but does not interact with the benzodiazepine-GABA receptor axis.[46] This compound interacts with serotonin sites and with the dopaminergic system, where it produces a mixed agonist-antagonist effect.[47] This compound and its congeners may help to clarify the connection between the neurochemical mechanism of anxiety and central dopamine and serotonin receptor activity.[46,47]

NEUROTRANSMITTER PRECURSORS
AS PSYCHOTROPIC DRUGS

Many psychiatric disorders, including depression, mania, and schizophrenia, result from defective neurotransmission. The defect may involve either decreased or increased neurotransmitter synthesis and release or, alternatively, defective function of the receptor site itself. Currently employed psychotropic drugs act by decreasing receptor site sensitivity or by impairing degradation of neurotransmitter substances. Cyclic and SSRI antidepressants produce a complex variety of actions, which include inhibition of neurotransmitter reuptake mechanisms, down-regulation of adrenergic and serotonergic receptors, and, in some cases, cholinergic receptor blockade. The multiple neurotransmitter systems within the brain may, in some cases, facilitate the action of one another and, in other instances, act in opposition to an alternative transmitter system. The complexity of these interactions appears, at this time, to preclude any simple solution to the variety of neurochemical defects underlying mental disorders.

Laboratory and clinical investigations at the Massachusetts Institute of Technology (MIT) and in other research centers have demonstrated that the administration of neurotransmitter precursors, including choline, and the amino acids tyrosine and tryptophan can enhance brain synthesis of neurotransmitters.[8] Prior to these findings, it was believed that neurotransmitter synthesis was regulated by the brain so as to prevent its enhancement by dietary manipulation.[8] Following the initial recognition of the ability of precursors to alter brain neurotransmitter synthesis, a large variety of clinical studies were conducted at MIT and elsewhere. Thus far, the clinical efficacy of neurotransmitter precursors in the treatment of psychiatric and neurologic disorders has been variable. Although some studies have been promising, many have yielded equivocal or negative results. Since precursors are naturally occurring substances, and have minimal side effects, they may be highly desirable therapeutic agents provided the technology is developed to administer them in ways that enhance their efficacy.

Choline and lecithin (phosphatidylcholine) are naturally occurring dietary substances which act as precursors for the synthesis of acetylcholine in the brain. A highly purified capsule form of phosphatidylcholine is currently being marketed. In some clinical studies, administration of 10 to 15 g of purified phosphatidylcholine per day has reduced early memory impairment in Alzheimer's disease.[8,9] In some studies, choline or lecithin has been administered along with the cholinesterase inhibitor physostigmine to Alzheimer's disease patients, with some improvement in cognitive function.[48] Patients with this disorder have increased sensitivity to anticholinergic drugs, impaired synthesis of acetylcholine, and possibly deterioration of cholinergic receptor sites. This disorder, however, also involves the development of neurofibrillary tangles and other structural brain changes, which would imply that a simple pharmacologic intervention is not likely to be curative. Increasing brain acetylcholine by the administration of choline, lecithin, or physostigmine has also been demonstrated to reduce manic symptoms.[19] However, the practical therapeutic application of cholinergic precursors in mania has not yet been extensively documented.

Tyrosine is the amino acid precursor for the synthesis of norepinephrine and other catecholamines. There have been isolated reports in the literature and several small studies which have shown an apparent antidepressant action when tyrosine is administered orally in doses of 50 to 100 mg/kg/day to depressed patients.[11,13] Other studies have failed to demonstrate a clinically significant antidepressant action with orally administered tyrosine. In some instances, tyrosine may produce mild elevation of blood pressure and this should be taken into account if the drug is employed clinically in hypertensive patients. Theoretically, it is possible that the administration of tyrosine to patients being treated with MAO inhibitors might provoke a hypertensive reaction, and therefore this combination of medications would appear to be inadvisable. It is conceivable that some depressed patients might benefit from the cautious administration of tyrosine in conjunction with a tricyclic antidepressant, particularly in those instances when the patient has shown limited responsiveness to conventional antidepressant drug therapy.

Preliminary clinical studies of depressed patients have in some cases found decreased plasma concentrations and urinary excretion of phenylacetic acid (PAA), the major metabolite of 2-phenylethylamine (PEA). One study suggested that these measurements may represent a state marker for depression.[49] L-Phenylalanine is an essential amino acid, which is converted in the body to tyrosine and PEA. Some studies have found that the oral administration of L-phenylalanine in daily doses of 500 mg to 14 g may exert a clinically useful antidepressant effect.[49] Not all studies of L-phenylalanine have shown it to be an effective antidepressant; nevertheless, cautious use of this substance may be appropriate in some depressed patients who do not tolerate or respond satisfactorily to conventional antidepressant drugs. Side effects experienced with phenylalanine administration may include transient headaches, nausea, insomnia, and increased anxiety. Hypomania may also occur as an adverse effect of phenylalanine administration. This pharmacologic use of phenylalanine as an antidepressant is not approved by the FDA, and clearly needs further clinical investigation to document safety and efficacy. Phenylalanine administration is contraindicated in patients with phenylketonuria.

Tryptophan is the amino acid precursor of the neurotransmitter serotonin. This compound has been extensively studied in psychiatric patients. Numerous controlled and uncontrolled studies have documented the ability of L-tryptophan to reduce sleep latency and facilitate patients falling asleep. This substance is not uniformly effective as a hypnotic, however, and many patients will fail to experience any sleep-inducing effect.[11,30] Other patients report falling asleep as easily following the administration of 1 g of L-tryptophan as they have previously experienced with conventional hypnotic drugs.[30] Tryptophan is useful in reducing sleep latency, but generally will not prevent nighttime awakening, nor will it be beneficial in eliminating early morning awakening. A large number of studies have employed tryptophan alone or in combination with MAO inhibitors or cyclic antidepressants in the treatment of depression.[8,11]

There have been reports of patients experiencing an antidepressant effect when treated with tryptophan in doses of 2 to 8 g/day as their sole therapeutic agent. Most carefully controlled studies, however, have failed to document clinically significant antidepressant efficacy with tryptophan. Some investigators have reported enhanced antidepressant efficacy when tryptophan is combined with a tricyclic or heterocyclic antidepressant.[8] The serotonin syndrome, characterized by restlessness, hyperreflexia, myoclonic movements, intense sweating, elevated temperature, elevated blood pressure, and irregular cardiac rhythm, has occurred in patients receiving tryptophan along with either an MAOI or an SSRI antidepressant.[50,51] Due to the occurrence of numerous cases of the potentially fatal eosinophilia-myalgia syndrome in patients receiving tryptophan, presumably due to impurities, all L-tryptophan has been withdrawn from the U.S. market, although it is likely that a purified standardized L-tryptophan may become available in the future.

REFERENCES

1. Weinberger DR (ed): SPECT imaging in psychiatry: a new look at depression. *J Clin Psychiatry* 1993;54(11, suppl):3-32.
2. Wong DF, Wagner HN Jr, Tune LE, et al: Positron emission tomography reveals elevated D_2 dopamine receptors in drug-naive schizophrenics. *Science* 1986;234:1558-1563.
3. Bloom FE: Neurohumoral transmission and the central nervous system. In Gilman AG, Rall TW, Nies AS, Taylor P (eds): *Goodman and Gilman's The pharmacological basis of therapeutics*, ed 8. New York, Pergamon Press, 1990, pp 244-268.
4. Coyle JT (section ed): Neuroscience; In Tasman A, Goldfinger SM (eds): *APA annual review of psychiatry;* Washington DC, American Psychiatric Press, 1991, vol 10, pp 397-528.
5. Taylor P: Cholinergic agonists. In Gilman AG, Rall TW, Neis AS, Taylor P (eds): *Goodman and Gilman's The pharmacological basis of therapeutics*, ed 8. New York, Pergamon Press, 1990, pp 122-130.
6. Hoffman BB, Lefkowitz RJ: Catecholamines and sympathomimetic drugs. In Gilman AG, Rall

TW, Neis AS, Taylor P (eds): *Goodman and Gilman's The pharmacological basis of therapeutics*, ed 8. New York, Pergamon Press, 1990, pp 187-220.

7. Baldessarini RJ: Drugs and the treatment of psychiatric disorders. In Gilman AG, Rall TW, Neis AS, Taylor P (eds): *Goodman and Gilman's The pharmacological basis of therapeutics*, ed 8. New York, Pergamon Press, 1990, pp 383-435.

8. Wurtman RJ, Wurtman JJ (eds): *Nutrients and the brain*. New York, Raven Press, 1986, vol. 7.

9. Blusztajn JK, Wurtman RJ: Choline and cholinergic neurotransmission. *Science* 1983;221: 614-620.

10. Milner JD, Wurtman RJ: Commentary: Catecholamine synthesis: physiological coupling to precursor supply. *Biochem Pharmacol* 1986;35:875-881.

11. Wurtman RJ: Nutrients affecting brain composition and behavior. *Integr Psychiatry* 1987;5: 226-251.

12. Cowen PJ: Psychotropic drugs and human 5-HT neuroendocrinology. *Trends Pharmacol Sci* 1987;8:105-108.

13. Gelenberg AJ, Wojcik JD, Gibson CJ, et al: Tyrosine for depression. *J Psychiatr Res* 1983;17:175-180.

14. Calne DB, Kelabian J, Silbergeld E, et al: Advances in the neuropharmacology of parkinsonism. *Ann Intern Med* 1979;90:219-229.

15. Granacher RP, Baldessarini RJ: Physostigmine in the acute anticholinergic syndrome associated with antidepressant and antiparkinsonism drugs. *Arch Gen Psychiatry* 1975;32:375-380.

16. Baldessarini RJ, Gelenberg AJ: Use of physostigmine in antidepressant-induced intoxication. *Am J Psychiatry* 1979;136:1608-1609.

17. Sitaran N, Weingartner H, Gillin JC: Human serial learning: enhancement with arecoline and choline, impairment with scopolamine. *Science* 1978;201:274-276.

18. Hollenberg MD, SARS: the receptor side of the coin. *Trends Pharmacol Sci* 1987;8:197-199.

19. Lefkowitz RJ, Hoffman BB, Taylor P: Neurohumoral transmission: the autonomic and somatic motor nervous systems. In Gilman AG, Rall TW, Nies AS, Taylor P (eds): *Goodman and Gilman's The pharmacological basis of therapeutics*, ed 8. New York, Pergamon Press, 1990, pp 84-121.

20. Stahl SM, Palazidou L: The pharmacology of depression: studies of neurotransmitter receptors lead the search for biochemical lesions and new drug therapies. *Trends Pharmacol Sci* 1987;7:349-354.

21. Green JP: Nomenclature and classification of receptors and binding sites: the need for harmony. *Trends Pharmacol Sci* 1987;8:90-94.

22. Creese I: Dopamine and antipsychotic medications. In Hales RE, Frances AJ (eds): *APA annual review*. Washington DC, American Psychiatric Press, 1985, vol 4, pp 17-36.

23. Enna SJ: γ-Aminobutyric acid (GABA) pharmacology and neuropsychiatric illness. In Hales RE, Frances AJ (eds): *APA annual review*. Washington DC, American Psychiatric Press, 1985, vol 4, pp 67-82.

24. Kosterlitz HW, Hughes J, Lord JAH, et al: Enkephalins, endorphins, and opiate receptors. *Soc Neurosci* 1977;2:291-307.

25. Pernow B: Substance P. *Pharmacol Rev* 1983;35:85-141.

26. Lewitt PA: New perspectives in the treatment of Parkinson's disease. *Clin Neuropsychopharmacol* 1986;9(suppl 1):S37-S46.

27. Snyder SH: Dopamine receptors, neuroleptics, and schizophrenia. *Am J Psychiatry* 1981;138: 460-464.

28. Creese I: Dopamine receptors explained. *Trends Neurosci* 1982;5:40-44.

29. Aghajanian GK, Wang RY: Physiology and pharmacology of central serotonergic neurons. In Lipton MA, Di Mascib A, Killam KF (eds): *Psychopharmacology: a generation of progress*. New York, Raven Press, 1978, pp 171-184.

30. Hartmann E, Cravens J, List S: Hypnotic effects of L-tryptophan. *Arch Gen Psychiatry* 1974;31:394-397.

31. Bernstein J: *Handbook of drug therapy in psychiatry*, ed 2. St Louis, Mosby, 1988.

32. Buchsbaum MS, Tang SW, Wu JC, et al: Effects of amoxapine and imipramine on cerebral glucose metabolism assessed by positron emission tomography. *J Clin Psychiatry* 1986;4:14-17.

33. Holman BL, Gibson RE, Hill TC, et al: Muscarinic acetylcholine receptors in Alzheimer's disease: in vivo imaging with iodine 123–labeled QNB. *JAMA* 1985;254:3063-3066.

34. Snyder S, Greenberg D, Yamamura HL: Antischizophrenic drugs and brain cholinergic receptors. *Arch Gen Psychiatry* 1974;31:58-61.

35. Snyder SH: Receptors, neurotransmitters, and drug responses. *N Engl J Med* 1979;300:465-472.

36. Snyder SH: The dopamine hypothesis of schizophrenia: focus on the dopamine receptor. *Am J Psychiatry* 1976;133:197-202.

37. Kety SS, Rosenthal D, Wender PH, et al: The biologic and adoptive families of adopted individuals who became schizophrenic: prevalence of mental illness and other characteristics. In Wynee LDC, Cromwell RL, Matthysse S (eds): *The nature of schizophrenia.* New York, John Wiley & Sons, 1978, pp 25-37.

38. Allen MG: Twin studies of affective illness. *Arch Gen Psychiatry* 1976;33:1476-1478.

39. Cadoret RJ, Winokur G, Clayton P: Family history studies. VII. Manic depressive disease vs. depressive disease. *Br J Psychiatry* 1970;166:625-635.

40. Whitlock FH, Evans LEJ: Drugs and depression. *Drugs* 1978;15:53-71.

41. Modigh K: Long term effects of electroconvulsive shock therapy on synthesis, turnover, and uptake of brain monoamines. *Psychopharmacology* 1976;49:179-183.

42. Mass JW: Biogenic amines and depression. *Arch Gen Psychiatry* 1975;32:1357-1361.

43. Janowsky DS, El-Yousef MK, Davis JM, et al: Parasympathetic suppression of manic symptoms by physostigmine. *Arch Gen Psychiatry* 1973;28:542-547.

44. Ortiz A, Dabbagh M, Gershon S: Lithium: clinical use, toxicology, and mode of action. In Bernstein JG (ed): *Clinical psychopharmacology,* ed 2. Littleton Mass, John Wright–PSG, 1984.

45. Paul SM, Marangos PJ, Goddwin FK, et al: Brain-specific benzodiazepine receptors and putative endogenous benzodiazepine-like compounds. *Biol Psychiatry* 1980;15:407-428.

46. Eison AS, Temple DL Jr: Buspirone: review of its pharmacology and current perspectives on its mechanism of action. *Am J Med* 1986;80(suppl 3B):1-9.

47. Taylor DP, Riblet LA, Stanton HC, et al: Dopamine and antianxiety activity. *Pharmacol Biochem Behav* 1982;17(suppl 1):25-35.

48. Thal LJ, Fuid PA, Masur DM: Oral physostigmine and lecithin improve memory in Alzheimer's disease. *Psychopharmacol Bull* 1983;19:454-456.

49. Sabelli HC, Fawcett J, Busovsky F, et al: Clinical studies on the phenylethylamine hypothesis of affective disorder: urine and blood phenylacetic acid and phenylalanine dietary supplements. *J Clin Psychiatry* 1986;47:66-70.

50. Insel TR, Roy BF, Cohen RM, et al: Possible development of the serotonin syndrome in man. *Am J Psychiatry* 1982;139:954-955.

51. Steiner W, Fontaine R: Toxic reaction following the combined administration of fluoxetine and L-tryptophan: five case reports. *Biol Psychiatry* 1986;21:1067-1071.

CHAPTER 2

Medicating the Psychiatric Patient

1. Rational pharmacotherapy requires decisions as to when and when not to medicate.
2. Emotional responses to ordinary life situations should generally not be medicated.
3. Psychiatric illnesses such as depression and psychosis generally require pharmacotherapy.
4. Failure to properly medicate may prolong the patient's illness and suffering.
5. Irrational use of medications may lead to simultaneous adverse reactions to multiple drugs.
6. Detailed medical and psychiatric history as well as patient attitudes toward medication are needed.
7. Appropriate medication must be carefully chosen.
8. The dose should be titrated according to response and adverse effects; the "standard dose" seldom is optimal.
9. All medications should be temporarily withheld if unexplained adverse response occurs.
10. It is generally advisable to start only one medication at a time, and to observe the patient before others are added.
11. Lack of desired response may indicate that the patient is not taking medication as directed.
12. The physician must be aware of the possible lack of bioequivalence among generic drug preparations.
13. The addicting potential of sedatives such as benzodiazepines should be kept in mind.
14. Interactions between various psychotropic drugs and between psychotropic and nonpsychotropic drugs, as well as potential interactions between alcoholic beverages and various medications, must be considered in prescribing medication.
15. Physicians must be aware of increased sensitivity and persistence of various drugs in elderly patients, and the interactions between underlying medical conditions and psychotropic drugs.

Continued.

16. Before prescribing medication, the potential risks and benefits of treatment must be discussed with patient.
17. The patient's consent for treatment, specific medications and dosages prescribed, and any changes in regimen must be documented in medical record.
18. The physician must be aware of legal ramifications of prescribing without the patient's consent, of undetected adverse drug reactions, and of complications of prolonged pharmacotherapy.

Physiologic and behavioral effects produced by a variety of chemical substances were recognized in biblical times.[1] The Book of Psalms states that alcohol gladdens the heart, and there are numerous biblical references to the disastrous effects of alcohol intoxication. Honey, a component of many ancient medicines, is mentioned in the Bible as a remedy used to revive a person who has fainted.[1] Indeed, neither mental illness nor psychotherapy was unknown in biblical times. In I Samuel we read about the depression and apparent psychotic symptoms experienced by King Saul. David demonstrated the temporary beneficial effects of psychotherapy in the form of the first recognized application of music therapy. Unfortunately, although David's therapeutic application of his ability to play the lyre provided some temporary lifting of King Saul's spirits, the king subsequently died by suicide, falling upon his own sword.[2] Thus, some of our views of psychiatry and the application of medications to modify mind and body are clearly not as recent in history as we tend to think. From the time of Hippocrates in the fifth century before the common era through the time of Galen in the second century of the common era, there was considerable thought about the emotions of man and even the connections among emotions, behavior, and bodily makeup. In this period a vast number of chemical remedies were concocted and administered to patients with a variety of illnesses.[3] The Talmud, the oral component of the Hebrew Bible that was compiled between the second and fifth centuries of the common era, includes a great deal of medical and psychiatric thought. The Talmud includes a discussion of what appears to be a toxic delirium, and describes a therapeutic regimen of red meat and diluted wine.[1]

Though experimental data are lacking, it is tempting for the modern pharmacologist to connect the apparent therapeutic efficacy of this remedy with the presence of tryptophan, a serotonin precursor found in red meat. One of the earliest known pharmacopoeias was issued by a hospital in Baghdad in the year 869 of the common era.[3] Over the next thousand years numerous remedies were proposed and utilized in the treatment of physical and psychiatric illness. With a few notable exceptions, such as digitalis and quinine, virtually all of those early remedies have been discarded from the practice of medicine.[3] Most medications in current use have been developed in very recent times. For most medical conditions, currently available newer therapeutic agents provide improvements on older remedies developed during the previous 2 or 3 centuries. Psychiatry, however, is unique, in that prior to the early 1950s there were no pharmacologic agents possessing proven therapeutic efficacy other than the brief benefits of sedation by barbiturates or stimulation by amphetamines.[4] Since psychiatry developed as a medical discipline prior to the availability of any effective pharmacologic treatments, it is not surprising that there has been a seeming disconnection between the understanding of psychiatric illness and the application of drug therapy. Ancient thought often connected the appearance of psychiatric illness to supernatural powers or possession by the devil.[1,3] More modern psychiatric theories invoked interactions between anatomically undefinable aspects of mental function — the id, the ego, and the superego — with derangements in mental function and behavior.[5] Much of modern psychiatry is an outgrowth of psychoanalytic thinking, and it is not surprising that the professional community within psychiatry was more attached to psychological concepts than to physiologically and biochemically based medicine. In the early years of electroconvulsive therapy and subsequent pharmacotherapy for the treatment of psychiatric illness, intense conflicts arose and persisted between the older established community within psychiatry and the renegades who proposed physical intervention as a means of controlling and alleviating conditions of an apparently psychological origin. In the early days of psychopharmacology — and even to some extent in the present era when drug therapy is becoming standard practice — it has often been felt that treatment by psychotherapy allows the patient to "work through" his problems, and that this is somehow superior to drug treatment wherein something is done *to* the patient to alleviate the problem.

The goal of the science of medicine is to diagnose diseases, treat them, and, wherever possible, prevent their occurrence. In the continuing evolution of psychiatry back to the mainstream of medicine, we are beginning to recognize disease entities more clearly and, perhaps, become less reliant on psychologic explanations of our patients' symptoms. In the mainstream of medicine, we recognize that any disease may exist at varying levels of severity and that a particular disease process may express itself by the presence of one or many physical signs and symptoms. The scientific understanding of medicine allows us to conceptualize the relationships between two or more seemingly disparate diseases. Indeed, a patient with heart disease may experience chest pain, shortness of breath, ankle edema, low blood pressure, and an abnormal ECG. These signs and symptoms may be seen as a composite, and may indeed represent the presence of a cardiomyopathy. The physician does not have to look to the chest wall as the source of pain, to the lungs as the cause of shortness of breath, to the feet as the source of the edema, to the peripheral vasculature as the cause of low blood pressure, and to the heart as the origin of the abnormal

ECG. These manifestations can be readily seen by the internist as coming from the dysfunctional state of one organ, the heart. An understanding of basic physiology allows the internist or practitioner in one of the subspecialties of internal medicine to integrate the various signs and symptoms, connect them to the dysfunctional organ, and understand them as different components of the same disease process.

In psychiatry, practitioners are less familiar with the relevant physiology and biochemistry of their organ, the brain. With increasing research and understanding of psychiatric illnesses, we must be ever more careful to focus on the brain, whose biochemistry and physiology will give us the clues to a better understanding and treatment of psychiatric disorders. We must not, however, lose sight of the patient whom we serve.

EDUCATING THE PATIENT

Many physicians who believe more strongly in psychotherapy than in pharmacotherapy feel that they have failed in their treatment of a patient when they include medication in the regimen.[6] Likewise, some patients feel that they have failed to respond as they should to psychotherapy when medication is prescribed. The physician may feel that he is "giving" something to the patient when he prescribes medication, and some patients interpret this therapeutic act as having "received" a specific treatment from the physician.[6] On the other hand, many patients maintain a negative attitude toward medication and feel that the physician prescribing medication for their emotional problems may be doing so because he is unskilled in his use of therapy or that they, the patients, are too ill to respond appropriately to psychotherapy.[6] Some patients are frightened of medication and will interpret a prescribed increase in the dosage as an indication that they are becoming worse, or a decrease in the dosage as an indication that they are recovering. The physician must recognize that different points of view exist among professionals regarding drug therapy, and that part of this difference is based on a lack of knowledge or understanding of the connection between pharmacotherapy and the nature of psychiatric illness. He must also recognize that similar conflicts exist in the mind of nearly every patient.[6] Most psychiatric patients and their families will connect abnormalities in mood and behavior with psychologic explanations of varying degrees of sophistication. Relatively few patients or family members will understand why medication should be given for what appears to be a state of emotional distress. The question we have all heard repeatedly is "If I am feeling depressed, how is a pill going to help me?"

In addition to the frequent lack of belief on the part of patients that medication can make a difference in how they feel emotionally, there are other commonly encountered clinical problems — such as the patient who is paranoid and believes that the medication is being given to poison him, or the patient who may be so grossly psychotic that he does not recognize there is anything wrong and tells the treating physician very plainly that he is feeling fine and does not need medication.[7] Until the physician manages to deal with these barriers to drug therapy, his sophisticated knowledge of the pharmacology of psychotropic drugs is of no therapeutic value. The most fundamental technique in the administration of medication to psychiatric patients is that of educating the patient.[8] Indeed, secrecy was a prime component of the practice of medicine from ancient times until quite recently.[24] Prescriptions were formerly written so that they could not be read by patients; Latin abbreviations and an illegible hand were somehow thought to be therapeutic by adding to the mystique and secrecy of the prescription. Furthermore, prior to the 1950s it was rare, and not considered good practice, for physicians to specify that prescription bottles include the name of the medication. Over the past 2 decades there has been such a dramatic change in this attitude that the majority of states have now enacted laws which require prescription bottles to be labeled with the generic name of the medication.

It is certainly important for patients to know the name of the medication that they are taking. Such information on prescription bottles adds to the safety of medication treatment by providing immediate information if the patient should develop an adverse reaction or take an overdose requiring emergency treatment by a physician other than the one who prescribed the medication. Giving the patient only the name of the medication which he is taking, however, provides rather limited education. In my own experience, and that of others who have conducted studies on medication compliance, there is evidence to support the contention that the better-informed patient is more likely to follow the prescribed therapeutic regimen.[9,10] It is not surprising that the average patient would have a hard time understanding the connection between taking a pill and achieving some relief of his depression. The patient has a right to know not only what medication he is taking and how to take it, but also why he is taking it, how it may alleviate his illness, and what adverse effects it may produce.[7,18]

Hundreds of volumes have been written on the techniques of psychotherapy, but unfortunately, relatively little has been written on the technique of pharmacotherapy. Providing adequate patient education is one of the fundamental techniques of good pharmacotherapy. The kind of information the patient needs involves a frank discussion of the nature of the illness being treated. Although it may or may not be appropriate in a particular situation to use a specific diagnostic label, it certainly is appropriate to explain to an individual that he is suffering from a psychosis, and that this may produce disturbances in the way he thinks and responds to others, that it may cause his imagination to play tricks on him so that he misperceives things in his environment, and that this may be expressed in the manifestation of hallucinations which he is experiencing. Likewise, an individual who is depressed has a right to know that there is a legitimate illness called depression and that his symptoms of sadness and lack of motivation, his loss of interest in those things he normally finds pleasurable, and his inability to eat or sleep may be symptoms of this illness. Many depressed patients who experience a profound weight loss become obsessed with the thought that they are suffering from cancer, but they are too frightened to even express this fear. Letting a depressed individual know that weight loss is a prominent component of depression and is not necessarily indicative of a serious or fatal physical illness can certainly reduce his fear and enable him to talk about some of his concerns.

In addition to reviewing with a patient the nature of his illness and the connection of this illness with some of the symptoms he is experiencing, it is certainly appropriate to discuss in greater or lesser detail with the individual our understanding of the connection between his psychiatric condition and underlying changes in brain function. With patients of average or above-average intellectual capacity, it would even be appropriate to discuss the concept of altered neurotransmitter activity.[8] Once a patient understands his symptoms and their connection with the illness, and understands further that the illness is in fact analogous to any other medical condition such as diabetes (wherein there is a biochemical defect), it is easier to discuss the role of medication in the prescribed treatment program. Allowing the patient to gain a biologic understanding of his illness makes it much easier to explain how a medication may benefit him. When appropriate, the physician should help the patient understand how the specific medication, whether it be an antipsychotic drug or an antidepressant drug, may actually modify the underlying neurotransmitter problem and thereby bring about relief of his distress. Such discussion often gives rise to questions about prognosis, and it is important to answer these questions as honestly as possible without being overly optimistic or overly bleak.

Any discussion of how the medication will work and its likelihood of benefiting specific symptoms should also include a discussion of some of the side effects that are likely to occur.[8] It is not necessary, nor is it clinically appropriate, to review exhaustively with the patient every side effect that may be found for a particular drug in a textbook of pharmacology or the *Physicians' Desk Reference*. On the other hand, those common side effects associated with psychotropic medication, such as blurred vision, dry mouth, constipation, drowsiness, and dizziness, occur commonly enough in patients receiving antidepressants and antipsychotic medications that they should be mentioned. When neuroleptics are prescribed, it is important to let the patient know that he may experience some muscular stiffness, a sensation of pulling in the neck or jaw, and tremor of the hands, so that if these reactions do occur he is not startled and frightened. Since tardive dyskinesia does not occur early in the course of antipsychotic treatment, it is probably not appropriate to discuss this complication at the outset of such treatment; discussion of this potential complication can be reserved until later in the treatment, after the patient recovers from the acute manifestations of psychosis, and the physician has decided on a course of treatment which may involve a more prolonged period of administration of the neuroleptic. Patients receiving phenothiazines should be alerted to the fact that they may become excessively sensitive to sunlight and burn more easily even when exposed to the sun for relatively short periods of time. These patients should be advised to use a sunscreen lotion even for brief sun exposure. Since many patients taking neuroleptic drugs will also receive prescriptions for antiparkinsonian medication, they should be advised that these medications may produce blurred vision, dry mouth, rapid pulse, constipation, and difficulty in urinating.[8]

When monoamine oxidase (MAO) inhibitor–type antidepressants are prescribed, the patient should be carefully informed about the potential of developing a headache or an elevation of blood pressure if stimulants, nasal decongestants, or tyramine-rich foods or alcoholic beverages are taken along with this medication. It is of utmost importance to give every patient taking MAO inhibitor–type antidepressants a printed list of instructions such as the one presented in Appendix A. Furthermore, it is good practice to advise these patients to contact the physician who prescribed the MAO inhibitor prior to taking any other medication.

When lithium carbonate is prescribed, the patient should be told that this medication may produce some stomach discomfort if taken on an empty stomach and should therefore always be taken with food. Patients taking lithium should also informed that if they develop fever, vomiting, or diarrhea, or if they restrict the salt content of their diet or take a diuretic, their lithium blood level may become excessive and they may develop a toxic reaction. It is important to advise patients who become ill while taking lithium to discontinue the medication temporarily, until their fever subsides and until the vomiting and diarrhea stop. They should also be told that lithium may produce diarrhea, and that the presence of this symptom while taking this medication indicates a need for a lithium blood level to be obtained before proceeding with this treatment.

When sedatives such as the benzodiazepines are prescribed, patients should be informed that they may experience drowsiness, fatigue, or loss of coordination, indicating that they may be taking an excessive dose. Patients taking these drugs should also be informed of the drugs' potential to induce addiction if they are taken regularly over a prolonged period of time.

Patients taking any psychotropic medication should be alerted to the fact that they may become drowsy or have difficulty concentrating at the outset of treatment. They should be advised not to operate machinery or motor vehicles until they have become accustomed to the medication and satisfactory medical evaluation has taken place to indicate that they can function adequately on the medication regimen. Since most psychotropic medications may have some influence on sexual performance, patients should be alerted to this possibility and encouraged to discuss sexual dysfunction with the physician should it arise during the course of treatment.[12] Many medication side effects diminish as the patient adjusts to the medication. Other side effects that are dose-related will diminish or disappear in response to dosage adjustment by the physician. For example, many patients will experience a tremor of the fingers when starting lithium therapy although this effect commonly disappears spontaneously. In some cases the tremor is persistent and will require intervention by the physician to change the lithium preparation prescribed, reduce the dose of lithium, or add propranolol to the regimen. Encouraging the patient to discuss medication side effects with the physician will increase the physician's ability to make appropriate adjustments of the treatment program and thereby minimize side effects.[13] Patients should be urged not to adjust their own dosage of medication either up or down since this may give rise to increased side effects or the loss of desired therapeutic benefit. Furthermore, patients receiving psychotropic medications should be strongly advised not to discontinue medication abruptly, since abrupt discontinuation of many medications will give rise to a variety of adverse effects.[14] Withdrawal symptoms associated with discontinuation of sedatives have already been mentioned.[15] Sudden discontinuation of antidepressants may lead to a worsening of the depression or occasionally to the precipitation of an acute manic episode. Abrupt withdrawal of neuroleptic drugs may produce a withdrawal dyskinesia which may appear virtually indistinguishable from tardive dyskinesia.[14] In addition to providing the initial education of the patient regarding the nature and goals of pharmacotherapy, it is important for the physician as he works with the patient to reinforce this educational program by periodically reviewing the goals of pharmacotherapy and attempting to ascertain that the patient is taking the prescribed medication in the proper dose.[11]

In reviewing some of the important techniques of pharmacotherapy, I have evolved what I call a bill of rights of drug prescribing:[16]

1. Right of the patient to know
2. Right drug
3. Right dose
4. Right schedule of administration
5. Right route of administration

CHOICE OF MEDICATION

The first item in this bill of rights — the right of the patient to know — is the cornerstone of good prescribing technique. The second involves the choice of the proper therapeutic agent. This choice can only be made based on a knowledge of the pharmacology of the various groups of psychotropic drugs and on variations in the characteristics in individual members in each of these groups. Although prescribing antianxiety agents such as the benzodiazepines might seem to be the easiest psychopharmacologic approach to a variety of conditions, it is often less beneficial than the choice of a specific psychotropic agent based on a satisfactory evaluation and diagnostic impression of the clinical situation being treated. The specific pharmacology of the various psychotropic drugs dictates their clinical application. As will be discussed elsewhere in this volume, only those agents which produce dopamine-receptor blockade have a true antipsychotic effect and are able to alleviate the delusions, hallucinations, and disordered thinking associated with psychotic illness.[17] Likewise, although antianxiety agents and neuroleptic drugs may produce a transient improvement in mood in depressed patients, a true antidepressant effect appears to depend upon the ability of the drug to affect neurotransmitter availability at neuronal junctions in the brain. There are a variety of drugs that exhibit a specific antidepressant effect.

DOSAGE

Choice of a medication with a mechanism of action appropriate to the clinical need is not likely to bring about a satisfactory therapeutic response unless the dosage prescribed is optimal. Since patients are neither computers nor mathematical models, it is not likely that a specific dose of a given therapeutic agent will be effective for every patient. Just as some patients will respond to one type of antidepressant and not to another, or to one antipsychotic agent better than to another, patients responsive to a given drug may require a different dosage than another seemingly similar patient. Throughout this volume I have endeavored to provide a range of therapeutic dosages for various medications, and to provide information regarding usual dosages without being dogmatic about the application of a specific dose of any particular drug. As a physician gains increasing clinical experience, he readily learns that dogmatism is generally incompatible with good medical practice. The effective therapeutic dose of a given agent will vary from patient to patient and is likely to be different at one point in time or state of illness than at another point in time or state of illness. Neither a carefully conducted double-blind research study nor a series of individual clinical observations gives the author the right to be dogmatic about dosage.

With any new therapeutic agent a wider range of effective dosage becomes apparent with increasing clinical experience. In the case of the neuroleptic haloperidol, the initial ceiling dose recommended was 15 mg/day; subsequently, in some patients it became apparent that at times during acute psychosis, much higher doses were required and well tolerated. There has been a wide swing of dosage recommendations for this agent, and currently somewhat lower doses seem more appropriate than the so called "megadoses" of a decade ago. Tricyclic antidepressants are generally recommended in a daily dose of 150 to 200 mg/day, yet some patients require double this dose, while others respond favorably and even achieve therapeutic serum concentrations with daily doses of 10 mg. The serotonin-selective reuptake inhibitors (SSRIs) are an excellent example of wide-ranging dosage requirements. Indeed, when fluoxetine was first marketed, a dosage of 20 to 60 mg daily was most commonly recommended. Subsequent research found that much lower doses were often equally effective and better tolerated, with fewer adverse reactions; indeed, one study demonstrated comparable efficacy between daily doses of 5 mg and 20 mg, with the lower dose being better tolerated.[18] Sertraline is a shorter-acting SSRI which was introduced with a daily dosage recommendation of 50 to 200 mg, although currently it is most widely used at a dosage of 50 mg daily, with many patients benefitting and having fewer side effects when employing doses as low as 12.5 to 25 mg daily.[19] While some depressed patients benefit from "super-low" doses of SSRIs, such as 1.25 to 2.5 mg of fluoxetine or 12.5 to 25 mg of sertraline, other patients, particularly those with severe obsessive compulsive disorder, may require fluoxetine doses in excess of 100 mg/day.[20]

There is no substitute for clinical experience in determining the appropriate dosage regimen — that is, the experience gained by the individual physician as well as the composite of clinical experience with a given pharmaceutical product in a particular clinical condition. Clinical experience repeatedly teaches the importance of individualizing the dosage of any given medication for the specific patient and clinical situation. In my own experience of seeing numerous patients in consultation because of their failure to respond to prescribed psychotropic medication, I have not infrequently found that this failure is directly related to the administration of improper dosage. At times the dosage prescribed is inadequate to produce a satisfactory response, and very often simply an increase in the dosage will bring about the desired clinical improvement. Frequently patients have been receiving excessive doses of medication and therefore have experienced a variety of unwanted side effects, which may have masked what would have been a favorable therapeutic response. Lowering the dosage diminishes the side effects and allows the intended therapeutic response to be observed.

Repeated studies of the willingness and ability of patients to take medication according to the prescribed regimen have demonstrated that many patients fail to follow the prescribed regimen.[9] Even when an appropriate dosage of the correct therapeutic agent is prescribed, there will not be a therapeutic response unless the medication is taken in an adequate dose with the necessary frequency of administration being followed. In talks with patients who have not taken their medication according to the prescribed regimen, several interesting pieces of information emerge. Many times the cost of medication presents a problem for the patient, and he chooses to take less of it in order to save money. When this situation is discovered, the physician needs to work with the patient to help him understand the necessity of following the prescribed program of drug administration. In some cases, perhaps, the physician might prescribe a less expensive product or provide samples of medication to defray the cost so that the patient can be adequately medicated.

SCHEDULE OF ADMINISTRATION

Although the cost may sometimes limit the patient's compliance with the prescribed regimen, perhaps the most common problem giving rise to noncompliance is that the prescribed regimen is too complicated. Thus the schedule of administration is often critical in facilitating proper medication compliance by patients. By schedule of administration, I refer to the frequency with which the patient must take medication. Studies of noncompliance have repeatedly suggested that simplification of the dosage schedule is likely to increase patient compliance.[9,13] Fortunately, most commonly used psychotropic medications may be given in a single daily dose. This is true of the neuroleptics, most antidepressants, and many benzodiazepine antianxiety agents. Although divided-dose regimens are useful when psychotropic medication therapy is initiated in order to properly titrate the dosage, in most situations the physician can rapidly move toward single daily-dose administration. Monoamine oxidase inhibitors and SSRIs should not be administered at bedtime because they are apt to disturb the patient's sleep. MAOs may, however, be administered in a regimen wherein half the dose is given in the morning and the other half at dinnertime, except in those patients who develop significant postural hypotension, to whom the MAO inhibitor may have to be administered in three or four divided doses. Lithium carbonate has a much shorter half-life than other psychotropic agents and should not generally be administered in a single-dose regimen, although this approach has been suggested by some psychopharmacologists. Any lithium preparation may be administered utilizing a schedule of half the medication at breakfast time and the other half in the evening, as long as some food accompanies each dose to reduce gastric irritation.

The simpler the medication schedule prescribed, the more likely it is that the patient will follow it. Furthermore, since many patients forget to take medication, it is useful to connect medication administration with specific events taking place during the day. If medication must be taken during the day, a mealtime schedule is useful; if a single dose is administered, a bedtime schedule allows the patient to keep his medication in a particular spot, which reminds him to take it in connection with that particular daily event.[13] If the patient is forgetful, or must take medication several times during the day, helping him construct a chart of required medication times may reinforce dosage scheduling.[9]

ROUTE OF ADMINISTRATION

The route of administration, whether oral or parenteral, is an important consideration in providing effective pharmacotherapy. All psychotropic medications may be administered orally, which is less invasive and less uncomfortable than IM injection. In the acute phase of psychotic illness when the patient is treated in the hospital setting, it may be advantageous to administer medication in liquid form—particularly when instituting treatment with antipsychotic medication in a patient who is likely to be paranoid. No attempt should be made to trick the patient into taking medication or make him believe that he is receiving fruit juice which does not contain medication.

Proper support and negotiation by the nurse administering medication to the hospitalized patient will often help even resistant patients and those who are paranoid to take oral medication. Where only tablets or capsules are available, it may be necessary for the nurse to observe the patient as he takes the medication and to check the mouth after the medication has been ostensibly swallowed to be certain that it is not hidden under the tongue. The added effort in ensuring proper consumption of oral medication will provide for less traumatic treatment of the patient and fewer complaints of involuntary medication than if medication is routinely given by the IM route. Although there is a slight increase in rapidity of onset with antipsychotic drugs administered IM, in most instances the time saved is not critical to a favorable therapeutic response, and may even be associated with greater trauma than if the medication is taken orally. Some psychotic individuals, however, are out of control and present considerable risk of harming themselves or others; such patients may need to be medicated on an emergency basis by the IM administration of appropriate antipsychotic medication. Repeatedly noncompliant schizophrenic patients may benefit from long-acting neuroleptic medications given by IM injection.

WILLINGNESS TO TAKE MEDICATION

The problem of administering medication against the patient's wishes must be considered in the context of the present climate of medicolegal activity and the patient's rights movement, wherein charges of assault and battery might result from involuntary medication.[7] Litigation in this area is continuing, and it is hoped that the question will be resolved in a more favorable way so that patients who are ill and need treatment may be treated even when they are not aware of their illness or their need for treatment. Most states permit emergency administration of medication against the patient's will when there is a documented issue regarding safety of the patient and others. Once the emergency has passed, however, there is the potential of legal problems arising when the patient is medicated involuntarily.[7] When such a situation is encountered clinically, it is advantageous for the physician to enlist the cooperation of the patient's family members in helping to convince the patient of his need for treatment and also in providing support for the physician in medicating the patient against his will. In most states, involuntary commitment of a patient to a hospital does not provide *carte blanche* for the administration of medication against the patient's wishes.[7] In addition to soliciting the support of the family, it may also be necessary to suggest that the family engage an attorney to arrange for the court's appointment of a temporary guardian who will be responsible for making decisions regarding hospitalization and medical treatment of the patient who does not wish to be medicated.

In addition to the patient's verbal message that he does not want to take medication in the acute stage of illness, a patient will often give other messages nonverbally regarding his unwillingness to take medication. The patient who is repeatedly hospitalized because of a recurrence of psychotic illness even though an appropriate antipsychotic regimen has been prescribed is giving such a nonverbal message. Patients with severe psychotic illnesses that recur repeatedly, necessitating multiple hospitalizations, may require the administration of a long-acting injectable antipsychotic medication such as fluphenazine decanoate or haloperidol decanoate which may be administered IM every 2 to 6 weeks and provide a slow release of medication over the interval of time between injections. Medicolegally a patient must give consent to receive long-acting antipsychotic medication, since there is the possibility of legal action arising out of the administration of long-acting medication against the patient's will. There may be an increased risk of tardive dyskinesia associated with the long-term administration of long-acting injectable preparations of antipsychotic drugs. There is, therefore, some suggestion that they may be somewhat less safe than orally administered antipsychotic medication. Likewise, the administration of long-acting injectable forms of medication is much more constraining than allowing the patient the freedom and responsibility to take his own medication, thus setting up a potential conflict between the patient and the force of the hospital or clinic, which he may see as controlling him. My preference is to use orally administered antipsychotic medication in patients with psychotic illness as opposed to the administration of long-acting IM preparations. Furthermore, if a patient is started on a long-acting injectable preparation, the physician should consider this therapeutic approach as temporary, and after a period of a few months provide the patient an opportunity to try taking his own medication in oral form. This practice may both reduce the risk of long-term neurologic complications of repeated administration of depot forms of the antipsychotic drug, as well as reduce the patient's feeling of being controlled by a medical adversary.

Since there are no long-acting forms of treatment for depression at this time, patients who repeatedly discontinue antidepressant medication and become depressed may be candidates for a course of electroshock therapy, which may provide a suitable mood improvement somewhat more long-lasting than an abruptly discontinued brief course of antidepressant medication. It should be recognized by all clinicians that a sizable proportion of patients suffering from recurrent mania actually enjoy their mania. Many manic individuals will feel worthless and inadequate, with or without associated depression, when they are not manic. This may explain why many manic patients will periodically discontinue lithium.[13] Psychotherapy may be usefully employed at times to help the patient learn to gain greater enjoyment out of life when he is not manic. Furthermore, even in the presence of lithium, many individuals with bipolar illness will experience depression. The willingness of the physician to recognize and treat the depression pharmacologically during the course of lithium maintenance may allow the patient to feel better and not crave a return to the manic state by discontinuing lithium.

One of the things that make prescribing drugs for psychiatric patients different from prescribing medication for nonpsychiatric patients is that, in general, patients suffering from medical and surgical illness are more apt to be aware that they are suffering from a medical problem, and more willing or enthusiastic to receive some treatment to either alleviate their discomfort or improve the long-term prognosis of their illness. Many psychiatric patients are unwilling to receive treatment, particularly medical treatment, in the acute phase of their psychiatric illness. As a result they may become belligerent or threaten legal action in an attempt to frighten the physician away. As has been previously stated, many patients suffering from psychiatric illness are unaware that there is anything wrong. If they are indeed psychotic, it becomes difficult to interpret reality for them until there is some improvement in their psychosis. Pharmacologic intervention may be necessary temporarily on an involuntary basis, until symptoms improve to the extent that the patient can recognize his condition and be willing to receive medical intervention. Even if a patient recognizes that he has a psychiatric illness such as depression where there may be considerable dysphoria, the physician is faced with the continuous challenge of helping the patient recognize the biologic as well as the psychologic and social dimensions of his psychiatric condition so that he becomes more willing to receive medical treatment. The process of repeatedly educating the patient is probably the most critical issue in providing good and effective ongoing psychopharmacologic treatment. Since psychiatric patients are somewhat more likely than nonpsychiatric patients to use excessive quantities of alcohol and to take nonprescribed drugs, it is important to help them recognize that both alcohol and a variety of other drugs may interfere with their favorable response to psychopharmacologic treatment, and may indeed enhance the risk of adverse effects of their medication treatment program. Because of the nature of psychiatric illness and the attitude of patients and their families toward the illness and its treatment, the psychiatrist is less apt to receive grateful words of appreciation from his patient than the physician treating other medical conditions. This, unfortunately, may add to the frustration of the psychiatrist; this frustration, coupled with the fear of legal action, may keep many psychiatrists from prescribing and maintaining the patient on an optimal pharmacologic regimen.

GENERIC DRUGS

In our age of increasing economic constraints and escalating consumerism, the physician is becoming a target of greater pressures to prescribe generic drugs in the interest of saving the patient money. For a number of years we have been exposed to extensive advertising by the major pharmaceutical manufacturers who have been the source of development of virtually all modern therapeutic agents. Although the style of pharmaceutical advertising has varied from time to time and from company to company, and has often been slick and at times overly glib,[21] by and large the advertising has been accurate, polite, and no more inappropriate or aggressive than the advertising campaign of any other major industry in the United States. This is in contradistinction to the pressure we have received in support of generic prescribing, which has not always been polite and which has often been aggressive and designed to induce guilt in the clinician who has tended to favor use of known established pharmaceutical preparations.[22]

If the pharmacologic action of a drug product depended solely on the quantity of the specific chemical present in the tablet, one might easily construct a convincing argument in favor of generic prescribing. The reality is that the actual effect of a medication on the patient is dependent not only on the quantity of chemical present in the tablet but also upon the technique of manufacturing the tablet and upon the inclusion of a variety of inert substances utilized in the manufacture of that dosage form of the pharmaceutical.[22] A simple chemical assay of several brands of amitriptyline would reveal no significant difference in the quantity of chemical among the brands tested. If a variety of amitriptyline preparations administered to patients and blood levels at different time intervals obtained, and there is no difference between the generic preparation and the standard brand, then bioequivalence exists, in that the preparations compared provide comparable bioavailability and blood levels at standard time intervals following dosage administration of the different preparations.[23] There are indeed generic preparations of tricyclic antidepressants which provide bioavailability data comparable with the standard-brand preparation of the same drugs. On the other hand, for many drug products, including the tricyclic antidepressants, there is not bioequivalence among all generic preparations and the standard reference compound. One Food and Drug Administration (FDA) study of bioequivalence of imipramine preparations reported in the *Federal Register* revealed that some generic preparations tested provided blood levels as low as 74% of the standard-brand preparation of imipramine.[24]

When an antidepressant drug or any other psychotropic or nonpsychotropic medication is prescribed by its generic name, the dispensing pharmacist has the option of dispensing any preparation of that drug that he wishes to purchase and sell. Most often the pharmacist will dispense a generic preparation that he is able to buy at the most advantageous price. Since the prices of generic pharmaceuticals fluctuate rapidly, and since there are so many companies manufacturing generic products, it is likely that from time to time the dispensing pharmacist will purchase different preparations of a given generic product manufactured by a variety of manufacturers. It is conceivable that if a patient has his antidepressant prescription refilled on a monthly basis, he may, over the course of a year of therapy, receive anywhere from two to 12 different products. My own policy is to always prescribe the standard brand of a given antidepressant preparation, because this at least will ensure that the patient is receiving the same medication over his course of treatment. If a patient asks me for a generic preparation in order to save money, I will advise him that I have no guarantee that the generic preparation will be equivalent but that I will be happy to prescribe it for him at his request as long as he accepts the responsibility for any adverse effects or failure to respond satisfactorily. Since I am so concerned about the possibility of inequivalence of generic preparations, I usually refuse to prescribe one during the first month of treatment with an antidepressant, because of my belief that the patient's failure to respond to the initial course of drug therapy may be dangerous to the patient by prolonging his depression. Also, the failure to respond to a trial of amitriptyline, for example, might lead me to conclude that the patient needs to be changed to a different antidepressant. If the failure to respond were not related to the specific pharmacologic agent, but rather to the preparation administered, that would produce an unnecessary complication in the patient's course of drug therapy. Once the patient has responded favorably to the standard preparation of an antidepressant, I will, on his request, prescribe the generic product.

During the last 15 years I have encountered a number of situations which have further established my negative view of generic prescribing. I have seen several patients who initially responded to Tofranil, and who subsequently appeared to lose their response when converted to generic imipramine, but regained their response following a return to the original Tofranil product. Likewise, in patients initially responding to Elavil, I have seen several who described a less favorable response to generic amitryptyline but who subsequently felt better as they resumed treatment with Elavil. Some patients in both antidepressant groups complained of greater anticholinergic effects with the generic preparation even though they felt less well from the standpoint of mood. This finding is difficult to explain, although the obvious technique that I should have employed to clarify the apparent generic inequivalence was to determine plasma tricyclic levels during the course of treatment with the standard preparation and the generic preparation. Tricyclic blood levels can be obtained periodically in patients taking generic tricyclic preparations in order to establish that they are maintaining adequate blood levels.

If the patient is unfortunate enough to receive a generic preparation which is not bioequivalent and thereby does become depressed, it is not unlikely that he could lose time from work, have a disturbance in his family life, or even contemplate suicide. Furthermore, it is likely that such an individual will require one or more extra visits to the psychiatrist to ascertain the nature of the problem and for suitable intervention. The cost of the extra visits might well exceed the money saved by the generic preparation, not to mention the potential of losing time from work, the disturbance in family life, and the unmeasurable cost of a suicide attempt.

In addition to data indicating a lack of bioequivalence between generic and brand-name antidepressants, there is growing evidence that this problem also exists for generic diazepam, antipsychotic drugs, and lithium carbonate preparations. Some clinicians and investigators have found that patients switched from brand-name Thorazine to generic chlorpromazine have required larger doses, have needed more frequent administration of prn doses, or have shown increased agitation while receiving the generic preparation. Similarly, generic thioridazine has been found to be less effective than brand-name

Mellaril by a number of investigators, who have reported the necessity to administer larger daily doses or more frequent prn doses of the generic product.[25] Several generic preparations of chlorpromazine and thioridazine have been withdrawn from the market because of the lack of bioequivalence. There have been anecdotal reports indicating that generic haloperidol preparations may be less effective in controlling psychotic symptoms and agitation, thus requiring the administration of larger daily doses of the generic product in comparison with brand-name Haldol. Although patients may be harmed and their recovery retarded by the use of less effective pharmaceuticals, it is also likely that the physician who prescribes generic products may be vulnerable to litigation as a result of adverse effects or lack of efficacy of these products.[22,26] The physician must be aware of a variety of clinical and nonclinical factors in arriving at his own decision regarding generic prescribing.[26]

ARE WE AN OVERMEDICATED SOCIETY?

As physicians we are continuously exposed to pharmaceutical advertising, which at times is overly zealous in urging the use of a particular product. We are simultaneously exposed to the lay press and to the media, which levy periodic attacks on the medical profession for producing an overmedicated society.[21] Rational pharmacotherapy is one of the most important and necessary aspects of the practice of medicine. Rational pharmacotherapy involves the thoughtful prescribing of the optimal medication for a particular clinical condition that can be expected to respond favorably to the intended treatment.[27] In properly considered drug therapy the benefits must exceed the risk of the medication. Optimal prescribing does not include the use of pharmaceutical products to modify our response to natural life events unless that response becomes pathologic and impairs our ability to function, as in the development of severe depression following the death of a spouse. On the other hand, an individual who suffers a loss needs to have a period of time in which to grieve and is not likely to benefit from the physician who too readily recommends a prescription of a sedative or tranquilizer.[21] The tendency of many patients who seek medication to help them deal with ordinary life events is one important component of the overmedication of our society. Unfortunately, some physicians are willing to medicate normal life events and thus become the instrument through which some individuals do become overmedicated.[21] The simultaneous use of multiple therapeutic agents by a physician in a given patient is another form of overmedication which may be associated not only with the administration of unnecessary drugs, but with the potential for multiple adverse drug reactions produced by the interaction of several medications.[27] Thus, another way to avoid the risk of overmedication is for the physician to be cautious in attempting to treat every patient with the least number of medications possible. The necessity to use the fewest number of medications in any given clinical situation does not absolutely state that the use of multiple medications is bad medical practice.

There are some clinical situations wherein several medications may need to be administered at any given time; this is true in medical illnesses such as hypertension, and in psychiatric conditions such as the major affective illnesses. Some patients suffering from affective illness may indeed require continued administration of lithium carbonate, a low-dose high-potency neuroleptic, and simultaneously an antidepressant drug. On the other hand, the simultaneous administration of two or more antipsychotic agents to a patient suffering from a psychotic illness is almost always irrational pharmacotherapy, since these drugs appear to exert their effect through one mechanism. Proper dosage adjustment of one neuroleptic should provide optimal therapeutic response and fewer adverse effects than if multiple neuroleptics are combined.

Despite concerns that we are an overmedicated society, my own observations and those of several other individuals interested in drug therapy suggest that we are at times undermedicated — not in the sense that we are not spending enough money for medication or that we are not taking enough medication, but in the sense that many patients who are suffering from medically treatable illnesses do not receive proper and necessary treatment.[28] Probably the best example of those who are undertreated are individuals suffering from depressive illness. Countless patients who suffer from prolonged depression are being treated by psychotherapy without the benefit of specific and highly effective antidepressant medication.[28] Other individuals suffering from depression may be receiving antianxiety agents such as the benzodiazepines, which do not exert a true antidepressant effect, and therefore produce only a Band-Aid effect rather than a true pharmacologic effect.

Increased awareness of the proper application of pharmacologic agents to the practice of psychiatry could lead to a reduction of much of the irrational overprescribing and equally irrational underprescribing of psychotropic medication. It remains easier to educate the professional community than it does the public, many of whom avoid professionally administered medical care and prefer to medicate themselves using readily obtainable over-the-counter products. Most laymen, and unfortunately many physicians, believe that medications sold without requirement of a prescription can be generally considered as relatively "weak" and safe. This is most definitely not true. There are a variety of over-the-counter products which contain phenylpropanolamine, a stimulant with weak amphetaminelike properties and considerable ability to produce tachycardia and hypertensive reactions.[29] The number of over-the-counter cold remedies, cough products, tranquilizers, and sedatives is vast. The one thing which all such products have in common is that antihistamines are invariably a major component; most often anticholinergic drugs are also included in the formula.[29] As discussed in chapter 12, anticholinergic drugs and antihistamines taken either individually or together can produce an acute toxic delirium if taken in excessive quantity by young healthy individuals. Elderly patients taking minute quantities of antihistamines or anticholinergic agents may develop a severe toxic delirium.[29]

Certainly if we are overmedicated, a good deal of the overmedication undoubtedly comes from the heavily advertised and promoted over-the-counter medications which so many patients take. Many people do not even consider over-the-counter products as medication, which is an extremely important consideration in gathering historical information from patients. Very commonly, unless the physician specifically asks about nonprescription pharmaceutical products, patients will deny that they take such products or will forget to mention them as they give a history of their current and previous experiences with drug therapy. Although it may be easier for physicians to regulate their own prescribing and attempt to achieve a rational approach to drug therapy, we are unable to control the use of nonprescribed medications, and illicit drugs, by our patients. Our own awareness that a variety of substances not prescribed by the physician may produce profound pharmacologic effects on the patient, and may also interact with prescribed pharmacologic agents, will help to increase the safety and efficacy of patient treatment and avoid therapeutic misadventures produced by such interactions.

RISK MANAGEMENT IN PSYCHOPHARMACOLOGY

Although in the past, litigation and malpractice actions were less frequent in psychiatry than in other fields of medicine, this problem is becoming more common and is a source of increasing anxiety for the practicing psychiatrist. No field of intellectual knowledge allows for accurate prediction of potential human behavior. Many patients will consult a psychiatrist because of thoughts of suicide. Under optimal conditions, proper diagnosis and treatment can prevent many suicides, though it would be unreasonable to think that any technique of suicide assessment or prevention could be foolproof. The physician must seriously consider hospitalization of any patient who appears to be suicidal. Working with the patient and responsible family members may allow a patient expressing suicidal ideation to be treated safely outside of the hospital setting. Since antidepressant drugs can become effective suicide weapons, these drugs should be prescribed in very limited quantities early in the course of treatment of a severely depressed patient.

Many of the most effective psychopharmacologic agents possess a variety of adverse effects. The physician's awareness of potential adverse effects, coupled with frequent and careful evaluation of the patient, can facilitate early diagnosis and treatment of adverse drug reactions. Failure to diagnose and properly treat an adverse drug reaction can lead to potentially serious medical complications for the patient and serious legal complications for the physician. In spite of our best efforts to provide optimal patient care, some adverse drug reactions are unavoidable. All currently available antipsychotic drugs have the potential of producing tardive dyskinesia with prolonged administration. Careful diagnostic assessment and the avoidance of neuroleptic drugs in patients for whom they are not clinically indicated can minimize the physician's liability.[30] The clinician must talk honestly with the patient about the nature of the illness and the potential risk of tardive dyskinesia associated with neuroleptic therapy when such treatment must be administered over a prolonged period of time.[30] During the course of follow-up care, it is important to periodically review with the patient the potential risks of long-term medication. Patients must be seen frequently enough to be certain that they are receiving an appropriate pharmacologic regimen and not experiencing inordinate or potentially dangerous side effects. It may be beneficial to the patient and to the physician to meet with family members on one or more occasions at the outset of treatment and periodically during the course of treatment in order to discuss the patient's progress and what effects, both favorable and adverse, can be anticipated from the program of pharmacotherapy.

Documentation is an extremely important component of good patient care as well as risk management. The physician should document in the medical record the names and dosages of all medications prescribed, and at each visit with the patient, document continuation of or changes in the pharmacologic regimen. The psychiatrist should also note in the record his discussions with the patient regarding any potential adverse effects of the medication prescribed. This documentation should also include comments regarding the patient's consent for treatment and any questions or problems that the patient raises regarding the treatment program. The record should also include documentation of the warnings given with respect to potential development of tardive dyskinesia with neuroleptic drugs. A caring physician who maintains an open and honest dialogue with the patient; a favorable doctor-patient relationship; and a well-documented medical record are the most important elements of risk management in the practice of psychopharmacology.

REFERENCES

1. Rosner F: *Julius Preuss' biblical and talmudic medicine.* New York, Sanhedrin Press, 1978.
2. Jewish Publication Society: *The prophets: I Samuel,* ed 2. Philadelphia, Jewish Publication Society of America, 1978, pp 133-164.
3. Major R: *A history of Medicine.* Springfield Ill, Charles C Thomas, 1954.
4. Ayd FJ, Blackwell B (eds): *Discoveries in biological psychiatry.* Philadelphia, JB Lippincott, 1970.
5. Ellenberger HF: *The discovery of the unconscious.* New York, Basic Books, 1970.
6. Gutheil TG: The psychology of psychopharmacology. *Bull Menninger Clin* 1982; 46:321-330.
7. Veliz J, James WS: Medicine court: Rogers in practice. *Am J Psychiatry* 1987;144:62-67.
8. Bernstein JG: The right to know: a patient's guide to psychotropic medications. In Bernstein JG (ed): *Clinical psychopharmacology.* Littleton Mass, PSG Publishing, 1978, pp 145-154.
9. Blackwell B: Drug therapy: patient compliance. *N Engl J Med* 1973;289:249-252.
10. Bursten B: Medication nonadherence due to feelings of loss of control in "biological depression." *Am J Psychiatry* 1985;142:244-246.
11. Goodwin FK, Jamison KR: Medication compliance (Chapter 25). In *Manic-depressive illness.* New York, Oxford University Press, 1990, pp 746-762.
12. Harrison WM, Rabkin JG, Ehrhardt AA, et al: Effects of antidepressant medication on sexual function: a controlled study. *J Clin Psychopharmacol* 1986;6:144-149.
13. Connelly CR, Davenport YB, Newberger JF: Adherence to treatment regimen in a lithium carbonate clinic. *Arch Gen Psychiatry* 1982;39:585-589.

14. Gardos G, Cole JO, Tarsy D: Withdrawal syndromes associated with antipsychotic drugs. *Am J Psychiatry* 1978;135:1321-1324.
15. Khantzian EJ, McKenna GJ: Acute toxic and withdrawal reactions associated with drug use and abuse. *Ann Intern Med* 1979;90:361-372.
16. Bernstein JG: Chemotherapy of psychosis. In Bernstein JG (ed): *Clinical psychopharmacology.* Littleton Mass, PSG Publishing, 1978, pp 40-51.
17. Creese I: Dopamine and antipsychotic medications. In Hales RE, Frances AJ (eds): *APA annual review.* Washington DC, American Psychiatric Press, 1985, vol 4, pp 17-36.
18. Wernicke JF, Dunlop SR, Dornseif BE, et al: Low-dose fluoxetine therapy for depression. *Psychopharmacol Bull* 1988;24:183-188.
19. Aguglia E, Casacchia M, Cassano GB, et al: Double-blind study of the efficacy and safety of sertraline versus fluoxetine in major depression. *Int Clin Psychopharmacol* 1993;8:197-202.
20. Stoll AL, Pope HG, McElroy SL: High-dose fluoxetine: safety and efficacy in 27 cases. *J Clin Psychopharmacol* 1991;11:225-226.
21. Lennard HL, Epstein LJ, Bernstein A, et al: *Mystification and drug misuse,* San Francisco, Jossey-Bass, 1971.
22. Carr EA Jr: Potential liabilities of generic drug prescribing. *Drug Ther* 1979;9:99-106.
23. Strom BL: Generic drug substitution revisited. *N Engl J Med* 1987;316:1456-1462.
24. Tricyclic antidepressants: proposed bioequivalence requirements, *Fed Reg* 1978;43:34, 2 CFR, §320.
25. Barone JA, Colaizzi JL: Critical evaluation of thioridazine bioequivalence. *Drug Intell Clin Pharm* 1985;19:847-858.
26. Dettelback HR: A time to speak out on bioequivalence and therapeutic equivalence. *J Clin Pharmacol* 1986;26:307-308.
27. Azarnoff DL: Do we achieve rational drug therapy? In Bochner F, Carruthers G, Kampmann J, et al (eds): *Handbook of clinical pharmacology.* Boston, Little Brown, 1978, pp 1-8.
28. Bernstein JG: Advances in the pharmacotherapy of depression. *Drug Ther* 1990;20:40-47.
29. Gardner ER, Hall RCW: Psychiatric symptoms produced by over-the-counter drugs. *Psychosomatics* 1982;23:186-190.
30. Appelbaum PS, Schaffner K, Meisel A: Responsibility and compensation for tardive dyskinesia. *Am J Psychiatry* 1985;142:806-810.

CHAPTER 3

Antianxiety Agents and Hypnotics

OVERVIEW

Management of Anxiety

1. Assess relationship of anxiety to life events and decide whether pharmacotherapy is indicated; consider relaxation training or psychotherapy.
2. Carefully evaluate severity, duration, and characteristics of anxiety symptoms to arrive at a specific *diagnosis*.
3. Medical disorders and affective illness may present as anxiety and be best remedied by specific pharmacotherapy or medical intervention.
4. In short-term situational anxiety or insomnia, intermittent benzodiazepines or sedating antihistamines may be effective.
5. Panic disorder, agoraphobia, and obsessive compulsive disorder should be treated with SSRIs, TCAs, or MAOIs with adjunctive clonazepam. High-dose prolonged courses of drugs such as alprazolam are to be avoided, and buspirone is likely to be ineffective.
6. Psychosis or mania should be treated with neuroleptics or lithium.
7. Neuroleptic-induced akathisia may be mistaken for anxiety and is best managed by reduced neuroleptic doses, antiparkinsonian drugs, benzodiazepines, or propranolol, which may also reduce physiologic symptoms of anxiety.
8. Neuroleptics should generally be avoided in nonpsychotic anxious patients.
9. Persistent severe anxiety may predispose to sedative abuse and dependency; buspirone may be useful, particularly in generalized anxiety, without the risk of drug dependency.
10. PTSD is difficult to treat but is often responsive to SSRIs or carbamazepine.

Continued.

Management of Insomnia

11. Avoid overuse of dependency-producing drugs; be aware of prolongation of sedative effect by co-administered drugs, including fluoxetine and alcohol; avoid triazolam and pharmacologically related hypnotics.

12. Consider sedating antihistamines, sedating cyclic antidepressants, clonazepam, chloral hydrate or melatonin and newer compounds when available.

Anxiety and insomnia are among the most common symptoms for which drug therapy is prescribed. Each of these symptoms may occur in association with a variety of psychiatric and medical illnesses. They may occur independently or simultaneously in the same individual. Either may occur suddenly, with or without an obvious cause, or may develop slowly from an imperceptible symptom recognizable only in the course of taking a detailed history. Anxiety may worsen gradually or come about abruptly to such a severe degree that an individual is incapacitated and cannot go about his daily routine. Insomnia may appear gradually and steadily worsen, or it may begin abruptly following a life crisis so that the individual quickly becomes exhausted and unable to function. Unfortunately there is often a tendency to quickly medicate the patient who suffers from anxiety or insomnia without an adequate clinical evaluation to recognize underlying emotional or physical causative factors that may respond to specific psychotherapy or pharmacotherapy. Such an evaluation may avoid the use of sedative drugs, most of which produce a rather generalized CNS depressant effect.

The history of the development of sedatives which have come to play a prevalent role in the treatment of anxiety and insomnia is long and complicated. Clearly, alcohol is the oldest known sedative used both medically and nonmedically. The development of sedative drugs throughout the ages has promised safety and efficacy, yet time has taught, often painfully, the dangers of dependency and the complications associated with sedative drugs. Generally, the history of newer sedatives has recapitulated the older well-known experience with alcohol. In Genesis, the first book of the Old Testament, we learn that when Noah left the ark after the flood he planted a vineyard. The Bible recounts the first known warning regarding the safety of the sedative alcohol: ". . . and he drank of the wine, and was drunken; and he was uncovered within his tent." This is perhaps the first documentation of an adverse drug reaction, as well as a statement regarding one of the risks of sedative drugs, including alcohol — the potential development of a state of intoxication wherein one may undergo a dramatic and perhaps embarrassing behavioral change. Following generations

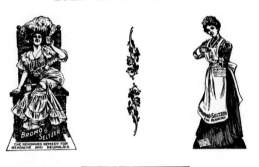

Fig. 3-1 Turn of-the-century Bromo-Seltzer advertisement.

of widespread use of alcohol as a sedative in medicine, a variety of other, presumably safer, sedatives were developed, including valerian and eventually the bromides, each with the promise of safety, which unfortunately was not fulfilled. A turn-of-the-century Bromo-Seltzer advertisement (Fig. 3-1) proclaims the absence of cocaine and morphine but of course fails to mention the risk of bromide dependency which became a serious complication, necessitating withdrawal of bromides from the therapeutic armamentarium.[1] The development of the barbiturates in the early 1900s was initially seen as a potentially safe and effective medical advance, which again, unfortunately, was followed by the recognition of some of the adverse effects of barbiturates, including their potential for addiction.[1]

DRUG DEPENDENCY

The first major advance following the barbiturates was the development of meprobamate in the mid-1950s. This drug was initially touted as effective and free of the addiction-producing liability of the barbiturates. Within a few years of the widespread initial clinical use of meprobamate, a number of individuals who had been using the drug regularly over a long period of time and who discontinued its use began to experience grand mal seizures and other symptoms similar to those seen with barbiturate withdrawal.[1,2] Following the meprobamate experience, the first benzodiazepine, chlordiazepoxide, appeared on the American market. Again, this drug was introduced with the promise of efficacy and safety, specifically the lack of risk of addiction. As greater experience was gained with chlordiazepoxide and related compounds such as diazepam, and alprazolam physicians began to report evidence of drug withdrawal not dissimilar from that seen with meprobamate and the barbiturates.[2] The physician must consider the problem of sedative addiction and its treatment as he contemplates prescribing sedative drugs, many of which do present a considerable liability for addiction. Furthermore, the potential of drug dependency raises important questions about the appropriateness of the large-scale clinical use of sedative drugs. This concern suggests a need to avoid the prolonged use of these drugs whenever possible, and to recognize that in many instances they can best be employed on an intermittent basis for a brief period of time.

Although many clinicians and even package inserts for many sedative drugs advise the physician against the excessive use of antianxiety and hypnotic drugs in the "addiction prone patient," it may be more appropriate to recognize that the potential for the development of addiction is more likely a function of the pharmacology of the drug than the personality of the patient.[2] Some individuals follow the physician's recommendation absolutely and others may tend to underuse or overuse a prescribed medication. It must be recognized, however, that the characteristics of a given drug or class of drugs may be more likely to facilitate or avoid addiction than the personality of the individual taking that drug. For example, there is no evidence that the use of any one of the antipsychotic medications, regardless of the dose, frequency, or duration of administration, will produce a true addiction syndrome; on the other hand, the evidence is overwhelming that with the administration of 400 to 600 mg pentobarbital per day for a period of 6 weeks at least 80% of individuals will show signs of withdrawal when the drug is discontinued.[3] Buspirone, a structurally unique non-benzodiazepine antianxiety drug, does not appear to produce tolerance, dependency, or withdrawal symptoms.

CLASSIFICATION OF ANXIETY

The most common form of anxiety, anticipatory anxiety, occurs when one approaches a situation or task in normal daily life and is indeed present in most everyone at some time or other. A person experiencing anticipatory anxiety is often described as "nervous" and usually does not require pharmacologic intervention, though occasionally small intermittent doses of benzodiazepines are clinically helpful. Indeed, this form of anxiety is so "normal" that it is not included in the official DSM-IV classification of anxiety disorders. Since the clinical forms of anxiety and their interrelationship with other disorders included in the affective spectrum are so variable, there is no uniform pharmacologic approach to anxiety, but rather specific approaches to rather distinct entities. Since many conditions—including obsessive-compulsive disorder, panic disorder, and phobic disorders, which are classified as anxiety disorders—rely heavily for their treatment on SSRIs and other drugs not classified as antianxiety agents, their management will be dealt with more extensively in later chapters.

The *Diagnostic and Statistical Manual of Mental Disorders,* fourth edition (DSM-IV), the most recent official guide to psychiatric disorders and their nomenclature, classifies the following forms of anxiety disorders:

1. Panic Disorder (with or without agoraphobia)
2. Specific Phobia
3. Social Phobia
4. Obsessive-Compulsive Disorder
5. Posttraumatic Stress Disorder
6. Acute Stress Disorder
7. Generalized Anxiety Disorder
8. Anxiety Disorder Due to a General Medical Condition
9. Substance-Induced Anxiety Disorder
10. Anxiety Disorder Not Otherwise Specified

According to the DSM-IV, posttraumatic stress disorder generally results following exposure to catastrophic events, which threaten the life or physical integrity of oneself, or others. In this disorder, the traumatic event is persistently reexperienced in at least one of the following ways:

1. Recurrent and intrusive distressing recollections of the event
2. Recurrent distressing dreams of the event
3. Sudden acting or feeling as if the traumatic event were recurring, including a sense of reliving the experience (illusions, hallucinations, and dissociative flashback episodes), which may occur upon awakening or when intoxicated
4. Intense psychological distress and exposure to events that symbolize or resemble an aspect of the traumatic event, including anniversaries of the trauma
5. Physiologic reactivity upon exposure to internal or external cue that symbolizes or resembles an aspect of the traumatic event

Patients with posttraumatic stress disorder attempt to avoid stimuli associated with the trauma. Patients also have persistent symptoms of increased arousal and may experience difficulty falling asleep or staying asleep, irritability or anger outbursts, difficulty concentrating, hypervigilance, exaggerated startle response, and difficulty recalling details of the traumatic event.[6]

Generalized Anxiety Disorder (GAD) as delineated in the DSM-IV consists of excessive anxiety and worry (apprehensive expectation) occurring more days than not for at least 6 months, about a number of events or activities. The person with GAD finds it difficult to control the worry and experiences at least three of the following symptoms:

1. Restlessness, feeling keyed-up or on edge
2. Easy fatiguability
3. Difficulty concentrating, mind going blank
4. Irritability
5. Muscle tension
6. Difficulty falling or staying asleep or restless unsatisfying sleep

The symptom complex now called GAD is consistent with what for many years has been termed chronic anxiety, due the pervasiveness and persistence of symptoms.

PHARMACOTHERAPY OF ANXIETY

An anxious patient will describe feeling nervous and uncomfortable with or without associated physiologic signs and symptoms. Most often, however, severe anxiety is accompanied by a variety of autonomic nervous system manifestations, including tachycardia, palpitations, irregular heart rhythm, dizziness, tremor, excessive sweating, dry mouth, diarrhea, abdominal pain, and headache.[5] These physiologic manifestations may be present regardless of the specific type of anxiety disorder. Administration of sedating drugs such as the benzodiazepines, either intermittently or during a prolonged regular course of therapy, may alleviate symptoms of nervousness and dysphoria, but generally provide only minimal blunting of the physiologic manifestations of anxiety. Numerous clinical studies, however, indicate that beta-adrenergic blocking drugs, such as propranolol, metoprolol, and atenolol, may dramatically inhibit the physiologic manifestations of anxiety, when administered alone or in conjunction with modest doses of benzodiazepines.[7-9] One major advantage of beta-adrenergic blocking drugs in the treatment of anxiety is their minimal risk of producing mental clouding and their absence of addiction potential. The anxious patient without prominent autonomic symptoms is less likely to benefit from beta-adrenergic blockade than is the patient who presents with significant tachycardia, palpitations, sweating, and gastrointestinal (GI) disturbance.

Patients who have a long-standing history of anxiety are likely, even with optimal pharmacologic response, to require persistent pharmacologic intervention. Since prolonged administration of benzodiazepines may be associated with drug dependency, it is important to make a specific diagnosis of the type of anxiety disorder and to utilize those pharmacologic treatments which provide optimal benefit with the lowest risk of adverse effects and drug dependency.[10] Obsessive compulsive disorder is most responsive to serotonin-selective reuptake inhibitors and to clomipramine and is discussed in detail in chapters 4 and 9. As discussed in chapter 9, patients suffering from agoraphobia and panic disorder are best treated with SSRIs, tricyclic antidepressants, or monoamine oxidase inhibitors (MAOIs). Individuals suffering from posttraumatic stress disorder may achieve a favorable therapeutic response when treated with SSRIs, tricyclic antidepressants, MAOIs, carbamazepine, or lithium, and may be at relatively high risk for developing drug dependency or disinhibition when treated with benzodiazepines.[11,12] Buspirone, which does not have specific antipanic or antiphobic activity, appears to be effective and clinically useful in the treatment of some patients with generalized anxiety disorder.[13]

Mechanisms of Action of Antianxiety Agents

Despite the lengthy history of the use of barbiturates, and the extensive experience with benzodiazepines and a variety of other sedative medications, the mechanisms of action of these agents are not fully understood.[1,10] Many sedatives used for the relief of anxiety and the induction of sleep exert a general CNS depressant effect, which is dose related.[1]

Benzodiazepines

The benzodiazepines compete for glycine receptors in the brain, and there are specific benzodiazepine receptors which appear to account for the selective action of these drugs on polysynaptic neuronal pathways throughout the CNS.[1] During barbiturate-induced anesthesia, there is an approximately 50% decrease in oxygen utilization by the brain and an increase in glycogen and high-energy phosphate content, probably secondary to the decrease in neuronal activity.[1] γ-Aminobutyric acid (GABA) is a naturally occurring inhibitory neurotransmitter. Low doses of barbiturates have been demonstrated to exert a GABA-like action or enhance the effects of GABA.[1]

The anxiolytic potency of various benzodiazepines correlates with their affinity for benzodiazepine receptors. GABA increases the affinity of benzodiazepines for their specific receptor sites. Benzodiazepines increase the frequency with which anion channels open in response to GABA.[14] Opening of anion channels produces hyperpolarization of the postsynaptic neuron, potentially decreasing the frequency of neuronal firing.[14] Since most of the effects of GABA are mediated through changes in anion channels, the anionic effects of benzodiazepine binding may be mediated at sites close to the channel. The ability of benzodiazepines to modulate the neurotransmitter activity of GABA in the brain is an important part of their action.[14] Pharmacologic actions of benzodiazepines may be blocked by the administration of inhibitors of GABA synthesis.[1] The relationship of GABA to the specific anxiolytic activity of benzodiazepines is suggested but not definitively proven.[1] It appears that the GABA-nergic action of the benzodiazepines may at least partially account for their anticonvulsant and muscle-relaxant effect.[1]

There is also some evidence that oxazepam, a commonly used benzodiazepine, may act in part by decreasing norepinephrine and serotonin turnover and that these mechanisms may account at least partially for the hypnotic and anxiolytic effects of the benzodiazepines.[1] Benzodiazepines have also been shown to increase the content of acetylcholine in certain brain areas.[1] Barbiturates may selectively abolish noradrenergic excitation and are also capable of decreasing the release and turnover of acetylcholine. It has been suggested that this interaction of barbiturates with acetylcholine may be a factor in the development of tolerance to these drugs.[1]

Buspirone

Buspirone is structurally and pharmacologically unrelated to the benzodiazepines. This drug is not a CNS depressant and does not produce significant sedative action, yet it alleviates many symptoms of generalized anxiety. This drug does not cross-react with benzodiazepines, and will not protect against benzodiazepine withdrawal symptoms, nor does it appear to produce tolerance or dependency of its own. Buspirone does not have anticonvulsant or muscle-relaxant properties, which are characteristic of the benzodiazepines. Buspirone does not displace radioactive benzodiazepine ligands from the benzodiazepine receptor complex, alter the effects of GABA on benzodiazepine binding, or interact directly with GABA receptors. Buspirone does not appear to effect monoamine uptake systems.[15] Buspirone appears to specifically block presynaptic rather than postsynaptic dopamine receptors.[15] Through this mechanism, buspirone markedly increases the firing rate of midbrain dopamine neurons.[15] Unlike neuroleptic drugs, which are postsynaptic dopamine antagonists, buspirone does not induce catalepsy in animals.[15] In fact, buspirone reverses neuroleptic-induced catalepsy, which suggests that it is unlikely to produce extrapyramidal side effects or tardive dyskinesia, which may occur with postsynaptic dopamine antagonists, such as the neuroleptic drugs.[15] Buspirone has also been shown to activate presynaptic 5-HT_{1A} serotonin receptors.[15] This mechanism appears to account for decreased striatal levels of serotonin and its metabolites following buspirone administration.[15] It is conceivable that decreased serotonin activity, which is produced both by buspirone and the benzodiazepines, may at least partially account for the anxiolytic effects of these drugs.[15]

Pharmacokinetic Aspects of Benzodiazepines

When benzodiazepines are administered for the treatment of anxiety or insomnia, it must be remembered that these drugs have long half-lives and the majority of them yield pharmacologically active metabolites, further extending the half-life of the parent compound[1] (Table 3-1). The half-life and duration of pharmacologic action of these drugs differ depending on whether a single dose is administered to an experimental subject or multiple doses are given

Table 3-1 Half-lives and dosage ranges of benzodiazepines

Benzodiazepine	Half-life (h)	Daily dosage range (mg)
Alprazolam (Xanax)*	12-19	0.25-5.0
Chlordiazepoxide (Librium)	12-48	5-100
Clonazepam (Klonopin)	18-28	0.5-5.0
Diazepam (Valium)	20-90	2-40
Estazolam (Prosom)*	10-24	0.5-2
Flurazepam (Dalmane)	24-100	15-30
Lorazepam (Ativan)	10-20	1-4
Oxazepam (Serax)	8-21	10-60
Quazepam (Doral)	39-73	7.5-15
Temazepam (Restoril)	12-24	15-30
Triazolam (Halcion)*	2.5-3.5	0.125-0.25

*Triazolobenzodiazepine dependency may be more difficult to treat.

throughout the day over a period of several days or weeks.[1] Thus the ability to observe drug effects and measure the blood and urine levels will be of longer duration in a patient receiving diazepam, a long-acting benzodiazepine, several times daily for a period of 2 weeks, than it would be if the same individual were to receive a single dose of the medication. Likewise, since these drugs tend to be very lipid-soluble, they may persist longer in an obese individual or in an individual whose fat-to-lean body mass is increased, as in the elderly.[1] Furthermore, reduced renal or hepatic function, related to disease or to aging, will likewise extend the duration of drug effect.

For these reasons, it is obviously advantageous to administer these drugs in the smallest possible dose, given as infrequently as possible over the shortest period of time, whatever the patient's clinical status or age. Furthermore, since even the "short-acting" benzodiazepines have lengthy half-lives, it is often preferable to use one of the shorter-acting drugs in this group. In evaluating the literature describing a new drug, the physician must recognize that the half-lives normally quoted are for single-dose administration, which may seem favorably short compared to actual data based on an extended period of drug administration. There are currently three benzodiazepines with relatively short durations of action. These drugs — alprazolam, lorazepam, and oxazepam — have half-lives of about 10 to 12 hours following administration of a single dose.[1,10] In one study of alprazolam, administered in a dose of 0.5 mg 3 times daily for 7 days, the elimination half-life increased from 11.7 hours after the first dose to 18.9 hours after the last dose.[16] With lorazepam and oxazepam, repeated administration over a period of a week produces a somewhat longer elimination half-life, and it would not be surprising to see elimination half-lives for any of these drugs approaching 48 hours when used extensively over a prolonged period of time. Triazolam, which is used in the short-term treatment of insomnia, has a half-life of 2.5 to 3.5 hours following single-dose administration; however, with prolonged administration, the half-life may become significantly longer.[1] The very short half-life of triazolam may increase risks for drug dependency and confusional states, particularly with prolonged use.

Anxiety Agents: Therapeutic Application and Adverse Effects

Benzodiazepines

One of the dangers in the use of diazepam is its disinhibiting effect; an individual prone to violence may become violent under the influence of the drug.[17] Even in persons who do not have a prior history of violence, loss of behavioral control or the occurrence of violent behavior may occur during benzodiazepine administration.[17,18] There is evidence to suggest that oxazepam is less likely to have a disinhibiting effect than the other drugs in this class.[19]

Alprazolam, estazolam, and triazolam are structurally unique among the benzodiazepines since their molecular configuration, which includes a triazolo ring, bears some similarity to the configuration of tricyclic antidepressants.[1] Alprazolam is also functionally unique among the benzodiazepines in that several studies have documented specific antidepressant and antipanic effects of this compound.[20,21] Alprazolam has been reported to induce manic symptoms.[22,23] In this respect, it differs from other benzodiazepines such as lorazepam and clonazepam, which may actually have an antimanic effect.[23,24] A number of reports have appeared regarding increased hostility, acute paroxysmal excitement, and behavioral dyscontrol among alprazolam-treated patients.[18,25,26] In some instances, this may be connected with the antidepressant action of alprazolam and represent a manic equivalent, while in other instances the effect may simply parallel the disinhibiting effect of other benzodiazepines.

It is well known that tricyclic antidepressants may produce stuttering. This has generally been attributed to their anticholinergic action, because it is less prominent among those agents with weaker anticholinergic activity. Although stuttering has not been associated with benzodiazepines, an interesting case report documented the occurrence of stuttering following 0.5 to 1.0 mg of orally administered alprazolam.[27] In that patient attempts to provoke stuttering by the oral administration of 10 mg of diazepam or 2 mg of lorazepam were unsuccessful. I have observed repeated instances of stuttering in one patient during treatment with alprazolam in a dosage range of 0.5 to 1.0 mg daily. This patient did not stutter at low doses of lorazepam or conventional doses of amitriptyline, though she did stutter on one occasion while taking 6 mg of lorazepam daily. Though most clinicians would suspect the tricyclic antidepressant when a patient develops a speech disturbance on a combined tricyclic-alprazolam regimen, the case cited above and my clinical experience suggest the necessity to consider alprazolam on an equal footing with the tricyclic drug as a potential cause of stuttering speech. Since alprazolam has only minimal anticholinergic effect, it is unlikely that this pharmacologic mechanism is responsible for the speech disturbance.

Benzodiazepines have well-known amnestic properties. This phenomenon may be observed during the clinical treatment of patients as well as in studies on normal volunteers. Diazepam has been shown to selectively impair anterograde episodic memory and attention, while sparing access to information in long-term memory in a study of normal volunteers.[28] Similar anterograde memory impairment has been observed in the clinical use of a variety of benzodiazepines, including the short-acting lorazepam and alprazolam.[29] Triazolam, which was introduced as an ultra–short-acting benzodiazepine for the short-term treatment of insomnia, has caused more nightmares for physicians and patients than any other benzodiazepine. Although this drug is still marketed in the United States, a complicated series of adverse experiences with it in the United Kingdom, Finland, and Argentina has led to its being withdrawn from those markets. Although the amnestic action of midazolam (Versed) is an important therapeutic benefit when this compound is used as a preanesthetic medication or for intravenous sedation during surgery, the rather frequent amnestic effect of triazolam is a decided disadvantage, when the patient receiving this drug for insomnia has impaired memory the following day. When it was initially released in 1983, the very short half-life of triazolam made it appear to be a useful hypnotic with less risk of hangover. However, subsequent reports of rebound insomnia, confusion, amnesia, bizarre behavior, agitation, and hallucinations have been dramatic and frightening. Indeed, an analysis of 260 adverse events reported to the FDA Spontaneous Reporting System through 1985[30] should make the FDA question why this agent is still marketed in the U.S. and should make the average physician question continuing to prescribe triazolam. I have observed episodes of amnesia and blackouts in four patients receiving short-term courses of 0.25 mg triazolam and in one patient receiving 0.5 mg for only 3 nights. Four of these patients were concurrently receiving MAOI antidepressants, and the fifth was receiving a tricyclic antidepressant; therefore a drug interaction may have occurred, although each patient failed to have similar symptoms when an alternate benzodiazepine was employed along with the antidepressant.

Several reports in the literature have found that concurrent administration of cimetidine decreases clearance of triazolam and increases its plasma concentration.[31] Cimetidine, like fluoxetine and paroxetine, is a potent inhibitor of the enzyme cytochrome P 450, which governs oxidative metabolism of a multitude of psychotropic and nonpsychotropic drugs, including tricyclic antidepressants and benzodiazepines; thus coadministration of any of these agents along with triazolam would be expected to increase its serum concentration, half-life, and risk of adverse events.

A similar interaction has been reported when oral contraceptives or the macrolide antibiotic erythromycin are administered concurrently with triazolam.[32,33] Concurrent administration of alcohol or the antituberculous drug isoniazid has also been shown to impair metabolic degradation of triazolam and other benzodiazepines as well. The ability of other medications to delay metabolism and increase plasma concentrations of triazolam is particularly important since this agent is the most potent and rapidly acting of currently available oral benzodiazepines. Nevertheless, when any drug is combined with a benzodiazepine regimen, the physician must seriously consider the potential of enhanced and prolonged benzodiazepine activity.

Although benzodiazepines with shorter half-lives and durations of pharmacologic action may be relatively more benign from the standpoint of cumulative pharmacologic effects, drugs with a shorter half-life may present a greater risk of dependency and addiction.[1] Triazolam, with a 2.5 to 3.5 hour half-life, appears to have a higher risk of addiction than other benzodiazepines, whose half-lives exceed 10 hours.[34,35] Psychosis and delirium have been reported following withdrawal of triazolam, and the addiction potential of this drug needs to be kept firmly in mind, even when it is employed for relatively short courses of therapy.[35] Withdrawal syndromes, including the occurrence of seizures, are known to occur following abrupt discontinuation or too rapid dosage reduction of alprazolam.[36,37,38] Case reports of patients experiencing withdrawal syndromes following discontinuation of triazolam and alprazolam, in spite of substitution of relatively large doses of other benzodiazepines, suggest that the dependency risk with triazolobenzodiazepines may be greater, perhaps due to greater affinity of these compounds, for the benzodiazepine receptor.[34,36] Since alprazolam is often used in high doses (3 to 6 mg/day or more in the treatment of panic disorder, agoraphobia, and depression), the potential for withdrawal reactions and the risk of seizures need to be emphasized. Furthermore, since patients receiving alprazolam for these latter indications may not achieve an adequate therapeutic response and may, subsequently, be treated with tricyclic antidepressants, which may lower seizure threshold, there is the potential for a significantly enhanced risk of withdrawal symptoms and seizures occurring when a patient is switched from alprazolam to a tricyclic antidepressant.

Good therapeutic technique dictates against the use of benzodiazepines in a manner that would be conducive to the development of addiction; if, however, one encounters a patient who has utilized these drugs excessively, it is important that they not be discontinued suddenly, but rather that their dosage be gradually tapered.[39,40] The same, obviously, applies for barbiturates, meprobamate, glutethimide, methaqualone, methyprylon, ethchlorvynol, and chloral hydrate.[1,2,41] When single bedtime doses of benzodiazepines are used to induce sleep, their lengthy duration of action may provide some continuing antianxiety effect during the course of the next day (see Table 3-1). These drugs tend to be more effective and safer if patients are encouraged to use them on an intermittent basis rather than every night. Because of the risk of addiction with barbiturates such as secobarbital and pentobarbital, these drugs probably have little place in the physician's battle against insomnia.[1] Methaqualone is an

Table 3-2 Half-lives and dosage ranges of sedatives

Sedative	Half-life (hr)	Daily dosage range (mg)
Barbiturates		
Amobarbital (Amytal)	8-42	100-500
Pentobarbital (Nembutal)	15-48	100-200
Phenobarbital (Luminal)	24-140	15-120
Secobarbital (Seconal)	19-34	100-200
Miscellaneous		
Chloral hydrate (Noctec)	4-9.5	500-2000
Meprobamate (Equanil)	6-17	200-800

addictive drug without therapeutic advantages. It is no longer available in the United States prescription market, although it is occasionally encountered as an imported illicit drug.

Non-benzodiazepines

Occasionally barbiturates such as phenobarbital and amobarbital may be of value in alleviating anxiety, if their dose and duration of administration are limited. Agitated psychotic patients receiving optimal doses of antipsychotic medication may experience a persistence of agitation during the day and at night, in which case the addition of amobarbital in a dose of 100 to 200 mg or lorazepam 1 to 2 mg may help produce some daytime calming and may also be used to encourage sleep at night.[1] Meprobamate, when used cautiously, may provide mild sedation and thereby improve anxiety and insomnia in nonpsychotic individuals.[1] Chloral hydrate is an effective nighttime sedative, and it is relatively safe if used intermittently. Chloral hydrate may produce GI irritation and considerable gastric distress in some people, however. The ability of chloral hydrate to displace anticoagulants such as warfarin from plasma protein–binding sites may produce excessive prolongation of prothrombin time and a risk of hemorrhage in anticoagulated patients; therefore, this drug should be avoided in patients receiving anticoagulants.[1] Fortunately, the benzodiazepines have minimal interaction with anticoagulants.

The high lipid solubility and risk of addiction with drugs such as ethchlorvynol, glutethimide, and methyprylon are good reasons for avoiding the therapeutic use of these drugs.[1] High lipid solubility makes it exceedingly difficult to remove the drugs by dialysis in the event of an overdose, and there is no clinical or scientific evidence to support the particular therapeutic advantage of any of these compounds.[1] Prescriptions for any sedative medication should strictly limit the quantity prescribed, and refill authorization must be limited to reduce the risk of overdose and drug abuse.[1,2]

Recognizing the potential risks of drug dependency associated with

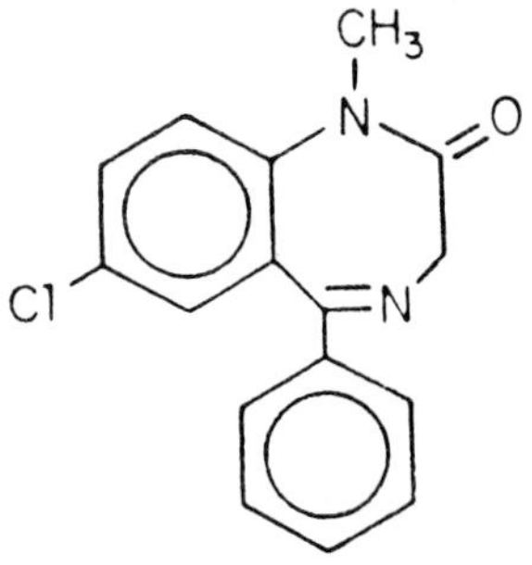

DIAZEPAM

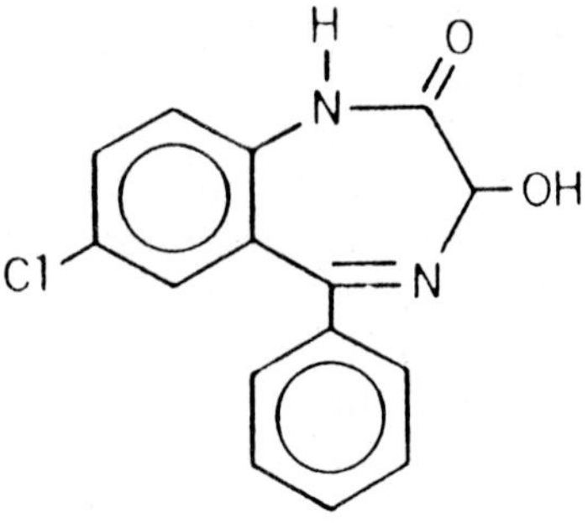

OXAZEPAM

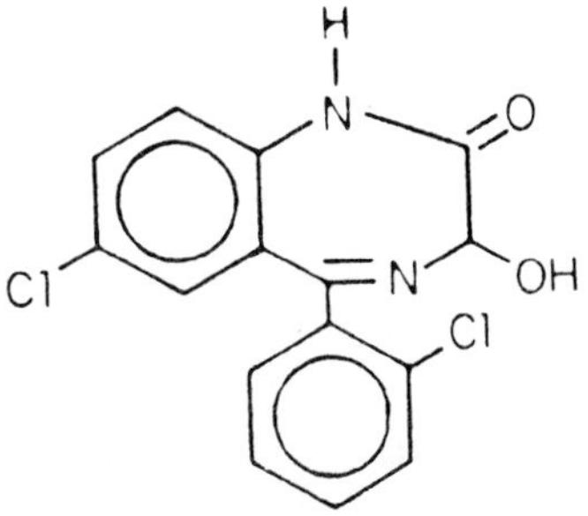

LORAZEPAM

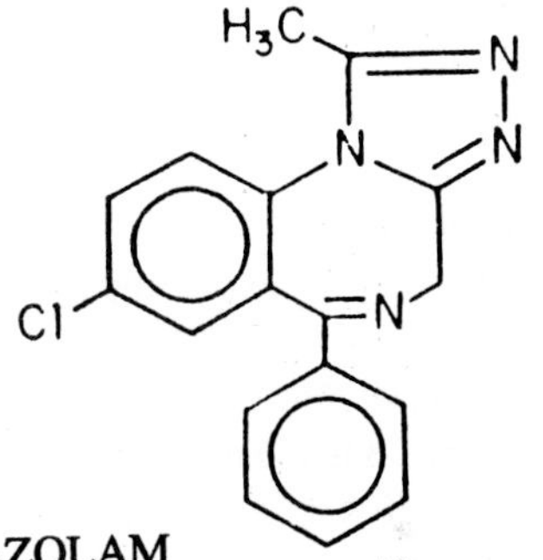

ALPRAZOLAM

$$NH_2COOCH_2\overset{\overset{\displaystyle CH_3}{|}}{\underset{\underset{\displaystyle CH_2CH_2CH_3}{|}}{C}}CH_2OOCNH_2$$

MEPROBAMATE

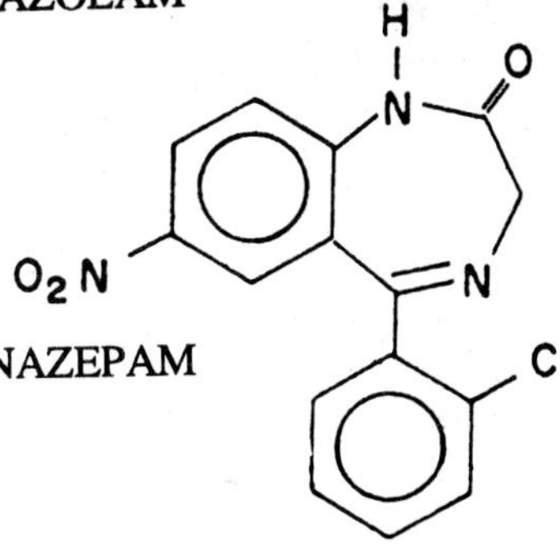

CLONAZEPAM

long-term use of benzodiazepines in the treatment of the chronically anxious patient who is likely to need prolonged drug therapy, several other agents are worthy of consideration. Patients who have discrete panic attacks and individuals with phobic anxiety should generally receive a therapeutic trial of a serotonin-selective reuptake inhibitor (SSRI), tricyclic antidepressant, or MAOI.[5] Among the tricyclics, imipramine has been widely studied and utilized in patients with phobic symptoms and panic disorder; however, since the late 1980s, the SSRIs have largely supplanted TCAs and MAOIs in these conditions.[13] In some anxious patients using more sedating tricyclic agents administered in divided doses throughout the day may be beneficial. Since patients with severe anxiety are apt to be particularly cognizant of medication side effects, it is preferable to choose those compounds with low anticholinergic potential. SSRIs and benzodiazepines lack anticholinergic effect, though the tricyclics can produce considerable cholinergic blockade. In studies comparing monoamine oxidase inhibitors to tricyclics in anxious patients, phenelzine has been the agent most widely studied and has generally been found to be more efficacious than either imipramine or amitriptyline.[13]

Because of the risk of tardive dyskinesia, neuroleptics should generally be avoided in the treatment of anxiety. Small doses, cautiously utilized for brief periods of time with adequate documentation and patient education, may be helpful when multiple more benign therapies have failed. When utilized for this indication, more sedating, less potent dopamine antagonists such as chlorpromazine or thioridazine would be preferable to more potent agents such as haloperidol.

Antihistamines

A variety of sedating antihistamines have been used for many years in the management of both anxiety and insomnia.[42] These compounds have the advantage of being nonaddicting.[42] They do, however, exert some anticholinergic effect, which may be only mildly apparent or may become troublesome, particularly in the elderly individual or a patient with organic dysfunction.[1] Among the antihistamines, diphenhydramine (Benadryl) has been widely used as a mild nighttime sedative, generally in a dose of 25 to 100 mg at bedtime. Smaller doses of 10 to 25 mg given several times throughout the day may be useful in some patients with relatively mild anxiety. Hydroxyzine (Atarax) is an antihistamine with moderate sedative action. Like the other antihistamines, it possesses significant anticholinergic effect and does not have addiction-producing potential. Hydroxyzine, in a dose of 10 to 25 mg 1 to 4 times daily, may be helpful in the relief of persistent anxiety with relatively minor side effects.[1,5] This compound may also be useful in helping patients with insomnia to fall asleep more easily when a dose of 25 to 100 mg is employed at bedtime.

HYDROXYZINE

Beta-blockers

Many patients with severe persistent anxiety have a physiologic component with associated tachycardia, palpitations, tremor, and sweating. Since these physical manifestations of anxiety are secondary to sympathetic nervous system hyperactivity, blockade of beta-adrenergic receptors by drugs such as propranolol, metoprolol, and atenolol will produce a slowing of the heart rate, decrease in palpitations, and a reduction in anxiety-associated sweating and tremor.[7-9] In one controlled study, propranolol was found to be as effective as chlordiazepoxide in the management of anxiety.[43] In some studies propranolol was found to be effective against the physiologic manifestations of anxiety, but not clearly effective in reducing patients' perceptions of anxiety. Clinical experience and research studies support the efficacy of β-blockers in the management of anxious patients, particularly those with pronounced physiologic manifestations of their anxiety.[44]

Many anxious individuals have associated physiologic symptoms that enhance the subjective perception of anxiety.[5] Beta-receptor antagonists are not CNS depressants, do not produce drug dependency, and are not generally associated with the development of drowsiness, which may occur with conventional antianxiety agents. Most patients whose anxiety responds favorably to propranolol require relatively small doses of this drug, specifically a range of 10 to 20 mg 3 to 4 times daily.

Although it is known that propranolol may produce or worsen depression, this effect tends most often to be associated with dosages in excess of those employed in the management of anxiety.[45] Propranolol may, in some sensitive individuals, produce a toxic organic brain syndrome which is not dose-dependent, and may occur regardless of the dose administered.[45] Propranolol generally has a dramatic effect in alleviating tremors associated with anxiety, as well as the rather common syndrome of essential (familial) tremor.[46] Likewise, propranolol is of considerable use in decreasing and generally obliterating the tremor which some patients experience while receiving therapeutic doses of lithium carbonate.[47]

Propranolol should not be used in patients with symptomatic bronchial asthma, in whom the drug may precipitate bronchospasm and also antagonize the therapeutic effects of commonly employed agents such as isoproterenol. Patients with congestive heart failure, or those individuals with poor myocardial function, may experience increasing congestive failure and decreased myocardial function when propranolol is administered. Although propranolol is an effective antihypertensive agent, it generally does not produce significant blood pressure lowering at the low doses employed in the management of the anxious patient.[5] This medication should not be prescribed by a psychiatrist who does not feel comfortable performing periodic physical examinations on his patients. Prior to instituting propranolol therapy, it is necessary to determine the patient's blood pressure and pulse rate and to listen to his heart; any irregularity in the cardiac rhythm or any evidence of gallop sounds should be documented. Likewise, auscultation of the lungs to determine the absence of bronchospasm, and evaluation of the patient for the presence of peripheral edema should be done prior to prescribing propranolol. During the course of treatment with this agent, periodic blood pressure determinations, auscultation of the heart and lungs, and evaluation for the presence of peripheral edema should be conducted.

With appropriate caution and medical evaluation, beta-adrenergic blocking drugs are safe and effective agents in the management of chronic anxiety with associated autonomic manifestations.[5,45] β-Blocking drugs such as metoprolol and atenolol are relatively cardioselective and less likely to produce bronchospasm and central nervous system side effects.

Anxious patients complaining of episodic tachycardia with or without sweating should be questioned regarding the possibility that they are suffering from panic disorder and would be better treated with low doses of SSRIs and benzodiazepines rather than a beta-blocker. These symptoms are also seen in social phobia, which is likewise often responsive to low-dose SSRIs along with low doses of benzodiazepines, such as clonazepam.

Buspirone

Buspirone is a selective 5-HT_{1A} mixed agonist-antagonist with weak dopamine blocking activity which is nonsedating and appears not to interfere with motor coordination or complex task performance.[48,49] Buspirone is not a benzodiazepine, lacks sleep-inducing effect, and appears not to induce tolerance, physical dependence, or withdrawal symptoms.[4,13] Patients taking this drug may experience relief of anxiety but generally do not feel a drug effect in contradistinction to the actions of benzodiazepines. Many patients who have been treated over prolonged periods of time with benzodiazepines miss the characteristic calming effect of these drugs when treated with buspirone. Buspirone has no anticonvulsant activity and will not protect a benzodiazepine-treated patient from withdrawal symptoms when the latter drug is discontinued. Indeed, it is often difficult to transition a patient from a benzodiazepine to buspirone, which is generally perceived by patients and physicians as a less effective agent. Some patients with generalized anxiety disorder do well with buspirone, although it is ineffective in panic disorder and phobias. One major disadvantage of buspirone is that it cannot be used

BUSPIRONE

on an as-needed basis and must be taken for at least 1 week or longer prior to the onset of any anxiety-relieving effect. The dosage must be individualized for the specific patient and it often requires persistence on the part of the patient and the physician to await the desired anxiolytic effect. Some patients, who have experienced mental clouding with benzodiazepines, feel greatly relieved to have their anxiety diminished without an accompanying feeling of being drugged. Patients that have been receiving benzodiazepines may have the dose of these medications gradually diminished following initiation of buspirone.

In general, the starting dose of buspirone should be 5 mg three times daily for the first week with gradual daily dose increments of 2.5 to 5 mg every 2 to 4 days until the desired response is achieved. Lightheadedness and dizziness are not infrequently encountered as side effects of buspirone. Other, occasional, side effects are dry mouth, nausea, decreased appetite, GI complaints, and restlessness. The usual effective daily dose ranges between 15 and 30 mg, though in some cases, divided-dose regimens of up to 60 mg/day may be required.[13] It appears that the primary area of utility for this drug is in the treatment of generalized anxiety disorder, wherein prolonged antianxiety therapy may be required and the potential lack of addictive qualities of buspirone would be advantageous.[13,49,50]

Management of Specific Types of Anxiety

In patients with intermittent anticipatory anxiety, low doses of short-acting benzodiazepines, such as alprazolam or lorazepam, appear to be the most effective therapeutic modality. If anticipatory anxiety is a frequent occurrence, patients may require a regularly administered benzodiazepine regimen; however, treatment with beta-adrenergic blocking drugs, low doses of an SSRI, or buspirone should also be considered.

Patients with agoraphobia or panic disorder may respond favorably to benzodiazepines such as alprazolam or clonazepam.[21,50,51] Generally, either drug should be started at a low dose with gradual upward titration as required to achieve symptomatic control. There is increasing evidence that clonazepam may be more effective than alprazolam.[50,51] There is also less likelihood of severe withdrawal symptoms following discontinuation of clonazepam, but in either case the dosage should be gradually titrated downward rather than abruptly discontinued since withdrawal syndromes can occur with any benzodiazepine, particularly when larger doses or more prolonged periods of administration have been employed. Generally, alprazolam requires a daily dose of 2 to 10 mg to achieve an antipanic effect, while similar effects are generally observed with clonazepam doses of 1 to 3 mg/day. Imipramine and the serotonin selective reuptake inhibitors such as sertraline have been shown to have prominent antipanic and antiphobic action. In some patients whose panic disorder is unresponsive to other agents, MAOIs such as phenelzine are often very effective.

Unfortunately, the FDA has approved the marketing of alprazolam 2 mg tablets and the indication for treatment of panic disorder with this compound in doses of up to 10 mg/day. What is known is that even at the middosage range a sizable percentage of panic patients will improve and most of them will have difficulty eventually discontinuing the drug after prolonged administration at doses of 3 mg daily or more. What remains unknown is which portion of patients receiving higher doses of alprazolam will be unsafe drivers or experience disinhibition.

Although numerous articles discuss the characteristics of posttraumatic stress disorder, relatively little has been written about the pharmacotherapy of this syndrome. Posttraumatic stress disorder has been primarily associated with combat experience; but it may also occur in civilian life among patients who have been exposed to a sudden and overwhelming stress, such as rape, robbery, or disaster affecting themselves, their families, or others with whom they have close relationships. Since episodic violence may occur, benzodiazepines, which may have a disinhibiting effect, are not desirable therapeutic agents. Since there are similarities between posttraumatic stress disorder and panic disorder, SSRIs, tricyclic antidepressants and MAOIs have been studied.[11,12,13] These drugs have been shown to be effective in patients who are willing to cooperate with the regimen, abstain from alcohol abuse, and take medication regularly. Lithium carbonate and carbamazepine have also been found to be effective in many patients with posttraumatic stress disorder.[12] Beta-adrenergic blocking drugs may blunt some of the autonomic symptoms and potentially reduce violence and impulsivity.

Generalized anxiety disorder is one of the most difficult forms of anxiety to treat, and has been most often treated with sedatives such as the benzodiazepines. If patients are carefully monitored and drug dosage escalation avoided, these agents alone or, very often, in combination with beta-adrenergic blocking drugs, may be useful therapeutic interventions. Neuroleptics which should be avoided, have occasionally been used for generalized anxiety disorder, but present a risk of tardive dyskinesia since therapy needs to be administered over a long period of time. Sedating antihistamines such as diphenhydramine and hydroxyzine used intermittently are sometimes effective in generalized anxiety disorder and have the advantage of avoiding dependency, even with long-term use. Buspirone appears to be the most promising agent in the treatment of generalized anxiety disorder, and should be considered prior to initiating benzodiazepine therapy for this condition.

EVALUATION AND MANAGEMENT OF INSOMNIA

One of the greatest risks of treating insomnia is that of prescribing medication without an adequate evaluation to rule out causes of insomnia which may respond to specific treatment other than sedation. Another obvious risk in the management of insomnia involves the potential for excessive drug use, with the eventual development of addiction or a state of continuous mental cloudiness due to the long half-life of the hypnotic agent. Whenever a sedative is prescribed there is the potential of an accidental or intentional overdose. Commonly used sedatives produce additive pharmacologic effects when taken in combination with alcohol and may be potentiated by drugs such as fluoxetine which may complicate the clinical picture and decrease the safety of prescribed medication.[1]

Patients complaining of insomnia may simply be stating that they do not like the way they sleep.[52] Medication may not improve satisfaction with the sleep pattern. Many geriatric patients complaining of insomnia may in fact be observing the natural decrement in their need for sleep, which is currently thought to reflect decreasing melatonin secretion with aging.[52,57] Insomnia may be manifested as requiring an excessive period before sleep occurs.[53] Difficulties falling asleep followed by a period of adequate sleep may require no therapy at all, or may respond to a relatively safe agent that will decrease sleep latency. The use of sedating antihistamines to speed the onset of sleep in a patient with an otherwise relatively normal sleep pattern may be quite satisfactory.[42]

The serotonin precursor, L-tryptophan, has been investigated extensively both in normal volunteers and in patients with insomnia.[54] L-Tryptophan produces a significant reduction in sleep latency time in normal subjects and in many individuals with insomnia characterized by difficulty in falling asleep.[54] In 1990 reports began to appear in the literature of a mysterious condition, eosinophilia-myalgia syndrome, appearing in patients who had used L-tryptophan to induce sleep.[55] The syndrome consisted of muscle pain and weakness, rash, mouth ulcers, abdominal pain, dyspnea, and eosinophilia.[55] Occurrence of this syndrome, which was later found to be the result of an impurity due to a bacterial fermentation product in batches of L-tryptophan manufactured by a Japanese chemical company, Showa Denko,[56] led to the removal of all L-tryptophan from the U.S. market, and ended what may have been a potentially useful nonaddicting sleep-inducing drug. Hopefully, in the future, the U.S. pharmaceutical industry, will be able to produce safe and reliable L-tryptophan, which may continue to have a useful place in the management of sleep disturbances and affective illness.

The pineal gland manufactures and releases serotonin, which is catalyzed in vivo to form melatonin. The pineal is the only site in the body which produces significant amounts of melatonin, which appears to be the natural endogenous regulator of sleep and light-dark accommodation.[57] Numerous studies have found that melatonin when exogenously administered can facilitate or induce sleep.[57-60] Although doses of melatonin studied have varied widely from 0.1 to 80 mg or more, all have been found to have sleep inducing activity.[59,60] Generally doses of 1 to 5 mg, administered between early evening and bedtime are capable of reducing sleep latency time in normal subjects and insomniacs.[57,58] Melatonin has also been found to be useful in managing sleep disturbances associated with jet lag.[57] From hundreds of studies of this compound over the last 30 years, it appears to be safe and to have minimal side effects, the most common of which is oversedation, which occurs rarely with lower doses. There is no apparent potential for addiction or physical dependency, a major problem with all commonly available hypnotic agents. Although work is ongoing to prove the safety and efficacy of melatonin and to ready this compound for FDA approval as a prescription pharmaceutical, it is currently available as a nutritional product in health food stores and may be worth considering in the management of patients whose insomnia is unresponsive to conventional agents or in whom there is concern about drug dependency. The one negative consideration regarding melatonin at this time is our awareness of the eosinophilia myalgia syndrome, which resulted from tainted batches of L-tryptophan, and concern as to whether a similar problem could surface with more extensive use of melatonin related not to the compound itself but rather to potential contaminants.

One common form of insomnia involves frequent awakening throughout the night, with difficulty returning to sleep; it is also often associated with early morning awakening and an inability to return to sleep. Patients experiencing nighttime or early morning awakening may or may not experience difficulty falling asleep initially when they go to bed. Although benzodiazepines may help an individual fall asleep initially, they generally have limited value in preventing nighttime and early morning awakening. If a benzodiazepine is necessary to induce sleep, a shorter-acting compound such as oxazepam in a dose of 15 to 30 mg may be useful without producing the morning hangover associated with longer-acting compounds. Although flurazepam (Dalmane) is marketed specifically as a hypnotic drug, it probably does not have any unique therapeutic value and, due to its very long half-life, is likely to produce a prolonged effect.[55] Clonazepam in a bedtime dose of 0.25 to 1.0 mg is often effective for inducing sleep, reducing nocturnal and early morning awakening while not producing significant daytime drowsiness; it is particularly useful in patients whose insomnia may be secondary to SSRIs or other antidepressants.

Temazepam (Restoril), a benzodiazepine with a reported single dose half-life of 10 hours, may be useful in inducing sleep with a far less pronounced cumulative effect than that seen with flurazepam when administered in comparable dosage.[55] As with other benzodiazepines, temazepam is not particularly useful in the patient with early morning awakening.

Quazepam, marketed as a benzodiazepine hypnotic, may be useful in some patients with nighttime and early morning awakening; used in a dose of 7.5 to 15 mg at bedtime for short periods, it is claimed to produce less rebound insomnia than other agents.[3] This compound and its major metabolite have a half-life of 39 hours, intermediate between those of flurazepam and temazepam or oxazepam, but has not been shown convincingly to be superior to the latter two compounds.[1]

Estazolam is a triazolobenzodiazepine, with a half-life of 10 to 24 hours, which in a dose of 1 to 2 mg may be effective in short term treatment of insomnia.[3] Considering evidence previously cited that triazolobenzodiazepines, such as alprozolam and triazolam, may be associated with more resistant withdrawal syndromes than other benzodiazepines, it may be prudent to avoid such compounds, which can bind more tenaciously to the benzodiazepine receptor.[36] Certainly there seems to be no good reason to utilize triazolam in the management of insomnia.

Zolpidem, an imidazopyridine, is not a benzodiazepine but binds selectively to the omega-1 benzodiazepine receptor, resulting in a sleep-inducing action without muscle-relaxant or anticonvulsant activity.[61] Its elimination half-life of 1.5 to 4.5 hours is similar to that of triazolam, which it also resembles in its ability to impair short- and long-term memory, psychomotor performance, and postural sway.[61] Though it has been marketed only relatively recently in the United States, the rapid appearance of reports of adverse events—including tolerance, confusion, memory and behavioral disturbances, and psychotic reactions—is alarming.[62] Although recommended in an initial bedtime dose of 10 mg with subsequent reduction to 5 mg at bedtime, it may have led one middle-aged woman whom I saw attempt to run her husband over after her first dose of only 5 mg. Though chemically unrelated to triazolam, zolpidem should be recognized as presenting similar risks.

Zopiclone, chemically unrelated to zolpidem or the benzodiazepines, binds to the benzodiazepine receptor complex and has anticonvulsant, muscle relaxant, and anxiolytic activity.[63] Marketed in Canada and Europe as Imovane, but not available in the U.S., it has a rapid onset of action and an elimination half-life of approximately 6 hours.[63,64] Its sleep-inducing effects have not been associated with significant adverse events or hangover, thus far, when employed for short periods at a nightly dose of 7.5 mg in adults and geriatric patients.[64]

Frequent nighttime awakening, with or without early morning awakening, should generally suggest that the patient may be suffering from an affective illness. This is the sleep disturbance pattern most often associated with depression, and in some cases may be the first or only symptom to suggest an affective illness. Even if the depression is not clinically obvious, such patients may respond quite favorably to an antidepressant. If a more sedating agent such as amitriptyline, doxepin, or trazodone is used, there may be a relatively prompt decrease in sleep latency, although a period of 2 to 3 weeks of treatment will be necessary before a significant improvement is made in the nighttime and early morning awakening pattern of sleep disturbance.[56] Less sedating antidepressant agents may likewise be of value in insomnia, but a waiting period is generally necessary prior to the onset of the antidepressant effect.

Meprobamate in a dose of 400 to 800 mg at bedtime may be useful in reducing sleep latency. Chloral hydrate in a dose of 500 mg to 1.5 g may also be useful in helping the patient who has difficulty falling asleep. Both of these agents have potential for creating addiction, and neither of them is particularly beneficial in alleviating the problem of nighttime or early morning awakening.[1,55]

The actions of benzodiazepines on the waking EEG are similar to those seen with other sedatives.[52,53] There is a decrease in alpha activity and an increase in low-voltage fast activity. Like the barbiturates, tolerance to the EEG effect of benzodiazepines is known to occur.[53] Unfortunately, most controlled sleep studies of these drugs have involved normal subjects rather than patients with insomnia or psychiatric illness. The benzodiazepines decrease sleep latency and diminish the number of awakenings.[1] Time spent in stage 1 is generally decreased by benzodiazepines, while time in stage 2 tends to increase. Benzodiazepines reduce the period of slow-wave sleep (stages 3 and 4). Decreasing stage 4 sleep is accompanied by a reduction in terrors and nightmares.[53] The duration of rapid eye movement (REM) sleep is usually shortened, though this may not occur when low doses of benzodiazepines are employed. Although the time in REM sleep is decreased, the number of cycles of REM sleep usually increases with benzodiazepines, mostly late in the period of sleep time. Overall, despite the shortening of stage 4 and REM sleep, the net effect of benzodiazepines is to increase total sleep time. This action is most prominent in the individual with the shortest baseline total sleep time, and is likely to be least apparent in those individuals who normally are able to sleep for a lengthy period of time.[1] The use of benzodiazepines tends to impart a feeling of deep and refreshing sleep but the correlation of this observation with actions on specific sleep parameters is not clear. Chronic use of benzodiazepines at night is generally associated with a decline in the effects of these drugs on the various stages of sleep.[1] Tolerance is more pronounced with respect to REM sleep than to non-REM sleep parameters. An increase in dreaming is generally experienced during chronic use, and after several weeks of nightly benzodiazepine use there may be a rebound in the amount and density of REM sleep when the drug is discontinued. Following withdrawal of benzodiazepines, the number of dreams occurring per night is likely to be similar to the number experienced before drug treatment, although dreams may take on a bizarre character.[53]

REFERENCES

1. Rall TW: Hypnotics and sedatives. in Gilman AG, Rall TW, Neis AS, Taylor P (eds): *Goodman and Gilman's The pharmacological basis of therapeutics*, ed 8. New York, Pergamon Press, 1990, pp 345-382.
2. Jaffe JH: Drug addiction and drug abuse. In Gilman AG, Rall TW, Neis AS, Taylor P (eds): *Goodman and Gilman's The pharmacological basis of therapeutics*, ed 8. New York, Pergamon Press, 1990, pp 522-573.
3. Wikler A: Diagnosis and treatment of drug dependence of the barbiturate type. *Am J Psychiatry* 1968;125:758-765.
4. Lader M: Assessing the potential for buspirone dependence or abuse and effects of its withdrawal. *Am J Med* 1987;82(suppl 5A):20-26.

5. Dubovsky SL: Generalized anxiety disorder: new concepts and psychopharmacologic therapies. *J Clin Psychiatry* 1990;51 (1 suppl):3-10.

6. American Psychiatric Association: *Diagnostic and statistical manual of mental disorders*, ed, revised [DSM-IV]. Washington DC, American Psychiatric Press, 1994.

7. Halstrom C, Treasden I, Edward JG, et al: Diazepam, propranolol, and their combination in the management of chronic anxiety. *Br J Psychiatry* 1981;139:417-421.

8. Noyes R, Anderson DJ, Clancy J, et al: Diazepam and propranolol in panic disorder and agoraphobia. *Arch Gen Psychiatry* 1984;41:287-292.

9. Mendels J, Chernoff RW, Blatt M: Alprazolam as an adjunct to propranolol in anxious outpatients with stable angina pectoris. *J Clin Psychiatry* 1986;47:8-11.

10. Hollister LE, Muller-Oerlinghausen B, Rickels K, Shader RI (eds): Clinical uses of benzodiazepines. *J Clin Psychopharmacol* 1993;13(suppl 1):1-169.

11. Falcon S, Ryan C, Chamberlain K, et al: Tricyclics: possible treatment for post-traumatic stress disorder. *J Clin Psychiatry* 1985;46:385-389.

12. Silver JM, Sandberg DP, Hales RE: New approaches in the pharmacotherapy of posttraumatic stress disorder. *J Clin Psychiatry* 1990;51(10 suppl):33-38.

13. Hollander E, Cohen LJ: The assessment and treatment of refractory anxiety. *J Clin Psychiatry* 1994;55(2 suppl):27-31.

14. Enna SJ: Role of gamma-aminobutyric acid in anxiety. *Psychopathology* 1984;17:15-24.

15. Sussman N: The potential benefits of serotonin receptor-specific agents. *J Clin Psychiatry* 1994;55(2 suppl):45-51.

16. Garzone PD, Kroboth PD: Pharmacokinetics of the newer benzodiazepines. *Clin Pharmacokinet* 1989;16:337-364.

17. Hall RCW, Zisook S: Paradoxical reactions to benzodiazepines. *Br J Clin Pharmacol* 1981;11:995-1045.

18. Rosenbaum JF, Woods SW, Groves JE, et al: Emergence of hostility during alprazolam treatment. *Am J Psychiatry* 1984;141:792-793.

19. Gardos G, DiMascio A, Salzman C, et al: Differential actions of chlordiazepoxide and oxazepam on hostility. *Arch Gen Psychiatry* 1968;18:757-760.

20. Feighner JP, Aden GC, Fabre LF, et al: Comparison of alprazolam, imipramine, and placebo in the treatment of depression. *JAMA* 1983;249:3057-3064.

21. Liebowitz MR, Fyer AJ, Gorman JM, et al: Alprazolam in the treatment of panic disorders. *J Clin Psychopharmacology* 1986;6:13-20.

22. Arana GW, Pearlman C, Shader RI: Alprazolam-induced mania: two clinical cases. *Am J Psychiatry* 1985;142:368-369.

23. Goodman WK, Charney DS: A case of alprazolam but not lorazepam, inducing manic symptoms. *J Clin Psychiatry* 1987;48:117-118.

24. Chouinard G, Young S, Annable L: Antimanic effect of clonazepam. *Biol Psychiatry* 1983;18:451-466.

25. Strahan A, Rosenthal J, Kaswan M, et al: Three case reports of acute paroxysmal excitement associated with alprazolam treatment. *Am J Psychiatry* 1985;142:859-861.

26. Gardner DL, Cowdry RW: Alprazolam-induced dyscontrol in borderline personality disorder. *Am J Psychiatry* 1985;142:98-100.

27. Elliot RL, Thomas BJ: A case of alprazolam-induced stuttering. *J Clin Psychopharmacol* 1985;5:159-160.

28. Wolkowitz OM, Weingartner H, Thompson K, et al: Diazepam-induced amnesia: a neuropharmacological model of an "organic amnestic syndrome." *Am J Psychiatry* 1987;144:25-29.

29. Kumar R, Mac DS, Gabrielli WF, et al: Anxiolytics and memory: a comparison of lorazepam and alprazolam. *J Clin Psychiatry* 1987;48:158-160.

30. Wysowski DK, Barash D: Adverse behavioral reactions attributed to triazolam in the Food and Drug Administration's spontaneous reporting system. *Arch Intern Med* 1991;151:2003-2008.

31. Britton ML, Waller ES: Central nervous system toxicity associated with concurrent use of triazolam and cimetidine. *Drug Intell Clin Pharm* 1985;19:666-668.

32. Kroboth PD, Smith RB, Stoehr GP, et al: Pharmacodynamic evaluation of the benzodiazepine–oral contraceptive interaction. *Clin Pharmacol Ther* 1985;38:525-532.

33. Phillips JP, Antal EJ, Smith RB: A pharmacokinetic drug interaction between erythromycin and triazolam. *J Clin Pharmacol* 1986;6:297-299.

34. Schneider LS, Syapin PJ, Pawluczyk S: Seizures following triazolam withdrawal despite benzodiazepine treatment. *J Clin Psychiatry* 1987;48:418-419.

35. Heritch AJ, Capwell R, Roy-Byrne PP: A case of psychosis and delirium following withdrawal from triazolam. *J Clin Psychiatry* 1987;48:168-169.

36. Fyer AJ, Liebowitz MR, Gorman JM, et al: Discontinuation of alprazolam treatment in panic patients. *Am J Psychiatry* 1987;144:303-308.

37. Breier A, Charney DJ, Nelson JC: Seizures induced by abrupt discontinuation of alprazolam. *Am J Psychiatry* 1984;141:1606-1607.

38. Mellman TA, Uhde TW: Withdrawal syndrome with gradual tapering of alprazolam. *Am J Psychiatry* 1986;143:1464-1466.

39. Noyes R, Garvey MJ, Cook BL, Perry PJ: Benzodiazepine withdrawal: a review of the evidence. *J Clin Psychiatry* 1988;49:382-389.

40. Rickels K, Case W, Schweizer EE, et al: Low dose dependence in chronic benzodiazepine users: a preliminary report on 119 patients. *Psychopharmacol Bull* 1986;22:407-415.

41. Smith DE, Wesson DR: Phenobarbitol technique for treatment of barbiturate dependence. *Arch Gen Psychiatry* 1971;24:56-60.

42. Carruthers SG, Shoeman DW, Hignite CE, et al: Correlation between plasma diphenhydramine level and sedative and antihistamine effects. *Clin Pharmacol Ther* 1978;23:375-382.

43. Wheatley D: Comparative effects of propranolol and chlordiazepoxide in anxiety states. *Br J Psychiatry* 1969;115:1411-1412.

44. Tanna VT, Penningroth RP, Woolson RF, et al: Propranolol in the treatment of anxiety neurosis. *Compr Psychiatry* 1977;18:319-326.

45. Bernstein JG: Drug interactions. In Cassem NH (ed): *Massachusetts General Hospital Handbook of general hospital psychiatry,* ed 3. St Louis, Mosby, 1991, pp 571-610.

46. Winkler GF, Young RR: Efficacy of chronic propranolol therapy in action tremors of the familial, senile, or essential varieties. *N Engl J Med* 1974; 290:984-988.

47. Lapiere YD: Control of lithium tremor with propranolol. *Can Med J* 1976; 114:619-624.

48. Jann MW: Buspirone: an update on a unique anxiolytic agent. *Pharmacotherapy* 1988;8;100-116.

49. Sussman N: *Buspirone: a review of the literature.* Princeton, Excerpta Medica, 1991.

50. Spier SA, Tesar GE, Rosenbaum JF, et al: Treatment of panic disorder and agoraphobia with clonazepam. *J Clin Psychiatry* 1986;47:238-242.

51. Pollack MH, Tesar GE, Rosenbaum JF, et al: Clonazepam in the treatment of panic disorders and agoraphobia: a one-year follow-up. *J Clin Psychopharmacol* 1986;6:302-304.

52. Fredrickson PA: The relevance of sleep disorders medicine to psychiatric practice. *Psychiatr Ann* 1987;17:91-100.

53. Kales A, Solsatos CR, Kales JD: Sleep disorders: insomnia, sleep walking, night terrors, nightmares, and enuresis. *Ann Intern Med* 1987;106:582-592.

54. Hartmann E: Insomnia: diagnosis and treatment. In Bernstein JG (ed): *Clinical psychopharmacology,* ed 2. Boston, John Wright–PSG, 1984, pp 177-188.

55. Hertzman PA, Blevins WL, Mayer J, et al: Association of the eosinophilia-myalgia syndrome with the ingestion of tryptophan. *N Engl J Med* 1990;233:869-873.

56. Raphals P: Disease puzzle nears solution. [News] *Science* 1990;249:619.

57. Grad BR, Rozencwaig R: The role of melatonin and serotonin in aging: update. *Psychoneuroendocrinology* 1993;18:283-295.

58. Dahlitz M, Alvarez B, Vignau J, et al: Delayed sleep phase syndrome response to melatonin. *Lancet* 1991;337:1121-1124.

59. Dollins AB, Lynch HJ, Wurtman RJ, et al: Effect of pharmacological daytime doses of melatonin on human mood and performance. *Psychopharmacology* 1993;112:490-496.

60. Dollins AB, Zhdanova IV, Wurtman RJ, et al: Effect of inducing nocturnal serum melatonin concentrations in daytime on sleep, mood, body temperature, and performance. *Proc Natl Acad Sci* 1994;91:1824-1828.

61. Berlin I, Warot D, Hergueta T, et al: Comparisons of the effects of zolpidem and triazolam on memory functions, psychomotor performances, and postural sway in healthy subjects. *J Clin Psychopharmacol* 1993;13:100-106.

62. Gelenberg AJ: Zolpidem-withdrawal reactions and CNS effects. *Biol Ther Psychiatry Newslett* 1993;16:46-47.

63. Goa KL, Heel RC: Zopiclone: review of its pharmacodynamic and pharmacokinetic properties and therapeutic efficacy as an hypnotic. *Drugs* 1986;32:48-65.

64. Musch B, Maillard F: Zopiclone, the third generation hypnotic: a clinical overview. *Int Clin Psychopharmacol* 1990;5(suppl 2):147-158.

CHAPTER 4

Antipsychotic Drugs

OVERVIEW

1. Clinical potency in controlling psychotic symptoms parallels dopamine receptor–blocking potency and may be facilitated by 5-HT$_2$ receptor antagonism.
2. More potent agents with low anticholinergic potential are more likely to produce acute extrapyramidal symptoms.
3. Occurrence of acute EPS does not predict greater likelihood of tardive dyskinesia.
4. Strongly anticholinergic antipsychotic agents may increase confusion or psychotic symptoms.
5. Low-potency agents are more likely to produce hypotension; patients may fall and sustain injury.
6. Avoid low-potency antipsychotic agents in elderly patients because of greater risk of hypotension.
7. Titrate antipsychotic dose gradually, depending on symptoms and response to medication.
8. Use oral route of administration whenever possible in acute and maintenance therapy.
9. Coadminister antiparkinsonian drugs or institute treatment if extrapyramidal symptoms occur.
10. Antipsychotic agents are indicated for acute treatment and maintenance in schizophrenia.
11. Antipsychotic agents are indicated in acute mania while awaiting response to lithium or other antimanic drugs.
12. Low-dose antipsychotic chemotherapy is useful in schizoaffective illness, psychotic depression, and a variety of other conditions including some patients with severe anxiety and OCD.
13. Avoid discontinuing antipsychotic agents too soon in schizophrenic patients.
14. Avoid prolonged administration of antipsychotic agents or their excessive use for trivial indications when they are not necessary.

Continued.

15. Taper dose gradually when discontinuing antipsychotic chemotherapy; abrupt discontinuation may provoke a withdrawal dyskinesia.
16. Antipsychotic drugs may provoke seizures in patients with convulsive disorders or those withdrawing from long-term use of sedatives.
17. Generally avoid simultaneous administration of two or more antipsychotic agents.
18. Risperidone and clozapine antagonize both D_2 and 5-HT_2 receptors and appear effective against both positive and negative schizophrenic symptoms, with significantly less risk of EPS and possibly lower risk of TD.

Psychosis is a form of mental illness wherein a person's ability to think, respond emotionally, remember, communicate, interpret reality, and behave appropriately is impaired to the extent that he is unable to meet the ordinary demands of life.[1] During the active phase of a psychosis an individual is generally unable to interact appropriately with others or to participate in normal activities at school, work, or within his family or social milieu. Psychotic illness is divided by various systems of psychiatric nomenclature into a variety of specifically defined mental disorders. Psychotic illnesses vary in their onset from sudden to gradual, and in their duration from a single episode to more serious illnesses such as schizophrenia, which tend to be lifelong. The most prevalent psychotic illness or, more likely, group of psychotic illnesses, is that commonly known as schizophrenia, wherein the patient may experience a variety of symptoms which severely impair his interaction with others. Box 4-1 presents the DSM-IV diagnostic criteria for schizophrenia.

In schizophrenia there are major disturbances in communication, thought, perception, and affect. The schizophrenic patient suffers from alterations of concept formation that may lead to misinterpretation and misperceptions of reality, and not infrequently, to the presence of delusions and hallucinations. In schizophrenia there is a blunting of affect, considerable uncertainty characterized as ambivalence, inappropriateness of behavior, and a loss of empathy with others.[2] The patient suffering from this illness may be withdrawn or may behave in a bizarre fashion. Most schizophrenic patients will at one time or other experience a profound degree of paranoia, frequently associated with hallucinations, which tend to be more often auditory than visual. The thinking process in schizophrenia is characterized by a loosening of associations, while the behavior which seemingly takes place without reference to surroundings is often characterized as autistic. In talking with a schizophrenic patient, the clinician most commonly has a feeling of being unable to connect emotionally with the

Box 4-1 Diagnostic criteria for schizophrenia

A. *Characteristic symptoms:* Two (or more) of the following, each present for a significant portion of time during a 1-month period (or less if successfully treated)
(1) Delusions
(2) Hallucinations
(3) Disorganized speech (e.g., frequent derailment or incoherence)
(4) Grossly disorganized or catatonic behavior
(5) Negative symptoms (i.e., affective flattening, alogia, or avolition)
Note: Only one Criterion A symptom is required if delusions are bizarre or hallucinations consist of a voice keeping up a running commentary on the person's behavior or thoughts, or two or more voices conversing with each other.

B. *Social/occupational dysfunction:* For a significant portion of the time since the onset of the disturbance, one or more major areas of functioning such as work, interpersonal relations, or self-care are markedly below the level achieved prior to the onset (or when the onset is in childhood or adolescence, failure to achieve expected level of interpersonal, academic, or occupational achievement).

C. *Duration:* Continuous signs of the disturbance persist for at least 6 months. This 6-month period must include at least 1 month of symptoms (or less if successfully treated) that meet Criterion A (i.e., active-phase symptoms) and may include periods of prodromal or residual symptoms. During these prodromal or residual periods, the signs of the disturbance may be manifested by only negative symptoms or two or more symptoms listed in Criterion A present in an attenuated form (e.g., odd beliefs, unusual perceptual experiences).

D. *Schizoaffective and Mood Disorder exclusion:* Schizoaffective Disorder and Mood Disorder With Psychotic Features have been ruled out because either (1) no Major Depressive, Manic, or Mixed Episodes have occurred concurrently with the active-phase symptoms or (2) if mood episodes have occurred during active-phase symptoms, their total duration has been brief relative to the duration of the active and residual periods.

E. *Substance/general medical condition exclusion:* The disturbance is not due to the direct physiological effects of a substance (e.g., a drug of abuse, a medication) or a general medical condition.

F. *Relationship to a Pervasive Developmental Disorder:* If there is a history of Autistic Disorder or another Pervasive Developmental Disorder, the additional diagnosis of Schizophrenia is made only if prominent delusions or hallucinations are also present for at least a month (or less if successfully treated).

Classification of longitudinal course (can be applied only after at least 1 year has elapsed since the initial onset of active-phase symptoms):

Episodic With Interepisode Residual Symptoms (episodes are defined by the reemergence of prominent psychotic symptoms); *also specify if* **With Prominent Negative Symptoms**

Episodic With No Interepisode Residual Symptoms

Continuous (prominent psychotic symptoms are present throughout the period of observation); *also specify if* **With Prominent Negative Symptoms**

Single Episode In Partial Remission; *also specify if:* **With Prominent Negative Symptoms**

Single Episode In Full Remission

Other or Unspecified Pattern

individual. The patient suffering from schizophrenia may be withdrawn, quiet, and regressed, or may present with considerable agitation, belligerence, and even combativeness. Schizophrenia, previously known as dementia praecox, has been divided into a number of subgroups, formerly seen by some as representing distinctly different illnesses. The etiology of schizophrenia is unknown; but by definition it is a nonorganic form of psychosis, and has been classified as "functional." In view of newer understandings of neurochemistry, and the interaction of a variety of psychotropic medications with the symptoms of schizophrenia, there is increasing evidence to suggest that schizophrenia is a manifestation of an abnormality in brain chemistry and neurotransmission.[3]

HISTORICAL PERSPECTIVES OF BIOLOGIC PSYCHIATRY

Earlier considerations of serious psychotic illness would have classified the spectrum known today as schizophrenia as madness or insanity. Human awareness of insanity is quite ancient and was known even in biblical times.[4] Ancient medicine was often divided regarding the etiology of this form of illness: whether it was of divine or supernatural origin, whether it was the result of social or psychological factors, or the product of some organic cause. Hippocratic teaching originating in ancient Greece argued against the more popular belief that insanity was of supernatural origin, and suggested what we now consider to be a more likely cause – namely, some abnormality in brain function. Throughout the generations this argument regarding the etiology of psychosis persisted. Approximately a century ago, the English physician and biochemist J.L.W. Thudichum began to study the chemical composition of the brain of cattle, which formed an early foundation of modern neurochemistry. Thudichum believed that many forms of insanity were caused by the generation of toxic substances within the body.[5] Approximately one half-century after the momentous hypothesis of this early neurochemist, other investigators began to conduct studies to find abnormal chemicals in the biologic fluid of psychotic individuals. One such early investigator was Herman Holland DeJong, who isolated a substance from the urine of schizophrenic patients which he termed "catatonin." He had hoped that this chemical would be a clue to the biochemical etiology of psychosis, but was later disappointed to find that the abnormal substances in the urine correlated with coffee and tobacco consumption by the patients, and could be more properly identified as metabolites of caffeine and nicotine rather than some specific psychototoxic substance. In the 1950s and 1960s a number of investigators identified abnormal substances in the blood and urine of psychotic individuals.[6] Again, the search for a naturally generated psychotogenic substance met with the unfortunate finding that the various chromatographic spots identified represented metabolites of, primarily, chlorpromazine, which the patients had been receiving.

R.G. Heath isolated a substance which he called "taraxein" from the blood of schizophrenic patients.[7] This substance, which was initially thought to have unique psychotomimetic qualities, and represented the long-awaited toxic metabolite responsible for psychotic behavior, unfortunately failed to reach this potentially important role in the understanding of schizophrenic illness.

Beginning in 1948 with the discovery of the hallucinogenic effects of lysergic acid diethylamide (LSD) and continuing for a period of nearly 20 years, investigations of chemically induced psychotic behavior in man and animals were central to the development of the embryonic science of biologic psychiatry.[8] Not only can psychotic behavior be observed in response to the administration of a number of chemical compounds, these hallucinogenic substances bear striking structural resemblances to naturally occurring neurotransmitters. LSD is an indole compound, chemically similar to the neurotransmitter serotonin. Mescaline, the most ancient of the hallucinogens, and adrenochrome, another psychotomimetic compound, were structurally related to the catecholamines (since there is also dopamine) norepinephrine and epinephrine.[6] Other early attempts to mimic or precipitate psychotic behavior in order to understand its biochemical mechanisms involved the administration of certain amino acids to schizophrenic patients who were clinically in remission. Administration of tryptophan, a serotonin precursor, and methionine, which facilitates neurotransmitter synthesis, was found to provoke acute psychotic symptoms in patients whose schizophrenic illnesses were in apparent remission.

Throughout the late 1950s and the 1960s a variety of investigators injected blood serum from schizophrenic patients into animals, in an attempt to observe modifications of behavior or interactions with a variety of administered neurotransmitter substances. Minz and Walaszek conducted some early studies on the effects of serum from schizophrenic patients on various physiologic and pharmacologic parameters in rabbits. These early investigations suggested a distinct difference between serum from normals and that from schizophrenics, but again failed to prove a distinct biochemical etiology for psychosis.[9]

A half-century ago, epidemiologic studies found an exceedingly low incidence of active allergic diseases during the course of acute psychotic illness. This finding led a number of investigators to administer histamine to schizophrenic patients to determine whether this chemical, which was thought to have a pivotal role in allergic disorders, would produce a differential response in psychotic patients compared with normal volunteers. The pharmacologic response to injected histamine as measured by gastric acid secretion was found to be markedly reduced in schizophrenics. Subsequently, in an attempt to explain this finding, I measured histaminase, the histamine-metabolizing enzyme, in the serum of schizophrenic patients and found the level of the enzyme to be approximately 2½-fold greater in these patients than in normal volunteers, suggesting a chemical correlation to the early finding of the reduced incidence of allergic disease and the subsequent physiologic finding of decreased histamine sensitivity in psychotic patients.[10] Although early investigations seeking a chemical etiology in schizophrenia were unsuccessful, they all contributed to our understanding of neurochemistry and psychopharmacology, and helped to pave the way for a modern view of psychosis as a manifestation of abnormal neurochemistry.

DEVELOPMENT OF ANTIPSYCHOTIC CHEMOTHERAPY

Probably the most fruitful area of investigation supporting our current thinking regarding the etiology of psychotic illness is an outgrowth of the administration of a variety of medications to medical and psychiatric patients. Among the earliest encouraging drug effects in psychosis was the finding of Pfeiffer and Jenney, who discovered that the potent cholinergic stimulant, arecoline, derived from the betel nut, could induce a short but dramatic lucid interval in schizophrenic patients following IV injection.[11] These investigators found that confused, hallucinating, paranoid individuals experienced a few minutes wherein there was virtual disappearance of psychotic symptoms following the injection of this substance, thus providing an early suggestion of the potential connection between neurotransmitters and behavior. Another early discovery that had a major impact on our understanding of the nature and treatment of psychosis was the repeated observation of the ability of reserpine, an antihypertensive drug, to induce severe depression in otherwise healthy hypertensive individuals.[12] The recognition that reserpine depleted brain stores of both norepinephrine and serotonin suggested a correlation between the production of depressed mood and the decrease in these neurotransmitters in the CNS. Reserpine was demonstrated to produce a calming effect and a reduction in psychotic symptoms when administered to individuals suffering from schizophrenia and other psychotic illnesses.[13] The ability of reserpine to produce profound depression and suicidal feelings led to its relatively short, although important, career as an early antipsychotic drug.

The modern era in our understanding and treatment of psychosis began with the synthesis of chlorpromazine in 1950.[14] A variety of barbiturates had been used to sedate agitated psychotic individuals, and although these drugs could produce pronounced sedative effects, the patients subsequently awakened with continuing psychotic symptoms. Likewise, in the preantipsychotic era, the primitive therapeutic approaches utilized included the application of cold packs, or actually placing patients in tubs of cold water, which at times seemed to improve agitation and other symptoms of psychosis. The recognition of chlorpromazine's ability to lower body temperature in animals contributed to the initial interest in this drug as a preanesthetic sedative, and also as an agent to potentially control agitated psychotic patients, some of whom seemingly responded favorably to what appeared to be the chemical induction of hypothermia. The initial administration of chlorpromazine to psychotic patients by Deniker and associates, at doses of 75 to 150 mg/day by injection, failed to produce significant changes in body temperature but were associated with a significant reduction in psychotic agitation.[14]

It is interesting that early observations of the antipsychotic effect of chlorpromazine occurred at dosages which produced minimal sedation, in contrast to the absence of a true antipsychotic action of barbiturates administered in doses which produced profound sedation. Early clinical experiments thus suggested the possibility that a chemical could reduce or alleviate psychotic symptoms without producing marked sedation and without lowering body temperature, which were presumed mechanisms of earlier effective treatments for psychosis. Chlorpromazine continued to be applied with increasing frequency in the treatment of psychosis, although neither its mechanism of action nor the biological etiology of psychosis were understood. The ability of chlorpromazine to lower blood pressure and to produce extrapyramidal and other unwanted side effects gave rise to the development of other chemical substances with similar beneficial therapeutic effects, hopefully with fewer adverse actions.

MECHANISM OF ACTION OF ANTIPSYCHOTIC DRUGS

A series of phenothiazine derivatives with antipsychotic effects followed the initial introduction of chlorpromazine. Compounds such as the thioxanthenes — closely related to the phenothiazines — and others such as the butyrophenones, dibenzoxazepines, and dihydroindolones were introduced in the 1960s for clinical use in the treatment of psychosis. Since there was a divergence in the chemical structure of substances that produced antipsychotic action clinically, the structure-activity relationships recognized in classical pharmacology could not be strictly applied to understanding the mechanism of action of these compounds. Extensive work from the laboratory of Snyder identified dopamine receptor blockade as the pharmacologic action critical to the ability of a given compound to alleviate psychotic symptoms.[3]

Furthermore, this work allowed for a close correlation between the in vitro antagonism of dopamine receptor sites and the antipsychotic potency demonstrable clinically.[15] Those compounds devoid of dopamine receptor–blocking activity likewise lack antipsychotic action. Drugs such as haloperidol, which produce specific and dramatic antagonism of dopamine receptors in vitro, likewise exhibit potent antipsychotic action in patients.[15] Agents relatively weak in dopamine receptor–blocking action (such as chlorpromazine) have lower clinical potency in the treatment of psychotic patients. The correlation of dopamine receptor–blocking potency and clinically observable antipsychotic action strongly suggested a relationship between the dopamine receptor and pathogenesis of psychotic symptoms.

During the 1970s and 1980s, research on the etiology of schizophrenia has focused on dopamine and its receptors, as well as the genetic predisposition to this disorder.[15,16] Dopamine D_2 receptors have been observed to be more numerous in the basal ganglia of postmortem brain samples from schizophrenic patients.[17] In a momentous investigation, utilizing positron emission tomography (PET), D_2-receptor density was found to be increased in the caudate nucleus of living patients with schizophrenia.[17] Dopamine D_2 receptor density was found to be increased by PET scanning in 10 schizophrenic patients who had never received antipsychotic chemotherapy and in five schizophrenic patients who had received prior neuroleptic medication in comparison to 11 normal volunteers.[17] Since PET scan studies of living non–drug-treated schizophrenic patients have identified increased numbers of dopamine receptors, similar to findings of numerous studies of postmortem material, there is strong support for a defect in dopamine neurotransmission as a major etiologic factor in schizophrenia.

Beginning in the 1960s, numerous studies of family members of schizophrenic patients and studies of identical twins reared apart have pointed to a genetic predisposition for schizophrenia.[16] There is indeed a much higher incidence of schizophrenia in close biological relatives of affected individuals and high statistical concordance for the existence of schizophrenia or a schizophrenialike syndrome in identical twins reared in different environments.[16] Though there is not yet a reliable genetic marker for schizophrenia, much work is moving in this direction. In all likelihood, the genetic predisposition leads to biochemical vulnerability, most likely involving dopamine synthesis or release, dopamine receptor binding, or other defects in neurotransmission.[18] Since there are a vast number of neurotransmitter systems within the brain that interact with one another and which may be modified by disease processes and pharmacologic interventions, it is likely that ultimately we will find schizophrenia to be etiologically connected, not only with dopamine neurotransmission, but with disturbances in a variety of other neurotransmitter systems.[19]

Although the connection between dopamine neurotransmission and the etiology and treatment of schizophrenia has been pivotal in our understanding of this aspect of psychopharmacology, two new drugs have been introduced in the treatment of psychotic disorders in the last decade in the United States which again emphasize the potential importance of other neurotransmitters in psychosis. Clozapine and, more recently, risperidone exert both dopamine (D_2) and serotonin (5-HT_2) antagonism.[21,22,23] Risperidone is a potent dopamine antagonist while clozapine is relatively weak in its dopamine receptor blocking activity.[21,22] Unlike earlier antipsychotic agents, including the highly potent standard, haloperidol, these new compounds not only improve positive symptoms of schizophrenia — including hallucinations, delusions, and thought disorder — but also exert unprecedented therapeutic action in alleviating negative symptoms including blunted affect, apathy, and social withdrawal.[21,23] It is likely that the 5-HT_2 antagonist actions of these new compounds account for their ability to alleviate negative schizophrenic symptoms and their ability to produce clinically significant antipsychotic action without significant extrapyramidal side effects, the latter being one major cause of patients discontinuing maintenance antipsychotic drug therapy.[21,22,23,23a] Unfortunately, clozapine can potentially produce serious leukopenia and agranulocytosis, which necessitates weekly white counts throughout therapy[21]; on a positive note, risperidone which is chemically unrelated to the former compound does not alter the white blood cell count and does not require hematologic monitoring.[24] One particularly interesting aspect of clozapine is its ability to suppress symptoms of tardive dyskinesia, making it the first agent with a potential benefit both in psychosis and in the major complication of antipsychotic drug therapy.[23a,25] Preliminary studies suggest that risperidone may also reduce abnormal movements of tardive dyskinesia.[23,23a] Clozapine and risperidone have both been found to benefit many schizophrenic patients who have been unresponsive to other neuroleptic drugs.[21,23]

INDICATIONS FOR ANTIPSYCHOTIC DRUGS

1. Schizophrenia—acute treatment and prophylaxis of recurrence
2. Schioaffective Disorder—acute treatment and prophylaxis
3. Schizophreniform Disorder and Brief Psychotic Disorder—acute treatment
4. Mania—acute treatment
5. Psychotic Depression—acute treatment and sometimes prophylaxis
6. Dementia—acute treatment, prophylaxis of recurrent psychotic symptoms
7. Drug-Induced Psychosis—acute short-term treatment
8. Tourette's Disorder (discussed in chapters 11 and 15)
9. Violence and Agitation—acute treatment
10. Obsessive-Compulsive Disorder and severe anxiety unresponsive to other agents

Although schizophrenia is less common than either anxiety or depression, it is certainly the most prevalent of psychotic illnesses and the psychiatric condition most often requiring treatment in the hospital setting. Schizophrenia is the first thought that comes to mind when psychosis is mentioned, but there are other psychotic disturbances which require pharmacologic intervention. Schizoaffective disorder, discussed in chapter 8, is an illness with both schizophrenic and affective features which responds to pharmacologic treatment. The DSM-IV includes the diagnosis of schizophreniform disorder, an illness resembling schizophrenia, but of brief duration without a specific precipitating psychosocial stress.[2] The DSM-IV mentions brief psychotic disorder which is associated with sudden onset, short duration, and often an identifiable precipitating stress.[2] The latter two psychotic disorders often require short-term pharmacologic intervention, and by definition do not generally entail long-term maintenance pharmacotherapy. Former diagnostic classifications included psychotic depression, involutional melancholia, and manic-depressive illness as forms of psychosis. DSM-IV classifies these conditions under the heading of major affective disorders. Patients with major affective disorders may experience psychosis with or without major depressive episodes. Certainly the role of antipsychotic medication is of major importance in the treatment of acutely manic patients, as mentioned in chapter 8 and as will be discussed in greater detail below. The discussion of tricyclic and heterocyclic antidepressants in chapter 5 comments on the application of antipsychotic agents in the treatment of patients with major depressive episodes, the current nomenclature for a variety of depressive illnesses previously classified as psychotic depression and involutional melancholia.

Dementia of the Alzheimer's type is a new diagnostic group appearing in DSM IV, which was included under organic mental disorders in DSM-III-R. Alzheimer-type Dementia (Alzheimer's disease), most commonly occurs in the elderly as a manifestation of age-associated anatomical and physiologic changes in the brain. The judicious use of low doses of high-potency antipsychotic agents in the treatment of organic brain dysfunction associated with aging is discussed in chapter 16 and is only briefly mentioned here. The DSM-IV includes substance-induced psychotic disorders that result from drug intoxication and withdrawal, as well as substance-induced delirium.[2] Application of antipsychotic agents in the treatment of drug intoxication and withdrawal will primarily be dealt with in chapter 18. The primary focus of this chapter is the pharmacology of antipsychotic drugs, with particular emphasis on their application to the treatment of schizophrenic and affective forms of psychotic illness.

INITIATING ANTIPSYCHOTIC THERAPY

The acutely psychotic patient, whether he presents in the hospital emergency room, ward consultation, physician's office, or psychiatric ward, represents a true medical emergency. These patients require careful and prompt evaluation. Treatment must be instituted rapidly to prevent the patient from harming himself or others and to relieve his own suffering. Acutely psychotic patients are generally very frightened and are often frightening to others. These patients may be agitated or belligerent, and may threaten verbally or be overtly violent. Some psychotic individuals, particularly those with long-standing schizophrenic illnesses, may be regressed and behaving in a most primitive manner, whereas other patients may be quiet and withdrawn and present a tremendous challenge to the clinician who attempts to speak to them and obtain even the most rudimentary information.[19,20]

Before initiating pharmacologic treatment, which is the cornerstone of therapy of these patients, as much historical information as possible must be obtained from the patient, family, and friends.[40] Although a proper history and physical examination are highly desirable and necessary, and should be obtained as early as possible upon making contact with the patient, it is often not possible to get an ideally detailed medical history or to perform a full and complete physical examination. Very often one can obtain only limited historical information. The following points are particularly important to clarify, even if only a limited history can be obtained.

1. Prior history of similar episodes
2. Previous psychotropic drug treatment
3. Favorable and adverse responses to any prior psychotropic medications

4. Any medical condition or recent treatment with medication for nonpsychiatric illnesses
5. Past and present alcohol history
6. Use of over-the-counter or illicit drugs (Having a friend or family member whom the patient trusts look through his pockets and personal belongings may be helpful in locating medication containers that may give clues to recent use of prescribed or illicit drugs.)

Having obtained the initial historical information, pharmacologic treatment should be started and continued with a single antipsychotic agent rather than using multiple medications or excessively changing from one neuroleptic to another.[19] As has been pointed out previously, the only psychotropic drugs that are useful in the treatment of psychotic symptoms such as paranoia, delusions, hallucinations, and disordered thinking are those agents termed neuroleptic or antipsychotic. All compounds in this group block dopamine receptor sites, which is believed to be responsible for their ability to alleviate psychotic symptoms.

Although dopamine receptor blockade is associated with the desirable clinical effect of neuroleptics, the alleviation of psychotic symptoms, this action also accounts for the production of extrapyramidal side effects of these drugs.[3,15] Following many years of attempts to separate antipsychotic action from extrapyramidal effects of these drugs has yielded two important newer antipsychotic drugs, currently available in the United States, clozapine and risperidone.[20,21,22] The former is a low-potency antagonist of D_2 dopamine sites while the latter has more potent D_2 blocking activity.[21,22] The most striking pharmacological difference of these newer drugs, which have been termed atypical antipsychotics, is their ability to block $5-HT_2$ serotonin receptors. Indeed both of these drugs bind more avidly to $5-HT_2$ sites than they do to D_2 receptors.[21,22] Although risperidone is a weaker D_2 antagonist than is haloperidol, which has generally been viewed as the most potent antipsychotic drug, the former compound appears to be clinically more potent than haloperidol.[22,23] It also appears that the ratio of high anti–$5-HT_2$ activity of risperidone and clozapine relative to their D_2 blocking activity may account for their dramatically lower potential to produce parkinsonian and other extrapyramidal side effects. Neither of these compounds is available for parenteral use. When used orally, however, risperidone has been demonstrated to produce rapid control of acute psychotic symptoms without significant extrapyramidal effects at doses of only 3 mg twice daily, making it a potential first-line drug in the treatment of acute psychosis and the prophylaxis of schizophrenic relapse.[23,24] Clozapine, which is of considerably lower potency, though excellent in avoiding extrapyramidal effects, does produce rather dramatic anticholinergic, sedative, and hypotensive side effects and has the potential for producing leukopenia and agranulocytosis.[21] Since agranulocytosis can have a potentially fatal outcome, patients receiving clozapine must have weekly white blood cell counts throughout therapy; thus clozapine can never be seen as a first-line drug in acute psychosis and is appropriately used in maintenance treatment, only after other less toxic antipsychotic drugs have proven ineffective or are not tolerated by the patient.[21] Risperidone is chemically unrelated to clozapine and appears to have no potential for adverse hematologic effects.[24] Studies of these newer antipsychotic drugs have focused on the differential responses of positive schizophrenic symptoms, including hallucinations, delusions and thought disorder, versus negative schizophrenic symptoms, such as blunted affect, apathy, and social withdrawal, to pharmacotherapy.[20,23] Indeed, standard antipsychotic drugs are highly effective against positive symptoms but lack efficacy in managing negative symptoms, while both respond to these newer neuroleptics.

Table 4-1 presents some important pharmacologic and clinical characteristics of the most commonly prescribed antipsychotic drugs. As can be seen from the table, which lists the neuroleptic drugs in descending order of clinical potency, there is an excellent correlation between clinically observable potency of the various drugs and their binding to tritiated haloperidol–labeled postsynaptic dopamine receptors in mammalian brain. Studies utilizing homogenates of fresh calf brain revealed that tritiated dopamine and tritiated haloperidol appeared to label distinct agonist and antagonist states of the receptor respectively.[15] Laboratory experiments utilizing this approach have facilitated our understanding of the interactions of a variety of drugs with receptor sites in the brain as well as in other tissues, and have added immeasurably to our clinical understanding of the actions and potency of numerous drugs, most notably the neuroleptics. Likewise, as shown in the third column of Table 4-1, the relative affinity of a number of neuroleptic drugs for muscarinic cholinergic receptors has been documented by laboratory investigation in several animal species.[26] The close correlation of cholinergic receptor binding affinities of various neuroleptic drugs with clinically observable anticholinergic action is notable, and helps us understand the pharmacologic basis of one of the most prominent adverse effects of neuroleptic and antidepressant drugs — their ability to produce anticholinergic side effects.

Since most research has linked antipsychotic activity of neuroleptic drugs to their ability to block dopamine receptors, and since excessive dopamine activity or increased sensitivity of dopamine receptors has been seen as playing an etiologic role in psychosis, higher-potency dopamine antagonists have generally been seen as the optimal therapeutic agents in acute psychosis and the preferred maintenance drugs in the prophylaxis of recurrence.[15,27,28] Conceivably, if the newer agents which antagonize 5-HT_2 serotonin receptors continue to prove effective and safe with widespread clinical use, agents such as risperidone may indeed revolutionize our thinking and clinical approach to treatment and prophylaxis of psychotic illness. The comparative potencies of orally administered antipsychotic drugs are shown in Table 4-2.

UNWANTED EFFECTS OF ANTIPSYCHOTIC DRUGS

Although efficacy is the most fundamental consideration in the choice of a specific therapeutic agent, all drugs have a variety of side effects, most of which

Table 4-1 Characteristics of commonly used antipsychotic drugs

Clinical potency of antipsychotic action (from most to least) [chemical class]	Inhibition of (^{3}H)-haloperidol binding K_1 (nmol)†	Relative affinity for muscarinic (cholinergic) receptor‡	Anticholinergic effects clinically observed	Parkinsonian effects clinically observed	Sedation clinically observed	Hypotension clinically observed
Risperidone (Risperdal) [benzisoxazole]	3.13 ± 1.30§	Negligible§	±	+	+	++
Haloperidol (Haldol) [butyrophenone]	1.5 ± 0.14	0.21	+	+++++	++	+
Fluphenazine (Prolixin) [piperazine-phenothiazine]	1.2 ± 0.12	0.83	++	+++++	++	++
Thiothixene (Navane) [piperazine-thioxanthene]	1.4 ± 0.11	0.78	++	++++	++	++
Trifluoperazine (Stelazine) [piperazine-phenothiazine]	2.1 ± 0.34	0.91	++	++++	+	++
Perphenazine (Trilafon) [piperazine-phenothiazine]			++	++++	+++	+++
Molindone (Moban) [dihydroindolone]			++	+++	+	++
Loxapine (Loxitane) [dibenzoxazepine]			++	+++	+++	++
Clozapine (Clozaril) [dibenzodiazepine]	100 ± 6	385	+++++	±	+++++	+++++
Chlorpromazine (Thorazine) [aliphatic-phenothiazine]	10.3 ± 0.2	10.0	++++	++	+++++	+++++
Thioridazine (Mellaril) [piperidine-phenothiazine]	14.0 ± 0.2	66.7	+++++	+	++++	+++++

*Drugs are listed in order of clinical potency, from most potent to least potent in their action against psychotic symptoms, based on my clinical experience and review of a wide range of published data. The likelihood of producing various side effects is likewise based on my observation of patients and a review of published information from numerous sources.

†From Creese I, et al: Science 1976; 192:481-483.

‡From Snyder S, et al: Arch Gen Psychiatry 1974; 31:58-61.

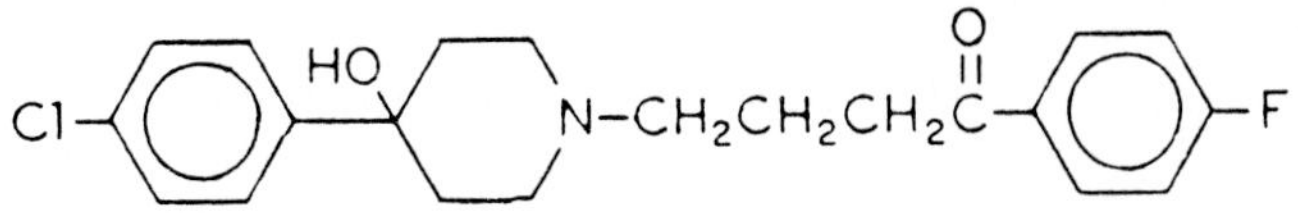

HALOPERIDOL

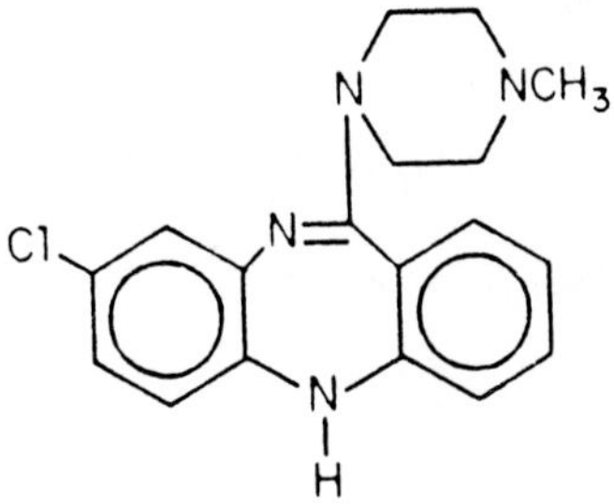

CLOZAPINE

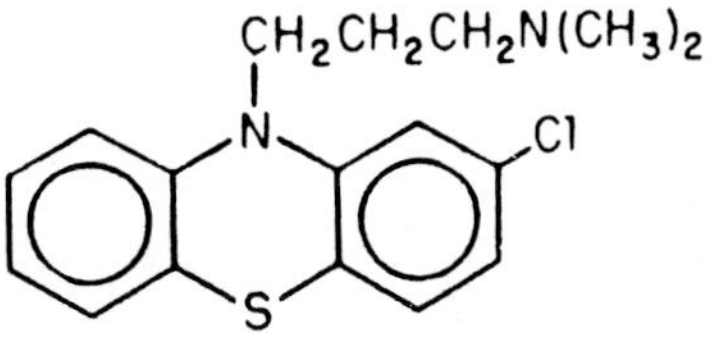

CHLORPROMAZINE

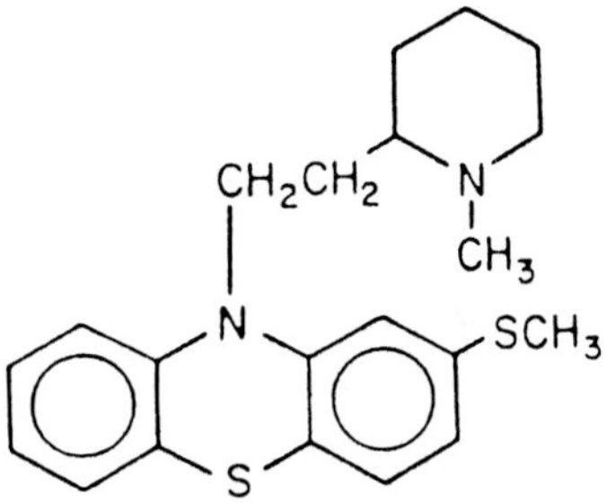

THIORIDAZINE

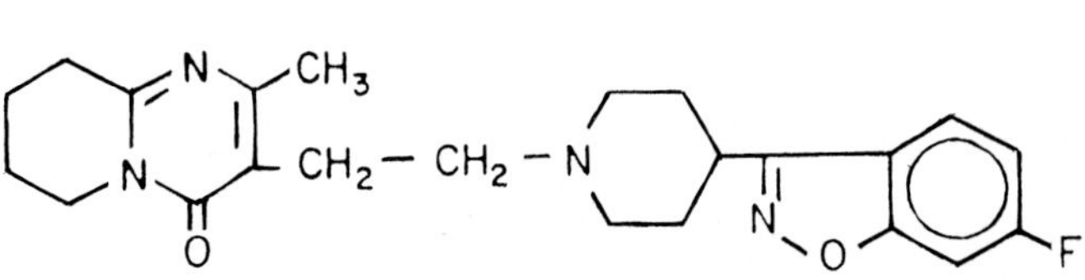

RISPERIDONE

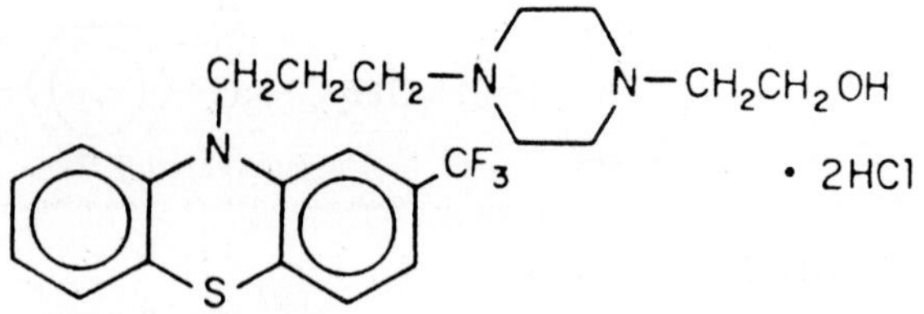

FLUPHENAZINE

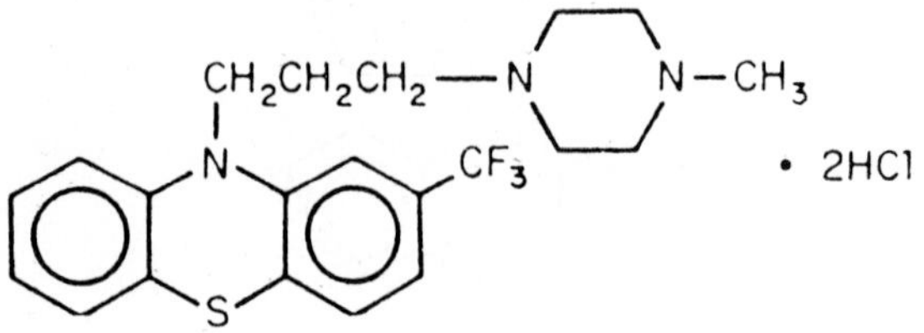

TRIFLUOPERAZINE

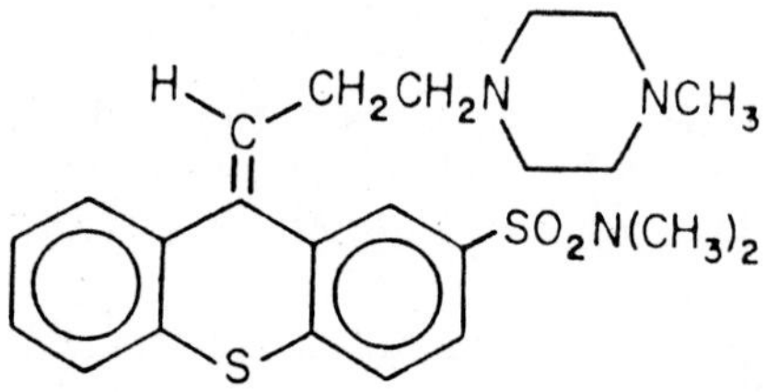

THIOTHIXENE

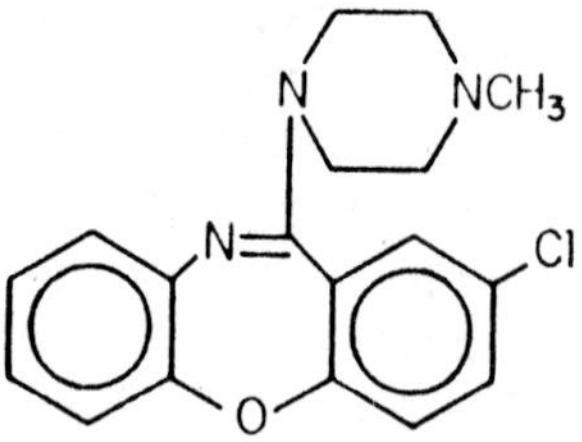

LOXAPINE

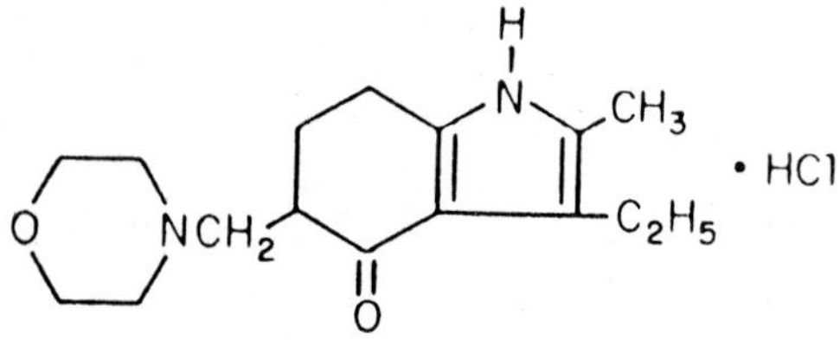

MOLINDONE

Table 4-2 Antipsychotic drugs —
approximate oral dosage equivalencies

Drug (trade name)	Equivalency (mg)
Chlorpromazine (Thorazine)	100
Clozapine (Clozaril)	50
Fluphenazine (Prolixin)	4
Haloperidol (Haldol)	4
Loxapine (Loxitane)	10
Molidone (Moban)	10
Perphenazine (Trilafon)	10
Risperidone (Risperdal)	1
Trifluoperazine (Stelazine)	5
Thiothixene (Navane)	5
Thioridazine (Mellaril)	100

are related directly to the pharmacology of the drug and may indeed be an extension of some of the mechanisms responsible for the therapeutic action of a given compound.[28] Among the antipsychotic drugs, variations in side effects are particularly prominent.[19,28] All available antipsychotic agents produce some anticholinergic action, which is responsible for the clinical appearance of blurred vision, dry mouth, decreased sweating, constipation, urinary retention, and tachycardia.[19,28] As can be seen from Table 4-1, there is considerable variation among the available antipsychotic agents in their likelihood of producing anticholinergic effects. Haloperidol is least anticholinergic, while clozapine, chlorpromazine, and thioridazine are most anticholinergic.[76]

Each of the currently available antipsychotic agents, with the possible exception of clozapine, is capable of producing acute extrapyramidal or parkinsonian effects. These actions of neuroleptic drugs are based on their ability to block dopamine receptors in the basal ganglia; and the likelihood of producing extrapyramidal effects is inversely proportional to the anticholinergic action of the drug.[26,28] Indeed, the anticholinergic effect of a given neuroleptic may be seen in some ways as protecting against acute parkinsonian effects. The acute effects of neuroleptic drugs on the extrapyramidal system may produce a variety of clinical findings: acute dystonic reactions, with tightening of facial and neck muscles; associated torticollis or retrocollis, with or without tightness in the jaw; and difficulty opening the mouth. Acute dystonic reactions are not uncommon in the early phase of treatment of a psychotic individual who is receiving therapeutic doses of any of the neuroleptic drugs. Other acute extrapyramidal manifestations of neuroleptic drug action include a parkinsonian syndrome characterized by flattening of facial expressions, stiffness of gait, muscular rigidity in the trunk and extremities, a pill-rolling tremor of the fingers, and at times excessive salivation.[28] It must be emphasized that extrapyramidal reactions to the neuroleptic drugs are more likely to occur in the first few weeks of therapy, and less likely to be present later in the course of antipsychotic maintenance treatment.[19]

The high anticholinergic potency of clozapine, alone, does not appear to account for its apparent virtual absence of extrapyramidal side effects, particularly when considering the minimal degree of extrapyramidal side effects seen with risperidone which lacks significant anticholinergic activity.[22] Both of these "atypical" antipsychotic agents have considerably greater ability to antagonize serotonin 5-HT$_2$ receptors than standard antipsychotic drugs. For comparison, clozapine has approximately 5 times greater affinity for the 5-HT$_2$ receptor than haloperidol does and risperidone is at least 50 times as potent as haloperidol in antagonizing 5-HT$_2$ receptors.[21,22] Current thinking suggests that the 5-HT$_2$ antagonism of these newer antipsychotic drugs may account in part for their greater antipsychotic efficacy, particularly with respect to negative symptoms, and their lower potential for producing extrapyramidal side effects.[20,21,22,23,24]

Although tardive dyskinesia, which is discussed in more detail in chapter 11, has occurred with all standard antipsychotic drugs, and has not been proven to be less of a risk with long-term treatment with low-potency antipsychotic agents, such as chlorpromazine, mesoridazine, and thioridazine, than with high-potency agents, such as haloperidol,[29,30,31] the perpetual hope is that effective antipsychotic chemotherapy can occur without this risk. If indeed the ability to antagonize 5-HT$_2$ sites with drugs such as clozapine and risperidone explains a new mechanism of minimizing acute extrapyramidal effects, different from that using conventional antipsychotic drugs, this could conceivably account for greater safety with respect to the development of tardive dyskinesia. Thus far, the virtual absence of extrapyramidal effects and dyskinesia with clozapine confers a major advantage to this otherwise relatively toxic drug.[20,21] Furthermore, both clozapine and risperidone appear to improve tardive dyskinesia induced by previous treatment with other antipsychotic drugs. Patients with affective disorders and elderly women appear to be at greater risk of developing tardive dyskinesia.[30] There is also evidence that patients who have experienced frequent, severe, or persistent drug-induced extrapyramidal symptoms may, with prolonged neuroleptic therapy, have an increased risk of developing tardive dyskinesia.[32] Thus, in these high-risk cases, there is reason to consider a therapeutic trial of agents such as risperidone or clozapine.

Certainly the goal of pharmacotherapy in psychiatry goes beyond the immediate need to suppress symptoms of the illness and extends, with even greater importance, to the need of the individual to return to a functional state in society.[19] Since it was demonstrated many years ago that sedation is not a necessary concomitant to the control of psychotic symptoms, it stands to reason that those neuroleptic drugs that produce greater sedation would place the patient at considerable disadvantage from the standpoint of being able to function alertly at school, at work, or within the family.[19] Furthermore, in the acute phase of treating the psychotic patient, whether in the hospital or in the outpatient setting, it is hoped that the individual will participate in a greater array of activities than simply taking medication. If the patient is excessively drowsy he will not be able to think clearly enough to interact satisfactorily with other persons socially, and will obviously be unable to participate in an active program of psychotherapy in the hospital or the physician's office. For this reason, the more strongly sedating antipsychotic drugs, such as clozapine, thioridazine, mesoridazine, and chlorpromazine, may present an added burden to the patient, who would likely be more alert and better able to function if treated with a compound with less sedative action, such as risperidone, haloperidol, a piperazine phenothiazine or thioxanthine, loxapine, or molindone.[7]

Of all the various adverse effects of the neuroleptic drugs, the ability to produce considerable lowering of blood pressure is the one most likely to be dangerous to the patient.[28] The ability of this group of drugs to block alpha-adrenergic receptors gives rise to peripheral vasodilation and a consequent fall in total peripheral resistance with an associated hypotensive reaction.[28] Although a hypotensive reaction will be most pronounced when the person changes from a sitting or reclining posture to the standing position, considerable blood pressure reduction can occur without postural change. Of the currently available agents, clozapine, chlorpromazine, thioridazine, and mesoridazine are most likely to produce significant hypotensive reactions.[19] Risperidone, loxapine, molindone, thiothixene, and the piperazine phenothiazines are much less likely to lower blood pressure.[33-35] Of all available antipsychotic agents, haloperidol has the least alpha-adrenergic blocking effect and is least likely to produce hypotensive reactions.[28,36,37] The IV administration of relatively large doses of haloperidol in a study of the treatment of agitation following open heart surgery was associated with minimal to nonexistent blood pressure changes.[38] Clozapine has pronounced hypotensive activity, comparable to thioridazine, while risperidone, which is a potent alpha-adrenergic receptor antagonist, exerts rather modest hypotensive responses clinically due to the low doses used and the recommended gradual dosage titration when initiating therapy.[24] As discussed elsewhere in this volume, the hypotensive action of neuroleptic drugs is of greatest consequence in patients with cardiovascular disease and in the elderly.

Phenothiazines, especially thioridazine and chlorpromazine, may produce ST and T wave changes on the ECG as well as cardiac conduction disturbances, which are discussed in chapter 10. Pimozide may also produce ECG changes and conduction disturbances while haloperidol does not produce ECG or conduction abnormalities.[35] The elderly are most likely to develop severe complications, including a worsening in mental status, when given antipsychotic agents that are strongly anticholinergic.[12] Elderly patients receiving modest doses of low-potency antipsychotic agents may become suddenly dizzy and fall, sustaining hip fractures and other physical injuries.[39] As discussed elsewhere in this volume, the administration of antipsychotic drugs to the elderly should almost always rely on high-potency antipsychotic agents with low potential for anticholinergic and hypotensive side effects.

Although acute extrapyramidal effects may be frightening both to the patient and the clinician, these are the pharmacologically induced actions of the neuroleptics that are perhaps the most easy to manage.[19] Although some controversy exists regarding the prophylactic use of antiparkinsonian medication along with neuroleptics, several clinical studies support the advantage of using these agents along with antipsychotic drugs, early in the course of treatment in young and middle-aged patients.[40-43] Prophylactic antiparkinsonian drugs should almost always be avoided in the elderly and in patients with organic brain dysfunction because of these patients' increased risk of developing acute confusional states or toxic deliria in response to anticholinergic medication.[41,42] Antiparkinsonian medications are not necessary with risperidone and clozapine therapy. According to studies with the recommended daily dose of 6 mg of risperidone, extrapyramidal effects are comparable to placebo.[23]

The relatively common occurrence of akathisia and restlessness during the early phase of antipsychotic drug treatment, and the likelihood of other extrapyramidal effects, including acute dystonic reactions in patients treated with high-potency neuroleptics, support the judicious use of antiparkinsonian medication.[41,42] During the first 2 to 4 weeks of antipsychotic chemotherapy, patients receiving 15 to 30 mg/day of a potent neuroleptic agent may benefit considerably by the coadministration of benztropine mesylate in a dose of 0.5 to 1.0 mg 3 to 4 times daily. Patients receiving these relatively small doses of antiparkinsonian medication are less likely to experience acute dystonic reactions and appear considerably less likely to develop stiffness, muscular rigidity, tremors, excessive salivation, and akathisia.[41-43] Benztropine appears somewhat more effective in reducing dystonia and rigidity, and somewhat less effective in reducing akathisia, than another commonly used antiparkinsonian agent, trihexyphenidyl, which is more effective in controlling akathisia. Although the IM or IV administration of benztropine is highly effective in controlling acute dystonic reactions, perhaps the most specific and beneficial acute treatment for drug-induced dystonic reactions is diphenhydramine (Benadryl), administered by the IM or IV route. If the latter route of administration is chosen, and 50 mg diphenhydramine is administered by slow injection, most often the dystonic reaction will be largely absent within 2 minutes following completion of the injection. Most patients who have been properly stabilized on antipsychotic medication and who continue to receive suitably reduced dosages during the maintenance phase of their treatment will have minimal to nonexistent extrapyramidal symptoms. Treatment with low-range maintenance dosage, if continued in such individuals, will most often not require continuation of antiparkinsonian medication, even though these persons continue to receive high-potency neuroleptic drugs.[41-43]

CLOZAPINE THERAPY: SPECIAL CONSIDERATIONS

Like other antipsychotic drugs, clozapine is capable of lowering seizure threshold and provoking grand mal convulsions, particularly in patients with previously known seizure disorders and when relatively high doses are employed.[21,35] Among standard neuroleptic drugs, chlorpromazine has the greatest potential for provoking seizures—although this risk appears to be greater with clozapine, which is reported to present a 1% to 2% risk at doses under 300 mg/day, a 3% to 4% risk at doses between 300 and 600 mg/day, and a 5% risk with doses exceeding 600 mg/day.[21] Patients with known seizure disorders should generally not be treated with clozapine if alternatives exist and should be carefully monitored and covered with anticonvulsants if the drug must be employed. Since a variety of other drugs, including antidepressants, particularly clomipramine, bupropion, and maprotiline, can provoke seizures, these agents should not be administered along with clozapine.[21] Drugs such as fluoxetine which inhibit drug metabolism by the cytochrome P-450 (IID6) enzyme system can increase blood levels of clozapine and other agents, potentially increasing the risk of seizures.[12]

In spite of its strong anticholinergic activity, clozapine paradoxically can produce hypersalivation which primarily occurs at night and can be voluminous, with potential complications if the saliva is aspirated. Up to 5% of patients may experience a 1° to 2° temperature elevation, particularly during the first 3 weeks of treatment, its occurrence needs to be evaluated as to whether it is an independent benign finding or related to infection secondary to agranulocytosis. Weight gain is a common side effect of antipsychotic drugs, particularly low-potency agents, and appears to be most common with clozapine, occurring in 4% or more of treated patients, perhaps related to potent histamine H_1 or serotonin receptor antagonism.[21]

The most serious potential complication of clozapine is agranulocytosis (granulocyte count of less than 500/cu mm) which can be fatal due to overwhelming sepsis. Less serious hematologic complications include neutropenia (neutrophil count of less than 1000/cu mm) and leukopenia (total white blood cell count of less than 3500/cu mm). As of 1991 in the U.S., 47 cases of agranulocytosis were documented among 7500 clozapine treated patients, all of which were detected on the required weekly white blood cell counts, with a fatal outcome in only one patient.[21] In the United States, white cell counts must be done weekly throughout clozapine treatment and for 4 weeks after its discontinuation, which allows for earlier diagnosis of leukopenia and prompt drug discontinuation, maximizing the chance for hematologic recovery. Of the 149 cases of agranulocytosis reported worldwide, prior to frequent hematologic monitoring 32% were fatal.[8]

Although agranulocytosis may begin as long as a year after initiating clozapine, 50% of 185 reported cases in one study began within 12 weeks and 75% within 6 months of starting clozapine.[21] Prior to initiating clozapine therapy, a white cell exceeding 3500/cu mm must be present. In the U.S., white counts must be done weekly, and the data reported to the dispensing pharmacy before the prescription, limited to a 1-week supply, can be filled. After initiating therapy, a white count below 3500, or a significant drop in the WBC, even if the total exceeds 3500/cu mm, requires a repeat count. If subsequent WBC counts are between 3000 and 3500 with a granulocyte count above 1500/cu mm, the drug may be continued with twice weekly WBC and differential counts. A WBC count below 3000 or a granulocyte count less than 1500/cu mm requires interruption of clozapine therapy and evaluation of the patient for signs and symptoms of infection. Therapy can be restarted if the WBC exceeds 3000 and the granulocyte count 1500, although blood counts must now be done twice weekly, until the WBC is 3500 or greater.[21] If the WBC is 2000/cu mm or less with a granulocyte count of 1000 or less, clozapine must be discontinued; the patient must have a thorough hematologic evaluation and may need protective isolation with evaluation and treatment for infectious complications. Although there are differences of opinion as to the appropriateness of rechallenge with clozapine following leukopenic events, I would strongly argue against rechallenge, from a medical and medicolegal standpoint. Particularly as other agents such as risperidone, with potentially equal efficacy but lacking hematologic and autonomic adverse effects, have become available, the number of patients appropriate for clozapine therapy is likely to diminish. Indeed, preliminary evidence suggests that risperidone at a daily dose of 4 to 8 mg may be approximately as effective as clozapine at a daily dose of 400 mg, with fewer side effects and no potential for leukopenia or agranulocytosis.[44]

ANTIPSYCHOTIC DRUGS AND SCHIZOPHRENIA

Regardless of which antipsychotic drug is chosen for the treatment of a given patient, the clinician must be fully familiar with the pharmacology of the drug, including its therapeutic and side-effects profile. It is not necessary for every clinician to use every drug in a given therapeutic class, but essential that each clinician be thoroughly knowledgeable about those drugs he does use so that he will be familiar with what he can expect of each drug. Proper dosage titration of any drug is one of the most critical issues in safe and effective therapeutics.

Combining multiple antipsychotic agents or making rapid changes from one antipsychotic to another is not rational pharmacotherapy.[19,28] The clinician's knowledge of the medications he employs, and his ability to titrate the dose in response to the clinical circumstances rather than looking for a new medication to administer, is certainly a more rational medical approach. Situations do arise wherein it is medically appropriate to change from one antipsychotic agent to another after the first agent has proved ineffective, or in the event that the patient has repeatedly had a particular side effect with one agent which might be avoided by changing to a different compound. As a general rule, when multiple medications are simultaneously administered or rapid changes are made from one to another, the clinician can expect an increased incidence of side effects, even if the new drug is likely to be more effective than the former one.[12] Based on my clinical observations, it appears that the simultaneous use of two or more neuroleptics or rapid switching from one agent to another may be a risk factor for the development of the potentially devastating complication of neuroleptic malignant syndrome,[45] which is discussed in detail in chapter 10. If chlorpromazine and haloperidol are both administered IM within 1 or 2 hours of each other, regardless of which agent is given initially, the patient may experience a pronounced hypotensive reaction resulting from haloperidol potentiation of chlorpromazine-induced alpha-adrenergic blockade. Having recognized hypotensive reactions in several patients who unfortunately received these drugs concomitantly by the IM route leads me to caution against this approach.[12] Although I have rarely administered these two agents by the oral route to the same individual within a short time period, I have not observed a similar additive hypotensive effect with orally administered medication.

PHASES OF ANTIPSYCHOTIC THERAPY

The treatment of the acutely ill schizophrenic patient with antipsychotic medication can be divided into three phases. In the *initiation* phase, the dosage should be gradually and steadily titrated upward over the first several days to reduce paranoia, delusions, and hallucinations. In view of the side effect profiles of the various antipsychotic drugs, my preference has been to use haloperidol as the standard agent in most acutely psychotic manic or schizophrenic patients. More recent work, demonstrating risperidone to benefit both positive and negative symptoms of schizophrenia, and its possible beneficial effects in tardive dyskinesia, along with a favorable side effect profile, suggests that risperidone could eventually replace haloperidol as the initial drug of choice in acute schizophrenia.[23,23a] The dosage of haloperidol may be titrated upwards, with little risk of excessive sedation or hypotension, and relatively mild anticholinergic effect. Although extrapyramidal symptoms occasionally occur, they can be easily managed.[43] Antipsychotic chemotherapy should generally be instituted using a divided-dose regimen. My preference is to administer haloperidol 5 mg orally 4 times/day in a healthy young or middle-aged individual, with additional 5 mg doses being administered on an intermittent basis as required to control agitation or other psychotic behavior. I routinely administer benztropine mesylate in a dose of 0.5 to 1.0 mg orally 4 times/day along with the haloperidol during the initial course of treatment. The patient's response to treatment during the acute phase of psychosis in the hospital setting should be evaluated once or twice daily, at which time the physician should evaluate the patient's necessity for receiving additional medication. The dose of haloperidol may be titrated upward depending on the patient's behavior, level of psychotic thinking, agitation, and sense of comfort.

During the initial phase of therapy, the dosage of haloperidol employed may range from 10 mg daily up to 40 mg daily, or infrequently higher. The initiation phase of treatment of the seriously ill schizophrenic or manic patient in the hospital generally requires a period of 3 to 10 days. When the patient improves, he will often complain of more drowsiness and experience an increase in extrapyramidal symptoms. At this point the clinician should be aware that probably considerable dopamine receptor blockade has been produced, resulting in an improvement in psychotic symptoms but also resulting in a need for decreased dosage of the antipsychotic agent.

At this point the patient enters what I have termed the *stabilization* phase of treatment, when the astute clinician should be gradually diminishing the dose of antipsychotic medication and observing the patient on a daily basis for evidence that he continues to be relatively free of psychotic symptoms. In the event that the gradual decrease in antipsychotic dosage is associated with an increase in psychotic symptoms, one needs to increase the dosage gradually upward until the symptoms are adequately controlled, observe the patient for several days, and again attempt to gradually titrate the dosage downward. The stabilization phase may last from one to 3 weeks, during which time the patient receives a gradually decreasing amount of medication and hopefully remains relatively free of psychotic symptoms.

As the dose of haloperidol is decreased to what appears to be the minimal effective dose, the patient enters the *maintenance* phase of antipsychotic chemotherapy.[20] Hopefully, if there has been any increase in drug-related side effects during the course of treatment, as the patient has begun to recover, these side effects are now diminishing during the dosage reduction that occurs during the stabilization and maintenance phases. As the patient enters the maintenance phase, the physician should bear in mind that the goal is to maintain the patient relatively symptom-free, utilizing the lowest possible dosage of antipsychotic medication. During the stabilization phase of chemotherapy, both the total daily dose of medication and the frequency of administration are decreased. During the stabilization phase, the patient may generally receive two doses daily, as opposed to four or more that he may have received during initiation. As the patient enters the maintenance phase, it is desirable in most circumstances to administer the antipsychotic medication as a single dose at bedtime, although in some circumstances it may be advantageous to administer a small portion of the daily dose in the morning and the majority at bedtime.

Most patients following the first weeks of antipsychotic chemotherapy, as their dose of medication is diminished, will no longer require continuous treatment with antiparkinsonian medication. The physician should be alert to this, and attempt to treat the patient during the maintenance phase without antiparkinsonian medication, if that is feasible.[41-43] If the patient is relatively free of psychotic symptoms but continues to complain of extrapyramidal symptoms, this may be an indication that he is receiving a larger dose of antipsychotic medication than is necessary. The striking thing that occurs in the treatment of the acute schizophrenic patient as he is followed through the phases of chemotherapy is the dramatic reduction in the amount of antipsychotic medication that he requires as he improves. Most patients whom I have treated successfully with large doses of haloperidol in the range of 60 mg/day are able to be discharged from the hospital after 2 to 3 weeks, receiving a daily dose of 15 to 20 mg haloperidol. Later during the course of maintenance chemotherapy, many individuals, even those who have required large doses during the acute phase of their illness, can be satisfactorily maintained with daily haloperidol doses of 5 to 10 mg. It can be administered as a single nighttime dose with minimal adverse effects and without the need for continuous antiparkinsonian medication.

Many acutely schizophrenic patients will not be fully cooperative in taking medication and will not infrequently attempt to conceal the medication under their tongue and later spit it out. For this reason I favor the liquid forms of antipsychotic medication during the first few days, until the patient's therapeutic response is established. Numerous studies have demonstrated potential benefits of a rapid treatment approach to acute psychosis, using high oral or IM doses of haloperidol or fluphenazine.[37,46] In previous years I often favored high-dose therapy, which is safe but, as recent studies show, not necessarily more effective.[47,48] Most current thinking favors moderate rather than high-dose medication.[47,48] The routine administration of haloperidol to acutely psychotic patients by the IM route may allow for a somewhat more rapid response, but the need for this rapid response must be balanced against the attitude of most psychotic patients toward receiving IM injections. Most individuals do not like injections, and the process of administration by this route is likely to be more traumatic psychologically. Nonetheless, one of the major advantages of haloperidol is that there is no pain or irritation at the injection site, in contradistinction to the local inflammation which occurs when chlorpromazine is injected.[37] Furthermore, the injection volume for 100 mg chlorpromazine is 4 ml, while an equally effective antipsychotic dose of haloperidol, 5 mg, represents an injection volume of only 1 ml. Intramuscular administration of the high-potency piperazine phenothiazines tends to be considerably more irritating than that of haloperidol. Thus it would appear both from its pharmacologic profile and its ease of administration that haloperidol is the ideal medication in most individuals who need acute treatment of psychotic illness. In treating acutely psychotic schizophrenic outpatients, I would start with 5 mg haloperidol 4 times daily, along with 1 mg benztropine mesylate 4 times daily. I would prefer to see the patient as frequently as possible, and titrate the dosage gradually upward to 10 mg orally 4 times daily, if required for control of psychotic symptoms. Most patients who are acutely psychotic and need relatively larger doses of antipsychotic medication, will need the added support and therapeutic environment of the hospital setting.

The careful reader will recognize that I am recommending lower doses of haloperidol for acute psychosis than those given in previous editions of this handbook. My current dosage recommendations are based on published research studies demonstrating the efficacy of low or moderate doses of haloperidol and fluphenazine in the treatment of acute psychosis.[19,47,48,50] My clinical experience with high-dose, orally administered haloperidol in acutely psychotic patients and studies of high-dose IV administered haloperidol to agitated cardiac patients at the Massachusetts General Hospital have not been associated with significant complications or serious adverse effects.[38] Nevertheless, the goal of any therapeutic intervention is to utilize the lowest effective dose of medication necessary to achieve the desired result. Dosage of medication must always be carefully adjusted to the specific patient, while monitoring the occurrence of both favorable and adverse drug effects. The physician's decision of the specific drug and dosage regimen to be followed must be governed by careful observation of the patient, rather than cookbook dosage recommendations or data from research studies.

Although a study comparing high- and low-dose haloperidol in the treatment of acute psychosis does not differentiate the degree and rapidity of symptom alleviation between the two dosage ranges employed, individual patients treated in a clinical setting often show differential responses to high- or low-dose neuroleptic regimens.[46] Rapid neuroleptization studies employing fluphenazine have failed to document more rapid improvement when higher doses are employed, although more extrapyramidal symptoms were seen with this drug in the high-dose groups.[47] Likewise, a study of oral versus IM administration of fluphenazine has failed to document a therapeutic advantage of parenteral administration.[47] My recommendations for individualized dosage adjustment of neuroleptic drugs have always focused on oral administration and gradual dosage adjustment in contradistinction to earlier studies, suggesting rapid parenteral neuroleptization.[37] I have also recommended the coadministration of prophylactic antiparkinsonian medication to reduce the risk of acute dystonic reactions and akathisia, a concept which has gained renewed support from continuing clinical investigations.[42,43]

Since agitation, restlessness, and insomnia often occur in the acutely psychotic patient, larger than optimal doses of dopamine-antagonist antipsychotic agents have often been employed in the past to control these symptoms, resulting in potentially increased extrapyramidal side effects with high-potency agents and excessive anticholinergic and hypotensive side effects when low-potency agents were utilized. Numerous clinical studies have confirmed the potential benefits of the judicial short-term use of benzodiazepines along with high-potency neuroleptics to control agitation, restlessness, and insomnia.[49] Although various benzodiazepines have been used to augment lower-dose antipsychotic chemotherapy, it appears that the optimal agent is either lorazepam given orally or intramuscularly or clonazepam administered orally. Generally the addition of 1 to 2 mg of lorazepam every 2 to 4 hours PO or IM along with usual doses of haloperidol has been shown to produce better behavioral control than either agent administered alone and to be equal or better than the effect obtained with larger doses of high-potency antipsychotic agents.[49] Clonazepam in a dose of 0.5 to 1 mg 2 to 4 times daily would be a suitable alternative to lorazepam.[50] It is inadvisable to employ excessive doses of benzodiazepines or to use triazolobenzodiazepines such as alprozolam since these approaches have repeatedly been reported to produce disinhibition and potentially serious behavioral dyscontrol.[51] Combinations of benzodiazepines with high-potency neuroleptics have also been shown to reduce the incidence and severity of akathisia, dystonia, and other extrapyramidal side effects. The combined use of benzodiazepines with low-potency neuroleptics (such as chlorpromazine and thioridazine) is generally to be avoided because of the potential for prolonged deep sedation.[12] Indeed, states of collapse and excessive sedation along with hypotension have occasionally been reported with the combined use of benzodiazepines and clozapine.[52]

Although the standard acute treatment of psychosis has been established with high-potency antipsychotic agents — including haloperidol, fluphenazine, and thiothixene — the recent availability of risperidone could dramatically alter this. Thus far several published studies indicate that risperidone has a rapid onset of antipsychotic action, within 24 hours when administered by the oral route, and exerts antipsychotic efficacy when administered in a daily dose of 6 mg, which is comparable to 20 mg of haloperidol, while producing minimal autonomic side effects and extrapyramidal side effects, comparable to placebo.[23] Certainly much additional clinical use of risperidone will be necessary to establish it as a standard in acute psychosis; however, this drug is most promising and a potential first-line therapeutic agent. Dosage is initiated at 1 mg twice daily, increased to 2 mg twice daily on the second day and 3 mg twice daily thereafter.

ANTIPSYCHOTIC AGENTS IN ACUTE MANIA

The treatment of acute mania is discussed in depth in chapter 8. Any one of the antipsychotic drugs may be used to control manic symptoms. In my experience and in the extensive literature of psychopharmacology, it seems rather clear that the antipsychotic agent of choice in the acutely manic patient is haloperidol. In a study comparing lithium, chlorpromazine, and haloperidol in acute mania, haloperidol clearly produced the most rapid control of manic symptoms.[53] In the acutely manic patient I institute treatment with lithium carbonate simultaneously with haloperidol, monitor lithium levels carefully, and gradually reduce the dose of haloperidol as symptoms become controlled and the lithium level reaches therapeutic range. Once the patient is stabilized on lithium and is showing definite improvement, the neuroleptic dose, is further diminished and discontinued.

OTHER CLINICAL APPLICATIONS OF ANTIPSYCHOTIC DRUGS

Major affective illness manifesting as depression with psychotic features is another important indication for the use of antipsychotic agents. Patients with these symptoms will generally require treatment with one of the antidepressant drugs or with electroconvulsive therapy (ECT), as discussed in chapter 7. Nevertheless, antipsychotic agents are very important in the proper management of these patients. A person who is psychotically depressed should have initial treatment with an antipsychotic agent, and subsequently the antidepressant should be added. If this patient is treated initially with an antidepressant, there may be an exaggeration of psychotic symptoms until the antidepressant is discontinued and a suitable response to an appropriate antipsychotic agent is obtained. Since these patients generally require a combination of an antidepressant with an antipsychotic agent, it is important to be aware of the similarities of some side effects of these two classes of drugs.[12] Tricyclic antidepressants and neuroleptic drugs both produce anticholinergic effects. Low-potency antipsychotic drugs with strong anticholinergic and hypotensive effects are to be avoided when the patient is receiving a tricyclic antidepressant which is likewise anticholinergic and may also lower blood pressure. Fluoxetine inhibits the metabolism of a wide variety of drugs, including antipsychotic agents, thus potentially increasing both therapeutic and adverse effects.[12] For agitated psychotic depressions, my preference is to institute treatment with haloperidol, generally in much lower doses than those used in schizophrenia or mania. I might initiate haloperidol at a dose of 1 to 5 mg orally 2 to 4 times daily and, after several days, as the psychotic symptoms diminish, add an appropriate antidepressant. In nonagitated patients who are depressed, other high-potency antipsychotic agents such as a piperazine phenothiazine, thiothixene, or loxapine may be employed, initially alone and then in combination with an appropriate antidepressant.

There is evidence from clinical studies that patients with borderline personality disorder may respond favorably to low dosages of high-potency neuroleptic agents such as haloperidol.[54] Neuroleptics, either alone or in combination with antidepressants, in addition to producing a favorable therapeutic response in many borderline patients, are particularly advantageous because of their safety: there is virtually no potential for serious complications of overdose; and no risk of addiction exists, in contrast to the benzodiazepines.

As discussed in chapter 8, schizoaffective illness is becoming recognized with increasing frequency. In this condition the patient bears both schizophrenic and affective symptomatology, and as the symptoms suggest, they respond best to a combined regimen of lithium and low-dosage high-potency neuroleptics.[55] Box 4-2 presents the DSM-IV criteria for schizoaffective disorder.

Transient psychotic disturbances may occur spontaneously, or as a result of drug intoxication or the withdrawal of certain addicting substances such as barbiturates and other sedatives. Patients with non–drug-induced acute psychotic episodes do not necessarily need pharmacologic intervention. However, in many instances short-term treatment with low-dosage high-potency antipsychotic agents will help the patient become more comfortable, as a result of the pharmacologically induced decrease in paranoia and other psychotic symptoms. Patients will often respond favorably to a course lasting 7 to 14 days and will not need further maintenance chemotherapy. Some follow-up treatment should be provided, however, if there is a recurrence of the psychotic symptoms. Although transient psychoses induced by drugs such as the hallucinogens are discussed in the chapter on drug abuse, it should be mentioned here that phencyclidine (PCP) is a long-acting hallucinogen which has high lipid solubility and is apt to produce series of recurring psychotic episodes over a period of 3 to 4 months after the initial episode takes place. There is some debate as to the proper treatment of PCP-induced psychoses. The recommendations of others to employ benzodiazepines seems particularly unwise to me, because these compounds may produce disinhibition and increase the risk of violence toward self or others that these patients may already possess as a result of their PCP psychosis. Furthermore, because of the profound effects of chlorpromazine on the autonomic nervous system and the simultaneous severe autonomic dysfunction associated with PCP, it is very clear that a low-potency antipsychotic drug should be absolutely avoided in patients who have taken PCP. Having successfully treated a large number of individuals who have had PCP-induced psychoses with haloperidol, it appears that this is the drug of choice because of the rather limited effects on the autonomic nervous system and its very high potency in counteracting the clinical symptomatology associated with PCP.[56] In a study of 30 men with PCP psychosis who were randomly assigned to receive either chlorpromazine, haloperidol, or pimozide, the latter two drugs, which are relatively specific antagonists of dopamine D_2 receptors, produced dramatic beneficial responses without major adverse effects. Scores of psychopathology were not improved by chlorpromazine.[57]

Psychoses with prominent visual hallucinations occur during the course of withdrawal from barbiturates, benzodiazepines, alcohol, and other sedative drugs.[56] These drug withdrawal psychoses should generally be treated by proper sedation. In the case of barbiturate and sedative addiction, the patient should undergo a pentobarbital tolerance test and gradual detoxification utilizing phenobarbital. In the event that a patient withdrawing from sedatives becomes

---

DSM-IV CRITERIA

Box 4-2 Diagnostic criteria for 295.70 schizoaffective disorder

A. An uninterrupted period of illness during which, at some time, there is either a Major Depressive Episode, a Manic Episode, or a Mixed Episode concurrent with symptoms that meet Criterion A for Schizophrenia.
  Note: The Major Depressive Episode must include Criterion A(1): depressed mood.
B. During the same period of illness, there have been delusions or hallucinations for at least 2 weeks in the absence of prominent mood symptoms.
C. Symptoms that meet criteria for a mood episode are present for a substantial portion of the total duration of the active and residual periods of the illness.
D. The disturbance is not due to the direct physiological effects of a substance (e.g., a drug of abuse, a medication) or a general medical condition.

Specify type:
Bipolar Type:
If the disturbance includes a Manic or a Mixed Episode (or a Manic or a Mixed Episode and a Major Depressive Episode)
Depressive Type:
If the disturbance only includes Major Depressive Episodes

From American Psychiatric Association: *Diagnostic and statistical manual of mental disorders,* ed 4 [DSM-IV]. Washington DC, American Psychiatric Press, 1994.

agitated and requires an antipsychotic medication, haloperidol is the safest drug to use because of its minimal likelihood of producing hypotension or other autonomic manifestations, and because of its minimal effect on seizure threshold.[12] Since patients withdrawing from sedatives are likely to have seizures, the administration of a drug such as chlorpromazine, which can lower seizure threshold and produce seizures, would be particularly dangerous. Thioridazine (Mellaril) has minimal effect on the seizure threshold; however its pronounced hypotensive and anticholinergic effect may produce unwanted effects in the patient who is already suffering from a sedative withdrawal delirium.[12]

CONSIDERATIONS REGARDING MAINTENANCE CHEMOTHERAPY IN SCHIZOPHRENIA

The most commonly asked question regarding treatment in the patient suffering from a schizophrenic illness is how long maintenance chemotherapy must continue. There is no definitive answer to this question. Since this illness is thought to be caused by changes in dopamine receptor site sensitivity or changes in the availability of dopamine at the receptor site, it is clear that initial treatment should almost always involve the administration of neuroleptic drugs. Since this biochemical abnormality most likely underlies the illness in question, the abnormality will probably persist, and therefore the continued administration of neuroleptic medication is necessary to prevent recurrence of the psychotic symptoms. Repeated studies have been done to document the long-term efficacy of continued administration of antipsychotic medications in patients suffering from schizophrenia.[19,58,59] The value and necessity of continuous neuroleptic maintenance therapy have been documented by studying relapse rates following drug discontinuation in patients who had been relatively symptom free during medication therapy. One study of first-episode patients found a relapse rate of 40% after drug discontinuation.[59] Another study of more seriously ill schizophrenics found a 62% relapse rate after stopping neuroleptics.[58] Studies of targeted neuroleptic treatment administered when signs of schizophrenic relapse appear have resulted in higher rates of relapse and hospitalization than were associated with continuous administration.[60]

Any clinician who treats a large number of patients has encountered some individuals whose schizophrenia initially responds to medication but who, as the years go by, continue to have some psychotic symptoms which seem unresponsive to pharmacotherapy. In individuals whose psychotic symptoms persist, even in the face of optimal chemotherapy, it may be appropriate to consider how long the patient should be maintained and to what extent the dosage should be increased in order to control symptoms and at what cost. Since the continued administration of excessively high doses of antipsychotic medication may produce a greater risk of tardive dyskinesia, the amount and duration of medication must be carefully considered.[19,58,59] Hopefully, medication will provide partial or complete control of psychotic symptoms in the majority of schizophrenic individuals, allowing them to lead more productive and rewarding lives.[19] However, those individuals whose response is less than optimal should be seen by their physician on a regular basis, and the possibility of discontinuing medication in order to ascertain the efficacy of treatment should be considered. There is, of course, the risk that symptoms will recur if medication is discontinued, and this must be weighed against the risk of long-term complications.

In most psychotic individuals who have had recurrent episodes of psychosis and have had a favorable response to chemotherapy, it will probably be necessary to continue maintenance over an indefinite period of time, utilizing the lowest dose of medication possible. The dosage should be reduced so that the individual is relatively free of side effects. A person who is receiving the minimal effective dose of antipsychotic medication may have some exacerbation of symptoms from time to time, which then can be managed by a temporary dosage increase.[19] An individual with an acute psychosis without a prior history of a psychotic disturbance and with a negative family history may require only short-term medication maintenance lasting for a period of several months. If, following that period, the medication is gradually decreased and there is a recurrence of psychotic symptoms, medication may need to be reinstituted and maintained over a prolonged period of time. Whenever antipsychotic medication is discontinued, there should be a gradual process of dosage reduction rather than an abrupt discontinuation.[61] Abrupt discontinuation may be associated with a neuroleptic withdrawal syndrome marked by autonomic symptoms and the appearance of a variety of extrapyramidal symptoms including abnormal movements of the face and mouth. This may be mistaken for tardive dyskinesia, but may be more properly termed a withdrawal dyskinesia, since the symptoms will gradually diminish and disappear several weeks or months after the medication has been discontinued.

In considering the choices of medications during the maintenance phase of chemotherapy in schizophrenia, the use of single nighttime oral doses of high-potency neuroleptics is generally preferable. These agents will produce less autonomic side effects and less sedation than will low-potency drugs.

Risperidone is a potent neuroleptic with considerable efficacy in the treatment and prophylaxis of schizophrenia. When employed at a dose of 2 to 3 mg twice daily, it is effective against both positive and negative schizophrenic symptoms, with minimal extrapyramidal and autonomic side effects and potentially decreased risk of tardive dyskinesia, making it an ideal maintenance medication.

The use of depot forms of neuroleptics such as fluphenazine enanthate or decanoate or haloperidol decanoate injection as a maintenance regimen should be considered in patients who refuse to take their medication regularly and who require repeated hospitalization.[19,62] The routine use of long-acting antipsychotic drugs by injection is not desirable in schizophrenic patients who are willing to cooperate and take medication. Medications that require administration by IM injection produce some discomfort to the patient. There is also the psychologic distress that the individual is somehow tied to a clinic or nurse who periodically administers "needles."

LONG-ACTING DEPOT NEUROLEPTICS

The first long-acting depot neuroleptic was fluphenazine enanthate, which was introduced for clinical use in the mid-1960s. Fluphenazine enanthate was then followed by fluphenazine decanoate, which produced somewhat more reliable and prolonged neuroleptic concentrations. Experience with various doses of fluphenazine decanoate has shown it to be a useful antipsychotic agent, whose efficacy is comparable to that achieved with maintenance doses of orally administered fluphenazine.[63] Prior to initiating depot neuroleptic treatment, the patient should first be stabilized on a comparable high-potency neuroleptic drug administered orally, following which the transition to depot medication can be made. In spite of a variety of proposals, no reliable formula yet exists to convert the dose of orally administered neuroleptic to the amount of depot medication that should be administered. Most often, 25 to 50 mg of fluphenazine decanoate is administered approximately every 3 weeks; however, some patients will require doses as high as 100 mg IM every week, and others may respond satisfactorily to doses of 5.0 to 12.5 mg every 3 to 6 weeks. Because of the general concept that the lowest possible maintenance dose of neuroleptics provides the greatest safety and the least risk of tardive dyskinesia, attempts have been made to compare various low- and ultralow-dose regimens to standard regimens of fluphenazine decanoate.[60] One study comparing low-dose and high-dose regimens of fluphenazine decanoate found that at the end of 1 year, 56% of the low-dose patients relapsed, compared with only 7% of the standard-dose patients.[64]

Many patients will require intermittent short-term use of orally administered antiparkinsonian medication during the first week following a depot neuroleptic injection, since increased extrapyramidal side effects may be present at the time the drug concentration reaches its peak. In general, side effects of depot neuroleptic treatment are comparable to those experienced by patients receiving effective doses of orally administered high-potency neuroleptics. The most agonizing question regarding long-acting injectable neuroleptics pertains to whether or not this form of treatment may carry with it an increased risk of complications, including neuroleptic malignant syndrome and tardive dyskinesia. A number of patients who have developed neuroleptic malignant syndrome were, indeed, receiving depot forms of fluphenazine. Further studies are needed before this form of antipsychotic drug therapy can be documented to be a particular risk factor or can be cleared of excess risk from the standpoint of this serious complication.[45] Some studies have suggested that patients maintained on long-acting injectable fluphenazine may have a greater risk of developing tardive dyskinesia than patients maintained on oral medication.[63]

Thus far, because of methodologic problems and insufficient data, it is not possible to impute a greater risk of tardive dyskinesia to depot neuroleptic administration. Since most patients maintained on oral neuroleptics periodically discontinue their medication, it is conceivable that through this means they are reducing their exposure to neuroleptics, and potentially, likewise, their risk of developing tardive dyskinesia, whereas patients maintained on depot therapy are less able to alter their intake of neuroleptics.

Haloperidol decanoate is an alternative long-acting injectable antipsychotic medication. Extensive experience with acute and maintenance, IM and oral, haloperidol confers a degree of predictability to the effects that we may encounter with the long-acting injectable form of this drug. Like fluphenazine, the decanoate form of haloperidol has been documented to produce effects that are comparable to orally administered haloperidol maintenance therapy.[62,65] Since oral and IM haloperidol have become standard treatments for acute psychosis, and since oral maintenance has continued to provide reliable prophylaxis against recurrent psychosis, the availability of the decanoate form of this drug is a significant advance, potentially extending the efficacy of acute phase treatment for many patients. Those patients who have responded favorably to haloperidol, but who periodically default from maintenance treatment by discontinuing medication, are the most suitable candidates for haloperidol decanoate therapy. The generally recommended dose is 50 mg IM every 4 weeks. Thus far, various formulas proposed to convert oral haloperidol dosage to IM decanoate dosage have proven to be similarly problematic to those utilized for fluphenazine treatment. Therefore it is my preference to give an initial haloperidol decanoate injection of 25 mg (0.5 mL), observe the patient while still maintaining oral haloperidol administration, and subsequently give a second IM dose 1 to 2 weeks after the first dose, with the second dose generally being 50 mg (1 mL). At this point, gradual downward dosage titration of the orally administered haloperidol should begin to take place as the patient is gradually in transition from oral to depot IM medication.

A dosage range of 50 to 450 mg haloperidol decanoate per month has been proposed. However, in the interest of minimizing chronic dosage of neuroleptic medication, most clinicians would favor starting the dosage low, titrating gradually, and employing the lowest effective dosage. Since all depot neuroleptics may have a cumulative effect, it is not uncommon during continuing depot administration to experience periodic exacerbation of drug-induced side effects, including akathisia, which may call for reducing the quantity of medication given per injection or, frequently, increasing the time interval between injections.[63,65,66]

ALTERNATIVE NEUROLEPTICS

Table 4-3 presents special characteristics and dosage ranges for the wide spectrum of currently marketed antipsychotic drugs. Mesoridazine is so closely comparable to thioridiazine that it is difficult to distinguish these two drugs

Table 4-3 Comparison of antipsychotic drugs: dosages and special characteristics

Chemical class and generic name (trade name)*	Daily dose range† (mg) (oral)	Special characteristics for clinical use
Phenothiazines		
Aliphatic		
Chlorpromazine (Thorazine)	100-2000	High sedation and hypotension risk, skin pigmentation, photosensitization Most likely to lower seizure threshold and produce convulsions, especially at higher dosage
Triflupromazine (Vesprin)	20-150	Similar to chlorpromazine
Piperidine		
Thioridazine (Mellaril)	100-600	Strongly anticholinergic and hypotensive, prominent ECG changes Retinal damage and visual loss may occur, especially at high dosage Minimal effect on seizure threshold
Mesoridazine (Serentil)	100-400	Strongly anticholinergic and hypotensive; avoid IM use because of risk of hypotension
Piperacetazine (Quide)	20-160	Similar to thioridazine
Piperazine		
Trifluoperazine (Stelazine)	5-60	Low sedation, high potency
Perphenazine (Trilafon)	8-64	Similar to trifluoperazine; somewhat less potent, somewhat more sedating
Fluphenazine (Prolixin)	5-30	Similar to trifluoperazine; may be used orally or IM for rapid neuroleptization Somewhat more painful at injection site than haloperidol Enanthate and decanoate are available as long-acting IM preparations
Butaperazine (Repoise)	30-100	Similar to trifluoperazine, but lower mg potency
Acetophenazine (Tindal)	20-100	Similar to trifluoperazine, but lower mg potency
Carphenazine (Proketazine)	100-400	Similar to trifluoperazine, but lower mg potency
Prochlorperazine (Compazine)	10-150	Somewhat less potent than trifluoperazine, with greater risk of hypotension and extrapyramidal effects; primarily used as an antiemetic, although its EPS make this use somewhat problematic

Thioxanthenes

Aliphatic

Thiothixene (Navane)	5-60	Therapeutic and adverse effects similar to trifluoperazine

Butyrophenone

Haloperidol (Haldol)	2-100	Somewhat more sedating and more potent than trifluoperazine; least pain when injected IM: available as deconoate for long-acting maintenance treatment
		Ideally suited to rapid neuroleptization by the oral or IM route
		Has been safely used IV in investigational studies
		Effective at low doses in maintenance, well tolerated by elderly and patients with cardiovascular disease

Dibenzoxazepine

Loxapine (Loxitane)	30-250	More potent, less sedating, and less hypotensive than chlorpromazine
		Less potent, produces less EPS than trifluoperazine
		May be effective in patients who do not tolerate high-potency agents and do not respond to low potency compounds.
		Low doses may be useful in anxiety and in depression

Dihydroindolone

Molindone (Moban)	10-225	Intermediate potency; least sedating neuroleptic
		Often will decrease appetite and allow weight loss in contradistinction to phenothiazines which promote weight gain
		May provoke motor seizures in susceptible patients even at low dosage

Continued.

Table 4-3 Comparison of antipsychotic drugs: dosages and special characteristics — cont'd

Chemical class and generic name (trade name)*	Daily dose range† (mg) (oral)	Special characteristics for clinical use
Benzisoxazole		
Risperidone (Risperdal)	1-6	High potency; low extrapyramidal, sedative, and autonomic side effects; potential rapid onset of action May reduce dyskinetic movements
Dibenzodiazepine		
Clozapine (Clozaril)	25-900	Low potency, low risk of EPS and TD; high sedative, hypotensive, and anticholinergic side effects; paradoxical hypersalivation; may reduce dyskinetic movements May provoke grand mal seizures, especially at higher doses Leukopenia and agranulocytosis may occur; requires weekly monitoring of white blood cell count throughout treatment

Modified from Bernstein JG: *Handbook of drug therapy in psychiatry*, ed 2. Chicago, Year Book Medical Publishers, 1988.
*The selected references at the end of this chapter provide documentation for the comments made regarding the specific drugs detailed above.
†The dose ranges presented are intended for medically healthy young or middle-aged adults. In some cases larger doses may be necessary, as in the acutely psychotic agitated patient who may require larger doses, especially when haloperidol is used in rapid neuroleptization or when doses up to 200 mg/day may need to be used. In elderly persons or those suffering simultaneously from severe medical or metabolic abnormalities, much lower doses should be used. The reader is directed to chapters 15 and 16 for additional dosage guidelines.

from the standpoint of either therapeutic or adverse effects. One caveat is that mesoridazine, unlike thioridazine, can also be given by IM injection, which may carry with it a significant risk of hypotension since this drug is a potent alpha-adrenergic blocking agent.

Loxapine is an effective neuroleptic drug whose potency is intermediate between the high-potency and low-potency agents. The therapeutic efficacy of orally or IM administered loxapine is generally greater than chlorpromazine, but less than more specific dopamine blockers classed as high-potency neuroleptics.[33,67] Loxapine has limited hypotensive activity and a relatively lower risk of extrapyramidal side effects than do high-potency neuroleptics. Loxapine, which has a mild sedative effect, has been useful in the treatment of some patients with borderline personality disorders and some with persistent severe anxiety who are unresponsive to other therapies. Like all other neuroleptics, long-term use of this drug in nonpsychotic individuals should be undertaken only with caution, and with careful monitoring of the patient for the development of abnormal movements.

Molindone tends to decrease appetite, in contradistinction to phenothiazines, which increase appetite, and may therefore be of value as a maintenance medication in patients concerned about weight gain during neuroleptic therapy. This drug appears to be less effective than piperazine phenothiazines, but is more potent than aliphatic phenothiazines. Occasionally, patients develop minor motor seizures during the initial phases of treatment with molindone.[12] In spite of claims that molindone does not produce tardive dyskinesia, this drug, like all others, has been associated with this complication. Indeed, I have seen a patient who had received molindone as his only neuroleptic agent over a period of 10 years develop tardive dyskinesia at a dose of approximately 20 mg daily. Molindone, which is available only for oral use, is the least sedating neuroleptic and has a relatively low hypotensive and extrapyramidal side effect profile.[34]

Prior to the phenothiazines, reserpine was the first drug to show promise as an antipsychotic agent. Reserpine has been found to be useful in studies of chronically disabled schizophrenic patients unresponsive to standard neuroleptic therapy.[68] Indeed, some patients who do not respond to conventional treatment may experience alleviation of some of their psychotic symptoms by the cautious combined use of neuroleptics and reserpine.[68]

Carbamazepine, which will be discussed in detail in chapter 8, may be a useful adjunct to neuroleptics in the management of agitated or refractory psychotic patients.[69] In spite of its potential therapeutic value in psychotic disorders, carbamazepine has also been demonstrated to potentially decrease serum concentration of haloperidol, which could impair the therapeutic utility of this drug.[70]

Amantadine, which has been useful in the treatment of neuroleptic-induced extrapyramidal side effects, has also been shown to decrease neuroleptic-induced hyperprolactinemia, galactorrhea, amenorrhea, and sexual dysfunction.[71] In addition to withdrawal dyskinesia, which may be associated with too rapid discontinuation of neuroleptic drugs, persistent severe vomiting may occur when these drugs are discontinued, which should alert the clinician to the necessity to establish a more gradual schedule of neuroleptic dose tapering.[72]

BLOOD LEVEL MONITORING OF ANTIPSYCHOTIC DRUGS

Periodic measurement of lithium blood level concentration is necessary in the proper management of patients being treated with this medication. There has been considerable application of laboratory techniques to monitor plasma concentration of a variety of antidepressant drugs; furthermore, platelet MAO levels can be measured with reasonable ease in patients taking MAO inhibitor–type antidepressants.

Although there are many reasons for the potential value of plasma level monitoring of antipsychotic drugs in increasing the efficacy and safety of this form of pharmacotherapy, the techniques available in the past were too complex or cumbersome. Furthermore, many antipsychotic agents such as chlorpromazine have numerous pharmacologically active metabolites. The previously developed techniques of monitoring plasma neuroleptic levels have involved complicated extraction procedures and the use of gas chromatography, fluorimetry, or radioimmunoassay, which entails the use of radiolabeled derivatives.[73] The use of these techniques has been complex, and it has been difficult to know which substance, the parent compound or the active metabolite, should in fact be monitored. A sensitive technique which involves competition for dopamine receptor binding has been developed and can be used to measure plasma neuroleptic concentration.[73] One advantage of this technique is that serum from patients may be utilized without extraction or purification procedures. This avoids complicated laboratory procedures and at the same time avoids the potential of erratic values based upon extraction techniques. It does not involve the administration of any radioactive material or other special compound other than the therapeutic agent the patient is receiving. Furthermore, since the results obtainable with this technique relate to the degree of dopamine receptor binding rather than a specific chemical assay technique, this approach is useful for a whole range of neuroleptic drugs, even though they vary considerably in their dosage, pattern of metabolism, and chemical structure.[73] Results obtained by radioreceptor assay (RRA) are comparable to those obtained utilizing more cumbersome radioimmunoassay techniques in patients receiving haloperidol.[73] Since RRA is not drug-specific, its usefulness is not limited to a single therapeutic agent, and its value is expressed in terms that may be more directly applicable to what is happening to the patient clinically. Since active metabolites as well as parent compound are measured by the RRA technique, the question of which active metabolites to measure for a compound such as chlorpromazine which has perhaps 100 metabolites becomes moot.

Unfortunately, in spite of advances in laboratory techniques, clinically useful correlations between serum neuroleptic concentrations and therapeutic response have not been adequately established.[74-76] Although the RRA is very sensitive, current techniques utilizing minimal effective doses of neuroleptic drugs often achieve plasma concentrations which approach the threshold of sensitivity of the assay.[74] Variations in drug metabolism from patient to patient may also alter observed plasma concentrations of drugs, and further complicate the relationship among dosage, blood level, and therapeutic response.[74,75] Although there are data to suggest that a therapeutic window exists for certain neuroleptic drugs, particularly haloperidol, the reports are conflicting.[76] A therapeutic window implies that below or above a certain plasma drug concentration, the therapeutic response would be less than within the range of the window. The clinical implications of this phenomenon, if it exists, would be extremely important in making decisions about drug dosage. Although serum drug monitoring has become useful in the application of a variety of other psychotropic agents, the routine clinical application of this technique in monitoring antipsychotic chemotherapy is generally not clinically useful in predicting optimal dosage.[19,77] Neuroleptic blood levels may be somewhat useful in assessing patient compliance, although variability of data raises questions about this use as well.

REFERENCES

1. American Psychiatric Association: *Psychiatric glossary.* Washington DC, American Psychiatric Press, 1984.
2. American Psychiatric Association: *Diagnostic and statistical manual of mental disorders,* ed 4 [DSM-IV]. Washington DC, American Psychiatric Press, 1994.
3. Synder SH, Banerjee SP, Yamamura HI, et al: Drugs, neurotransmitters and schizophrenia. *Science* 1974;184:1243-1253.
4. Rosner F: *Julius Preuss' biblical and talmudic medicine.* New York, Sanhedrin Press, 1978.
5. Kety S: The biological bases of mental illness. In Bernstein JG (ed): *Clinical psychopharmacology.* Littleton Mass, PSG Publishing, 1978, pp 1-13.
6. Sankar DVS (ed): Some biological aspects of schizophrenic behavior. *Ann NY Acad Sci* 1962;96:1-490.
7. Silva F, Heath RG, Rafferty T, et al: Comparative effects of administration of taraxein, d-LSD, mescaline, and psilocybin to human volunteers. *Compr Psychiatry* 1976;1:370-376.
8. Hollister LE: Human pharmacology of lysergic acid diethylamide (LSD). In Efron DH (ed): *Psychopharmacology: review of progress, 1957-1967.* Washington DC, US Public Health Service, 1968, pp 1253-1261.
9. Walaszek EJ: Brain neurohormones and cortical epinephrine pressor responses as affected by schizophrenic serum. *Int Rev Neurobiol* 1960;2: 137-173.
10. Bernstein J, Mazur WP, Walaszek EJ: The histaminolytic activity of serum from schizophrenic patients. *Med Exp* 1960;2:239-244.
11. Pfeiffer CC, Jenney EH: Lucid intervals induced by arecoline in schizophrenic patients. *Ann NY Acad Sci* 1957;66:753-757.
12. Bernstein JG: Drug interactions. In Cassem NH (ed): *Massachusetts General Hospital handbook of general hospital psychiatry,* ed 3. St Louis, Mosby, 1991, pp 571-610.
13. Sulser F, Bass AD: Pharmacodynamic and biochemical considerations on the mode of action of reserpine-like drugs. In Efron DH (ed): *Psychopharmacology: a review of progress 1957-1967.* Washington DC, US Public Health Service, 1968, pp 1065-1075.
14. Deniker P: Introduction of neuroleptic chemotherapy into psychiatry, in Ayd FJ, Blackwell B (eds): *Discoveries in biological psychiatry.* Philadelphia, JB Lippincott, 1970, pp 155-164.
15. Creese I: Dopamine and antipsychotic medications. In Hales RE, Frances AJ (eds): *APA annual review.* Washington DC, American Psychiatric Press, 1985, vol 4, pp 17-36.

16. Schulz SC: Genetics of schizophrenia: a status report. In Tasman A, Goldfinger SM (eds): *American Psychiatric Press Review of psychiatry.* Washington DC, American Psychiatric Press; 1991, vol 10, pp 79-97.

17. Wong DF, Wagner HN, Tune LE, et al: Positron emission tomography reveals elevated D_2 dopamine receptors in drug-naive schizophrenics. *Science* 1986;234:1558-1563.

18. Wyatt RJ: The dopamine hypothesis: variations on a theme. II. *Psychopharmacol Bull* 1986;22:923-927.

19. Kane JM, Marder SR: Psychopharmacologic treatment of schizophrenia. *Schizophr Bull* 1993;19:287-302.

20. Brier A, Buchanan RW, Kirkpatrick B, et al: Effects of clozapine on positive and negative symptoms in outpatients with schizophrenia. *Am J Psychiatry* 1994;151:20-26.

21. Baldessarini RJ, Frankenburg FR: Clozapine: a novel antipsychotic agent. *N Engl J Med* 1991;324:746-754.

22. Leysen JE, Gommeren W, Eens A, et al: Biochemical profile of risperidone, a new antipsychotic. *J Pharmacol Exp Ther* 1988;247:661-670.

23. Chouinard G, Jones B, Remington G, et al: A Canadian multicenter placebo-controlled study of fixed doses of risperidone and haloperidol in the treatment of chronic schizophrenic patients. *J Clin Psychopharmacol* 1993;13:25-40.

23a. Chouinard G: Effects of risperidone in tardive dyskinesia: an analysis of the Canadian multicenter risperidone study. *J Clin Psychopharmacol* 1995;15(1):36S-44S.

24. Borison RL, Pathiraja AP, Diamond BI, Meibach RC: Risperidone: clinical safety and efficacy in schizophrenia. *Psychopharmacol Bull* 1992;28:213-218.

25. Small JG, Milstein V, Marhenke JO, et al: Treatment outcome with clozapine in tardive dyskinesia, neuroleptic sensitivity, and treatment-resistant psychosis. *J Clin Psychiatry* 1987;48:263-267.

26. Snyder S, Greenberg D, Yamamura HI: Antischizophrenic drugs and brain cholinergic receptors. *Arch Gen Psychiatry* 1974;31:58-61.

27. Donlon PT, Hopkin J, Tupin JP: Overview: Efficacy and safety of the rapid neurolepticication method with injectable haloperidol. *Am J Psychiatry* 1979;136:273-278.

28. Baldessarini RJ: Drugs and the treatment of psychiatric disorders. In Gilman AG, Rall TW, Nies AS, Taylor P (eds): *Goodman and Gilman's The pharmacologic basis of therapeutics,* ed 8. New York, Pergamon Press, 1990, pp 383-435.

29. APA Task Force: *Tardive dyskinesia.* Washington DC, American Psychiatric Press, *1992.*

30. Jeste DV, Wyatt RJ: *Understanding and treating tardive dyskinesia.* New York, Guilford Press, 1982.

31. Baldessarini RJ: Clinical and epidemiological aspects of tardive dyskinesia. *J Clin Psychiatry* 1985;46(4, sec 2):8-13.

32. Chouinard G, Annable L, Mercier P, et al: A five-year follow-up study of tardive dyskinesia. *Psychopharmacol Bull* 1986;22:259-263.

33. Tuason VB, Escobar JI, Garvey M, et al: Loxapine versus chlorpromazine in paranoid schizophrenia: a double-blind study. *J Clin Psychiatry* 1984; 45:158-163.

34. Claghorn JL: Review of clinical and laboratory experiences with molindone hydrochloride. *J Clin Psychiatry* 1985;46(8, sec 2):30-33.

35. Kane JM, Lieberman JA (eds): *Adverse effects of psychotropic drugs.* New York, Guilford Press, 1992.

36. Settle EC Jr, Ayd FJ Jr: Haloperidol: a quarter century of experience. *J Clin Psychiatry* 1983;44:446-448.

37. Anderson WH, Kuehnle JG: Diagnosis and management of acute psychosis. *N Engl J Med* 1981;305:1128-1130.

38. Tesar GE, Murray GB, Cassem NH: Use of high-dose intravenous haloperidol in the treatment of agitated cardiac patients. *J Clin Psychopharmacol* 1985;5:344-347.

39. Ray WA, Griffin MR, Schaffner W, et al: Psychotropic drug use and the risk of hip fracture. *N Engl J Med* 1987;316:363-369.

40. Keepers GA, Clappison VJ, Casey DE: Initial anticholinergic prophylaxis for neuroleptic-induced extrapyramidal syndromes. *Arch Gen Psychiatry* 1983;40:1113-1117.

41. Rifkin A, Quitkin F, Kane J, et al: Are prophylactic antiparkinsonian drugs necessary? *Arch Gen Psychiatry* 1978;35:483-489.
42. Winslow RS, Stillner V, Coons DJ, et al: Prevention of acute dystonic reactions in patients beginning high-potency neuroleptics. *Am J Psychiatry* 1986;143:706-710.
43. Boyer WF, Bakalar NH, Lake CR: Anticholinergic prophyalxis of acute haloperidol-induced acute dystonic reactions. *J Clin Psychopharmacol* 1987;7:164-166.
44. Heinrich K, Klieser E, Lehman E, et al: Experimental comparison of the efficacy and compatibility of risperidone and clozapine in acute schizophrenia. In Kane JM (ed): Risperidone: major progress in antipsychotic drugs. Proceedings of satellite symposium, Collegium Internationale Neuro-Psychopharmacologicum, Kyoto Japan, 1990, pp 37-39.
45. Pearlman CA: Neuroleptic malignant syndrome: a review of the literature. *J Clin Psychopharmacol* 1986;6:257-273.
46. Neborsky R, Janowsky D, Munson E, et al: Rapid treatment of acute psychotic symptoms with high- and low-dose haloperidol. *Arch Gen Psychiatry* 1981;38:195-199.
47. Coffman JA, Nasrallah HA, Lyskowski J, et al: Clinical effectiveness or oral and parenteral rapid neuroleptization. *J Clin Psychiatry* 1987;48:20-24.
48. Remington G, Pollock B, Voineskos G, et al: Acutely psychotic patients receiving high-dose haloperidol therapy. *J Clin Psychopharmacol* 1993;13:41-45.
49. Bodkin JA: Emerging uses for high potency benzodiazepines in psychotic disorders. *J Clin Psychiatry* 1990;51(5 suppl):41-46.
50. Altamura AL, Mauri MC, Mantero M, et al: Clonazepam/haloperidol combination therapy in schizophrenia: a double-blind study. *Acta Psychiatr Scand* 1987;76:702-706.
51. Dietch JT, Jennings RK: Aggressive dyscontrol in patients treated with benzodiazepines. *J Clin Psychiatry* 1988;49:184-188.
52. Sassim N, Grohmann R: Adverse drug reactions with clozapine and simultaneous application of benzodiazepines. *Pharmacopsychiatry* 1988;21:306-307.
53. Shopsin B, Gershon S, Thompson H, et al: Psychoactive drugs in mania. *Arch Gen Psychiatry* 1975;32:34-42.
54. Brinkley JR, Beitman BD, Friedel RO: Low dose neuroleptic regimens in the treatment of borderline patients. *Arch Gen Psychiatry* 1979;36:319-326.
55. Biederman J, Lerner Y, Belmaker RH: Combination of lithium carbonate and haloperidol in schizo-affective disorder. *Arch Gen Psychiatry* 1979; 36:327-333.
56. Khantzian EJ, McKenna GJ: Acute toxic and withdrawal reactions associated with drug use and abuse. *Ann Intern Med* 1979;90:361-372.
57. Giannini AJ, Nageotte C, Loiselle RH, et al: Comparison of chlorpromazine, haloperidol, and pimozide in the treatment of phencyclidine psychosis: DA-2 receptor specificity. *Clin Toxicol* 1984-1985;22:573-579.
58. Chung HK: Schizophrenics fully remitted on neuroleptics for 3-5 years: to stop or continue drugs? *Br J Psychiatry* 1981;139:490-494.
59. Kane JM, Rifkin A, Quitkin F, et al: Fluphenazine versus placebo in patients with remitted, acute first episodes of schizophrenia. *Arch Gen Psychiatry* 1982;39:70-73.
60. Marder SR, Wirshing WC, Van Putten T, et al: Fluphenazine vs placebo supplementation for prodromal signs of relapse in schizophrenia. *Arch Gen Psychiatry* 1994;51:280-287.
61. Gardos G, Cole JO, Tarsy D: Withdrawal syndromes associated with antipsychotic drugs. *Am J Psychiatry* 1978;135:1321-1324.
62. Davis JM, Andrinkaitis S: The natural course of schizophrenia and effective maintenance drug treatment. *J Clin Psychiatry* 1986;6:65-105.
63. Kane JM: The use of depot neuroleptics: clinical experience in the United States. *J Clin Psychiatry* 1984;45(5, sec 2):5-12.
64. Kane JM, Rifkin A, Woerner M, et al: Low dose neuroleptic treatment of outpatient schizophrenics. I, Preliminary results for relapse rates. *Arch Gen Psychiatry* 1983;40:893-896.
65. Vasavan Nair NP, Suranyi-Cadotte B, Schwartz G, et al: A clinical trial comparing intramuscular

haloperidol decanoate and oral haloperidol in chronic schizophrenic patients: efficacy, safety, and dosage equivalence. *J Clin Psychopharmacol* 1986;6:305-375.

66. Kane JM: Dosage strategies with long-acting injectable neuroleptics, including haloperidol decanoate. *J Clin Psychopharmacol* 1986;6(suppl):20-23.

67. Tuason VB: A comparison of parenteral loxapine and haloperidol in hostile and aggressive acutely schizophrenic patients. *J Clin Psychiatry* 1986;47:126-129.

68. Berlant JL: Neuroleptics and reserpine in refractory psychoses. *J Clin Psychopharmacol* 1986;6:180-184.

69. McAllister TW: Carbamazepine in mixed frontal lobe and psychotic disorders. *J Clin Psychiatry* 1985;46:393-394.

70. Kidron R, Averbuch I, Klein E, et al: Carbamazepine-induced reduction of blood levels of haloperidol chronic schizophrenia. *Biol Psychiatry* 1985;20:199-228.

71. Correa N, Opier LA, Kay SR, et al: Amantadine in the treatment of neuroendocrine side effects of neuroleptics. *J Clin Psychopharmacol* 1987;7:91-95.

72. Grob CS: Persistent supersensitivity vomiting following neuroleptic withdrawal in an adolescent. *Biol Psychiatry* 1986;21:398-401.

73. Creese I, Snyder SH: A simple and sensitive radioreceptor assay for antischizophrenic drugs in blood. *Nature* 1977;270:180-182.

74. Zohar J, Shemesh Z, Belmaker RH: Utility of neuroleptic blood levels in the treatment of acute psychosis. *J Clin Psychiatry* 1986;47:600-603.

75. Contreras S, Alexander H, Faber R, et al: Neuroleptic radioreceptor activity and clinical outcome in schizophrenia. *J Clin Psychopharmacol* 1987;7:95-98.

76. Volauka J, Cooper TB: Review of haloperidol blood level and clinical response: looking through the window. *J Clin Psychopharmacol* 1987;7:25-30.

77. Koreen AR, Lieberman J, Alvir J, et al: Relation of plasma fluphenazine levels to treatment response and extrapyramidal side effects in first-episode schizophrenic patients. *Am J Psychiatry* 1994;151:35-39.

SELECTED REFERENCES

Chlorpromazine
Rivera-Calimlin L, Nasrallah H, Strauss J, et al: Clinical response and plasma levels: effects of dose, dosage schedules, and drug interactions on plasma chlorpromazine levels. *Arch Gen Psychiatry* 1976;133:636-642.

Thioridazine
Smith GR, Taylor CW, Linkous P: Haloperidol versus thioridazine for the treatment of psychogeriatric patients: a double-blind clinical trial. *Psychosomatics* 1974;15:134-138.

Trifluoperazine
Wijsenbeek H, Steiner M, Goldberg SC: Trifluoperazine: a comparison between regular and high doses. *Psychopharmacologia* 1974;36:147-150.

Perphenazine
Vestre ND, Dehnel LI, Schiele BC: A sequential comparison of amitriptyline, perphenazine, and the amitriptyline-perphenazine combination in recently admitted anergic schizophrenics. *Psychosomatics* 1969;10:269-303.

Fluphenazine
Rifkin A, Quitkin F, Carrillo C, et al: Very high dosage fluphenazine for nonchronic treatment-refractory patients. *Arch Gen Psychiatry* 1971;25:398-403.

Groves JE, Mandel MR: The long-acting phenothiazines. *Arch Gen Psychiatry* 1975;32:893-900.

Butaperazine
Simpson GM, Lament R, Cooper TB, et al: The relationship between blood levels of different forms of butaperazine and clinical response. *J Clin Pharmacol* 1973;13:288-297.

Thiothixene
Ban TA (ed): *Psychopharmacology of thiothixene*. New York, Raven Press, 1978.

Haloperidol
Ayd FJ Jr (ed): *Haloperidol update:* 1958-1980. Baltimore, Ayd Medical Communications, 1980.
Loxapine
Zisook S, Click MA Jr: Evaluations of loxapine succinate in the ambulatory treatment of acute schizophrenic episodes. *Int Pharmacopsychiatry* 1980;15:365-378.
Molindone
Binder R, Glick I, Rice M: A comparative study of parenteral molindone and haloperidol in the acutely psychotic patient. *J Clin Psychiatry* 1981;42:203-206.
Clozapine
Yesavage J: *Clozapine: a compendium of selected readings.* East Hanover NJ, Sandoz Pharmaceuticals, 1992.
Risperidone
Addington DE, Jones B, Bloom D, et al: Reduction of hospital days in chronic schizophrenic patients treated with risperidone: a retrospective study. *Clin Ther* 1993;15:917-926.
Borison RL, Diamond BI, Pathiraja A, Meibach RC: Clinical overview of risperidone. In Meltzer HY (ed): *Novel antipsychotic drugs.* New York, Raven Press, 1992, pp 233-239.
General
Kurland AA, Hanlon TE, Tatom MH, et al: The comparative effectiveness of six phenothiazine compounds, phenobarbital and inert placebo in the treatment of acutely ill patients: global measures of severity of illness. *J Nerv Ment Dis* 1965;133:1-18.
Zavodnick S: A pharmacological and theoretical comparison of high and low potency neuroleptics. *J Clin Psychiatry* 1978;38:332-336.
Sriwatanakul K, Weis O: Using antipsychotic drugs during pregnancy. *Drug Therapy* 1982;12: 97-100.
Kane JM: The current status of neuroleptic therapy. *J Clin Psychiatry* 1989;50:322-328.
Neurotransmitters and receptors
Richelson E, Nelson A: Antagonism by neuroleptics of neurotransmitter receptors of normal human brain in vitro. *Eur J Pharmacol* 1984;103:197-204.
Meltzer HY, Matsubara S, Lee JC: Classification of typical and atypical antipsychotic drugs on the basis of dopamine D-1, D-2, and serotonin pK_1 values. *J Pharmacol Exp Ther* 1989;241:238-246.

CHAPTER 5

Tricyclic, Heterocyclic, and Serotonin Selective Antidepressants

OVERVIEW

Chemotherapy of Depression

1. Severity and duration of depression are major indicators of necessity for pharmacotherapy.
2. Depression results from disorder of neurotransmission.
3. Antidepressants prescribed in adequate doses correct abnormal neurotransmission.
4. Choice of antidepressants (do not require blood level monitoring).
5. Neuotransmitter action (major/minor reuptake inhibition):

S = serotonin; N = norepinephrine.

High-sedating	*Low-sedating*	*Low-sedating*
Amitriptyline	Desipramine	*Not-anticholinergic*
(S/N)	(N)	*SSRIs*
Doxepin	Amoxapine	Fluoxetine
(S/N)	(N/S)	Fluvoxamine
Maprotiline	Imipramine	Paroxetine
(N)	(S/N)	Sertraline
Trazodone		
(S)		*SSRI + N + DA*
Trimipramine		Venlafaxine
(S/N)		
Clomipramine		*Dopaminergic*
(S/N)		Bupropion

High-anticholinergic	*Low-anticholinergic*
Amitriptyline	Desipramine
(S/N)	(N)
Imipramine	
(S/N)	
Trimipramine	Amoxapine
(S/N)	(N/S)
Clomipramine	Maprotiline (N)
(S/N)	Trazodone (S)

Continued.

6. Nortriptyline has "therapeutic window"; requires blood level monitoring; may produce less postural hypotension.
7. Amoxapine has rapid onset of action and weak neuroleptic effect.
8. In psychotic depression start high-potency neuroleptic first, then add antidepressant.
9. Cyclic antidepressant side effects include drowsiness, dry mouth, constipation, tremor, speech blockage, sexual dysfunction, increased sweating, postural hypotension, tachycardia, and cardiac arrhythmias.
10. SSRI side effects include nervousness, insomnia, nausea, diarrhea, headache, and sexual dysfunction.
11. Therapy should continue for 6 to 12 months after complete recovery from depression, then taper dose gradually; should never be abruptly discontinued.
12. If patient fails to respond, consider the following:
    A. Dosage adjustment
    B. Trial of drug that acts on alternative neurotransmitter; cyclic vs SSRI
    C. Addition of lithium, triiodothyronine, carbamazepine, or low dose of neuroleptic
    D. Trial of MAOI alone or in combination with tricyclic
    E. If patient is suicidal and does not respond to initial adequate medication trial, consider a course of electroconvulsive therapy

The severity of depression varies considerably, from sadness and depression in response to a loss or disappointment, to the other end of the spectrum, wherein an individual becomes incapacitated and unable to function because of a severe depressive illness which appears spontaneously and is not triggered by a major life event.

The symptoms of depression may be seen along a continuum. The milder end is represented by a person who feels sad in response to a personal loss, while the other end is represented by an individual who, for no apparent reason, becomes suddenly depressed, hopeless, and suicidal.[1] Most persons who seek treatment for depression present with symptoms that are more extensive than simple sadness. Many depressed individuals have already contemplated suicide or perhaps have made an attempt prior to consulting a physician. It is of utmost importance in evaluating an individual with depression to ask very specific questions about suicidal thoughts, attempts, or plans. Contrary to popular opinion, this component of the interview does not enhance the risk of self-destructive behavior, but may indeed reduce its risk of occurrence by allowing the patient to discuss such thoughts and feelings frankly.[1]

In addition to feeling sad, down, and hopeless, many depressed patients have lost interest in their usual work and leisure activities. Furthermore, most depressed individuals experience the loss of pleasure associated with previously enjoyable pursuits. Loss of appetite, with or without weight loss, is extremely common in depression, although some depressed patients give a history of excessive eating and weight gain.[2] Insomnia, particularly associated with frequent nighttime or early morning awakening, is extremely common. In addition, many depressed patients will also describe difficulty falling asleep. Some depressed individuals have a tendency to sleep excessively, going to bed early at night or awakening very late in the morning; they may also take multiple naps throughout the day. Decreased sexual interest, associated with reduced frequency of sexual relations or impaired enjoyment of sexual activity, commonly occurs in depression. Most depressed patients will describe a loss of energy and a feeling of fatigue, and they may commonly demonstrate either psychomotor retardation (being slowed down) or agitation and restlessness.[1,2]

Depressed individuals tend to feel excessively guilty, because of perceived personal inadequacies or minor legal or moral infractions. Many depressed patients have difficulty thinking and concentrating, show memory impairment, and are indecisive.[2] Recurrent thoughts of death, the desire to be dead, or frank thoughts of suicide occur more commonly in depressed patients than many clinicians realize. Patients without prior psychiatric histories may present with subtle or even grossly overt evidence of an active psychotic process during their depressive illness. Severely depressed individuals may be obsessed with the fact that they are evil and deserve to be punished or even to die. Depressed patients who are psychotic may present with persecutory delusions and feel that people are out to kill them. Such individuals may describe hearing voices that tell them they are bad and deserve to suffer.[1,2] Figure 5-1 lists some of the common symptoms of depression.

In the early days of antidepressant chemotherapy it was commonly taught

---

Affect — flattened or labile
Mood — dysphoric, depressed, sad, blue, anxious, irritable
Psychomotor — agitation, retardation
Energy — impaired, feelings of fatigue
Feelings — worthlessness, helplessness, hopelessness
Guilt — self-reproach, loss of interest, loss of pleasure
Concentration — thinking and memory impaired, indecisive
Inability — to carry out daily routine
Insomnia — or hypersomnia
Anorexia — with weight loss, or hyperphagia with weight gain
Loss of libido and decreased sexual function
Somatic symptoms — constipation, headache, atypical pain
Suicidal thoughts — plans, or attempts
Psychotic thinking — auditory hallucinations, persecutory delusions

---

Fig. 5-1 Common symptoms of depression.

DSM-IV CRITERIA

Box 5-1 Criteria for major depressive episode

A. Five (or more) of the following symptoms have been present during the same 2-week period and represent a change from previous functioning; at least one of the symptoms is either (1) depressed mood or (2) loss of interest or pleasure.
Note: Do not include symptoms that are clearly due to a general medical condition, or mood-incongruent delusions or hallucinations.

   (1) Depressed mood most of the day, nearly every day, as indicated by either subjective report (e.g., feels sad or empty) or observation made by others (e.g., appears tearful). **Note:** In children and adolescents, can be irritable mood.
   (2) Markedly diminished interest or pleasure in all, or almost all, activities most of the day, nearly every day (as indicated by either subjective account or observation made by others)
   (3) Significant weight loss when not dieting or weight gain (e.g., a change of more than 5% of body weight in a month), or decrease or increase in appetite nearly every day. **Note:** In children, consider failure to make expected weight gains
   (4) Insomnia or hypersomnia nearly every day
   (5) Psychomotor agitation or retardation nearly every day (observable by others, not merely subjective feelings of restlessness or being slowed down)
   (6) Fatigue or loss of energy nearly every day
   (7) Feelings of worthlessness or excessive or inappropriate guilt (which may be delusional) nearly every day (not merely self-reproach or guilt about being sick)
   (8) Diminished ability to think or concentrate, or indecisiveness, nearly every day (either by subjective account or as observed by others)
   (9) Recurrent thoughts of death (not just fear of dying), recurrent suicidal ideation without a specific plan, or a suicide attempt or specific plan for committing suicide
B. The symptoms do not meet criteria for a Mixed Episode.
C. The symptoms cause clinically significant distress or impairment in social, occupational, or other important areas of functioning.
D. The symptoms are not due to the direct physiological effects of a substance (e.g., a drug of abuse, a medication) or a general medical condition (e.g., hypothyroidism).
E. The symptoms are not better accounted for by Bereavement (i.e., after the loss of a loved one, the symptoms persist for longer than 2 months or are characterized by marked functional impairment, morbid preoccupation with worthlessness, suicidal ideation, psychotic symptoms, or psychomotor retardation).

From American Psychiatric Association: *Diagnostic and statistical manual of mental disorders*, ed 4 [DSM-IV]. Washington DC, American Psychiatric Press, 1994.

that only the more severe forms of depression, particularly those with psychotic features, should be treated pharmacologically. Psychotherapy was often suggested as the preferred form of treatment for milder forms of depression, which, until the advent of DSM-III and DSM-IV nomenclature, were generally referred to as "depressive neurosis." Newer work in psychiatry has made the term depressive neurosis obsolete; likewise, our modern knowledge of antidepressant medications is making obsolete the concept that only the most severe forms of depression should be treated pharmacologically.[1,3] This does not imply that every person who becomes mildly depressed following some personal loss should receive antidepressant chemotherapy. On the other hand, it would be equally wrong to delay pharmacologic treatment until an individual becomes so severely immobilized by his depression that he cannot work or enjoy his leisure activities. It is even worse for an individual who is receiving nonpharmacologic treatment for depression to experience a suicide attempt before receiving definitive medical management.

BIOLOGIC BASIS OF DEPRESSION AND ITS TREATMENT

Although a detailed discussion of depressive illness is beyond the scope of this chapter, it is important to review some aspects of its classification and etiology. The DSM-IV criteria for major depression and dysthymic disorder, the two most common forms of depression, are shown in Boxes 5-1, 5-2 and 5-3. This approach to diagnostic nomenclature emphasizes a greater continuity and connection between various forms of depressive illness than did the former DSM-III. The newer nomenclature also implies a greater understanding of the biochemical factors which appear to be important in the etiology of depressive illness. Most contemporary clinicians and investigators believe that a functional

---

DSM-IV CRITERIA

Box 5-2 Criteria for melancholic features specifier

Specify if:
With Melancholic Features (can be applied to the current or most recent Major Depressive Episode in Major Depressive Disorder and to a Major Depressive Episode in Bipolar I or Bipolar II Disorder only if it is the most recent type of mood episode)
A. Either of the following, occurring during the most severe period of the current episode:
   (1) Loss of pleasure in all, or almost all, activities
   (2) Lack of reactivity to usually pleasurable stimuli (does not feel much better, even temporarily, when something good happens)
B. Three (or more) of the following:
   (1) Distinct quality of depressed mood (i.e., the depressed mood is experienced as distinctly different from the kind of feeling experienced after the death of a loved one)
   (2) Depression regularly worse in the morning
   (3) Early morning awakening (at least 2 hours before usual time of awakening)
   (4) Marked psychomotor retardation or agitation
   (5) Significant anorexia or weight loss
   (6) Excessive or inappropriate guilt

From American Psychiatric Association: *Diagnostic and statistical manual of mental disorders*, ed 4 [DSM-IV]. Washington DC, American Psychiatric Press, 1994.

Box 5-3 Diagnostic criteria for 300.4 dysthymic disorder

A. Depressed mood for most of the day, for more days than not, as indicated either by subjective account or observation by others, for at least 2 years. **Note:** In children and adolescents, mood can be irritable and duration must be at least 1 year.

B. Presence, while depressed, of two (or more) of the following:
   (1) Poor appetite or overeating
   (2) Insomnia or hypersomnia
   (3) Low energy or fatigue
   (4) Low self-esteem
   (5) Poor concentration or difficulty making decisions
   (6) Feelings of hopelessness

C. During the 2-year period (1 year for children or adolescents) of the disturbance, the person has never been without the symptoms in Criteria A and B for more than 2 months at a time.

D. No Major Depressive Episode has been present during the first 2 years of the disturbance (1 year for children and adolescents); i.e., the disturbance is not better accounted for by chronic Major Depressive Disorder, or Major Depressive Disorder, In Partial Remission.

   Note: There may have been a previous Major Depressive Episode provided there was a full remission (no significant signs or symptoms for 2 months) before development of the Dysthymic Disorder. In addition, after the initial 2 years (1 year in children or adolescents) of Dysthymic Disorder, there may be superimposed episodes of Major Depressive Disorder, in which case both diagnoses may be given when the criteria are met for a Major Depressive Episode.

E. There has never been a Manic Episode, a Mixed Episode, or a Hypomanic Episode, and criteria have never been met for Cyclothymic Disorder.

F. The disturbance does not occur exclusively during the course of a chronic Psychotic Disorder, such as Schizophrenia or Delusional Disorder.

G. The symptoms are not due to the direct physiological effects of a substance (e.g., a drug of abuse, a medication) or a general medical condition (e.g., hypothyroidism).

H. The symptoms cause clinically significant distress or impairment in social, occupational, or other important areas of functioning.

Specify if:
   Early Onset: if onset is before age 21 years
   Late Onset: if onset is age 21 years or older
Specify (for most recent 2 years of Dysthymic Disorder):
   With Atypical Features

From American Psychiatric Association: *Diagnostic and statistical manual of mental disorders,* ed 4 [DSM-IV]. Washington DC, American Psychiatric Press, 1994.

deficiency of norepinephrine, dopamine, or serotonin, or an abnormality of their receptors, is an etiologic factor in depression.[4,5] Drugs such as reserpine, which can induce depression, are known to deplete brain stores of norepinephrine, dopamine, and serotonin. Monoamine oxidase inhibitors increase the availability of these neurotransmitters in the brain and alleviate depression.[6] The tricyclic (TCA) and heterocyclic (HCA) antidepressants block nerve reuptake of both serotonin and norepinephrine, thereby increasing the availability of these biogenic amines at receptor sites in the brain and other tissues.[6]

Serotonin-selective reuptake inhibitors (SSRIs) inhibit the reuptake of serotonin, with minimal effect on other transmitters (except for venlafaxine, which also inhibits the reuptake of norepinephrine and to some extent dopamine). The differential effects of antidepressant drugs on serotonin, dopamine, or norepinephrine reuptake may account for their differential efficacy in individual patients. Maas classified depression into two groups and correlated different metabolic patterns and drug responses for each group.[4] Group A patients have low pretreatment urinary methoxyhydroxyphenylglycol (MHPG) excretion, suggestive of a norpinephrine metabolic disorder, and respond best to antidepressants which preferentially inhibit norepinephrine reuptake. These patients have normal or high spinal fluid concentrations of 5-hydroxyindoleacetic acid, (5-HIAA) and fail to respond to amitriptyline, which preferentially inhibits serotonin reuptake. These patients also show an improvement in mood when given a test dose of dextroamphetamine. According to the classification of Maas group B patients have normal or high pretreatment urinary MHPG and low spinal fluid concentrations of 5-HIAA. These patients, whose metabolic disorder involves serotonin, respond best to antidepressants such as amitriptyline which preferentially inhibit reuptake of this transmitter.

Group B patients respond rather poorly to drugs which primarily inhibit norepinephrine reuptake, and they fail to show an improvement in mood when given a test dose of dextroamphetamine. Although numerous investigators, beginning with the work of Schildkraut, have attempted to classify and predict treatment response of depression by measuring blood, CSF, and urinary metabolites of biogenic amines, these techniques have not proved reliable in making diagnostic or therapeutic predictions.[42] Table 5-1 presents the pharmacologic profiles of TCAs and HCAs and indicates their comparative antagonism of neurotransmitter reuptake mechanisms.

According to estimates by the National Institute of Mental Health, in any given year, 15% of adults between the ages of 18 and 74 will suffer a serious depression. Fewer than 5% of depressed patients receive treatment by a psychiatrist. Many depressed persons are treated by nonpsychiatric physicians or non-physician psychotherapists. Approximately one fourth of admissions to psychiatric hospitals are for depression, while 30% of psychiatric admissions to general hospitals are for depression. Approximately 15% of patients with primary affective illness eventually die by suicide. Women have a higher incidence of depression than men, and the incidence of suicide attempts by women is higher than that for men although men are more likely to succeed in their attempts.[1]

Table 5-1 Pharmacologic profiles of tricyclic and heterocyclic antidepressants

	Postural hypotension*	Anticholinergic effect*	Sedative effect*	Reuptake/inhibition	
				Norepinephrine†	Serotonin†
Tricyclic					
Tertiary amines					
Amitriptyline (Elavil)	+ + + +	+ + + + +	+ + + + +	+	+ + + +
Imipramine (Tofranil)	+ + +	+ + + +	+ + +	+ +	+ + +
Clomipramine (Anafranil)	+ + +	+ + + +	+ + + +	+	+ + + +
Trimipramine (Surmontil)	+ + +	+ + + +	+ + + +	+ +	+ + +
Doxepin (Sinequan)	+ + +	+ + +	+ + + +	+ +	+ + +
Secondary Amines					
Desipramine (Norpramin)	+ +	+	+	+ + + + +	0
Protriptyline (Vivactil)	+ + +	+ + +	+	+ + +	+ +
Nortriptyline (Pamelor)	+ +	+ + +	+ +	+ + +	+ +
Dibenzoxazepine					
Amoxapine (Asendin)	+ +	+ +	+ +	+ + + +	+
Heterocyclic					
Tetracyclic					
Maprotiline (Ludiomil)	+ + +	+ +	+ + + +	+ + + + +	0
Triazolopyridine					
Trazodone (Desyrel)	+ + +	+ +	+ + + + +	0	+ + + +
Aminoketone					
Bupropion (Wellbutrin)	0	+	+	+/+ DA	0

*Relative hypotensive, anticholinergic, and sedative potencies are based on a composite of multiple published clinical studies of each drug.
†Relative effects of the various antidepressant drugs on nerve reuptake of norepinephrine, dopamine, and serotonin are based on published laboratory and clinical investigations.

Compiled from the following: Richelson E: *Mayo Clin Proc* 1990; 65:1227-1236. Brogdon RN, et al: *Drugs* 1981; 21:401-409. Greenblatt EN, et al: *Arch Int Pharmacodyn Ther* 1978; 233:107-135. Maitre L, et al: *J Int Med Res* 1975; 3 (suppl 2):2-15. Ferris RM, Cooper BR: *J Clin Psychiatr Monogr* 1993; 11:2-14. Synder SH, Yamamura HI: *Arch Gen Psychiatry* 1977; 34:236-239.

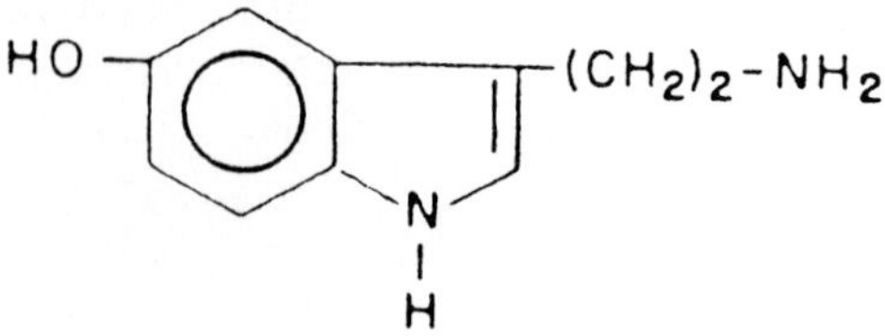

HO—[benzene ring fused to pyrrole]—$(CH_2)_2-NH_2$
N
H

SEROTONIN

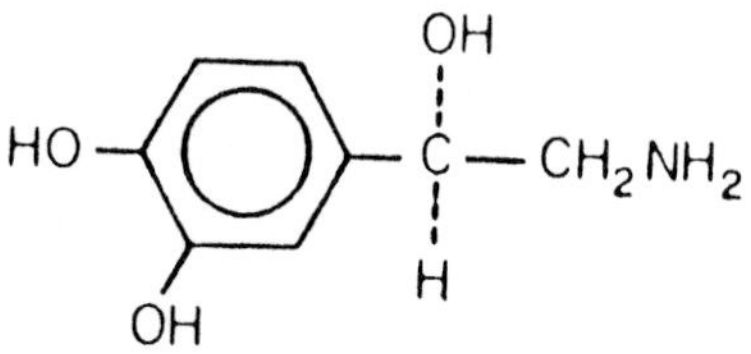

OH
HO—[benzene ring]—C—CH_2NH_2
H
OH

NOREPINEPHRINE

OH
HO—[benzene ring]—$CH_2-CH_2-NH_2$ · HCl

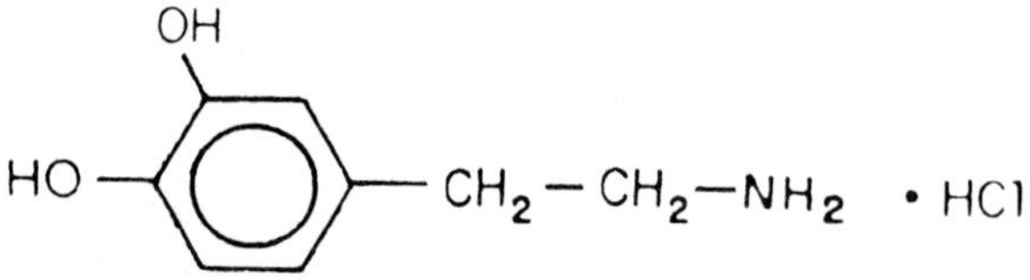

DOPAMINE

Prior to the advent of somatic therapies, including medications and electroshock therapy, the median length of a depressive episode was 8 months.[8] There is no controlled evidence to suggest that nonsomatic treatment shortens the length of an acute endogenous affective episode.[8] On the other hand, about 30% of patients fail to respond to the initial course of somatic therapy. Furthermore, a severe depressive episode may require 6 to 8 weeks of pharmacotherapy to achieve significant improvement.[8]

Electroconvulsive therapy (ECT), the first effective treatment for severe depression, was developed in the late 1930s. However, antidepressant drugs have revolutionized our thinking about the etiology and treatment of depressive illness, and allowed thousands of people with depression to function normally and lead productive lives. In dealing with a severe depression it should be remembered that despite adverse publicity in the lay press, ECT remains an effective and safe modality for treatment. Depressions that fail to respond to pharmacotherapy, and patients who are acutely suicidal are situations in which ECT may be both effective and potentially lifesaving.

Following the initial development of ECT, amphetamines were the first pharmacologic agents capable of improving mood and alleviating depression. These compounds were widely used from the late 1940s until the early 1960s, and may still be useful alone or as an adjunct to other pharmacologic treatment of depression.[9] The amphetamines have the disadvantage of producing relatively short-term beneficial effects, and also have the risk of inducing tolerance and physical dependency. They are generally less effective than other more widely used antidepressant compounds.

The monoamine oxidase inhibitors, whose antidepressant actions were discovered by accident in the early 1950s, were the first drugs to have a true mood-elevating effect. They are important not only because of their therapeutic role, but also because they opened the door for psychopharmacologists to observe and correlate changes in brain chemistry with changes in mood and behavior, helping us to begin to understand some of the important factors in the biological etiology of psychiatric illness.[6]

ANTIDEPRESSANT DRUG THERAPY

The first effective antidepressant developed in the 1950s was iproniazid, initially employed as an antituberculous drug. Tricyclic antidepressants, which are chemically related to the phenothiazines were discovered in the 1950s and 1960s during attempts to produce more effective and safer analogs of chlorpromazine. The first highly potent and selective inhibitor of serotonin reuptake (SSRI), fluoxetine, was developed in the 1970s and initially marketed in the United States in 1987. One of the most important principles of clinical psychopharmacology is that newer drugs should not necessarily supplant the clinical use of older established therapeutic agents. Since the advent of SSRI antidepressants, many psychiatrists have begun to virtually ignore previously used and still clinically useful drugs. Indeed, monoamine oxidase inhibitors and tricyclic antidepressants have not been made obsolete by the newer serotonin selective reuptake inhibitors. Many patients who do not tolerate or respond adequately to SSRIs will achieve the desired therapeutic response when treated with an appropriate MAOI or tricyclic or heterocyclic antidepressant. The favorable side effect profile of SSRIs has made these agents generally the drugs of first choice when initiating antidepressant chemotherapy. Although it is true that some patients will respond more favorably to one SSRI than to another, the practice of some clinicians to use SSRIs almost exclusively and to change from one agent to another of the same group when the initial response is unsatisfactory is often not the best approach. Indeed failure to respond to or tolerate an SSRI should make the clinician think about using an alternative antidepressant of the TCA, HCA, or MAOI groups rather than slavishly going through a long sequence of one SSRI after another. As will be discussed later, there are indications for considering the use of a tricyclic, monoamine oxidase inhibitor, or bupropion rather than an SSRI as the initial therapeutic agent.

In the early days of psychopharmacology there was considerable controversy regarding the role of drug therapy in depression. There were implications that drug therapy was not as good as the long and painful process of psychotherapy. It was commonly felt that milder, so-called neurotic, depression should be treated without medication and that medication should be reserved for more

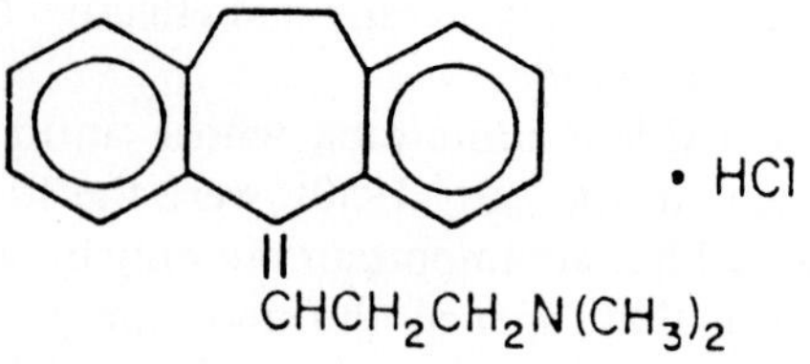

$\bullet$ HCl

$\overset{\|}{C}HCH_2CH_2N(CH_3)_2$

AMITRIPTYLINE

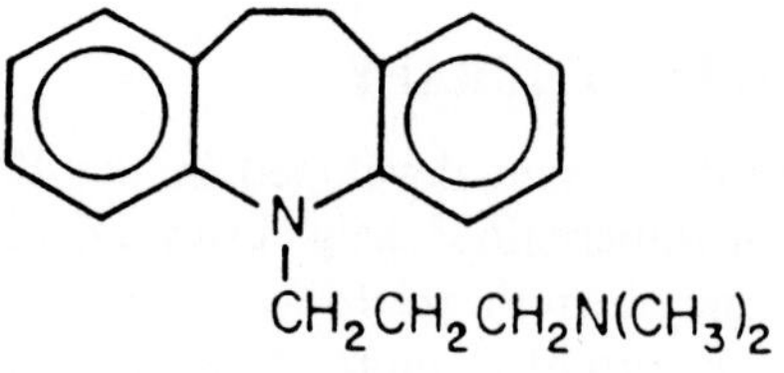

$CH_2CH_2CH_2N(CH_3)_2$

IMIPRAMINE

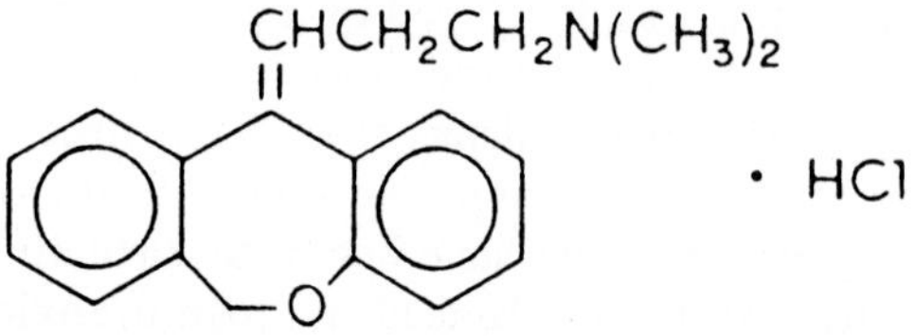

$CHCH_2CH_2N(CH_3)_2$

$\bullet$ HCl

DOXEPIN

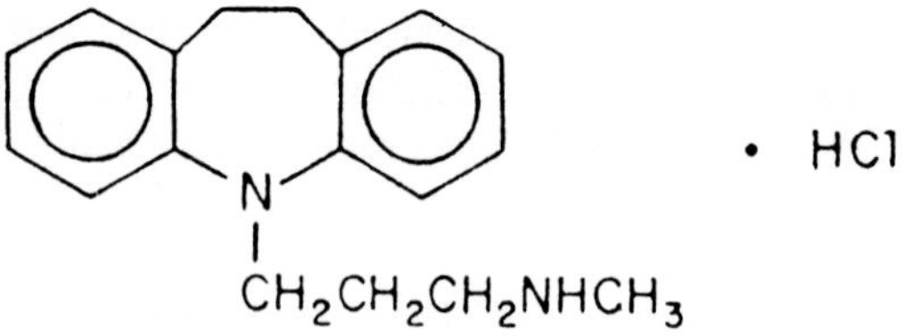

$\bullet$ HCl

$CH_2CH_2CH_2NHCH_3$

DESIPRAMINE

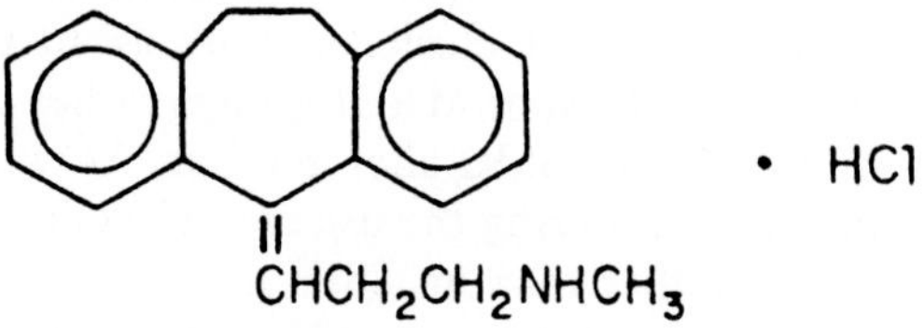

$\bullet$ HCl

$\overset{\|}{C}HCH_2CH_2NHCH_3$

NORTRIPTYLINE

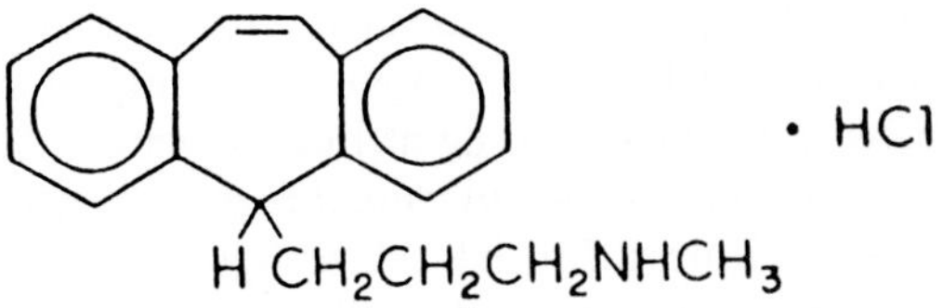
• HCl
H CH2CH2CH2NHCH3

PROTRIPTYLINE

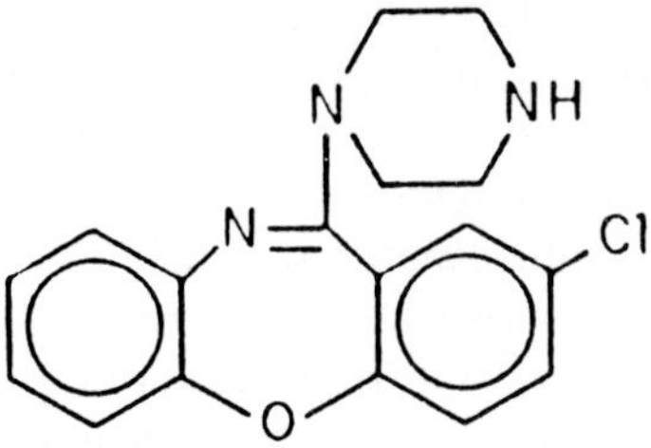
N
NH
N
Cl
O

AMOXAPINE

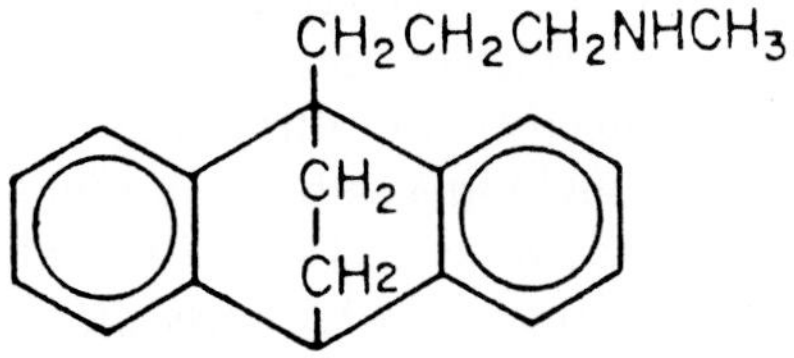
CH2CH2CH2NHCH3
CH2
CH2

MAPROTILINE

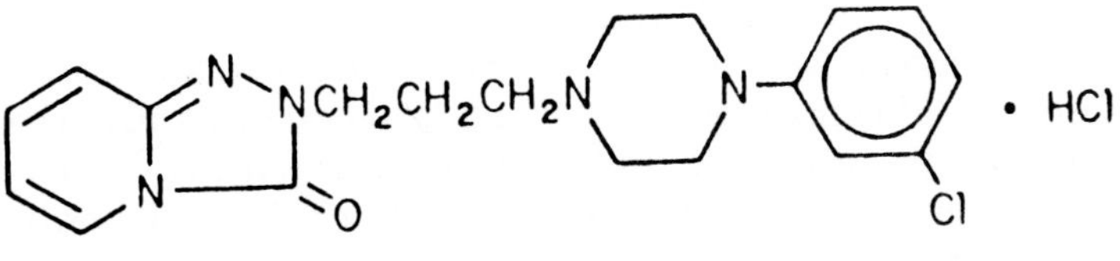
N
NCH2CH2CH2N
N
• HCl
N
O
Cl

TRAZODONE

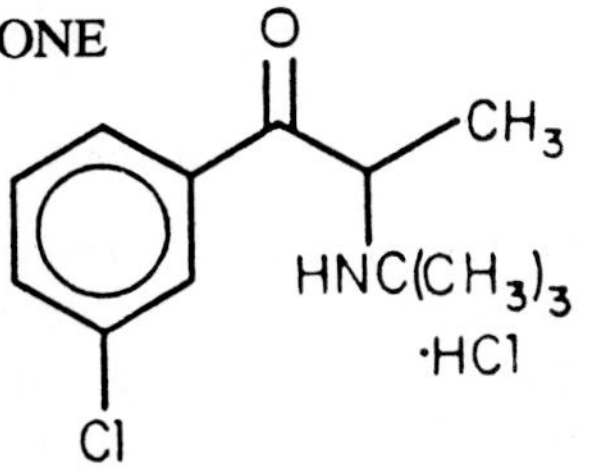
O
CH3
HNC(CH3)3
·HCl
Cl

BUPROPION

severe depressive illnesses such as psychotic depression. Research over the past 3 decades strongly supports the value of pharmacologic intervention, not only in major depression and depression associated with bipolar illness, but also in milder forms of depression which may impair the ability of an individual to be productive and enjoy life. The changing attitude toward the pharmacotherapy of depression is a manifestation of advancement in our knowledge of the etiology and course of depressive illness. Indeed, the recognition of the high incidence of depression, and the considerable potential for a favorable outcome, has yielded a more definitive therapeutic approach for this serious health problem. The DSM-III, published in 1980 and the new (1994) DSM-IV have changed the diagnostic categorization of depression in a direction that is more consistent with a biological understanding of psychiatric illness.[2]

Depressive illness, though it may be categorized in a number of ways, most likely exists along a continuum, from mild to more severe forms, with varying degrees of functional impairment. There is clearly a tendency of depressive illness to run in families; thus, genetic factors appear to be important. Extensive research suggests that the clinical manifestations of depression are related to changes in neurotransmitter function in the brain.[5,6] Reserpine, which depletes brain serotonin and norepinephrine, can induce severe depression and even suicidal behavior.[8] Methyldopa, a widely used antihypertensive which impairs brain neurotransmitter function, can likewise induce depression.[10]

Antidepressants are highly effective in alleviating the symptoms of depressive illness and melancholia, including sadness and hopelessness as well as anorexia and insomnia. These drugs reduce feelings of worthlessness and guilt and improve the patient's ability to engage in formerly pleasurable activities, including work and leisure pursuits. As the depressive symptoms subside, patients generally experience an improvement in their energy level, a decrease in fatigue and psychomotor symptoms, and the disappearance of suicidal thoughts.[8] For more than 3 decades, the psychiatric literature has documented the high degree of efficacy of tricyclic and heterocyclic antidepressant drugs.

Throughout the history of antidepressant chemotherapy, three problems repeatedly encountered with antidepressants have been the following:

1. With any given drug, a significant percentage of patients fail to respond.
2. Response to antidepressants usually requires 2 to 3 weeks of treatment.
3. Side effects are common and increase with increasing dosage.

In spite of claims to the contrary, studies of antidepressants since the 1950s indicate that with any given drug in virtually any depressed population, approximately two thirds of patients respond and a third fail to achieve therapeutic benefit. This finding is well documented and is as true of the latest SSRIs as it is of imipramine, the first tricyclic antidepressant. Thus the long-term goal of finding a nearly universally effective antidepressant has not yet been achieved. Since many depressed patients experience suicidal feelings and make suicide attempts, the goal of finding a rapidly effective agent, not requiring prolonged treatment before a response is seen, is extremely important.

Table 5-2   SSRI side effects contrasted with TCA side effects

Advantages of SSRIs vs. TCAs/HCAs	Disadvantages (side effects) of SSRIs
Not anticholinergic	Nervousness
Not antihistaminic	Agitation
Not alpha$_1$-adrenergic antagonists	Insomnia
Unlikely to cause	Tremor
Postural hypotension	Nausea
Tachycardia	Diarrhea
Delayed cardiac conduction	Headache
Blurred vision	Decreased libido
Dry mouth	Erectile dysfunction
Sedation	Anorgasmia

Again, we have not yet adequately met this goal, though progress has been made with the development of some drugs which in many (not all) patients can produce a more rapid response. Psychostimulants, including dextroamphetamine and methylphenidate, often produce a rapid, though not always sustained, mood improvement. In some patients tranylcypromine, a nonselective MAOI, will reduce depressive symptoms within the first few days of administration — perhaps due in part to its direct amphetamine-like stimulating activity. Amoxapine, a noradrenergic tricyclic antidepressant with dopamine-blocking activity, often produces some initial improvement within 4 to 7 days of initiating treatment, quite likely due to its dopamine antagonism.[11] Venlafaxine, which has prominent serotonin and noradrenergic activity, appears to produce an initial therapeutic response in some patients within the first week of therapy.[12] Since there is generally a lag time of 2 to 3 weeks from the start of medication until a response is seen, many patients experience initial side effects and discontinue medication before achieving the desired therapeutic goal. Indeed, the long delay of the initial response and the common occurrence of side effects are the major reasons for noncompliance with pharmacotherapy. The most common side effects of tricyclic and heterocyclic antidepressants include drowsiness; anticholinergic activity with associated dry mouth, constipation, and memory impairment; and cardiovascular changes including postural hypotension, tachycardia, and altered cardiac rhythm and conduction, which (as shown in Table 5-2) are essentially absent with the SSRIs. Indeed, it is the absence of these prominent TCA/HCA side effects which has accounted probably more than anything else, for the popularity of the SSRIs.[10]

SIDE EFFECTS OF ANTIDEPRESSANTS

As previously mentioned, the TCAs have variable effects in blocking the reuptake of norepinephrine and serotonin.[4,6,13] The other major difference between the drugs in this therapeutic class is their variability in side effect profile.[13,14] They vary greatly in their anticholinergic potential[15-17] as can be

---

**Box 5-4 Adverse effects of tricyclic
and heterocyclic antidepressants***

Allergic
  Rash (rare) — somewhat more frequent with maprotiline
Anticholinergic
  Blurred vision (common) — narrow angle glaucoma may worsen
  Dry mouth (common)
  Constipation (common)
  Urinary retention (occasional)
  Sweating — increased or decreased (infrequent)
  Sinus tachycardia (common)
  Speech blockage, mental clouding (occasional), confusion, delirium (rare)
Cardiovascular
  Postural hypotension, dizziness (occasional)
  Hypertension (rare)
  Sinus tachycardia (common) — anticholinergic effect
  Premature atrial or ventricular beats (infrequent)
  Antiarrhythmic effect, myocardial depression (additive with antiarrhythmic
    drugs)
  Pedal edema (occasional) — may worsen congestive heart failure
  ECG — ST segment depression, T wave flattened or inverted, QRS prolongation
Gastrointestinal
  Constipation (common) — anticholinergic effect
  Nausea, vomiting, heartburn (infrequent)
Neurologic
  Central anticholinergic effects as above — vary considerably with different drugs
  Drowsiness — varies considerably with different drugs
  Muscle tremors, twitches, jitteriness (occasional)
  Extrapyramidal symptoms (rare)
  Paresthesias, fatigue, weakness, ataxia (infrequent)
  Seizures — with overdose or in patient with known seizure disorder
  Hallucinations, delusions, activation of schizophrenic or manic psychosis

---

*Adverse effects may decrease or disappear with use of a lower-dosage or divided-dosage regimen, or by changing to a different antidepressant, based on the pharmacologic profile, as shown in Table 5-1.

seen from the data presented in Table 5-1. Anticholinergic effects are manifested clinically by dry mouth, blurred vision, constipation, difficulty urinating, and tachycardia (see Box 5-4). Since these drugs must enter the brain to exert their therapeutic effect, their anticholinergic actions may also be manifested centrally.[10,14] Elderly persons and those with organic brain dysfunction are much more sensitive to the central anticholinergic effects of these drugs.[10,14,16] Young healthy persons may also become quite uncomfortable as a result of anticholinergic effects. The CNS manifestations of cholinergic blockade include impaired memory and impaired concentrating ability, both of which may also be seen in untreated depressed patients.[14,16] Occasionally, patients receiving antidepressants experience difficulties expressing their thoughts verbally.[18] Speech blockage and stuttering may occur with cyclic antidepressants, particularly those which are more strongly anticholinergic, and have been reported as a rare side effect of MAOI antidepressants and alprazolam, which have minimal anticholinergic activity.[18-20] Persons who are particularly sensitive to cholinergic blockade or who have taken excessive dosages of antidepressants, may experience confusion, disorientation, disorganized thinking, and visual or auditory hallucinations.[10,14] Toxic psychoses can occur in response to centrally acting anticholinergic drugs.[10] In patients with an underlying psychosis or history of bipolar illness, antidepressants may exacerbate the psychotic or manic condition, probably as a result of central anticholinergic, noradrenergic, and serotonergic mechanisms.[8] In choosing an antidepressant for a patient with a prior history of sensitivity to anticholinergic effects, it is preferable to utilize a drug with lower potential for cholinergic blockade such as an SSRI, desipramine, bupropion, or trazodone.[10,13] This is particularly true in the elderly, especially those with organic brain dysfunction.[16,21,22] Likewise, in a patient with cardiovascular disease, a drug with lower anticholinergic potential may be advantageous since it will be less likely to increase heart rate and alter cardiac conduction.[21-23] Postural hypotension is a rather common unwanted effect of tricyclic antidepressants, which is probably related to the drugs' ability to relax vascular smooth muscle.[21-23] Bupropion, amoxapine, nortriptyline, and maprotiline are less likely to produce significant postural hypotension than are imipramine and amitriptyline.[14,22-25]

Sedation is another pharmacologic parameter that differentiates the various antidepressants. In a depressed patient who has difficulty sleeping it is often advantageous to utilize a more strongly sedating antidepressant in a single dose at bedtime. If the patient is not likely to have difficulty with a strongly anticholinergic agent, amitriptyline, (the most sedating TCA) would be an appropriate choice. If, on the other hand, there is need to avoid cholinergic blockade and at the same time a desire for a drug with more prominent sedating qualities, doxepin, maprotiline, nefazodone, or trazodone in a single bedtime dose would be desirable.[26,27,28] If the patient tends to be excessively drowsy during the day, it is often preferable to utilize one of the antidepressants with lower sedative potential. Desipramine, which has little sedative effect, and amoxapine, whose sedative action is likewise relatively mild, are both well tolerated if given in divided doses throughout the day. Since amoxapine has some ability to inhibit serotonin reuptake as well as a primary effect on norepinephrine reuptake, it may be more effective than desipramine, which only inhibits norepinephrine reuptake.[24] The serotonin-selective antidepressants— including fluoxetine, fluvoxamine, paroxetine, sertraline, and venlafaxine—are devoid of anticholinergic, hypotensive, cardiovascular, and sedative side effects.[14,23]

Decreased libido, reduced sexual arousal, and impaired orgasmic function may all be associated with depressive illness. Unfortunately, various antidepressants can also impair sexual function and it is often difficult to determine whether the illness or its treatment is the cause.[29] Tricyclic and heterocyclic compounds can all impair sex drive and function, although sexual dysfunction is more frequently associated with MAOI antidepressants, and most common with serotonin selective antidepressants.[30] In up to one third of patients, SSRI antidepressants can reduce libido, arousal, and orgasmic function, which can improve with dosage reduction but often requires discontinuing the SSRI medication and a change to an unrelated antidepressant.[30,31] However, many individuals maintain very robust orgasmic function during use of SSRIs, and there have been isolated reports in the literature of spontaneous orgasms associated with SSRI use.[30] Fluoxetine and other SSRIs have been extremely useful in the management of premature ejaculation, often when employed in very low doses.[30,31] Of all marketed antidepressants, bupropion has the least potential for inhibiting sexual function and will generally significantly improve sexual function if administered in low doses along with SSRIs or cyclic antidepressants.[30] In many patients who have had impairment of sexual drive, arousal, or orgasmic function with other antidepressants, sexual function can be restored when antidepressant therapy is changed to bupropion.[30] Over the years of pharmacotherapy various mechanisms — including anticholinergic effect, alpha-adrenergic antagonism, and excess serotonergic function — have been implicated in the etiology of sexual dysfunction.[29,31] Just as there is no certainty as to mechanism, there is no definitive treatment; yet a variety of remedies have at times been shown to be effective. Neostigmine, which inhibits cholinesterase and increases cholinergic function, has been given in doses of 7.5 to 15 mg 1/2 to 1 hour prior to intercourse in order to improve erectile and ejaculatory function.[30] By a similar mechanism, bethanechol, a direct-acting cholinomimetic drug, administered at a dose of 10 to 25 mg 3 times daily, or by a single oral dose of 25 to 50 mg 1 hour before intercourse, may also be helpful.[30] Cyproheptadine, a serotonin antagonist, has been shown to alleviate orgasmic dysfunction due to cyclic and MAOI antidepressants when administered in a dose of 4 mg nightly or 1 hour prior to intercourse.[32] There are many disadvantages to cyproheptadine, including drowsiness and increased appetite, but the major problem is the likelihood that this drug will block the antidepressant efficacy of SSRIs, which I feel essentially contraindicates this pharmacologic approach to sexual dysfunction.[33]

Some clinicians have found that changing from a mixed serotonergic-noradrenergic antidepressant to a pure noradrenergic drug such as desipramine may alleviate antidepressant-induced sexual dysfunction.[14] Trazodone and its congener, nefazodone, antagonize $5-HT_2$ receptors and inhibit serotonin reuptake; the former may improve erectile function in men and has been shown to improve sexual arousal in women.[28,34] Based on their structural similarity, we can assume that the clinical efficacy and side effects of trazodone and nefazodone will likewise be similar. Prolonged painful erections, known as priapism, have been reported in a number of men during trazodone treatment.[35,36] The mechanism of drug-induced priapism may relate to both alpha$_1$-adrenergic and 5-HT$_2$ receptor antagonism by trazodone.[31,36] Priapism has also been reported as a rare complication of neuroleptic medications, fluoxetine, and MAOIs, but apparently does not occur with lithium.

Tricyclic and heterocyclic antidepressants have a quinidine-like effect and through this mechanism may depress intraventricular conduction and myocardial contractility, as will be discussed in chapter 10.[22,23] The electrophysiologic, noradrenergic, and anticholinergic activity of cyclic antidepressants accounts for their ability to both provoke and suppress cardiac arrhythmias, depending on the patient's clinical condition, drug dosage, and coadministration of other medications.[22,23]

Bupropion and the SSRI antidepressants do not alter cardiac rhythm or automaticity, or blood pressure, and they lack arrhythmogenic and antiarrhythmic activity.[57,62]

Occasionally, cyclic antidepressants may interfere with sleep, producing nightmares and hypnagogic phenomena.[14] Sleep disturbances occur more commonly with MAOIs and serotonin selective antidepressants. Changing the regimen from one type of antidepressant to another, or the short-term use of 1 to 2 mg of trifluoperazine at bedtime, often alleviates antidepressant-induced sleep disturbances. Appetite stimulation, carbohydrate craving, and weight gain are common side effects of cyclic and MAOI antidepressants, but generally not of bupropion and the SSRIs, as discussed in detail in chapter 10.

Convulsions are a rare complication of antidepressant drug therapy.[37] If seizures do occur, they are most likely the result of an overdose, an excessively high therapeutic dosage, or the exacerbation of a dormant seizure disorder by the convulsive threshold–lowering effect of the antidepressant. All tricyclic and heterocyclic antidepressants can provoke seizures, at a rate of 0.3% to 0.6%.[37] With careful choice of drug, and, where indicated, plasma drug concentration monitoring, antidepressants can be safely used even in patients with previous seizure disorders. Monoamine oxidase inhibitors and SSRIs are less likely than cyclic drugs to provoke convulsive events.[37] Bupropion, clomipramine, and maprotiline are more likely to lower seizure threshold and provoke convulsions at therapeutic dosage, when high doses are employed, or when the patient has a previous convulsive disorder.[37,38] As the dose of maprotiline is titrated above 150 mg/day, caution should be employed and prolonged use of dosages exceeding 200 mg/day should generally be avoided.[22] Maprotiline should not be used in the treatment of any patient with a previously known convulsive disorder and should be discontinued and not restarted in any patient who develops seizure activity during maprotiline treatment. Bupropion is contraindicated when there is a prior history of seizures, head injury, or bulimia; however, in the absence of these findings, it probably does not present an excessive seizure risk when given in divided doses, not exceeding a total of 450 mg/day. Clomipramine has a greater seizure risk in susceptible patients or when excessive blood levels are achieved.[37] Clozapine lowers seizure threshold and should not be used along with these agents in seizure-prone patients. Fluoxetine and some other SSRIs increase blood levels of these drugs, further increasing seizure risk.[10]

Fine high-frequency tremors are occasionally seen in patients receiving SSRIs, TCAs and HCAs, particularly when higher doses are employed or lithium is coadministered.[14] Tremors may improve or disappear when the antidepressant dosage is decreased. Persistent tremors may be managed by the addition of propranolol in a dose of 10 to 20 mg 2 to 4 times daily. Low doses of benzodiazepines, such as 0.25 to 0.5 mg of Lorazepam 2 to 4 times daily may also help minimize antidepressant-induced tremor.[14] Myoclonus is a well-known side effect of MAOIs, which also occurs occasionally with SSRIs and tricyclic and heterocyclic antidepressants.[39] It may be an incidental finding which does not require specific remediation. On the other hand, if it is troubling to the patient, reduction in antidepressant dosage, change to a different antidepressant, or the addition of clonazepam, carbamazepine, or valproate may be useful remedies.[39]

Extrapyramidal side effects have occasionally been reported with a variety of antidepressant drugs, including the SSRIs. Amoxapine, which is the N-desmethyl derivative of the neuroleptic loxapine, has weak dopamine-blocking activity, which may account for its more rapid onset of antidepressant action.[24] Dopamine blockade by amoxapine also yields occasional extrapyramidal side effects, including parkinsonian reactions and akathisia.[40] I have observed only five instances of akathisia in approximately 300 patients whom I have treated with amoxapine in a dosage range of 50 to 200 mg/day. In each case the akathisia disappeared promptly with dosage reduction or discontinuation. Although I have never observed any form of dyskinesia during treatment or following discontinuation of amoxapine, there have been approximately 30 cases of dyskinesia reported to the manufacturer in association with amoxapine therapy. Nearly all of these cases have occurred in association with sudden dosage reduction or discontinuation, and abnormal movements, in most cases, persisted only for brief periods of time, and subsequently completely disappeared.

Trimipramine is a tricyclic with weak dopamine-blocking activity. Trazodone binds to dopamine receptors with an affinity comparable to that of chlorpromazine.[41] Chorea and myoclonus have been reported in a patient receiving high-dose therapy with trazodone.[42] I have observed one patient who developed akathisia with associated myoclonus while receiving trazodone 100 mg daily. In this patient, gradual increase of trazodone dosage up to 150 mg/day was associated with worsening akathisia, which subsequently resolved when trazodone was discontinued.

With the advent of newer antidepressant drugs that are more potent serotonin uptake inhibitors, including clomipramine and the SSRIs, a serotonin syndrome has been described[43,44] (see Box 5-5). This syndrome is characterized by restlessness, diaphoresis, hyperreflexia, myoclonus, nausea, diarrhea, abdominal cramps, and insomnia.[43,44] Depending on the severity of the syndrome, the patient may experience one, several, or all of these symptoms. If the patient

---

Box 5-5 Drug interactions of SSRIs
due to excess CNS serotonin

SEROTONIN SYNDROME likely to occur if SSRI combined with
  MAO inhibitors — phenelzine, tranylcypromine
  MAOI (selective) — selegiline, moclobemide
  Tryptophan (serotonin precursor)
Signs and symptoms of SEROTONIN SYNDROME (most to least frequent)
  Mental status changes — including confusion or hypomania
  Restlessness or agitation
  Myoclonus
  Hyperreflexia
  Diaphoresis
  Shivering (or shaking chills)
  Tremor
  Diarrhea, abdominal cramps, nausea
  Ataxia or incoordination
  Headache

---

is acutely uncomfortable, the symptoms may be alleviated by administration of the serotonin antagonist cyproheptadine. This syndrome is more likely to occur when the serotonin precursor tryptophan is administered in conjunction with a potent serotonin reuptake inhibitor or when a serotonergic antidepressant is used in conjunction with an MAOI. The occurrence of these symptoms may necessitate changing the therapeutic regimen to an antidepressant with weaker serotonergic activity.

Peripheral edema is a fairly common side effect of cyclic antidepressant drugs. The mechanism of edema appears to involve increased capillary permeability.[21] Amitriptyline is somewhat more likely than other tricyclic drugs to induce edema. However, this side effect is also known to occur with trazodone administration.[45] Unfortunately, all cyclic antidepressants can result in a fatal outcome when employed as a weapon of suicide. It appears, however, that trazodone is relatively safer when taken in overdose than other cyclic antidepressants.[46]

At the conclusion of a course of antidepressant therapy, medication dosage must be gradually reduced; to reduce the risk of depressive recurrence, treatment should never be abruptly discontinued. Sudden withdrawal of cyclic antidepressants may be associated with anorexia, nausea, vomiting, abdominal pain, diarrhea, increased salivation, headaches, muscular pains, dizziness, and sleep disturbance.[47,48] Withdrawal symptoms associated with cyclic antidepressants are virtually identical to those seen when antiparkinsonian drugs are abruptly discontinued.[47] These symptoms can be promptly alleviated by the administration of an anticholinergic drug. Similar symptoms can be provoked by the administration of cholinomimetic drugs such as bethanechol or cholinesterase inhibitors such as physostigmine.[48] It appears that withdrawal symptoms associated with TCAs and antiparkinsonian drugs are due to rebound increased activity of the cholinergic system in the absence of the anticholinergic effect of these therapeutic agents.

TECHNIQUES OF CYCLIC ANTIDEPRESSANT THERAPY

In initiating cyclic antidepressant medications it is often advantageous to employ divided doses throughout the day, so that the patient can gradually accommodate to side effects. Once the optimal therapeutic dosage is achieved and the patient is tolerating medication satisfactorily, any of the currently available TCAs or HCAs can be given as a single bedtime dose with equal therapeutic efficacy. Single bedtime doses may not be desirable in elderly patients who are likely to be sensitive to anticholinergic and cardiovascular side effects.[10] Anxious patients may benefit from a divided-dosage schedule, which may help to alleviate anxiety without the need for additional medication. Most tricyclic antidepressants exert their therapeutic effect only after 2 to 3 weeks of treatment, and it may be necessary at the outset to coadminister a benzodiazepine or a low dose of trifluoperazine (1 to 2 mg 2 to 4 times daily) while awaiting the therapeutic response of the antidepressant.[49] If a rapidly acting tricyclic such as amoxapine is chosen, the need to coadminister an additional agent in a nonpsychotic depressed patient is generally obviated by the ability of amoxapine to diminish anxiety and also produce a rapid antidepressant response. In the event that the clinician wishes to administer a benzodiazepine concurrently at the outset of antidepressant drug therapy, alprazolam would be a good choice because of its relatively short half-life and the fact that it may exert its own antidepressant action.[50]

In the depressed patient who presents with paranoid ideation and delusional thinking, it is usually preferable to initiate treatment with a potent antipsychotic agent such as haloperidol or trifluoperazine prior to starting treatment with the antidepressant. Low-potency antipsychotic agents such as chlorpromazine and thioridazine should be avoided in such individuals. These drugs are strongly anticholinergic and they may cause postural hypotension that will add to similar pharmacologic effects produced by cyclic antidepressant agents.[10] Amoxapine has been found to be effective in treating psychotic depression without the need for simultaneous administration of a neuroleptic drug.[51]

The two most common errors made in prescribing antidepressants are failure to utilize adequate dosage and failure to continue treatment long enough to allow the patient to recover from the depressive episode and to provide a period of prophylaxis to reduce the risk of recurrence.[52] Table 5-3 presents dosage guidelines for the currently available cyclic antidepressant compounds. As a general rule, antidepressant treatment should be started by utilizing a

Table 5-3   Tricyclic and heterocyclic antidepressant dosages

	Usual adult daily dose (mg)*	Range (mg)
Tertiary amine — tricyclic		
Amitriptyline (Elavil)	150-200	50-300
Imipramine (Tofranil)	150-200	50-300
Trimipramine (Surmontil)	150-200	50-300
Doxepin (Sinequan)	150-250	50-300
Clomipramine (Anafranil)	150-250	25-300
Secondary amine — tricyclic		
Desipramine (Norpramin)	150-250	50-300
Protriptyline (Vivactil)	30-40	15-60†
Nortriptyline (Pamelor)	75-100	30-100†
Dibenzoxazepine — tricyclic		
Amoxapine (Asendin)	150-200	50-300
Tetracyclic		
Maprotiline (Ludiomil)	150-200	50-225
Triazolopyridine derivative		
Trazodone (Desyrel)	100-250	50-400

*Elderly patients should generally be treated with approximately one half of the usual adult dosage of any of the above antidepressants.
†Therapeutic window effect implies the possibility of reduced therapeutic response if excessive dosage and blood levels are attained.

divided-dose regimen, gradually building to the desired level and then converting to a single bedtime dose or, alternately, a regimen which gives a portion of medication during the daytime and the remainder at bedtime. For example, if one were utilizing amitriptyline or imipramine, it would be reasonable to start an ambulatory patient on 25 mg 3 times daily, gradually increasing the total dose to 150 to 200 mg/day over the first 3 to 7 days and then gradually moving to a single daily dose once the patient demonstrates that he is tolerating the medication satisfactorily. It is important to underscore the fact that elderly patients require approximately 50% of the usual adult dosage for each of the antidepressants listed in Table 5-3. Although some elderly people will tolerate, and indeed require, larger-than-predicted doses of these medications, well-documented studies have demonstrated that elderly persons attain blood levels approximately twice as high as younger patients at comparable dosage of tricyclic antidepressants.[53]

One of the continuing problems in achieving a prompt and therapeutically satisfactory response to antidepressant drugs is the inability to predict which patient will respond optimally to which type of antidepressant. As mentioned earlier, attempts to utilize blood, CSF, and urine tests of neurotransmitter metabolites to predict responsiveness to specific antidepressant drugs have been unsuccessful. Most often, the process of arriving at an optimal antidepressant response involves considerable trial and error employing different antidepressant drugs until a satisfactory therapeutic response is established with a tolerable level of side effects. Several investigators have employed the stimulant drugs dextroamphetamine and methylphenidate as predictive tests of antidepressant responsiveness. Different methods have been employed utilizing single or multiple doses of stimulant administered on one day or several days in succession. Most commonly, methylphenidate 5 to 20 mg as a single dose or a twice-daily regimen, or dextroamphetamine 5 to 20 mg as a single dose or a twice-daily regimen, have been employed. Most studies have found that those patients who experience a prompt mood improvement following stimulant drug administration will be responsive to noradrenergic antidepressants such as desipramine.[54,55] Patients who experience a dysphoric response to the stimulant test generally do not respond well to noradrenergic-type antidepressants, but do achieve a favorable therapeutic response to serotonergic-type drugs, such as amitriptyline or one of the SSRIs.[54,55]

TECHNIQUE FOR USE OF BUPROPION

Bupropion has the advantage of producing minimal sedative, anticholinergic, and cardiovascular side effects and presenting little risk of appetite stimulation and sexual dysfunction.[56,57] This agent, which has dopaminergic and noradrenergic effects, may be particularly useful in withdrawn, anergic, depressed patients.[58,59] There is also some evidence that bupropion may help to stabilize mood when used along with lithium in bipolar patients.[60] The major adverse event risk is that it may be somewhat more likely than most cyclic antidepressants to provoke seizures in susceptible individuals. Bupropion is contraindicated in patients with a history of a seizure disorder, head injury, or bulimia. The maximum daily dose recommended is 450 mg, with no more than 150 mg given in a single dose, each dose being separated by approximately 8 hours. If these precautions are followed and the drug is initiated at a low dose with gradual dosage titration, the risk of seizures is not significantly different from that for standard TCA compounds.[61] I generally initiate bupropion with 75 mg given twice daily for the first 2 days, followed by 75 mg 3 times daily for approximately 1 week. If there is evidence of an initial response at this point, I would often continue this dose for at least 1 additional week before further dosage increase. If there is no apparent response with no evidence of nervousness or insomnia after the initial week at the low dose, I would then increase to 100 mg 3 times daily for 1 to 2 weeks. If there is still no response and the patient is tolerating bupropion well, I would then, over the next week or 2, gradually increase the dose to 150 mg 3 times daily. Failure to respond to the dose of 450 mg daily after a period of 2 to 3 weeks would indicate that the patient is not likely to respond to this agent at accepted and safe dosage and would therefore indicate the appropriateness of changing to an alternative antidepressant, or a trial of lithium augmentation.

TECHNIQUE OF THERAPY WITH
SEROTONIN-SELECTIVE ANTIDEPRESSANTS

Although fluoxetine is the oldest and most widely used SSRI,[62] there are now several other agents (as delineated in Table 5-4), including fluvoxamine, paroxetine, and sertraline.[63,64,65] I have also placed venlafaxine in that table since its potency as a serotonin reuptake inhibitor is comparable to that of fluoxetine, although in addition it has rather potent ability to inhibit reuptake of norepinephrine,[66,67] thus it may be termed an atypical serotonin reuptake inhibitor with additional noradrenergic activity. The contribution of dopamine reuptake inhibition to the clinical activity of venlafaxine and sertraline is unknown at this time.

Clomipramine is chemically a tricyclic antidepressant with greater serotonin reuptake inhibitory potency than fluoxetine; the primary active metabolite of clomipramine, desmethylclomipramine, is a potent norepinephrine reuptake inhibitor. Individual patients will vary in their metabolism of clomipramine, which may account for its variation in clinical response, relative to increased brain availability of serotonin and norepinephrine. Unlike SSRIs, clomipramine has the usual tricyclic side effects, including sedation, hypotension, cardiac conduction delay, and anticholinergic action, all of which are absent with the SSRI compounds. In addition, clomipramine can lower seizure threshold, and provoke convulsions in susceptible individuals, to a somewhat greater extent than other tricyclics, while the SSRIs do not alter seizure threshold. Clomipramine is primarily used in the treatment of obsessive-compulsive disorder[68] and will be discussed in more detail in chapter 9.

In considering the standard SSRI antidepressants, there are variations in potency and dosage, in their likelihood to yield pharmacologically active metabolites, and in their ability to inhibit cytochrome P-450 IID6, which governs the oxidative metabolism of many psychotropic and nonpsychotropic drugs (as shown in Table 5-4). A critical difference between the various SSRI drugs is their half-life and that of any active metabolites which are generated. This latter characteristic is extremely important, since it governs how long the drug remains active following its discontinuation. As a general principle, five half-lives must elapse before one can be relatively certain that the drug is absent and there is no risk of interaction with an incompatible substance. In practical terms, SSRI interactions with MAOI antidepressants are the most dangerous psychotropic drug interactions, resulting in the serotonin syndrome, with potentially fatal results.[43,44] When fluoxetine has been administered in a standard dose of 20 mg daily, at least 5 weeks must elapse following its discontinuation before a monoamine oxidase inhibitor can be safely administered.[43] If the patient had been receiving sertraline, paroxetine, or fluvoxamine, it would be reasonably safe to initiate MAOI therapy 2 weeks after their discontinuation.[63] Based on half-life data, it would most likely be safe to start MAOI antidepressants 1 week following discontinuation of venlafaxine.[66] Probably 3 weeks should elapse after stopping clomipramine prior to starting an

Table 5-4 Comparison of serotonin-selective reuptake inhibitors

	Half-life* (mean)	Half-life (metabolite)	Activity of metabolite	Cytochrome inhibition	Impairment of drug metabolism*	Reuptake inhibition (K_i)		
						Serotonin	Norepinephrine	DA
Fluoxetine (Prozac)	2-3 days	7-9 days	Equal to F	++++	+++++	25	500	4200
Fluvoxamine (Luvox)	15 hr	Inactive	0	+	+++	6.2	1100	>10,000
Paroxetine (Paxil)	21 hr	Inactive	0	+++++	+++	1.1	350	2000
Sertraline (Zoloft)	26 hr	2-4 days	Minimal	+	+	7.3	1400	230
Venlafaxine (Effexor)	5 hr	11 hr	Equal to V	±	±	21	64	280
Clomipramine‡ (Anafranil)	32 hr	69 hr	CM/serotonin DCM/NEPI	±	+	7.4	96	91

Key: F = fluoxetine; V = venlafaxine; CM = clomipramine; DCM = demethylclomipramine; NEPI = norepinephrine;
*Impairment of drug metabolism parallels the potency of cytochrome P-450 inhibition and drug half-life (DeVane CL: *J Clin Psychiatry* 1992; 53[2, suppl]:13-20).
†Smaller numbers indicate higher potency (Tulloch IF, Johnson AM: *J Clin Psychiatry* 1992; 53[2, suppl]:7-12).
‡Clomipramine-TCA (not SSRI) presented for comparison. The parent compound, clomipramine, is primarily serotonergic; the metabolite, desmethyl-clomipramine, is primarily noradrenergic. The half-life shown is for single-dose administration; it may be 2 to 4 times higher with continuous or high-dose regimens.

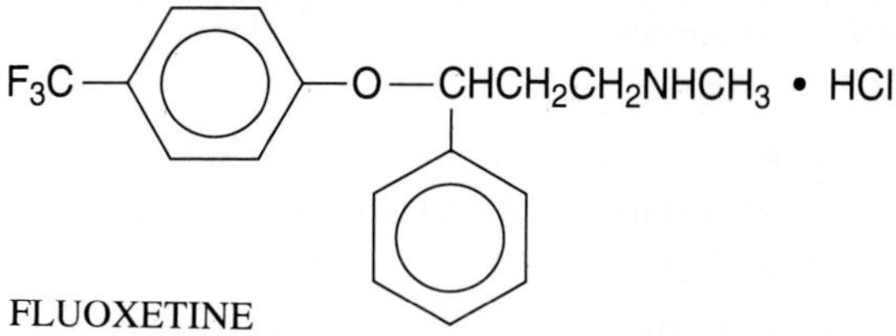
F3C
O
CHCH2CH2NHCH3 • HCl

FLUOXETINE

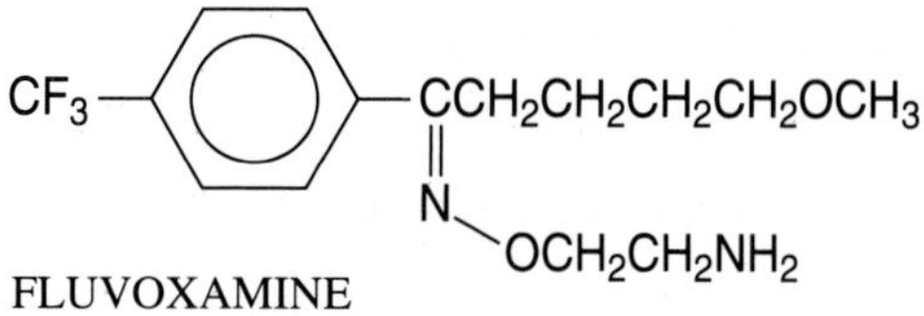
CF3
CCH2CH2CH2CH2OCH3
N
OCH2CH2NH2

FLUVOXAMINE

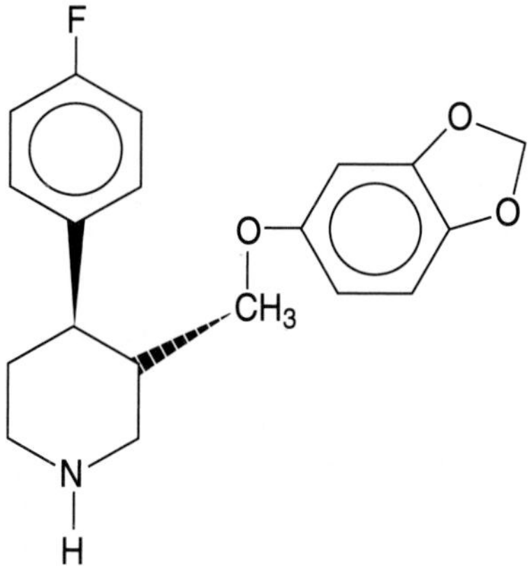
F
O
O
O
CH3
N
H

PAROXETINE

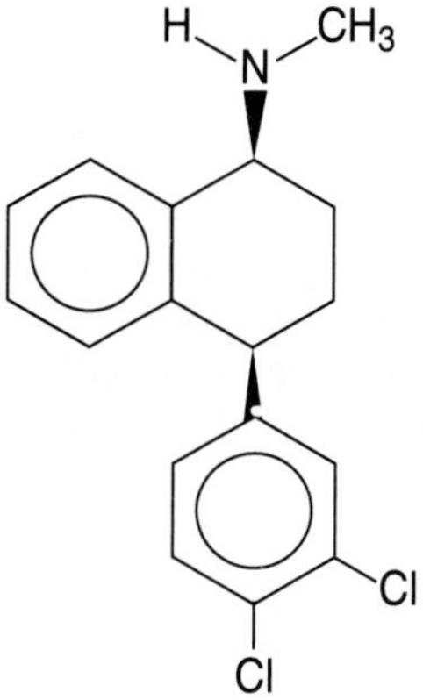
H
N
CH3
Cl
Cl

SERTRALINE

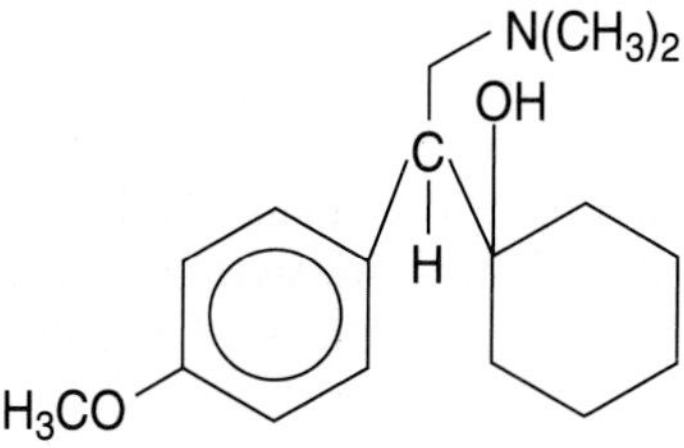
N(CH3)2
OH
C
H
H3CO

VENALAFAXINE

Box 5-6 Drug interactions of SSRIs due
to cytochrome P-450 inhibition (SSRIs:
fluoxetine, fluvoxamine, paroxetine)

Blood levels and adverse effects of the following are increased:
  Antidepressants — tricyclics and trazodone
  Barbiturates
  Benzodiazepines — except lorazepam and oxazepam
  Carbamazepine
  Narcotics — particularly pentazocine, dextromethorphan, and meperidine
  Neuroleptics
  Nifedipine
  Phenytoin
  Valproate
  Verapamil

MAOI. The SSRIs, including fluoxetine, fluvoxamine, paroxetine, sertraline, and venlafaxine, have no affinity for muscarinic, histamine H_1, 5-HT_1, 5-HT_2, or alpha$_1$- or alpha$_2$-adrenergic receptors[63] and therefore do not induce anticholinergic side effects, sedation, appetite stimulation, or postural hypotension, which are common with TCAs and HCAs.[14]

Inhibition of drug metabolism, through inhibition of the cytochrome P-450 enzyme system, is extremely important, since serum concentrations and therapeutic as well as toxic effects of a variety of coadministered drugs will be increased[69] (Box 5-6). Although discussed in greater detail in chapter 12, it must be strongly stated here that if fluoxetine, fluvoxamine, or paroxetine are coadministered with tricyclic antidepressants, blood levels and potentially toxic effects of the latter will be increased, quite possibly as much as 10-fold in the case of the interaction between fluoxetine and a TCA.[70,71] Furthermore, the extent and duration of the effect on drug metabolism will depend on the potency of cytochrome P-450 inhibition as well as the half-life of the drug and its dose and duration of administration. Indeed, the relatively short half-lives of paroxetine and fluvoxamine relative to that of fluoxetine would make the latter drug much more active as an inhibitor of metabolism of a coadministered substance. Since the former two SSRIs have relatively short half-lives, their ability to inhibit the metabolism of other drugs would become insignificant within several days of their discontinuation; but this effect of fluoxetine may persist for as much as a month or more after it is stopped.[72] Patients who have been treated with higher doses of fluoxetine, 40 to 80 mg/day for several months, may have an altered ability to metabolize other drugs including tricyclics and most benzodiazepines for much longer.[73] Indeed, switching from fluoxetine to a tricyclic antidepressant may yield adverse effects or highly toxic effects to conventional doses of TCAs. Patients who have been treated with fluoxetine within the previous month may have a very serious or even fatal result from a relatively modest overdose of tricyclic antidepressants.[74]

In prescribing SSRI antidepressants, it is preferable to employ those agents with less ability to impair metabolism of coadministered drugs and those agents with shorter half-lives.[71] My preference is to use sertraline, generally starting at a dose of 25 mg each morning, and to gradually increase the dose as required to achieve the desired antidepressant or antiobsessional effect.[75] Patients with social phobia or panic disorder most often achieve an optimal response at low doses of 25 to 50 mg daily, while depressed patients may require a somewhat higher dose (50 to 150 mg/day) and those with obsessional disorders most often require relatively higher doses (150 to 200 mg daily). Most often 2 to 3 weeks will be required to obtain an initial therapeutic effect, although not uncommonly the maximal therapeutic action of any SSRI may require 6 or occasionally 8 weeks of continuous administration.[62,75] Except for their pharmacokinetic differences, most of the SSRIs behave similarly therapeutically, although occasional patients respond better to one SSRI than to another.[65,67,75] Patients who do not respond favorably to sertraline may be given a therapeutic trial of either a tricyclic antidepressant or another SSRI such as paroxetine, fluvoxamine, or fluoxetine, although the greater potential for drug interactions of these compounds must be considered as well as the considerably longer half-life of the latter drug.[70,71,72] Some patients will respond preferentially to one but not another SSRI antidepressant, and some will experience less restlessness, insomnia, or appetite suppression with one but not another of these compounds.[65] In practical terms, I generally find it more fruitful to change to a different type of antidepressant if the initial SSRI has been tried in adequate dosage for a long enough period of treatment (approximately 6 weeks). Not infrequently patients who fail to tolerate or respond to a given dose of a specific SSRI will have fewer side effects and a better therapeutic response if the dosage is lowered, provided a long enough period elapses (2 to 4 weeks) to allow the patient to equilibrate to the lower dose. An important case in point is fluoxetine, which is often very effective with minimal to absent side effects at a daily dose of 5 mg in patients who previously appeared not to respond to doses of 20 to 40 mg/day or who had intolerable side effects with the more usually employed larger dose.[76] Most often when I use fluoxetine, I will initiate therapy at 5 mg/day and treat for 2 to 3 weeks at this dose before increasing, except in patients with obsessive-compulsive disorder, who generally require higher doses.

Venlafaxine is a very promising addition to our antidepressant armamentarium, in that it has potent serotonergic and noradrenergic activity.[66] This pharmacologic aspect of venlafaxine resembles the dual neurotransmitter action of imipramine but with greater potency and without anticholinergic, sedative, or hypotensive side effects.[67] It should be noted, however, that venlafaxine, particularly in higher doses, may cause a modest increase in systolic and/or diastolic pressure, usually not more than 5 to 10 mm. This drug also is a weak inhibitor of dopamine reuptake, which, along with its noradrenergic effect, may make it more activating, particularly in patients whose energy level is diminished.[66,67] Restlessness and insomnia, which can occur with any of the SSRIs, may be somewhat more common with venlafaxine, which (like other drugs in this group) is best not administered at bedtime.[67] The effective dosage range for venlafaxine is 75 to 375 mg/day, although most often doses above 225 mg/day are not necessary and some patients will respond to doses of less than 75 mg/day; this drug, however, due to its short half-life, needs to be administered in two or three divided doses each day, while other SSRIs may generally be given in a single dose each morning.[12] Since venlafaxine is a potent inhibitor of serotonin uptake as well as norepinephrine uptake and has dopaminergic activity, it is often effective and better tolerated in patients who have not responded to selective serotonin drugs.[77] Side effects of venlafaxine are similar to those of the selective serotonin reuptake inhibitors, with somewhat more risk of nausea, particularly with higher doses or rapid dose titration, and somewhat lower potential to cause sexual dysfunction in men as well as women.[77] Patients being changed from fluoxetine to any drug, including venlafaxine, need to be followed as the new antidepressant dosage is adjusted, since prolonged metabolic inhibition by fluoxetine will increase the blood level and potential therapeutic and adverse effects of the new drug for at least a month after fluoxetine discontinuation.[70,72]

When a patient has not responded satisfactorily to an SSRI, bupropion, a tricyclic or a monoamine oxidase inhibitor should next be considered, generally in that order, keeping in mind the need to allow an adequate SSRI-free period prior to initiating MAOI therapy. If the patient is unable to tolerate a drug-free interval between the SSRI and the next antidepressant, it is often most reasonable to change from the SSRI to imipramine or another tricyclic (*not* clomipramine), since TCAs can be administered simultaneously with SSRIs and with MAOIs.[10] Thus I speak of using the TCA as a bridge between the SSRI and the MAOI, or in the reverse direction, while allowing the previous incompatible medication to dissipate before initiating the new medication. Utilizing this bridge function often results in a patient's responding well to the initial combination of tricyclic with SSRI or the tricyclic with an MAOI and achieves

Table 5-5   Serotonin-selective reuptake inhibitor dosages

	Usual adult daily dose (mg)	Range (mg)
Fluoxetine (Prozac)	5-20	1-100
Fluvoxamine (Luvox)	50-150	25-300
Paroxetine (Paxil)	20-30	10-50
Sertraline (Zoloft)	25-100	12.5-200
Venlafaxine (Effexor)	75-225	25-375

the desired therapeutic result even before making the transition to another class of antidepressant.[10] (Table 5-2 contrasts common side effects of cyclic and SSRI antidepressants.) The range of dosage of SSRIs is shown in Table 5-5.

ROLE OF BLOOD LEVEL MONITORING IN ANTIDEPRESSANT THERAPY

Since TCAs have been widely used and effective therapeutic agents for many years prior to the availability of plasma level monitoring, it is clear that routine measurement of plasma concentration is generally not necessary for effective therapy. Amitriptyline and imipramine have been the most widely used for the longest period of time, and current research substantiates a linear dose-response relationship for both of these compounds.[78] One recent study has, however, supported a possible therapeutic window for amitriptyline.[79] If a patient fails to respond to a particular dosage of amitriptyline or imipramine, and is indeed taking the medication, it is generally appropriate to increase the dosage and evaluate the response, rather than make the patient incur the considerable expense of plasma level determinations. The effective plasma level for amitriptyline is expressed as the sum of this compound and its major metabolite, nortriptyline.[78] Plasma concentrations of imipramine, as applied clinically, also represent the sum of the parent compound plus its major metabolite, desipramine.[78] Most evidence supports a linear relationship between plasma concentration and therapeutic response when desipramine is used as the therapeutic agent, although one study has suggested a therapeutic window for desipramine wherein plasma concentrations above 155 ng/mL may produce a diminished response.[80] There is considerable variability in the relationship between plasma concentration and therapeutic response for doxepin and its major metabolite, desmethyldoxepin; therefore measurement of serum levels are not likely to be clinically useful. Nortriptyline produces a curvilinear dose-response curve; beyond a plasma concentration of 150 mg/mL, a diminished clinical response is likely to be observed. Although less well established, there may be a similar curvilinear dose-response curve for protriptyline. Thus when an antidepressant with a nonlinear dose-response curve is utilized, increasing the administered dose may decrease the therapeutic response; therefore, the proper clinical application of these later compounds generally requires intermittent monitoring of plasma tricyclic concentration. Table 5-6 presents the generally accepted therapeutic range of plasma levels of some commonly prescribed tricyclic antidepressant drugs.

Since increased plasma concentrations of tricyclic drugs have been well documented in the elderly, occasional plasma level measurements may be useful in geriatric patients if the expected therapeutic response is not achieved at the geriatric dosage level.[53] Most elderly patients do not need tricyclic plasma level monitoring. This technique may at times be useful, however, and facilitate both the safety and the efficacy of treatment.

Table 5-6 Tricyclic antidepressant blood levels

Drug	Range (ng/mL)	Relationship
Imipramine and desipramine (combined levels)	150-250	Linear
Desipramine	150-250	Linear; plateau above 250 ng/mL
	100-155	?Therapeutic window
Amitriptyline and nortriptyline (combined levels)	100-250	Linear
	130-220	?Therapeutic window
Nortriptyline	50-140	Curvilinear; therapeutic window
Protriptyline	80-240	Linear; ?therapeutic window
Doxepin and desmethyldoxepin	120-250	Linear; ?therapeutic window
Maprotiline	150-250	Linear

Clinical application of plasma tricyclic level monitoring is as follows:

1. Not necessary in routine treatment with imipramine and amitriptyline where a linear relationship exists
2. Useful in elderly patients who achieve higher levels with standard doses
3. Useful in nonresponders who may not be taking medication properly
4. Necessary in titrating dosage of tricyclic drugs such as nortriptyline, where curvilinear therapeutic window exists
5. Inadequate data to reliably correlate plasma drug concentration with therapeutic response for amoxapine, trimipramine, and trazodone

Patients of any age who fail to respond to standard tricyclic dosages may benefit from the measurement of plasma tricyclic concentrations. Some individuals will appear to have a dramatic therapeutic response to a tricyclic dose which is far below the standard dose; in such cases it may be both interesting and useful to measure plasma tricyclic concentration. One patient whom I saw in consultation responded very favorably to imipramine at a dose of 10 mg daily, while she was unable to tolerate higher daily dosage. This patient, a middle-aged woman, had a plasma level of approximately 150 ng/ml on her 10 mg daily dose.

Since many patients fail to take their medication according to instructions, or indeed fail to take their medication altogether, in appropriate clinical situations plasma tricyclic monitoring may help to point out the noncompliant patient and give added impetus to a restructuring of the therapeutic relationship. Furthermore, plasma tricyclic level monitoring may be useful in pointing out previously unrecognized drug interactions. It is well known that phenothiazines tend to increase plasma tricyclic concentrations.[10] This may be of therapeutic value in enhancing the therapeutic response to the antidepressant, but could conceivably also facilitate the development of an adverse reaction due to excessive plasma level of the tricyclic.

At this time there are inadequate data to support the correlation of therapeutic response and plasma level for SSRIs, bupropion, amoxapine, trimipramine, or trazodone.

There is evidence that not all drugs are created equal; that is to say, differences in plasma concentration between a standard brand of a given antidepressant and a generic preparation have been recorded in some instances.[81] The differences in therapeutic response and plasma concentrations to different preparations of imipramine were presented before a government hearing. I have treated several patients who have responded initially to a particular brand of either amitriptyline or imipramine; they subsequently lost their beneficial response when they chose to take a generic preparation, and then regained the favorable response when they returned to the initial brand of medication. I have encountered a few patients who complained of greater anticholinergic effect when utilizing a generic preparation, which I have been able to explain by finding higher serum concentration with some generic drugs. When initiating antidepressant drug therapy, it is preferable to utilize a standard preparation, and once the therapeutic response has been established to continue treatment with the same preparation unless the patient requests a generic product. In that case, the response to the generic product may be compared by the patient and physician to the prior response. Unfortunately, the availability of large numbers of generic preparations of amitriptyline, desipramine, and imipramine may cause a situation wherein the patient may receive a product from a different manufacturer each time the prescription is filled, giving rise to considerable potential for unevenness in the therapeutic response.

STIMULANTS AND ALTERNATIVE DRUGS IN DEPRESSION

Dextroamphetamine and methylphenidate are often useful in initiating antidepressant drug therapy, particularly in hospitalized medical patients, in whom it is desirable to achieve an initial mood improvement in a short period of time, which is not possible with conventional antidepressants.[9] These drugs when used in limited dosage for brief interventions present little risk of dependency, yet they are generally underutilized, largely because they are Class II controlled substances, and physicians are often uncomfortable prescribing them. In general, stimulants are not good long-term alternatives to the conventional antidepressants, yet they can be highly beneficial or occasionally lifesaving when there is not time to achieve a response with other agents. These psychostimulants can also be useful adjuncts which may be employed in conjunction with cyclic or SSRI antidepressants to enhance therapeutic response. When more long-term psychostimulant therapy is indicated, magnesium pemoline (Cylert), which like the amphetamines and methylphenidate has dopamine agonist activity, may be a useful agent, particularly since it is a Class IV controlled substance, the prescription of which may be less stigmatizing to the physician.[9] The risk of tolerance and dependence when higher doses of stimulants are employed is likely to be less with pemoline.[9] When using methylphenidate or dextroamphetamine, generally doses of 5 to 10 mg of the former or 5 mg of the latter may be administered 1 to 3 times daily, while with pemoline a dose of 37.5 mg once or twice daily is most reasonable.

Recent antidepressant development has focused heavily on serotonergic compounds, although in former times relatively more attention was given to norepinephrine or dopamine active drugs, which include the amphetamine derivatives and the TCA desipramine. Pharmacologically oriented clinicians have come to recognize correlations between certain behavioral abnormalities and apparent alterations of various neurotransmitters, including serotonin, norepinephrine, dopamine, and acetylcholine.[5] Nomifensine, which is no longer available in the United States due to its association with serious medical complications (including fever and hemolytic anemia), had prominent dopaminergic activity and often produced rapid and dramatic mood improvements. Bupropion is often somewhat beneficial in former nomifensine responders but has much less potent dopaminergic activity. Minaprine, a French drug, has potent dopaminergic and serotonergic as well as weak cholinomimetic activity and demonstrates considerable antidepressant action, although, its patent has expired and it is not likely to be marketed in the United States.[79]

Carbamazepine (Tegretol) has been used for many years in the treatment of trigeminal neuralgia and seizure disorders. Since the late 1970s, numerous studies have found that carbamazepine, which structurally resembles the TCAs, has utility in the treatment of a wide variety of affective disorders, which will be discussed in more detail in chapters 8 and 13. Carbamazepine has been shown to have an antimanic effect acutely and as a maintenance medication. Carbamazepine also has been found to be useful in the treatment and prophylaxis of recurrent depression.[83,84]

TREATMENT-RESISTANT DEPRESSION

Not all patients respond easily and quickly to antidepressant medication. One major cause of antidepressant drug failure is the use of inadequate dosage.[85] The first step in evaluating an apparent treatment-resistant patient is to measure the plasma tricyclic concentration, assess patient compliance, and consider appropriate dosage adjustment of the prescribed medication. Studies have found that patients failing to respond to cyclic antidepressants in spite of adequate plasma level concentration tended to be individuals who have had more previous episodes of depression and higher anxiety scores on the Hamilton Rating Scale.[86]

As previously discussed, some cyclic antidepressants act more specifically on norepinephrine pathways, whereas others exert more potent effects on serotonin neurotransmission. A patient that has failed to respond to one or more norepinephrine-active drugs should generally be given a trial of a serotonergic antidepressant. Unfortunately, the process of choosing the appropriate antidepressant often involves trial and error and may necessitate therapeutic trials of several antidepressants before a satisfactory response is achieved. Some nonpsychotic depressed patients will have a more favorable response when a low dose of a neuroleptic such as trifluoperazine 2 to 6 mg/day is added to the antidepressant regimen.[87]

Although much controversy has surrounded the use of L-triiodothyronine in conjunction with antidepressants, there is considerable literature and clinical experience demonstrating that the use of 25 μg/day of this compound, in conjunction with conventional tricyclic antidepressants, may enhance the speed or magnitude of response to the antidepressant.[88] I have treated patients who, having failed to respond to adequate trials of tricyclic medication, showed, within a matter of several days following addition of 25 μg of L-triiodothyronine, a dramatic improvement in mood. In these patients and in others reported in the literature, measurements of thyroid function were found to be normal prior to initiating therapy.[88] In most instances, triiodothyronine (T$_3$) may be discontinued within several weeks of achieving the desired response, and the patient will continue to do well. However, in some cases, T$_3$ must be continued over a prolonged period of time, along with the antidepressant, in order to achieve a continued therapeutic benefit.

Although there is not total agreement as to the antidepressant efficacy of lithium carbonate (the FDA has not approved this drug as an antidepressant), some studies have indicated its beneficial effect in patients with depressed mood.[89] Although some investigators have found that lithium administered alone may exert an antidepressant effect, this has rarely been my experience. I have, however, used lithium carbonate in conjunction with SSRIs, TCAs, or MAOIs in many patients who have failed to respond to adequate trials of the antidepressant alone. In the majority of these patients, most of whom had recurrent unipolar depression, there was a good-to-dramatic and generally rapid antidepressant response, even though the patient had failed to respond previously to adequate doses of the same antidepressant in the absence of lithium. Controlled studies have confirmed the ability of lithium to augment therapeutic response to a variety of TCAs and MAOI-type antidepressants.[90,91] According to a controlled clinical study, as well as my own extensive clinical experience, the combination of tranylcypromine and lithium carbonate frequently will produce a dramatic clinical improvement in severely treatment-refractory depression.[91]

Carbamazepine 200-600 mg/day may improve depressed mood when used alone or in combination with a cyclic or MAOI-type antidepressant.[92] Furthermore, carbamazepine is worth trying in a patient who has a history of impulsive behavior and recurrent depression, and in whom lithium therapy is either not feasible or not well tolerated.[92] Prior to starting carbamazepine, a complete blood count (CBC), differential white blood count (WBC), and liver function tests should be done. These laboratory procedures should be repeated weekly during the first month of treatment, subsequently at monthly intervals, and eventually, every 2 months if a prolonged course of carbamazepine is employed. Although carbamazepine has been reported to produce leukopenia and agranulocytosis, the incidence of these findings is exceedingly low in comparison to the fears that many physicians have regarding this drug.

Patients that have failed to respond to adequate trials of SSRI or cyclic

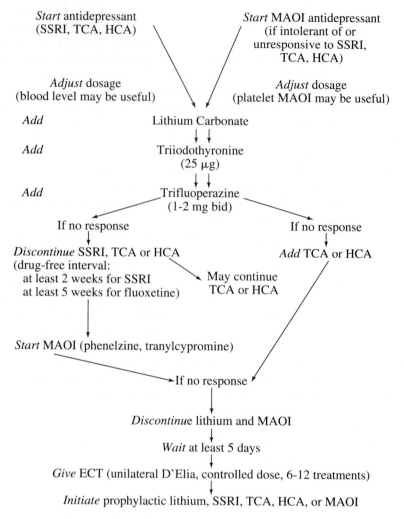

Fig. 5-2 Flowchart for treatment-resistant depression.

antidepressants alone or in combination with one of the above-mentioned augmenting agents should receive an MAOI, which should be initially admininstered alone or in conjunction with lithium carbonate. Many patients who fail to respond to other antidepressants will achieve a satisfactory therapeutic response when treated with adequate doses of an MAOI.[6] Any of the previously mentioned augmenting agents may be used in conjunction with MAOIs and can potentially enhance the therapeutic response. A patient that has not responded satisfactorily to treatment with a single antidepressant agent should next receive a course of combined MAOI–cyclic antidepressant therapy.[93] Since the late 1970s, numerous controlled clinical studies employing combinations of a wide variety of cyclic antidepressants with each of the available MAOIs have been reported.[93] The conclusion of virtually all of these studies has been that the incidence and severity of adverse drug reactions with the combined regimen was comparable with that experienced by patients receiving any one of the antidepressant drugs singly. The major exception is that when SSRIs or clomipramine are combined with MAOI-type antidepressants, the potentially fatal serotonin syndrome may result.[43,44] Less strongly serotonergic drugs such as amitriptyline or trazodone have been safely and effectively combined with MAOIs.

Although there is general agreement about the safety of combined cyclic-MAOI therapy, there are less substantial data from controlled studies supporting enhanced antidepressant efficacy. In my own series of over 200 patients treated with a variety of cyclic antidepressants in conjunction with MAOIs, I have encountered no serious adverse reactions and a very high incidence of favorable therapeutic responses among patients whose depression did not respond to moderate or high-dose treatment with single antidepressant agents. In a retrospective chart review study, the most favorable response to combined antidepressant drug therapy was achieved during simultaneous administration of amitriptyline and tranylcypromine, in which 51% of patients achieved a "very good" response and 27% experienced a "good" response.[93] Specific techniques for the employment of combined cyclic-MAOI regimens are discussed in more detail in chapter 6. Patients whose depression fails to respond to pharmacologic treatment should undergo a course of ECT, after which they should be stabilized on an appropriate prophylactic regimen consisting of a cyclic antidepressant, SSRI, MAOI, or lithium. In some cases, combined lithium-antidepressant drug therapy provides the most effective prophylaxis against recurrent depression. Alternative pharmacologic approaches for treatment-resistant depression are illustrated in Figure 5-2.

UNSUSPECTED DEPRESSIONS

Depression in latency-age children and adolescents is now becoming more commonly recognized. Many youngsters who are depressed will not present with classical symptoms, but rather with behavioral changes which may include obstinance at home and difficulties at school. Not infrequently these children are seen as "acting out," and receive either no treatment or counseling by a nonphysician therapist. These patients often become involved with drugs or sexual activity at an early age and will fail to respond to limit setting, support, or counseling. Many of them are suffering from depressive illness, even though classical vegetative signs are commonly lacking. A therapeutic trial of an SSRI or tricyclic antidepressant in conjunction with individual supportive therapy and family therapy may turn what was previously a nightmare into a therapeutic success.[94] The dosage of antidepressants should initially be somewhat lower than in adults, although generally adolescents will require and respond to conventional adult doses of standard antidepressants. A therapeutic trial of 6 to 8 weeks may be necessary before a favorable response is seen. These medications are generally quite safe and have no known long-term complications. These drugs have been well studied in phobic school children with favorable results.[94] If there is no clear clinical improvement, the medication may be discontinued by gradual tapering without anything having been lost in the treatment of the youngster. On the other hand, failure to treat such individuals with medication may allow the depression to become more severe, with the development of increasing behavioral disturbances and the potential for suicide attempts. We are increasingly recognizing that more severe forms of affective illness, such as bipolar illness, often begin in childhood or adolescence, and considerable experience has demonstrated that lithium may be necessary and therapeutically beneficial in these younger patients.

The diagnosis of depression is too frequently missed in the elderly, who are more apt to be labeled as senile or presenile dementia. Although elderly persons may be demented and may not respond to therapeutic intervention, the failure to treat them may consign them to a less full life than they deserve or are capable of having. The pharmacotherapy of depression in the elderly requires caution and dosages that are generally below the standard adult dosages. Special considerations regarding the application of antidepressants in the elderly are discussed in chapter 16.

DURATION OF TREATMENT AND DISCONTINUATION OF ANTIDEPRESSANTS

Premature discontinuation of antidepressant chemotherapy is a common cause for relapse in depressed patients.[52] In an individual with no prior history and no family history of depressive illness, a 3- to 6-month course of medication is appropriate for the first episode of depression. If an individual has a positive family history or has experienced repeated episodes of depression, it is more reasonable to plan for at least a 12-month course of antidepressant medication followed by cautious tapering of dosage rather than abrupt discontinuation. In general, antidepressant medication should never be withdrawn abruptly; the dose should always be gradually tapered, preferably over a period of several weeks. As the dose is being gradually tapered, recurrence of depressive symptoms should alert the clinician to the need for a continued period of medication maintenance, which can be promptly instituted, allowing for a minimal delay in reestablishing the desired therapeutic effect. In addition to the use of tricyclic, heterocyclic, and SSRI drugs in the maintenance of depressed individuals, some persons with recurrent episodes of depression, even in the absence of mania, may benefit from maintenance lithium therapy alone or in conjunction with an appropriately chosen antidepressant medication.

As our knowledge of the biologic basis of depressive illness becomes more firmly established and as we begin to recognize that for some patients depression is indeed a chronic or lifelong illness with the potential for recurrence, we become better prepared to accept the necessity of more long-term medication maintenance. Indeed, some patients will suffer repeatedly from episodes of severe depression. Clinicians must become increasingly aware of the fact that many such individuals may require maintenance with antidepressant drugs or lithium, or the two agents in combination, for many years or, in some cases, throughout the lifetime of the patient. The willingness of the physician to accept this concept may spell the difference between a functional human being taking a regular daily dose of medication as opposed to a chronically ill patient unable to pursue the occupational and social goals that many of us take for granted. Indeed, medicine has advanced to the point that few physicians would have adverse feelings about prescribing insulin for their diabetic patient or medication for the patient with hypertension throughout the lifetime of the individual. Hopefully, the medical specialty of psychiatry is progressing to the point that practitioners can begin to recognize that many of the concepts of therapeutics applied to other medical problems need not be foreign to the psychiatrist treating the patient who is subject to chronic or recurrent depressive illness.

REFERENCES

1. Dunner DL: Affective disorder: Clinical features. In Michels R, Cavenar JO, Brodie HKH, et al (eds): *Psychiatry*. Philadelphia, JB Lippincott, 1985, vol 1, pp 1-15.
2. American Psychiatric Association: *Diagnostic and statistical manual of mental disorders*, ed 4 [DSM-IV]. Washington DC, American Psychiatric Press, 1994.
3. Covi L, Lipman RS, Derogatis LR, et al: Drugs and group psychotherapy in neurotic depression. *Am J Psychiatry* 1974;131:191-198.
4. Maas JW, Koslow SH, Katz MM, et al: Pretreatment neurotransmitter levels and response to tricyclic antidepressant drugs. *Am J Psychiatry* 1984;141:1159-1171.
5. van Praag HM, Asnis GM, Kahn RS, et al: Monoamines and abnormal behaviour: a multi-aminergic perspective. *Br J Psychiatry* 1990;157:723-734.
6. Potter WZ, Rudorfer MV, Manji H: The pharmacologic treatment of depression. *N Engl J Med* 1991;325:633-642.
7. Janicak PG, Davis JM, Chan C, et al: Failure of urinary MHPG levels to predict treatment response in patients with unipolar depression. *Am J Psychiatry* 1986;143:1398-1402.
8. Klein DF, Gittelman R, Quitkin F, et al: *Diagnosis and drug treatment of psychiatric disorders: adults and children*, ed 2. Baltimore, Williams & Wilkins, 1980.
9. Chiarello RJ, Cole JO: The use of psychostimulants in general psychiatry. *Arch Gen Psychiatry* 1987;44:286-295.
10. Bernstein JG: Drug interactions. In Cassem NH (ed.): *Massachusetts General Hospital Handbook of general hospital psychiatry*, ed 3, St Louis, Mosby, 1991, pp 571-610.
11. McNair DM, Rizley R, Kahn RJ: Amoxapine and speed of onset: new antidepressant faces old methodology. *J Clin Psychiatry Monogr Ser* 1986;4:18-22.
12. Mendels J, Johnston R, Mattes J, et al: Efficacy and safety of b.i.d. doses of venlafaxine in a dose-response study. *Psychopharmacol Bull* 1993;29:169-174.
13. Richelson E: Antidepressants and brain neurochemistry. *Mayo Clin Proc* 1990;65:1227-1236.
14. Kane JM, Lieberman JA (eds): *Adverse effects of psychotropic drugs*. New York, Guilford Press, 1992.

15. Tollefson GD, Senogles SE: A comparison of first and second generation antidepressants at the human muscarinic cholinergic receptor. *J Clin Psychopharmacol* 1983;3:231-234.
16. Bernstein JG: Pharmacologic management of the elderly patient. In Bernstein JG (ed): *Clinical psychopharmacology*, ed 2. Boston, John Wright–PSG, 1984, pp 233-256.
17. Snyder SH, Yamamura HI: Antidepressants and the muscarinic cholinergic receptor. *Arch Gen Psychiatry* 1977;34:236-239.
18. Schatzberg AF, Cole JO, Blumer DP: Speech blockage: a tricyclic side effect. *Am J Psychiatry* 1978;135:600-601.
19. Goldstein DM, Goldberg RL: Monoamine oxidase inhibitor–induced speech blockage. *J Clin Psychiatry* 1986;47:604.
20. Elliot RL, Thomas BJ: A case of alpraxolam-induced stuttering. *J Clin Psychopharmacol* 1985;5:159-160.
21. Jefferson JW: A review of the cardiovascular effects and toxicity of tricyclic antidepressants. *Psychosom Med* 1975;37:160-179.
22. Salzman C: Pharmacologic treatment of depression in the elderly. *J Clin Psychiatry* 1993;54 (2 suppl):23-28.
23. Glassman AH, Preud'homme XA: Review of the cardiovascular effects of heterocyclic antidepressants. *J Clin Psychiatry* 1993;54(2 suppl):16-22.
24. Bernstein JG: Amoxapine: rapid onset and clinical use. *J Clin Psychiatry Monogr Ser* 1986;4:3-8.
25. Goldman LS, Alexander RC, Luchins DJ: Monoamine oxidase inhibitors and tricyclic antidepressants: comparison of their cardiovascular effects. *J Clin Psychiatry* 1986;47:225-229.
26. Bernstein JG: Pharmacotherapy of geriatric depression. *J Clin Psychiatry* 1984;45(10, sec 2):30-34.
27. Montgomery I, Oswald I, Morgan K, et al: Trazodone enhances sleep in subjective quality but not in objective duration. *Br J Clin Pharmacol* 1983;16:139-144.
28. Feighner JP, Pambakian R, Fowler RC, et al: A comparison of nefazodone, imipramine, and placebo in patients with moderate to severe depression. *Psychopharmacol Bull* 1989;25:219-221.
29. Segraves RT: Overview of sexual dysfunction complicating the treatment of depression. *J Clin Psychiatry Monogr* 1992;10(2):4-10.
30. Segraves RT: Treatment-emergent sexual dysfunction in affective disorder: a review and management strategies. *J Clin Psychiatry Monogr* 1993;11(1):57-60.
31. Zajecka J, Fawcett J, Schaff M, et al: The role of serotonin in sexual dysfunction: fluoxetine-associated orgasm dysfunction. *J Clin Psychiatry* 1991;52:66-68.
32. DeCastro R: Reversal of MAOI-induced anorgasmia with cyproheptadine. *Am J Psychiatry* 1985;142:783.
33. Goldbloom DS, Kennedy SH: Adverse interaction of fluoxetine and cyproheptadine in two patients with bulimia nervosa. *J Clin Psychiatry* 1991;52:261-262.
34. Gartrell N: Increased libido in women receiving trazodone. *Am J Psychiatry* 1986;143:781-782.
35. Scher M, Frieger JN, Juergens S: Trazodone and priapism. *Am J Psychiatry* 1983;140:1362-1363.
36. Warner MD, Peabody CA, Whiteford HA, et al: Trazodone and priapism. *J Clin Psychiatry* 1987;48:244-245.
37. Rosenstein DL, Nelson JC, Jacobs SC: Seizures associated with antidepressants: a review. *J Clin Psychiatry* 1993;54:289-299.
38. Dessain EL, Schatzberg AF, Woods BT, et al: Maprotiline treatment in depression. *Arch Gen Psychiatry* 1986;43:86-90.
39. Garvey MJ, Tollefson GD: Occurrence of myoclonus in patients treated with cyclic antidepressants. *Arch Gen Psychiatry* 1987;44:269-272.
40. Gaffney GR, Tune LE: Serum neuroleptic levels and extrapyramidal side effects in patients treated with amoxapine. *J Clin Psychiatry* 1985;46:428-429.
41. Seeman, P: Neuroleptics. In Kalant H, Roschlau HE, Sellers EM (eds): *Principles of medical pharmacology*, ed 4. Toronto, University of Toronto Press, 1985, p 329.
42. Demuth GW, Breslow RE, Drescher J: The elicitation of a movement disorder by trazodone: case report. *J Clin Psychiatry* 1985;46:535-536.
43. Sternbach H: The serotonin syndrome. *Am J Psychiatry* 1991;148:705-713.

44. Beasley CM Jr, Masica DN, Heiligenstein JH, et al: Possible monoamine oxidase inhibitor-serotonin uptake inhibitor interaction: fluoxetine clinical data and preclinical findings. *J Clin Psychopharmacol* 1993;13:312-320.

45. Barrnett J, Frances A, Kocsis J, et al: Peripheral edema associated with trazodone: a report of ten cases. *J Clin Psychopharmacol* 1985;5:161-164.

46. Gamble DE, Peterson LG: Trazodone overdose: four years of experience from voluntary reports. *J Clin Psychiatry* 1986;47:544-546.

47. Lawrence JM: Reactions of withdrawal of antidepressants, antiparkinsonian drugs, and lithium. *Psychosomatics* 1985;26:869-875.

48. Dilsaver SC, Kronfol Z, Sackelaves JC, et al: Antidepressant withdrawal syndrome: evidence supporting the cholinergic over-drive hypothesis. *J Clin Psychopharmacol* 1983;3:157-164.

49. Robertson MM, Trimble MR: Major tranquilizers used as antidepressants. *J Affective Disord* 1982;4:173-193.

50. Mendels J, Schless AP: Comparative efficacy of alprazolam, imipramine, and placebo administered once a day in treating depressed patients. *J Clin Psychiatry* 1986;47:357-361.

51. Anton RF, Hitri A, Diamond BI: Amoxapine treatment of psychotic depression: dose effect and dopamine blockade. *J Clin Psychiatry Monogr Ser* 1986;4:32-36.

52. Kupfer DJ, Frank E, Perel JM, et al: Five-year outcome for maintenance therapies in recurrent depression. *Arch Gen Psychiatry* 1992;49:769-773.

53. Nies A, Robinson DS, Friedman MJ, et al: Relationship between age and tricyclic plasma levels. *Am J Psychiatry* 1977;134:790-793.

54. Van Kammen DP, Murphy DL: Prediction of imipramine antidepressant response by a one-day *d*-amphetamine trial. *Am J Psychiatry* 1978;135:1179-1184.

55. Sabelli HC, Fawcett J, Javaid JI: The methylphenidate test for differentiating desipramine-responsive from nortriptyline-responsive depression. *Am J Psychiatry* 1983;140:212-214.

56. Settle EC: Bupropion: general side effects. *J Clin Psychiatry Monogr* 1993;11(1):33-39.

57. Roose SP, Dalack GW, Glassman AH, et al: Cardiovascular effects of bupropion in depressed patients with heart disease. *Am J Psychiatry* 1991;148:512-516.

58. Ferris RM, Cooper BR: Mechanism of antidepressant activity of bupropion. *J Clin Psychiatr Monogr* 1993;11(1):2-14.

59. Zisook S: Efficacy of bupropion. *J Clin Psychiatry Monogr* 1993;11(1):20-29.

60. Haykal RF, Akiskal HS: Bupropion as a promising approach to rapid cycling bipolar II patients. *J Clin Psychiatry* 1990;51:450-455.

61. Johnston JA, Lineberry CG, Ascher JA, et al: A 102-center prospective study of seizure in association with bupropion. *J Clin Psychiatry* 1991;52:450-456.

62. Stokes PE: Fluoxetine: a five-year review. *Clin Ther* 1993;15:216-243.

63. Wilde MI, Plosker GL, Benfield P: Fluvoxamine: an updated review of its pharmacology and therapeutic use in depressive illness. *Drugs* 1993;46:895-924.

64. Nemeroff CB: Paroxetine: an overview of the efficacy and safety of a new selective serotonin reuptake inhibitor in the treatment of depression. *J Clin Psychopharmacol* 1993;13(suppl 2):10-17.

65. Aguglia E, Casacchia M, Cassano GB, et al: Double-blind study of the efficacy and safety of sertraline versus fluoxetine in major depression. *Int Clin Psychopharmacol* 1993;8:197-202.

66. Muth EA, Moyer JA, Haskins JT, et al: Biochemical, neurophysiological, and behavioral effects of Wy-45,233 and other identified metabolites of the antidepressant venlafaxine. *Drug Dev Res* 1991;23:191-199.

67. Schweitzer E, Feighner J, Mandos LA, Rickels K: Comparison of venlafaxine and imipramine in the acute treatment of major depression in outpatients. *J Clin Psychiatry* 1994;55:104-108.

68. Benkelfat C, Murphy DL, Zohar J, et al: Clomipramine in obsessive-compulsive disorder: further evidence for a serotonergic mechanism of action. *Arch Gen Psychiatry* 1989;46:23-28.

69. Shen WW, Lin KM: Cytochrome P-450 monooxygenases and interactions of psychotropic drugs. *Int J Psychiatry Med* 1991;21:47-56.

70. Ciraulo DA, Shader RI: Fluoxetine drug-drug interactions. I, Antidepressants and antipsychotics. *J Clin Psychopharmacol* 1990;10:48-50.

71. Preskorn SH, Alderman J, Chung M, et al: Pharmacokinetics of desipramine coadministered with sertraline and fluoxetine. *J Clin Psychopharmacol* 1994;14:90-98.

72. Pato MT, Murphy DL, DeVane CL: Sustained plasma concentrations of fluoxetine and/or norfluoxetine four and eight weeks after fluoxetine discontinuation. [Letter to the editor.] *J Clin Psychopharmacol* 1991;11:224-225.

73. Ciraulo DA, Shader RI: Fluoxetine drug-drug interactions. II, *J Clin Psychopharmacol* 1990;10:213-217.

74. Rosenstein DL, Takeshita J, Nelson JC: Fluoxetine-induced elevation and prolongation of tricyclic levels in overdose. [Letter to the editor.] *Am J Psychiatry* 1991;148:807.

75. Cole JO: New directions in antidepressant therapy: a review of sertraline, a unique serotonin reuptake inhibitor. [Academic Highlights.] *J Clin Psychiatry* 1992;53:333-340.

76. Wernicke JF, Dunlop SR, Dornseif BE, et al: Low-dose fluoxetine therapy for depression. *Psychopharmacology Bull* 1988;24:183-188.

77. Montgomery SA: Venlafaxine: a new dimension in antidepressant pharmacotherapy. [Academic Highlights.] *J Clin Psychiatry* 1993;54:119-126.

78. Perry PJ, Pfohl BM, Holstad SG: The relationship between antidepressant response and tricyclic antidepressant plasma concentrations. *Clin Pharmacokinet* 1987;13:381-392.

79. Boyer WF, Lake CR: Initial severity and diagnosis influence the relationship of tricyclic plasma levels to response: a statistical review. *J Clin Psychopharmacol* 1987;7:67-71.

80. Coryell W, Turner RD, Sherman A: Desipramine plasma levels and clinical response: evidence for curvilinear relationship. *J Clin Psychopharmacol* 1987;7:67-71.

81. Tricyclic antidepressants: proposed bioequivalence requirement. *Fed Reg* 1978;43:34.

82. Amsterdam JD, Dunner DL, Fabre LF, et al: Double-blind, placebo controlled, fixed dose trial of Minaprine in patients with major depression. *Pharmacopsychiatry* 1989;22:137-143.

83. Ballenger JC, Post RM, Bunney WE: Carbamazepine in manic-depressive illness: a new treatment. *Am J Psychiatry* 1980;137:782-790.

84. Stuppaeck CH, Barnas C, Schwitzer J, et al: Carbamazepine in the prophylaxis of major depression: a 5-year follow-up. *J Clin Psychiatry* 1994;55:146-150.

85. Lydiard RB: Tricyclic-resistant depression: treatment resistance or inadequate treatment? *J Clin Psychiatry* 1985;46:412-417.

86. Roose S, Glassman AH, Walsh BT, et al: Tricyclic non-responders: Phenomenology and treatment. *Am J Psychiatry* 1986;143:345-358.

87. Stern SI, Mendels J: Drug combinations in the treatment of refractory depression: a review. *J Clin Psychiatry* 1981;42:368-373.

88. Goodwin FK, Prange AJ Jr, Post RM, et al: Potentiation of antidepressant effects by L-triiodothyronine in tricyclic non-responders. *Am J Psychiatry* 1982;139:34-38.

89. Ortiz A, Dabbagh M, Gershon S: Lithium: clinical use, toxicology, and mode of action. In Bernstein JG (ed): *Clinical psychopharmacology,* ed 2. Boston, John Wright–PSG, 1984, pp 111-144.

90. Heninger GR, Charney DS, Sternberg DE: Lithium carbonate augmentation of antidepressant treatment: an effective prescription for treatment-refractory depression. *Arch Gen Psychiatry* 1983;40:1335-1342.

91. Price LH, Charney DS, Heninger GR: Efficacy of lithium-tranylcypromine treatment in refractory depression. *Am J Psychiatry* 1985;142:619-623.

92. Folks DG: Carbamazepine treatment of selected affectively disordered inpatients. *Am J Psychiatry* 1982;139:115-117.

93. Schmauss M, Kapfhammer HP, Meyr P, et al: Combined MAO-inhibitor and tri-(tetra)cyclic antidepressant in therapy resistant depression: a retrospective study. *Pharmacopsychiatry* 1986;19:251-252.

94. Gittelman R, Kanner A: Overview of clinical psychopharmacology in childhood disorders. In Bernstein JG (ed): *Clinical psychopharmacology,* ed 2. Boston, John Wright–PSG, 1984, pp 189-210.

CHAPTER 6

Monoamine Oxidase Inhibitors

OVERVIEW

Guidelines for Monoamine Oxidase Inhibitor Therapy

1. Carefully evaluate patient; assess potential interaction of medical conditions or other treatments with MAO inhibitor.
2. Assess patient's ability to understand and follow the important dietary and medication restrictions.
3. Carefully instruct patient orally, and use printed format regarding food and medication restrictions.
4. MAOIs cannot be combined with SSRIs or clomipramine. Fluoxetine must be discontinued at least 5 weeks before starting MAOI; other SSRIs should be stopped 2 weeks before starting MAOIs. Three weeks should elapse between clomipramine and MAOIs. MAOIs must be stopped at least 2 weeks before starting SSRI.
5. If a patient is to be changed from an MAOI to a tricyclic, approximately 10 days will be required to return monoamine oxidase enzyme levels to normal; thus, either wait between medications or start low doses of tricyclic with gradual titration.
6. Combined MAOI-tricyclic antidepressant therapy is safe and may add to efficacy. Generally the MAOI is added gradually to an established tricyclic drug regimen. Patients already taking MAOIs may have a tricyclic such as imipramine or amitriptyline added cautiously, with gradual dosage increase.
7. Phenelzine is often the best MAOI to start with in the anxious depressed patient, or the patient with panic disorder.
8. Tranylcypromine is preferable in the nonanxious, withdrawn, depressed patient and may produce some initial antidepressant response as early as the second or third day of treatment.
9. Lithium carbonate and low-dose haloperidol or trifluoperazine may be used safely with an MAOI.

Continued.

153

10. Postural hypotension is the commonest side effect of MAOI treatment; it will be worsened by chlorpromazine and thioridazine. Advise patient to change position slowly, increase dietary salt intake, or use salt tablets. Tranylcypromine may produce less postural hypotension than phenelzine.

11. Hypertensive reactions generally respond to lying down in a quiet darkened environment; mild sedatives may be useful. Moderate to severe reactions may be treated with sublingual nifedipine or IV phentolamine. Chlorpromazine and thioridazine may produce uncontrolled hypotension and should not be utilized.

12. MAOI therapy may be beneficial in mild, moderate, and severe depression with or without neurovegetative signs. MAOIs should be employed cautiously if at all in patients with psychotic symptoms. Patients with panic disorder, anxiety, phobias, obsessions, hypochondriasis, somatization, fatigue, and anergia and those with atypical depression often respond exceedingly well to MAOI therapy.

The antidepressant effect of iproniazid was initially observed through a fortunate therapeutic accident. This compound, which closely resembles isoniazid, was initially utilized to treat tuberculosis in the mid-1950s. Some of the early patients to receive this drug were observed to become energized and, indeed, hyperactive.[1] As investigators assessed the response of these tuberculous patients, who had sustained lengthy inactive stays in sanitoria, it became apparent that many of these persons had been depressed and were experiencing an improvement in mood in response to this new therapy. Other patients had become manic in response to iproniazid. These observations, and the recognition that this compound inhibits the enzyme monoamine oxidase (MAO), led to some early correlations between brain chemistry and mood. These observations sparked a series of clinical studies on the antidepressant efficacy of iproniazid, and also gave rise to a new therapeutic agent which, along with reserpine, the first antipsychotic drug, became a cornerstone in the development of what has become a major field in medicine, psychopharmacology.[2]

The early clinical trials of iproniazid yielded encouraging results with respect to its ability to alleviate depressed mood. Many attempts to confirm therapeutic efficacy by double-blind control studies were less convincing. Indeed, many of the early controlled studies of the efficacy of the MAO inhibitors (MAOIs) were discouraging.[3] We now recognize that the dosages of MAOIs employed often produced inadequate levels of MAO inhibition.[4,5]

Newer technology has allowed us to correlate clinical efficacy not only with the dosage of these compounds, but also with the degree of platelet MAO inhibition.[5]

In addition to the controversies regarding therapeutic efficacy, two more serious problems arose. Unfortunately, they have continued to this day to color the thinking of physicians with regard to the safety of this group of therapeutic agents. Some of the earlier MAOIs, including iproniazid, which was eventually removed from the market, produced hepatocellular damage.[2] The more widely known and feared adverse effect of the MAOIs, however, was the ability to produce a hypertensive reaction, which in a number of instances did culminate in a full-blown cerebrovascular accident.[2] It is important for clinicians to realize that MAOIs were rather widely employed in the treatment of depression for a number of years before the cause of these hypertensive reactions was recognized. In the early years, clinicians were unaware of the interaction between tyramine-rich foods and MAOIs, or the more serious potential of an adverse hypertensive reaction when MAO inhibitors were utilized simultaneously with stimulants such as the amphetamines or with vasoconstrictors used as nasal decongestants. Once the interaction between MAO inhibitors and tyramine or phenylethylamine compounds was recognized it became standard clinical practice to warn all patients taking MAOIs of this risk.[2] The proper warning regarding which foods and medications to avoid has significantly decreased the incidence of hypertensive reaction so that it rarely occurs in a properly instructed and reasonably cooperative patient. Nevertheless, the fears generated by the early therapeutic misadventures have continued to persist and indeed have caused many physicians to avoid prescribing MAOIs. The persistence of these fears has caused many physicians and pharmacists to tell patients who are receiving MAOIs that the person recommending this treatment is doing them an injustice. The persistence of these old fears has generated frightening statements which continue to be carried in package inserts and *Physicians' Desk Reference* monographs on these drugs. The removal from the market of the more hepatotoxic MAOIs has contributed to the safety of this form of treatment.[2] Although the SSRI compounds have become the most popular antidepressants, they have not made the clinical use of MAOIs obsolete; yet they have introduced a serious risk, their potentially fatal interaction with MAOIs, which all clinicians must be aware of and guard against.

INFORMING PATIENTS ABOUT MONOAMINE OXIDASE INHIBITORS

The most important information that needs to be imparted to any clinician learning about MAOIs is that they are far more effective and safer than earlier experiences indicated. At the same time, it is essential for any clinician who prescribes MAOIs to provide thorough information in printed form regarding the safe use of these drugs and the dietary and medication restrictions which

Table 6-1 Tyramine content of cheeses

Type of cheese	Tyramine (µg/g)	Reference(s)
Argenti (imported)	168	7
Blue (Danish)	31-256	6
Brick (Canadian)	524	6
Brie	0-260	8
Camembert (American)	86	9
Camembert (Danish)	23-1340	6
Cheddar, fresh (Canadian)	120	6
Cheddar, center cut (Canadian)	192	6
Cheddar, old center (Canadian)	1530	6
Cheddar, New York State	1416	7
Cheddar (25 samples)	25-2330 (average 384)	8
Colby	100-560	8
Cream cheese	<0.2	7
Cottage cheese	<0.2	7
Edam	300-320	8
Emmenthaler	225-1000	7
Gouda	20-670	8
Gruyere (American)	516	7
Gruyere (British)	11-1184	10
Limburger	204	7
Liederkranz	1226; 1683	7
Mozzarella	410	6
Munster	110	7
D'Oka (imported)	310; 158	7
Parmesan (American)	4-290	6
Parmesan (Italian)	65	6
Processed (American)	50	9
Processed (Canadian)	26	6
Provolone	38-150	13
Romano	80-238	8
Roquefort (French)	27-520	6
Swiss	50-1800	8
Stilton	460-2170	8
Yogurt	<0.2	10

From DaPrada M, Zurcher G: *Psychopharmacology* 1992; 106 (suppl):32-34.

must be followed. Tables 6-1, 6-2, and 6-3 provide data on the tyramine content of various cheeses,[6-10] other foods,[10-15] and alcoholic beverages,[7,10,13,16,17] and will serve as a guide to the physician when discussing dietary restrictions with the patient receiving MAOI therapy. The warning the patient receives about the potential interactions of these drugs must be clear, but must not

Table 6-2 Tyramine content of selected
foods and alcoholic beverages

	Tyramine (µg/g)	Reference(s)
Food		
Avocado (fresh)	23	11
Banana peel	65 (dopamine 70 µg/g)	10, 11
Banana pulp	7	11
Broad beans, pods	dopamine	10
Cocoa powder	0.1-2.8	12
Eggplant	3	11
Grapes, raisins	0	11
Herring, pickled	Up to 3030	10
Liver, chicken (not refrigerated)	94-113	10
Liver, chicken, fresh	0	10
Liver, beef, spoiled	274	10
Liver, beef, fresh	5.4	10
Marmite (yeast extract)	1639-1807	13
Meat extracts (soup, gravy bases)	95-304	9, 13
Orange	10	11
Plum (red)	6	11
Potato	1	11
Raspberries	12.8-95.5	10
Raspberry jam	Up to 38.4	10
Sauerkraut	20-95	10
Sausage, Belgian dry-fermented	101.8-1506	10
Sausage, dry-fermented	244	10
Sausage, semi–dry-fermented	85.5	10
Soybean paste	0.2-169.5	14
Soy sauce, chemically hydrolyzed	1.8	10
Soy sauce, Japanese	136.6-882	14
Soy sauce, Tamari	466	15
Spinach	1	11
Tomato	4	11
Yeast extract	2057-2256	13
Alcoholic beverage		
Ale	Average 8.8	13
Beer (various types)	0.6-11.2	7, 13
Beer (tap)	26-113	21
Distilled spirits	Negligible	10, 17
Wines		
Chianti	25.4	7, 10
Port	0.2	7
Red	0.3-1.3	16
Riesling	0.6	7
Sauterne	0.4	7
Sherry	3.6	7
Vermouth	High	10

Table 6-3 Tyramine content of some typical oriental and far eastern foods

Food (country)	Tyramine (mg/100 g)
Vegetarian curd, cooked (Taiwan)	4.8
Duck, dried, breast (China)	3.53
Sausages	3.06
Tofu, dehydrated mix (Japan)	0.009
Tofu, fried (Hong Kong)	0.066
Soya bean (miso) soup (Japan)	0.182
Bean curd with vegetables (China)	0.48
Soya bean salad (China)	0.12
Noodles, fried (China)	1.06
Bean sprouts (China)	0.48
Spring roll (China)	0.138
Wonton soup (China)	0.102
Soup, bean curd base (Korea)	0.439
Glass noodles and mushrooms (Korea)	3.36
Hot vegetable pickles (Korea)	3.14
Sweet and sour beef (Korea)	2.18
Korean beer (Korea)	4.00
Malasian curry (Indonesia)	3.84
Dry curry (India)	1.27
Rice, basmati (India)	0.043
Papaya salad (Thai)	0.358
Fried rice, beef (Thai)	0.165
Chicken and coconut sauce (Thai)	6.31
Fried chicken and ginger (Thai)	1.08
Chicken and bamboo curry (Thai)	2.25

From DaPrada M, Zurcher G: *Psychopharmacology* 1992; 106 (suppl):32-34.

frighten the patient away from utilizing these highly effective therapeutic agents.[10] The printed instructions which I use for patients taking MAOIs are reproduced in Appendix A, and may be photocopied for distribution to MAOI-treated patients.

FOOD AND DRUG INTERACTIONS OF MONAMINE OXIDASE INHIBITORS

Although it may seem unconventional to begin the discussion of a class of therapeutic agents by considering drug interactions, this is the first problem that many clinicians think of when MAOI antidepressants are mentioned. Indeed, the incidence of hypertensive crises during treatment with MAOIs is very low and virtually nonexistent among patients who are carefully instructed and followed by their physician. Nevertheless, if a hypertensive reaction occurs, the consequences may be serious in that a dramatic, persistent rise in blood pressure that is undetected and untreated may be associated with the occurrence of intracranial hemorrhage. Most hypertensive reactions are quite minor and produce only a 20 or 30 mmHg rise in systolic blood pressure associated with headache, flushing, and sweating. Mild hypertensive reactions can occur following the consumption of 6 mg of tyramine while receiving an MAOI.[10,18] Moderate to severe hypertensive reactions generally require the consumption of 10 to 25 mg or more of tyramine orally.[10,18] Cerebrovascular accidents resulting from an MAOI-associated hypertensive reaction are rare.[18] Studies have found that a significant proportion of MAOI-treated patients follow their diet rather casually, yet do not experience hypertensive reactions.[19] Patients who are given a less restrictive diet and thorough instructions regarding the foods that must be absolutely avoided and those which may be consumed cautiously and in limited quantity are more likely to comply with these restrictions.[20] Surveys have been conducted of the various MAOI instructions provided to patients, and a considerable diversity of foods, both permitted and restricted, has been found.[17] Indeed, the list provided in the *Physicians' Desk Reference,* and in patient instruction sheets provided by pharmaceutical manufacturers, as well as in various lay books on drug therapy, proscribe many substances which are in fact not hazardous to the MAOI-treated patient.[18,20]

Tyramine provokes the release of norepinephrine from endogenous stores in the body, and through this mechanism may provoke a hypertensive reaction in the absence of the body's ability to degrade ingested tyramine and endogenous catecholamines.[10,18] Although most dietary instructions advise against consumption of beans and bananas, these foods do not contain significant amounts of tyramine. The pod of the Italian broad (fava) bean and the peel of the banana contain large amounts of dopamine, a potent pressor substance, which may provoke a hypertensive reaction, although consumption of the beans themselves and the pulp of the banana carries no risk.[10] Most lists warn against chocolate, raisins, and canned figs, none of which are likely to produce a hypertensive reaction. Much of the information that led to MAOI dietary restrictions resulted from single, often not well-documented, case reports. Since patients may discover on their own that they can eat many of the items on their restricted list, they may explore further dietary indiscretions and eventually eat a substance that is truly dangerous.[18,19]

Alcoholic spirits, including bourbon, scotch, rum, gin, and vodka, contain no significant amounts of tyramine, and therefore will not produce a hypertensive reaction, although they may produce excessive CNS depression as a result of their pharmacologic actions being potentiated by MAOIs.[10,18] Hypertensive reactions produced by wine have generally resulted from the consumption of Chianti; occasional reports have incriminated vermouth.[10,18] Some publications have indicated a lower tyramine content in white wine than in red wine; others, however, have reported just the opposite.[10,13] As can be seen from Table 6-1, the tyramine content of wine is relatively low and not greatly different between red and white wine. If the volume of wine or beer consumed is kept to about 3 oz daily and other tyramine-rich foods are not consumed, it is highly unlikely that a hypertensive reaction will result. One of the greatest difficulties in assessing the relative dangers of different foods is that the same food subjected to different fermentation or storage conditions may have widely divergent levels of tyramine, as in the case of chicken liver and sausage.[10] Samples taken from different places in the same block of cheese may show dramatically different tyramine concentrations.[10] Increasing clinical experience with MAOIs over the years of their use indicates that most dietary constituents produce a lesser risk of a severe hypertensive reaction than formerly believed.[17] A case in point is that bottled beer or canned beer seems to be relatively safer than previously thought, although tap beer is more likely to raise blood pressure.[21]

The best advice that can be given regarding dietary precautions with MAOI therapy is that any protein food subjected to fermentation during its processing or storage may present the risk of a hypertensive reaction. Foods that are likely to be high in tyramine content, such as cheeses, Chianti, sausages, pickled herring, yeast extracts, and meat extracts, should be avoided. Foods containing small amounts of tyramine may be eaten cautiously in small quantities once the patient has stabilized on an MAOI regimen. Some foods contain histamine, which may provoke headache, dizziness, flushing, and sweating, but will not produce a hypertensive reaction.[8] Many patients taking MAO inhibitors will experience postural hypotension related to the drug therapy but unrelated to simultaneous consumption of foods or other medication.[18] The symptoms of hypotensive reactions may be quite similar to those of a hypertensive reaction and may be confused with the latter by the patient and the physician.[17,18] Alerting patients to the possibility of postural hypotension in association with MAOI therapy is of clinical importance since it may minimize the risk of a patient being frightened and suspecting that he has experienced a hypertensive crisis.

The artificial sweetner aspartame is metabolized to phenylalanine and aspartic acid. The former amino acid could provoke a hypertensive reaction in an MAOI-treated patient, and is more likely to enter the brain if consumed in conjunction with carbohydrates such as bread or other starches or sweets. A hypertensive reaction has been reported in an MAOI-treated patient who used large quantities of aspartame-sweetened beverages along with carbohydrate-containing food.[22] MAOI-treated patients should be advised to consume no more than 1 g of aspartame per day. Although a clinical study found no evidence that the flavor-enhancing substance monosodium glutamate elevates blood pressure in MAOI-treated patients,[23] I have seen a number of patients experience dizziness and headache after consuming monosodium glutamate during MAOI therapy.

Prior to the advent of serotonin selective reuptake inhibitors, the most dangerous interaction was the coadministration of an MAOI with the narcotic meperidine, which is known to provoke hypertension, hyperpyrexia, seizures, and potentially death.[2,18] It is generally believed that this potentially fatal interaction with meperidine is due to a combination of massive catecholamine and serotonin activity.[2] The meperidine-MAOI interaction closely resembles the serotonin syndrome, which may result when an MAOI is administered along with the serotonin precursor tryptophan, an SSRI antidepressant, or clomipramine. In view of the widespread use of the large variety of SSRIs currently available, their coadministration with MAOIs represents the most common dangerous interaction of MAOI therapy. The serotonin syndrome consists of confusion or hypomania, accompanied by restlessness, myoclonus, hyperreflexia, diaphoresis, shivering, hyperpyrexia, and tremor, and may be fatal.[24] Symptoms of the serotonin syndrome vary in severity, and not all symptoms need be present to make a diagnosis. This syndrome bears a striking similarity to neuroleptic malignant syndrome as discussed in chapter 10. Prior to initiating MAOI therapy, the patient must have discontinued fluoxetine at least 5 weeks previously (longer if daily doses exceeded 20 mg), other SSRIs should be discontinued approximately 2 weeks before starting an MAOI,[24,25] and 3 weeks should elapse after clomipramine before starting an MAOI.[24,25] Generally 2 weeks should elapse after discontinuing MAOI therapy prior to initiating SSRI medications. Although it was initially thought that the selective MAO-B inhibitor selegiline and the reversible selective MAO-A inhibitor moclobemide did not require these precautions, clinical experience has yielded significant interactions between selegiline and SSRIs and dangerous interactions have been observed when moclobemide and an SSRI were coadministered.[26,27] I generally recommend that my MAOI treated patients wear a MedicAlert identification indicating that they are receiving MAOI drugs and that this identification specifically state that they are "allergic to meperidine and selective serotonin drugs" since I am not always confident that the physician they encounter in an emergency situation will be familiar with these potentially serious drug interactions. Although there have been occasional reports in the literature of interactions between dextromethorphan, propoxyphene, and other narcotic-derived drugs with MAOIs, these reactions have rarely been serious when opiates other than meperidine have been administered at relatively low doses.[28,29] There is substantial evidence that morphine can be safely used for severe pain during MAOI treatment.[29] Furthermore, I routinely allow MAOI-treated patients to use cough syrups containing 5 mg of dextromethorphan up to 4 times daily when needed, and have never encountered an adverse reaction.

Phenylethylamine compounds, including amphetamine, phenylpropanolamine, phenylephrine, and related stimulants, decongestants, and bronchodilators may all provoke hypertensive reactions in MAOI-treated patients. The hypertensive reactions provoked by these compounds result from the release of catecholamines from endogenous stores.[2,18] Patients receiving MAOI therapy should be informed that they must avoid stimulants, appetite suppressants, decongestants, and bronchodilators, which may all provoke hypertensive reactions. Generally, asthmatic patients, who must continuously or intermittently receive bronchodilator therapy, should not receive MAOIs. Those with mild bronchial asthma who require MAOI therapy should use a beclomethasone inhaler rather than one containing isoproterenol or other beta-adrenergic bronchodilator. Patients must be urged to tell any physician whom they may consult that they are receiving an MAOI prior to receiving a prescription for any medication. I encourage my patients to contact me prior to taking any other medication while they are receiving MAOI therapy.

COMPARISON OF MONOAMINE OXIDASE INHIBITORS

There are currently only two monoamine oxidase inhibitor antidepressants marketed in the United States—phenelzine, which is a hydrazine compound, and tranylcypromine, a nonhydrazine. The hydrazine nucleus implies some potential for hepatotoxicity, as in the case of iproniazid (the first-marketed MAOI). Although the risk of hepatotoxicity with phenelzine is very low, its use should generally be avoided in patients with liver disease. Isocarboxyzid is a hydrazine MAOI which has not been widely used in recent years and is no longer being marketed in the United States. Pargyline, a nonhydrazine, relatively selective, MAO-B inhibitor, which was formerly used primarily in the treatment of hypertension, has likewise been removed from the U.S. market due mainly to small volume sales. Selegiline is a selective inhibitor of MAO-B used primarily in the treatment of Parkinson's disease and secondarily in depression. Moclobemide is a reversible inhibitor of MAO-A (RIMA) which is marketed throughout the world; however, it remains an investigational drug in the United States, its primary virtue being its relative safety in the absence of dietary restrictions, yet it cannot be combined with meperidine, clomipramine, or SSRIs. Table 6-4 shows some characteristics of currently employed MAOIs.

Phenelzine

Phenelzine (Nardil) is the MAOI which has been most widely studied and used clinically and is the subject of the most extensive clinical study.[5,30-36] It has a mild sedating effect and appears to have specific antianxiety activity.[50,65,69] In addition to its antidepressant effect, this compound is very effective in controlling panic attacks, as well as phobic and obsessive symptoms.[5,37-39] When compared with tricyclic and SSRI antidepressants, phenelzine is often superior in controlling agoraphobia, and has revolutionized the treatment of this condition.[37-39] In addition, many depressed patients who do not respond satisfactorily to SSRI or tricyclic compounds will have a considerable mood improvement with this agent.[40] Earlier studies of phenelzine found it to be no better than placebo in severely depressed patients.[3] However, in the past 2 decades numerous investigators have correlated antidepressant efficacy with the

Table 6-4   Monoamine oxidase inhibitors*

Drug	Class	Dosage range (mg/day)	MAOI diet	Special characteristics
Phenelzine (Nardil)	Nonselective (hydrazine)	30-90	Yes	Atypical depression; anxious, phobic, obsessional patients Effect may be enhanced when combined with TCAs or lithium
Tranylcypromine (Parnate)	Nonselective (nonhydrazine)	20-60	Yes	Direct stimulant effect, often rapid onset Useful in fatigued anergic patients Effect may be enhanced when combined with TCA or Li
Selegiline (Eldepryl)	Selective MAO-B (nonselective)	5-15	No	20 mg/day or more requires dietary restriction
		20-50	Yes	Stimulant, energizing properties; tolerated and effective in some who cannot take other MAOIs
Moclobemide	Selective MAO-A (reversible [RIMA])	300-600	No	Minimal hypotension, excitation, and sexual effects Efficacy similar to that of other MAOIs but terminate more rapidly after discontinuation

*It must be noted that none of these MAOIs can be safely combined with clomipramine or any SSRI.

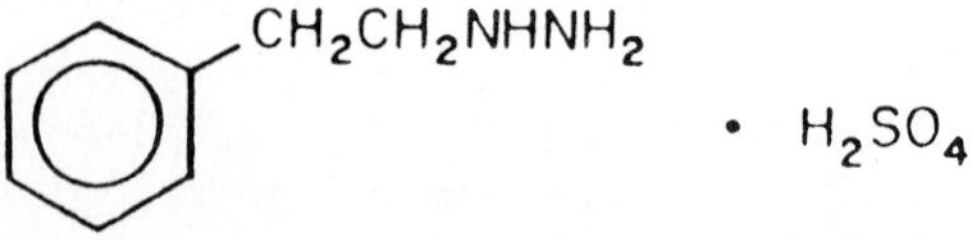

$CH_2CH_2NHNH_2$

$\bullet \ H_2SO_4$

PHENELZINE

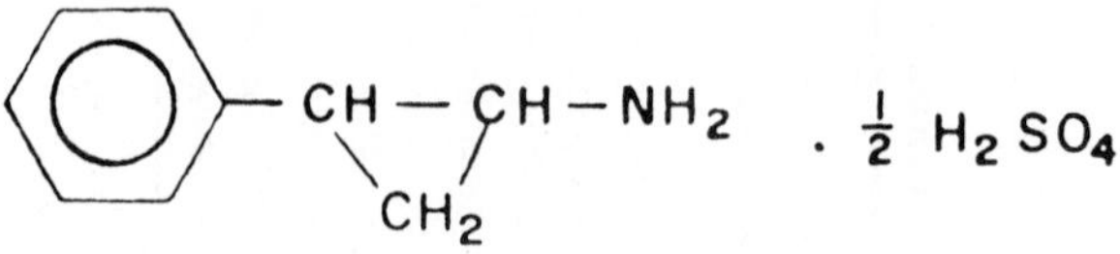

$CH-CH-NH_2$ $\cdot \ \frac{1}{2} \ H_2SO_4$

CH_2

TRANYLCYPROMINE

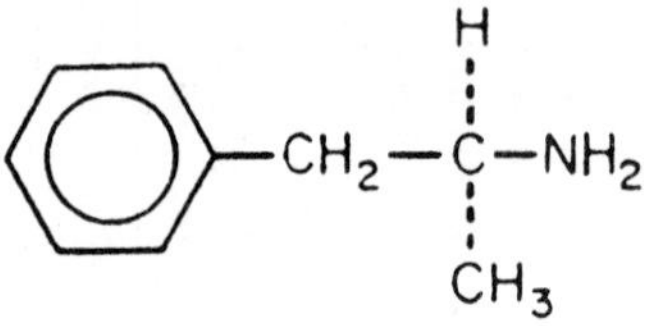

H

$-CH_2-\overset{\underset{CH_3}{|}}{C}-NH_2$

DEXTRO-AMPHETAMINE

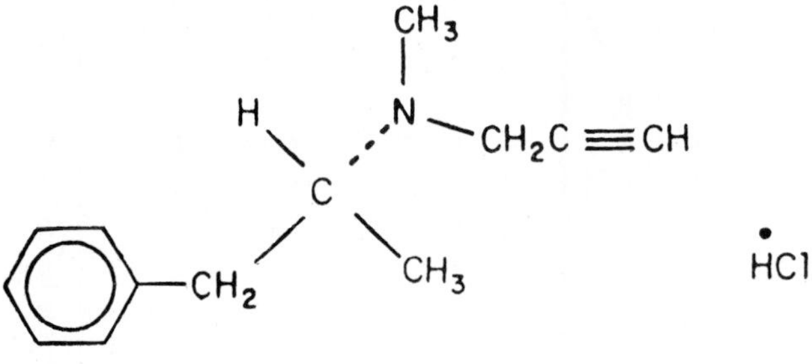

CH_3

$\overset{H}{\underset{CH_2}{\diagdown}} \ \overset{N-CH_2C \equiv CH}{\underset{CH_3}{C}}$

$\overset{\bullet}{HCl}$

SELEGILINE

$Cl-\underset{}{}\overset{}{}-\underset{\underset{O}{\|}}{C}-NH-CH_2-CH_2-N\overbrace{}O$

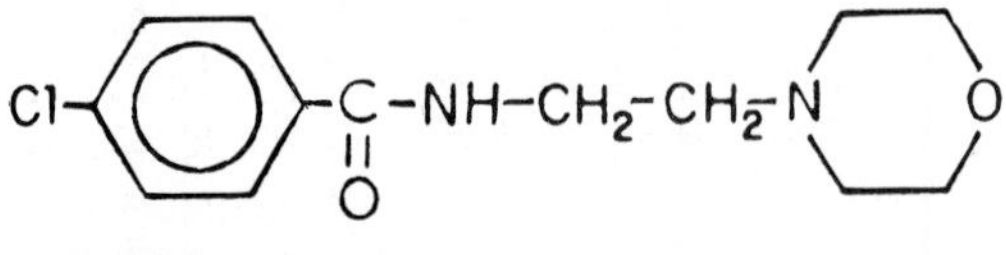

MOCLOBEMIDE

extent of platelet MAO enzyme inhibition.[5,30] The dosages employed for phenelzine in the earlier work were generally inadequate to produce significant enzyme inhibition.[5] Clinical studies have demonstrated that 30 mg/day of phenelzine produces less than 60% MAO inhibition.[5] We have learned that in man and rats, for brain concentrations of dopamine, norepinephrine, and serotonin to be significantly increased, there must be at least 85% inhibition of MAO.[5] Studies indicate that phenelzine at a dosage of 60 mg daily will produce a mean MAO inhibition exceeding 80%. Thus there is a correlation between the level of platelet MAO inhibition and the currently accepted effective dose of phenelzine, which is 60 mg/day.[5] In the majority of patients being treated with MAOIs, these data can be applied clinically without the need to monitor platelet MAO inhibition levels.

In patients who fail to respond to conventional dosages of phenelzine, it may be useful to measure platelet MAO.[5,30] Some individuals are able to rapidly acetylate MAOIs such as phenelzine and thereby inactivate them. Fast acetylators generally require larger doses whereas slow acetylators respond to lower doses.[41] Postural hypotension is commonly associated with phenelzine and occurs to a lesser extent with tranylcypromine, but may require dosage reduction.[42,43] If postural hypotension is pronounced, patients should be advised to change position slowly and to increase salt intake by drinking tomato juice, adding salt to their food or by taking four to six tablets of sodium chloride (0.5 g per tablet) daily.[44] In some cases 25 µg/day of triiodothyronine or 0.1 mg/day of fludrocortisone acetate may be necessary to control postural hypotension.[44]

Tranylcypromine

Tranylcypromine (Parnate) is a nonhydrazine MAOI with structural similarity to the amphetamines. It often produces a stimulant effect and is particularly useful in withdrawn, anergic depressed patients.[45] Perhaps as the result of its stimulant action, it is less likely to cause postural hypotension than phenelzine.[43,46] Likewise, as a result of its stimulant activity, tranylcypromine may produce a more rapid antidepressant response than other MAOIs.[2,31,47] I have seen some individuals who feel slightly better after the first few doses and some who feel less depressed after 3 days of treatment with tranylcypromine.

Tranylcypromine is more likely to cause insomnia than phenelzine, although the latter, which is more sedating, may also interfere with sleep. It is preferable to advise patients not to take MAO inhibitors after 6 P.M. and to take their doses earlier in the day if a sleep disturbance occurs.[46] Generally MAOIs should be given in a divided-dose regimen—in the case of tranylcypromine 10 to 20 mg 2 to 3 times daily, with phenelzine being given in a dose of 15 to 30 mg 2 or 3 times daily. The lesser likelihood of postural hypotension with tranylcypromine may allow relatively larger individual doses of this drug than of phenelzine.[43,46] Although many patients will respond and tolerate phenelzine or tranylcypromine equally well, I have seen a great number who will respond well to one agent and not at all to the other. It is not uncommon to have a patient fail to respond to a tricyclic or SSRI antidepressant and achieve an outstanding therapeutic benefit when given a monoamine oxidase inhibitor. The major caution, which cannot be stated too frequently, is the need for an adequate SSRI-free time interval before starting MAOI therapy. Furthermore, prescription of tranylcypromine immediately after discontinuing phenelzine may be associated with a hypertensive crisis; thus 2 weeks should separate phenelzine from tranylcypromine, although a shorter waiting time is satisfactory in making the change in the other direction. MAOIs may be so uniquely effective in some patients that these agents, particularly tranylcypromine (often in conjunction with lithium), should be considered before embarking on electroconvulsive therapy in a seemingly refractory patient, based upon my clinical experience and published controlled studies.[32,47]

ALTERNATIVE MAO INHIBITORS

Both phenelzine and tranylcypromine are irreversible nonselective inhibitors of both types of the monoamine oxidase enzyme, MAO-A and MAO-B. MAO-A primarily is involved in the metabolic degradation of serotonin and norepinephrine, while the primary substrates for the B form are phenylethylamine and benzylamine.[48,49] Dopamine and tyramine are substrates for both forms of the enzyme.[49] The A form is found primarily in catecholaminergic neurons while MAO-B is primarily in serotonergic neurons. The dominant enzyme form in cells of the intestinal wall is MAO-A. The ability to selectively inhibit MAO-B, which is characteristic of low doses of selegiline, allows this drug to be used without restricting dietary tyramine; however, at doses of 20 mg/day or greater the selectivity is lost and both MAO-A and MAO-B are inhibited, thus necessitating dietary precautions.[49,50] Moclobemide and brofaromine, which are investigational drugs in the United States, also may be used without the need to restrict dietary tyramine — through a different mechanism, namely the fact that both are reversible selective inhibitors of MAO-A known as RIMAs. Although it may take up to 2 weeks to regenerate normal levels of MAO after discontinuing an irreversible inhibitor, discontinuation of a RIMA is followed by prompt return of metabolically adequate levels of MAO enzyme. Furthermore, consumption of moderate amounts of tyramine during treatment with a RIMA such as moclobemide or brofaromine will result in displacement of the RIMA from the MAO enzyme and prompt attenuation of its inhibitory effect.[48,51] Although these newer approaches decrease the impact of dietary factors on MAOI therapy, they by no means should be seen as conferring safety on combined treatment with SSRIs and either selegiline or RIMAs.

Selegiline

Selegiline (Eldepryl), formerly known as L-deprenyl, is a selective inhibitor of MAO-B at doses up to 10 or 15 mg daily, leaving MAO-A available for metabolic degradation of dietary tyramine and thus not requiring dietary restrictions. At higher doses this drug loses isoenzyme selectivity and dietary tyramine must be limited. Selegiline is metabolized to three active compounds, including amphetamine and methamphetamine, which may contribute to its pharmacologic activity; furthermore, these compounds are known to interfere with neuronal uptake and to enhance release of norepinephrine, dopamine, and serotonin, which may also play a role in the antidepressant effect of selegiline. The metabolites of selegiline may contribute to the stimulating effect often seen with this drug and may also partially account for anxiety which is occasionally encountered as a side effect.

Studies of the antidepressant activity of selegiline (deprenyl) dating back to the 1960s have revealed conflicting results as to efficacy.[49,50] Many studies have concluded that antidepressant efficacy was associated with larger doses, in the range of 30 to 50 mg daily, wherein MAO-B selectivity was lost, while smaller doses which maintain isoenzyme selectivity exhibit little or no antidepressant response.[50,52] Clinically I have used selegiline in many patients at doses of 5 to 15 mg daily, with a favorable antidepressant response, without the necessity to employ a low-tyramine diet and without the occurrence of postural hypotension or sexual dysfunction, which are so commonly encountered with standard nonselective MAOI agents. I generally start with 2.5 mg twice daily and gradually increase first to 5 mg twice daily and then to a maximum of 5 mg 3 times daily. In the event that higher doses are employed, patients must be instructed regarding dietary restriction. Selegiline is particularly useful in patients who have anergic depressions, even if they have been unresponsive to or intolerant of other MAOIs, TCAs, or SSRIs. Fluoxetine must be discontinued at least 5 weeks prior to starting selegiline, while 2 weeks must elapse between other SSRIs and selegiline. Lithium may be safely combined with selegiline, as with other MAOIs, and may enhance therapeutic efficacy. Depressed bipolar II patients often respond extremely well to the combination of lithium and selegiline.

Moclobemide

Although not yet marketed in the United States, moclobemide (available as Manerix in Canada and Aurorex in Mexico) is a reversible inhibitor of MAO-A with antidepressant efficacy comparable to amitriptyline and fluoxetine.[53,54] Clinical studies indicate that moclobemide may produce fewer adverse effects than either of these drugs and is less likely to produce postural hypotension, sexual dysfunction, and hypertensive reactions to dietary tyramine than are standard nonselective MAOIs.[51,53,54] Moclobemide is generally given in divided doses, with a total of 300 to 600 mg daily. At this time it appears that the nonselective MAOIs may be somewhat more effective. Like all other MAOI antidepressants, moclobemide cannot be safely administered with SSRIs or in close time-proximity to these drugs. Brofaromine, another reversible inhibitor of MAO-A, is similar to moclobemide; however, in addition, it inhibits serotonin reuptake. Although it is currently an investigational drug, questions may be raised about the safety of brofaromine, which possesses these two characteristics, since it is known that simultaneous administration of SSRIs along with MAOIs may produce a fatal outcome.

One of the advantages of the MAOI antidepressants is their absence of anticholinergic action compared with the tricyclic antidepressants. Since the anticholinergic effect of TCAs and HCAs is one of the major complications of their use in the elderly, MAOIs have proved to be useful and safe in this population.[55,56] Again, the fears many clinicians have about MAO inhibitors has undoubtedly diminished their clinical application in geriatric patients. Nevertheless, some very favorable observations have been made on the safety and efficacy of MAOIs in the elderly.[55] Studies have documented improvement in depression in patients suffering from dementia.[56,57] The greater risk of postural hypotension to the elderly patient would sound a note of caution regarding treatment of these patients; however, cautious use of tranylcypromine would be less likely to produce postural hypotension.[46] In the elderly, starting at a single 10 mg dose daily, tranylcypromine may be gradually titrated upward to 10 mg 3 times daily as required to control depression. Older individuals as well as younger patients may develop psychotic symptoms in response to MAOIs, and a prior history of psychosis should put the clinician on notice to be cautious in the use of MAOIs regardless of the patient's age. Low-dose high-potency antipsychotic agents such as haloperidol or trifluoperazine may be used safely along with MAOIs in the elderly as well as in younger patients, although the likelihood of postural hypotension with MAOIs should warn physicians against combining chlorpromazine or thioridazine with MAOIs regardless of the patient's age.

MANAGEMENT OF SIDE EFFECTS

Postural hypotension is the most common side effect of MAOIs and may produce symptoms of light-headedness, dizziness, coldness, and headaches in approximately 50% of patients.[44,46] Less frequently, patients receiving MAOIs whose blood pressure is not carefully monitored may experience fainting episodes, particularly when salt or fluid intake is restricted. Management of postural hypotension should begin by the clinician's utilizing the lowest daily dose of medication in a divided-dose regimen. In some cases patients who experience postural hypotension with one MAOI may be cautiously switched to another agent, which may result in a reduction of postural symptoms. Tranylcypromine is less hypotensive than phenelzine.[42,43] I have, however, seen some patients who developed postural hypotension on tranylcypromine subsequently stabilized without significant blood pressure changes on phenelzine. Since changing from phenelzine to tranylcypromine may be associated with a hypertensive reaction, hyperpyrexia, and a potentially fatal outcome, patients should have a 1- to 2-week drug-free interval before initiating tranylcypromine.[58] This reaction appears to be due to the direct stimulant action of the latter MAOI. Adverse reactions are not likely to occur when a patient receiving tranylcypromine is switched to phenelzine.

If dosage reduction or a change to a different MAOI does not satisfactorily control postural hypotension, the next step is to increase the patient's salt intake. Obviously, in a patient with poorly compensated congestive heart failure this procedure cannot be safely undertaken. When there are no contraindications, the patient may be advised to salt his food heavily, drink tomato juice, or consume table salt by taking one-fourth teaspoonful in a glass of water 2 to 3 times daily. Alternatively, commercially available salt tablets, containing 0.5 g of sodium chloride, may be employed in a dosage of one to two tablets 2 to 3 times daily. I have found that some patients with postural hypotension will respond favorably to the addition of triiodothyronine in a dose of 25 μg daily. If these regimens are unsuccessful, the salt-retaining steroid fludrocortisone (Florinef) may be employed in a dose of 0.1 mg once or twice daily.[44] Yohimbine, a central alpha$_2$-adrenergic antagonist which elevates blood pressure in non–MAOI-treated patients, has been used unsuccessfully to treat MAOI-induced postural hypotension.[59]

Although hypertensive reactions to tyramine-rich foods and phenylethylamine-derived drugs do occur in patients receiving MAOIs, these reactions are usually mild and respond to nonpharmacologic treatment. Patients suspected of having a reaction should be taken into a quiet relatively dark room, allowed to lie down, and have their blood pressure measured. If the blood pressure elevation is modest, the patient may be monitored for 1 to 2 hours without the administration of specific blood pressure lowering drugs. Such patients may benefit from small doses of a short-acting benzodiazepine such as lorazepam. If the blood pressure is found to be significantly elevated, a standard treatment is to administer phentolamine IV in a dose of 5 mg. Since phentolamine is a relatively short-acting alpha-adrenergic blocking drug, the patient will require periodic blood pressure monitoring and may need further doses of this medication. Slow IV infusions of sodium nitroprusside or trimethaphan have also been found to be useful in managing hypertensive crises. Alternatively, IV administered β-blockers, including propranolol, metoprolol, and labetalol, may be used in the treatment of MAOI-associated hypertensive crises.

Orally administered thioridazine or chlorpromazine administered orally or parenterally has also been used in treating MAOI-associated hypertension. These drugs, however, should be avoided because they may produce serious and uncontrolled hypotensive reactions. The calcium channel–blocking drug nifedipine, administered sublingually, is effective in controlling MAOI-associated hypertensive reactions without producing hypotension.[60] Its ease of administration and the unlikelihood of provoking a severe hypotensive reaction make it a highly desirable intervention. Indeed, some patients may be taught to monitor their own blood pressure and self-administer nifedipine. A 10 mg capsule of nifedipine may be punctured with a needle, placed under the tongue and allowed to slowly release its content. Alternatively, the capsule may be placed in the mouth, chewed briefly, and then swallowed.

One significant advantage of MAOIs is that, in spite of their potential for producing postural hypotension or a hypertensive reaction in association with improper foods or drugs, they are relatively free of cardiovascular side effects. Indeed, when compared to conventional tricyclic antidepressants, the MAOIs have less likelihood of cardiovascular toxicity.[61] In contradistinction to the tricyclic antidepressants, MAOIs have little effect on heart rate, do not prolong cardiac conduction, and do not depress myocardial function.[61] Indeed, the absence of adverse electrophysiologic effects of MAOIs may make them safer antidepressants in patients that have recently had a myocardial infarction. It should be noted, however, that atrial fibrillation has been reportedly precipitated by tyramine-containing foods, and therefore careful dietary and medication restriction is important in the cardiac patient receiving MAOIs.[62]

A variety of neurologic side effects may occasionally occur during treatment with MAOIs. These drugs have been used in conjunction with tryptophan to enhance their antidepressant action. However, this combination regimen has been reported to produce an adverse effect, which may include sweating, tremor, drowsiness, and delirium.[63]

Delirium may occur as a consequence of excessive dosage of MAOIs and may occur in some patients who, for unknown reasons, are excessively sensitive to MAO inhibition. Parkinsonian side effects, which have been infrequently reported with tricyclic antidepressants, have occurred in a 75-year-old depressed woman during phenelzine treatment.[64] MAOI-associated delirium and parkinsonism both disappeared following drug discontinuation. Tinnitus is a rare side effect of tricyclic and MAOI antidepressant therapy. I have observed two instances during phenelzine treatment. One of the patients was receiving a brief course of chloroquine at the time that tinnitus appeared. In that patient the tinnitus diminished following chloroquine discontinuation but persisted during continuing treatment with phenelzine, 22.5 mg/day, which could not be discontinued. In another patient the tinnitus disappeared following reduction of the MAOI dosage. Although the relationship of tinnitus to pyridoxine deficiency is unclear, the administration of 100 to 200 mg/day of pyridoxine has been reported anecdotally to benefit some patients who experience this symptom while receiving MAOIs.

Hydrazine drugs, such as isoniazid and hydralazine, are capable of producing pyridoxine deficiency. Phenelzine has also been documented to produce pyridoxine deficiency.[65] Pyridoxine deficiency can result in peripheral neuropathy, stomatitis, ataxia, anemia, hyperacusis, hyperirritability, depression, and, in extreme cases, convulsions and coma.[65] There is evidence that carpal tunnel syndrome may result from pyridoxine deficiency, and the occurrence of this syndrome or other symptoms suggestive of vitamin B_6 deficiency should alert the physician to prescribe supplemental pyridoxine in a dosage of 100 to 300 mg/day. Many patients taking hydrazine-type MAOIs complain of "electric shocks" or jumping movements of their extremities, which may be manifestations of pyridoxine deficiency.[66] Not uncommonly, patients receiving therapeutic doses of MAOI antidepressants will experience hyperactive deep tendon reflexes, which may be associated with clonus.[66] The occurrence of increased reflexes is not necessarily an indication of a neurologic side effect of the drug; however, it should alert the physician to the potential need for treatment with supplemental pyridoxine or for a dosage reduction of the MAOI. Indeed, at high doses of MAOIs patients may be more apt to experience exaggerated reflexes and may, on occasion, experience a delirium, even in the absence of any drug or food interaction or the occurrence of a hypertensive crisis.[66] Although speech blockage is a known side effect of tricyclic antidepressants, it has been reported to occur also with alprazolam and with MAOIs. The occurrence of this side effect may necessitate dosage reduction or discontinuation of medication.[67]

Sexual dysfunction is a well-known side effect of MAOIs. Decreased libido has been reported in both men and women receiving phenelzine and other MAOIs.[68,69] These drugs may also impair sexual arousal in both men and women. Difficulties achieving or maintaining erection not uncommonly occurs in men being treated with MAOIs. Slowed or impaired ability to ejaculate may occur, and women have been reported to experience orgasmic dysfunction while receiving MAOIs.[70] Although seemingly contradictory to phenelzine inhibition of erectile function, a case of priapism has been reported in a man receiving this medication. Sexual dysfunction associated with MAOIs may be treated by reducing antidepressant dosage to the minimal effective level. If this is unsuccessful, some patients have experienced improved sexual function while receiving the serotonin antagonist cyprohepatidine in a dose of 2 to 4 mg once or twice daily. This drug has the disadvantage, however, of producing drowsiness and may also stimulate appetite and carbohydrate craving. Perhaps the best treatment for MAOI-induced sexual dysfunction is a cooperative and committed partner, who will employ time and ingenuity to induce satisfactory and mutually rewarding sexual achievement in the MAOI-treated patient. In some cases, male sexual dysfunction may be benefited by the co-administration of methyltestosterone either orally on a daily basis or monthly by depot injection.

One rare side effect of MAOI antidepressants is the occurrence of excessive flatus. Although these drugs are relatively selective inhibitors of the enzyme monoamine oxidase, they also inhibit a variety of other enzymes, including disaccharidases, that are necessary for the digestion of a variety of foods, including milk, complex carbohydrates, and beans. The presence of these substances in undigested form appears to contribute to the development of flatus.[71] In some cases oral administration of lactase in tablet form prior to meals may significantly reduce the inconvenience and embarrassment of drug-associated flatus.

Peripheral edema is occasionally encountered as an MAOI side effect. It appears to occur more frequently with phenelzine than with tranylcypromine. Although its mechanism is uncertain, it appears to be related to increased capillary permeability, perhaps contributed to by decreased venous return.[44,46]

MAOI-induced peripheral edema may improve with dosage reduction and in some cases, responds favorably to the simultaneous use of diuretics, which must be used cautiously to avoid hypotension.

Perhaps the rarest side effect of MAOIs is a lupuslike reaction, which has been reported with phenelzine in a 66-year-old woman who had taken the drug for 8 months.[72] The clinical and laboratory abnormalities disappeared following discontinuation of the drug. I have seen two young women, both of whom developed peripheral edema and mild joint swelling, who on laboratory testing were found to have a positive antinuclear antibody (ANA). In both cases, phenelzine was discontinued and both the peripheral edema and the joint swelling disappeared. In one case the antinuclear antibody reverted to negative 2 months following discontinuation of phenelzine. In the other it remained positive at 2 months following discontinuation and the patient failed to return for a follow-up laboratory determination, though she reported by telephone that she was well and free of any joint or other autoimmune symptoms. Similar immunologic abnormalities and clinical symptoms of a lupuslike syndrome are known to occur with other hydrazine-type drugs, including hydralazine, isoniazid, and procainamide, which is a structurally different compound. These autoimmune phenomena and laboratory evidences of immunologic abnormality have not been reported in patients receiving non–hydrazine-type MAOIs, such as tranylcypromine. Patients who have lupus, rheumatoid arthritis, or other immunologic disorders should be treated with tranylcypromine rather than with phenelzine if MAOI therapy is required.

SELECTION OF PATIENTS FOR THERAPY

One of the puzzling aspects of treating depression is that some patients will respond to one particular drug and not to another. The variety of effects on neurotransmitter reuptake of the different tricyclic drugs may explain the variation in response to this group of therapeutic agents. Also, some patients will respond well to one MAOI and not to another. Some time after the introduction of tranylcypromine (Parnate) some observers suggested it was more likely to produce hypertensive reactions than other MAOIs, and the FDA removed it from the market.[2] Following this, there were reports of "Parnate-specific patients," who had a favorable therapeutic response to this drug but who became depressed and failed to respond to any other antidepressant when the drug was no longer available.[2] When the drug was returned to the U.S. market, with no proof of its greater likelihood of producing toxicity, several of these patients were again noted to achieve a favorable therapeutic response. The fact that some patients respond to one antidepressant and not to others suggests that the dictum held by many clinicians and by the *Physicians' Desk Reference* — that the MAO inhibitors be reserved for patients who fail to respond to other antidepressants — should be reevaluated since it may add to the discomfort of patients who may have to suffer through prolonged periods of therapeutic trial of other agents before receiving the MAOI that might be beneficial for them.

Although it is difficult to predict in advance which patients are most likely to respond to MAOIs and may therefore be better treated with an initial course of one of these agents rather than a conventionally used SSRI or tricyclic drug, several guidelines may be of value. Nonpsychotic depressed patients with or without neurovegetative signs are more apt than psychotically depressed patients to respond to an MAOI.[73] Patients whose depression is accompanied by anxiety, somatization, and hypochondriasis generally respond favorably to MAOIs, though they may also respond favorably to SSRIs or tricyclic drugs.[73] Patients with persistent fatigue often respond well to MAOIs while those with major personality disorders often do not.[73] Obsessional patients and those with phobic disorders, with or without associated depression, may have a more dramatic improvement with MAOIs than with tricyclic antidepressants.[38] With the advent of SSRI antidepressants, I have changed a number of patients from MAOI therapy to an SSRI drug, and have often found the MAOI to be more efficacious.

Although earlier studies suggested that severely depressed patients with melancholia were unresponsive to MAOIs, more recent studies utilizing adequate doses have demonstrated a response rate in excess of 80% in melancholic depressed patients treated with either phenelzine or tranylcypromine.[35,74] These latter findings are consistent with my clinical experience with these drugs in severely depressed melancholic patients. Previously it was felt that patients with major depressive disorder were more likely to respond to tricyclics than to MAOIs. However, controlled studies have found comparable efficacy between phenelzine and imipramine in these patients.[34] Chronically depressed patients meeting DSM-IV criteria for dysthymic disorder have also been found to respond more favorably to treatment and maintenance on phenelzine.[36] In my experience many patients with severe refractory depressions achieve their best antidepressant response, with prolonged recovery, on a combined regimen of tranylcypromine and lithium. This finding has been confirmed by other clinicians and investigators.[31,32,47,75]

Atypical depression is a syndrome meeting Research Diagnostic Criteria for either major or minor depression, in association with mood reactivity while depressed, and two or more of the following: increased appetite or weight gain, oversleeping or spending more time in bed while depressed, severe fatigue, creating a sensation of leaden paralysis or extreme heaviness of arms or legs while depressed, and rejection sensitivity as a trait throughout adulthood. Atypical depression has been shown to be dramatically responsive to MAOI therapy.[33] Generally, the response of these patients to phenelzine is superior to their response to tricyclics such as imipramine.[33] A related atypical form of depression with hysteroid dysphoria is likewise generally more responsive to phenelzine than to tricyclics.[76]

There has been extensive documentation indicating a specific therapeutic response of patients suffering from agoraphobia and social phobias to the MAOIs.[38,39,77] Although habitual use of alcohol would often recommend against a trial of an MAOI because of the potential difficulty in getting the patient to abstain from alcohol, many alcohol abusers do have affective illnesses; they may suffer from social phobias and persistent anxiety which contribute to their alcohol use, so that a potentially effective therapeutic agent might mitigate against their continued excessive alcohol intake. The selection of a particular patient for a therapeutic trial of an MAOI should be made with consideration of his intellectual level and ability to understand and follow the dietary and medication restrictions. Obviously an individual suffering from a medical condition that might require the use of a nasal decongestant or bronchodilator (which may interact with the MAOI) should lead the clinician to serious thought and discussion with the patient prior to instituting MAOI therapy.

A patient who is prone to impulsive suicide attempts calls for special caution if MAOIs are being considered, since theoretically that patient would have a greater chance of a successful suicide, not only by using an overdose of the prescribed medication but by combining various foods or other medications in order to make a more serious and potentially fatal suicide attempt. Although suicidal ideation does not specifically call for treatment with an MAOI or avoidance of these drugs, it does suggest considerable caution and ongoing evaluation of the patient's suicidal status if the MAOI is prescribed. During many years of prescribing MAOIs for patients, I have not yet encountered anyone who made a suicide attempt by ingesting substances which he had been instructed would be dangerous to take with the drug. Several patients have consumed large quantities of alcohol while taking MAOIs, but in no case were these identifiable suicide attempts nor did they result in serious complications of a hypertensive nature. One patient who drank a considerable quantity of alcohol and took cocaine while on MAOI therapy did become transiently psychotic but recovered and returned to his previous level of functioning in a demanding profession within 72 hours.

In instructing patients regarding the precautions to be considered during treatment with an MAOI, I ask them to contact me before taking any patent medication or medication prescribed by another physician. Although I do not wish to encourage arrogance, I would urge physicians prescribing MAOIs to assume that other health care professionals do not understand these drugs. I learned this 20 years ago when a patient taking an MAOI asked the pharmacist who dispensed this product to him to also give him a cough syrup that would be safe to use. The pharmacist dispensed a decongestant-containing cough syrup and the patient experienced a brief period of "feeling high" along with a rapid pulse. The patient saw me the next day and I sent him to the emergency ward of a major hospital with a note about the medication restrictions necessary because of his tranylcypromine therapy. The patient was given an ephedrine-containing tablet by the emergency physician; the next day he reported symptoms similar to those he had experienced with the cough syrup he had previously received.

Although dietary restrictions should be followed as strictly as possible, the most important items to avoid are strong cheeses, red wine, tap beer, sauerkraut, and fermented meat and fish products. Most critical of these restrictions is the avoidance of any serotonin-selective reuptake inhibitor (such as fluoxetine and similar drugs), meperidine, nasal decongestants, cocaine, and stimulant drugs. Patients should be advised that they can safely take aspirin and acetaminophen and can use cetylpyridium (Cepacol) or Chloraseptic as a gargle for sore throat. Cough syrups containing small amounts of alcohol are safe, provided they do not contain decongestants. I generally recommend plain guaifenesin (Robitussin) or Benylin DM for cough; the latter contains 10 mg of dextromethorphan per teaspoonful, which may be used 4 times daily. Although occasional reports of adverse interactions between MAOIs and dextromethorphan have appeared, this reaction is unlikely when limited doses of the latter are used. Since MAOIs may potentiate the pharmacologic action of narcotics and sedatives, these drugs should be used cautiously and in limited doses in MAOI-treated patients.

COMBINED THERAPY WITH MONOAMINE OXIDASE INHIBITORS AND TRICYCLIC ANTIDEPRESSANTS

Several years ago most psychopharmacologists would not have combined tricyclic and MAOI antidepressants. The package inserts and *Physicians' Desk Reference* monographs continue to warn against this usage, in accordance with the FDA's lack of approval of this form of treatment. Therefore, if combined therapy seems clinically necessary it is of utmost importance to discuss the proposed treatment with the patient and a responsible family member if there is any question of the patient's competence. It would also be good practice to include a note in the medical record describing the patient's prior response to other therapies and the need for utilizing the combined drug treatment approach. Although an additional caution may at this point seem redundant, it must be restated that the combination of serotonin-selective reuptake inhibitors with MAOIs is never safe or acceptable.

Despite these cautions and the anxiety generated in the clinician whenever a new form of therapy is tried, there is considerable literature now accumulating to document the safety of this therapeutic approach.[78-81] One of the most striking studies documenting the safety of a combined regimen found that the incidence and severity of side effects among patients receiving a tricyclic in combination with an MAOI was essentially the same as observed in 150 patients receiving an MAOI alone[78] and another 150 patients receiving a tricyclic antidepressant alone.[34] With increasing experience utilizing the combined regimen, some data support its superior therapeutic efficacy in selected patients; however, the increased efficacy of the combined regimen is less well documented than is the safety of the regimen.[78-81] Assuming the regimen is safe, and recognizing that many depressed patients do not respond when treated appropriately with a single antidepressant agent, there seems to be little reason not to try the combined regimen in healthy persons whose lives are significantly impaired by depression. The regimen which has been most widely utilized and reported involves the addition of phenelzine to a previously established regimen of amitriptyline.[78] Other well-controlled studies have utilized a combination of tranylcypromine and amitriptyline, wherein patients were started on either drug or a combination of the two agents simultaneously.[79,80] In one study the combination treatment produced a non-significantly higher frequency of minor side effects, none of which required discontinuation of treatment.[79]

Less frequently, imipramine and other tricyclic antidepressants have been combined with MAOIs.[81] Because of the greater degree of norepinephrine effect of imipramine as compared with amitriptyline, there has been some concern about a greater potential for adverse effects.[81] However, having utilized at different times both of these tricyclic agents with phenelzine or tranylcypromine, I have not observed a difference in the pattern of adverse effects when these agents are used in any combination as compared with single-agent therapy. The combined regimen may be more likely to uncover psychotic symptoms; therefore, screening patients for the absence of a psychotic illness as well as for their ability to cooperate and follow instructions, would be a primary requirement when combined therapy is considered.

It is well known that tricyclic, heterocyclic, and MAOI antidepressants can provoke mania when single-drug therapy is employed. The use of cyclic antidepressants in combination with MAOIs has also been demonstrated to provoke manic responses.[82] Theoretically it would seem that combined regimens may be more likely to produce mania than single-agent therapy. However, adequate data to support or refute this construct are not yet available. Since lithium has been demonstrated to enhance the antidepressant response of cyclic drugs as well as MAOIs and since it may protect against a drug-induced manic response, lithium may be a beneficial adjunct when combination therapy is considered, particularly in a patient with a prior manic history.[75] One group has reported on the successful treatment of 16 patients with treatment-resistant depression with regimens combining either dextroamphetamine or methylphenidate with MAOIs, and in some patients, a third drug, a tricyclic antidepressant.[83] Although this type of regimen is not for the faint-hearted (doctor or patient), a favorable antidepressant effect was achieved in one study without serious life-threatening complications.[83] In that series, some patients experienced blood pressure elevations which in some cases resulted in alleviation of MAOI-induced hypotension. Indeed, some clinicians have utilized very small doses of dextroamphetamine or methylphenidate along with MAOI therapy to counteract postural hypotension, although I would advise extreme caution and careful patient monitoring if this treatment approach is employed. I have seen the rewards of combined TCA-MAOI regimens in a number of patients who have described histories of up to 20 years of depression unresponsive to a variety of single-agent therapies. The need to perform physical examinations and to monitor blood pressure, pulse, and ECG in patients receiving pharmacotherapy, particularly with complicated regimens, should be underscored. It should also be pointed out that, if a combined regimen is utilized, titration of the second drug should begin at a lower than usual dosage level and proceed more slowly than if single-agent therapy is being administered.[81]

REFERENCES

1. Bloch RG, Dooneief AS, Buchberg AS, et al: The clinical effects of isoniazid and iproniazid in the treatment of pulmonary tuberculosis. *Ann Intern Med* 1954;40:881-900.
2. Klein DF, Gittelman R, Quitkin F, et al: *Diagnosis and drug treatment of psychiatric disorders: adults and children*, ed 2. Baltimore, Williams & Wilkins, 1980.
3. Medical Research Council. Clinical Psychiatry Committee: Clinical trial of the treatment of depressive illness. *Br Med J* 1965;1:881-886.
4. Robinson DS, Nies A, Ravaries CL, et al: The monoamine oxidase inhibitor, phenelzine, in the treatment of depressive-anxiety states. *Arch Gen Psychiatry* 1973;29:407-413.
5. Ravaris CL, Nies A, Robinson DS, et al: A multiple-dose, controlled study of phenelzine in depression-anxiety states. *Arch Gen Psychiatry* 1976;33:347-350.
6. Rizack MA, Hillman CDM (eds): *The Medical Letter handbook of adverse drug interactions*. New Rochelle NY, The Medical Letter, 1993, pp 176-179.
7. Horwitz D, Lovenberg W, Engelman K, et al: Monoamine oxidase inhibitors, tyramine and cheese. *JAMA* 1964;188:1108-1110.
8. Rice SL, Eitenmiller RR, Koehler PE: Biologically active amines in food: A review. *J Milk Food Technol* 1976;39:353-358.
9. Blackwell B, Marley E, Price S, et al: Hypertensive interaction between monoamine oxidase inhibitor and foodstuffs. *Br J Psychiatry* 1967;113:349-365.
10. McCabe BJ: Dietary tyramine and other pressor amines in MAOI regimens: a review. *J Am Diet Assoc* 1986;76:1059-1064.
11. Udenfriend S, Lovenberg W, Sjoerdsma A: Physiologically active amines in common fruits and vegetables. *Arch Biochem Biophys* 1959;85:487-490.
12. Jalon M, Santos-Buelga C, Rivas-Gonzalo JC, et al: Tyramine in cocoa and derivatives. *J Food Sci* 1983;48:545-547.
13. Sen NP: Analysis and significance of tyramine in foods. *J Food Sci* 1969;34:22-26.
14. Yamamoto S, Wakabayashi S, Makita M: Gas-liquid chromatographic determination of tyramine in fermented food products. *J Agric Food Chem* 1980;28:790-793.
15. Chin KDH, Koehler PE: Identification and estimation of histamine, tryptamine, phenylethylamine and tyramine in soy sauce by TLC of dansyl derivatives. *J Food Sci* 1983;48:1826-1828.
16. Rivas-Gonzalo JC, Santos-Hernandez JF, Marine-Font A: Study of the evolution of tyramine content during the vinification process. *J Food Sci* 1983;48:417-418.
17. Shulman KI, Walker SE, MacKenzie S, et al: Dietary restriction, tyramine, and the use of monoamine oxidase inhibitors. *J Clin Psychopharmacol* 1989;9:397-402.
18. Folks DG: Monoamine oxidase inhibitors: reappraisal of dietary considerations. *J Clin Psychopharmacol* 1979;40:33-37.
19. Neil JF, Licata SM, May SJ, et al: Dietary non-compliance during treatment with tranylcypromine. *J Clin Psychiatry* 1979;40:33-37.
20. McCabe B, Tsuang MT: Dietary consideration in MAO inhibitor regimens. *J Clin Psychiatry* 1982;43:178-181.
21. Tailor SAN, Shulman KI, Walker SE, et al: Hypertensive episode associated with phenelzine and tap beer: a reanalysis of the role of pressor amines in beer. *J Clin Psychopharmacol* 1994;14:5-14.

22. Ferguson JM: Interaction of aspartame and carbohydrates in an eating-disordered patient. *Am J Psychiatry* 1985;142:271.

23. Balon R, Pohl R, Yeragani VK, et al: Monosodium glutamate and tranylcypromine administration in healthy subjects. *J Clin Psychiatry* 1990;51:303-306.

24. Beasley CM, Masica DN, Heiligenstein JH, et al: Possible monoamine oxidase inhibitor-serotonin uptake inhibitor interaction: fluoxetine clinical data and preclinical findings. *J Clin Psychopharmacol* 1993;13:312-320.

25. Tackley RM, Tregaskis B: Fatal disseminated intravascular coagulation following a monoamine oxidase inhibitor/tricyclic interaction. *Anesthesia* 1987;42:760-763.

26. Suchowersky O, deVries JD: Interaction of fluoxetine and selegiline. *Can J Psychiatry* 1990;35:571-572.

27. Dingemanse J: An update of recent moclobemide interaction data. *Int Clin Psychopharmacol* 1993;7:167-180.

28. Zornberg GL, Hegarty JD: Adverse interaction between propoxyphene and phenelzine. *Am J Psychiatry* 1993;150:1270-1271.

29. Browne B, Linter S: Monoamine oxidase inhibitors and narcotic analgesics: a critical review of the implications for treatment. *Br J Psychiatry* 1987;151:210-212.

30. Bresnahan DB, Pandey GN, Janicak PG, et al: MAO Inhibition and clinical response in depressed patients treated with phenelzine. *J Clin Psychiatry* 1990;51:47-50.

31. Martin L, Bakish D, Joffe R: MAOI treatment of depression. In Kennedy SH (ed): *Clinical advances in monoamine oxidase inhibitor therapy*. Washington DC, American Psychiatric Press, 1994, pp 147-180.

32. McGrath PJ, Stewart JW, Nunes EV, et al: A double-blind crossover trial of imipramine and phenelzine for outpatients with treatment-refractory depression. *Am J Psychiatry* 1993;150:118-123.

33. Quitkin FM, Harrison W, Stewart JW, et al: Response to phenelzine and imipramine in placebo nonresponders with atypical depression. *Arch Gen Psychiatry* 1991;48:319-323.

34. Davidson J, Raft D, Pelton S: An outpatient evaluation of phenelzine and imipramine. *J Clin Psychiatry* 1987;48:143-146.

35. McGrath PJ, Steward JW, Harrison W, et al: Phenelzine treatment of melancholia. *J Clin Psychiatry* 1986;47:420-422.

36. Stewart JW, McGrath PJ, Quitkin FM, et al: Chronic depression: response to placebo, imipramine, and phenelzine. *J Clin Psychopharmacol* 1993;13:391-396.

37. Johnson MR, Lydiard RB, Ballenger JC: MAOIs in panic disorder and agoraphobia. In Kennedy SH (ed): *Clinical advances in monoamine oxidase inhibitor therapy*. Washington DC, American Psychiatric Press, 1994, pp 205-224.

38. Gitow A, Liebowitz MR, Schneier FR: MAOI therapy of social phobia. In Kennedy SH (ed): *Clinical advances in monoamine oxidase inhibitor therapy*. Washington DC, American Psychiatric Press, 1994, pp 225-253.

39. Buigues J, Vallejo J: Therapeutic responses to phenelzine in patients with panic disorder and agoraphobia with panic attacks. *J Clin Psychiatry* 1987;48:55-59.

40. Schatzberg AF: Evaluation and treatment of the refractory depressed patient. In Bernstein JG (ed): *Clinical psychopharmacology*, ed 2. Boston, John Wright–PSG, 1984, pp 77-92.

41. Davidson J, McLeod MN, Blum MR: Acetylation phenotype, platelet monoamine oxidase inhibition, and the effectiveness of phenelzine in depression. *Am J Psychiatry* 1978;135:467-469.

42. Kronig MH, Roose SP, Walsh BT, et al: Blood pressure effects of phenelzine. *J Clin Psychopharmacol* 1983;3:307-310.

43. O'Brien S, McKeon P, O'Regan M, et al: Blood pressure effects of Tranylcypromine when prescribed singly and in combination with amitriptyline. *J Clin Psychopharmacol* 1992;12:104-109.

44. Rabkin JG, Quitkin FM, McGrath P, et al: Adverse reactions to monoamine oxidase inhibition. II, Treatment correlates and clinical management. *J Clin Psychopharmacol* 1985;5:2-9.

45. Himmelhoch JM, Thase ME, Mallinger AG, et al: Tranylcypromine versus imipramine in anergic bipolar depression. *Am J Psychiatry* 1991;148:910-916.
46. Rabkin J, Quitkin FM, Harrison W, et al: Adverse reactions to monoamine oxidase inhibitors. I, A comparative study. *J Clin Psychopharmacol* 1984;4:270-278.
47. Thase ME, Mallinger AG, McKnight D, et al: Treatment of imipramine-resistant recurrent depression. IV, A double-blind crossover study of tranylcypromine for anergic bipolar depression. *Am J Psychiatry* 1992;149:195-198.
48. Freeman H: Moclobemide. *Lancet* 1993;342:1528-1532.
49. Yu PH, Boulton AA: Clinical pharmacology of MAO-B inhibitors. In Kennedy SH (ed): *Clinical advances in monoamine oxidase inhibitor therapies*. Washington DC, American Psychiatric Press, 1994, pp 61-82.
50. Knoll J: Deprenyl (selegiline): the history of its development and pharmacological action. *Acta Neurol Scand* 1983 (suppl) 95:57-80.
51. Waldmeier PC, Amrein R, Schmid-Burgk W: Pharmacology and pharmacokinetics of brofaromine and moclobemide in animals and humans. In Kennedy SH (ed): *Clinical advances in monoamine oxidase inhibitor therapies*. Washington DC, American Psychiatric Press, 1994, pp 33-59.
52. Mann JJ, Aarons SF, Wilner PJ, et al: A controlled study of the antidepressant efficacy and side effects of (-)- deprenyl: a selective MAOI. *Arch Gen Psychiatry* 1989;46:45-50.
53. Bakish D, Bradwejn J, Nair N, et al: A comparison of moclobemide, amitriptyline, and placebo in depression: a Canadian multicentre study. *Psychopharmacology* 1992;106(suppl):98-101.
54. Williams R, Edwards RA, Newburn GM, et al: A double-blind comparison of moclobemide and fluoxetine in the treatment of depressive disorders. *Int Clin Psychopharmacol* 1993;7:155-158.
55. Jenike MA: *Handbook of geriatric psychopharmacology*. Littleton Mass, PSG Publishing 1985.
56. Jenike MA: Monoamine oxidase inhibitors as treatment for depressed patients with primary degenerative dementia (Alzheimer's disease). *Am J Psychiatry* 1985;142:763-764.
57. Ashford JW, Ford CV: Use of MAO inhibitors in elderly patients. *Am J Psychiatry* 1979;136:1466-1467.
58. Bazire SR: Sudden death associated with switching monoamine oxidase inhibitors. *Drug Intell Clin Pharm* 1987;48:249-250.
59. Lin SC, Hsu T, Fredrickson PA, et al: Yohimbine and tranylcypromine-induced postural hypotension. *Am J Psychiatry* 1987;144:119.
60. Clary C, Schweizer E: Treatment of MAOI hypertensive crisis with sublingual nifedipine. *J Clin Psychiatry* 1987;48:249-250.
61. Goldman LS, Alexander RC, Luchins DJ: Monoamine oxidase inhibitors and tricyclic antidepressants: comparison of their cardiovascular effects. *J Clin Psychiatry* 1986;47:225-229.
62. Jacob LH, Carron DB: Atrial fibrillation precipitated by tyramine containing foods. *Br Heart J* 1987;57:205-206.
63. Page HG, Jonas JM, Hudson JI, et al: Toxic reactions to the combination of monoamine oxidase inhibitors with tryptophan. *Am J Psychiatry* 1985; 142:491-492.
64. Teusink JP, Alexopoulos GS, Shamoian CA: Parkinsonian side effects induced by a monoamine oxidase inhibitor. *Am J Psychiatry* 1984;141:118-119.
65. Steward JW, Harrison W, Quitkin F, et al: Phenelzine-induced pyridoxine deficiency. *J Clin Psychopharmacol* 1984;4:225-226.
66. Lieberman JA, Kane JM, Reife R: Neuromuscular effects of monoamine oxidase inhibitors. *J Clin Psychopharmacol* 1985;5:221-228.
67. Goldstein DM, Goldberg RL: Monoamine oxidase inhibitor–induced speech blockage. *J Clin Psychiatry* 1986;47:604.
68. Rapp MS: Two cases of ejaculatory impairment related to phenelzine. *Am J Psychiatry* 1979;136:1200-1201.
69. Barton JL: Orgasmic inhibition by phenelzine. *Am J Psychiatry* 1979;136:1616-1617.

70. Harrison WM, Rabkin JG, Ehrhardt AA, et al: Effects of antidepressant medication on sexual function: a controlled study. *J Clin Psychiatry* 1986;6:144-149.
71. Olson AC, Gray GM, Gumbmann MR, et al: Flatus causing factors in legumes. In Ory RL (ed): *Antinutrients and natural toxicants in foods.* Westport Conn, Food & Nutrition Press, 1981.
72. Swartz C: Lupus-like reaction to phenelzine. *JAMA* 1978;239:269.
73. Tyrer P: Towards rational therapy with monoamine oxidase inhibitors. *Br J Psychiatry* 1976;128:354-360.
74. McGrath PJ, Quitkin FM, Harrison W, et al: Treatment of melancholia with tranylcypromine. *Am J Psychiatry* 1984;141:288-289.
75. Price CH, Charney DS, Heninger GR: Efficacy of lithium-tranylcypromine treatment in refractory depression. *Am J Psychiatry* 1985;142:619-623.
76. Kayser A, Robinson DS, Nies A, et al: Response to phenelzine among depressed patients with features of hysteroid dysphoria. *Am J Psychiatry* 1985;142:486-488.
77. Liebowitz MR, Fyer AJ, Gorman J, et al: Phenelzine in social phobia. *J Clin Psychopharmacol* 1986;6:93-98.
78. Spiker DG, Pugh DD: Combined tricyclic and monoamine oxidase inhibitor antidepressants. *Arch Gen Psychiatry* 1976;33:828-830.
79. White K, Pistole T, Boyd JL: Combined monoamine oxidase inhibitor-tricyclic antidepressant treatment: a pilot study. *Am J Psychiatry* 1980;137:1422-1425.
80. Razani J, White KL, White J, et al: The safety and efficacy of combined amitriptyline and tranylcypromine antidepressant treatment. *Arch Gen Psychiatry* 1983;40:657-661.
81. White K, Simpson G: The combined use of MAOIs and tricyclics. *J Clin Psychiatry* 1984;45(7,sec 2):67-69.
82. De La Fuente JR, Berlanga C, Leon-Andrade C: Mania induced by tricyclic-MAOI combination therapy in treatment-resistant bipolar disorder: case reports. *J Clin Psychiatry* 1986;47:40-41.
83. Feighner JP, Herbstein J, Damlouji N: Combined MAOI, TCA, and direct stimulant therapy of treatment-resistant depression. *J Clin Psychiatry* 1985;46:206-209.

CHAPTER 7

Electroconvulsive Therapy

OVERVIEW

Indications

Primary: Severe depression with any of the following:
1. Unresponsive to adequate trial of medication
2. Inability to tolerate antidepressant drugs
3. Immediate risk of suicide

Secondary: Unresponsiveness to pharmacotherapy in patients with:
4. Mania
5. Schizophrenia

Contraindications
1. Brain tumor
2. Recent myocardial infarction or cerebrovascular accident
3. Inability to tolerate general anesthesia

Pre-ECT Evaluation
1. Medical history and complete physical examination
2. ECG
3. Chest, cervical, and thoracolumbar spine x-ray
4. EEG
5. CT scan and neurologic examination if clinically indicated
6. CBC, urinalysis, automated blood chemistry, and electrolytes

Preparation for Treatment
1. Discontinue lithium at least three days before treatment.
2. Evaluate other medications and reduce dosage or discontinue as clinically indicated.
3. Explain procedure fully to patient.
4. Have patient sign consent form; if patient is not fully able to understand it, family member should also sign.
5. Patient should be NPO after midnight the night before each treatment.
6. Administer anticholinergic IM, preferably glycopyrrolate 0.2 to 0.6 mg, 30 to 45 minutes before each treatment.

Continued.

> **Treatment**
> 1. The unilateral D'Elia electrode technique is preferable.
> 2. Use a low-energy ECT machine such as MECTA or Thymatron with ECG and EEG monitoring.
> 3. Usual course is six to eight treatments; ECT is given every second or third day, with general anesthesia (methohexital 1 mg/kg) and muscle relaxant (succinylcholine 1 mg/kg). Twelve treatments may be required.
>
> **Posttreatment**
> Prophylactic maintenance with lithium carbonate or antidepressant.

Although the origin of convulsive therapy in psychiatry was pharmacologic, present use employs electrically induced convulsions rather than those induced by drugs. The origin of this form of treatment was based on the observation that epileptic patients rarely had schizophrenia and schizophrenics rarely suffered from seizures. Although this finding was later not supported by research data, it did give rise to the use of a variety of chemicals, including camphor, pentylenetetrazol, and flurothyl (Indoklon), to induce seizures initially in schizophrenic patients.[1] This early work of Meduna led Cerletti and Bini to induce seizures, initially in animals and subsequently in human patients, through the use of an electrical stimulus.[2] Convulsive therapy, used initially in schizophrenia, appeared to show more promise in patients suffering from depression, and depression has become the primary indication for convulsive therapy. Electrically induced seizures are generally more reliable and controllable than those induced chemically.[2] Since chemically induced convulsions, including the use of insulin shock, are primarily of historical interest rather than clinically useful techniques, they will not be discussed in this chapter.

Optimal clinical practice of psychiatry, including the best pharmacotherapy, does yield some patients with limited therapeutic responses. Some depressed patients will have an inadequate response to the most expert application of pharmacotherapy, and some who are acutely suicidal will not allow a long-enough interval for treatment to take place without the risk of a serious suicide attempt.[3] For these reasons, ECT still has an important role in clinical practice. Although its primary use is in the treatment of depression,[2] there are other clinical conditions which may respond, such as refractory mania[4] and, at times, schizophrenia[5] when a suboptimal response to pharmacologic treatment has been achieved.

It is important for clinicians to recognize that there are interactions between pharmacotherapy and ECT.[6-8] These may be favorable, as in medications used prophylactically following a satisfactory course of ECT.[8] There are also adverse interactions between pharmacotherapy and ECT, such as increased confusion and memory disturbance associated with the administration of ECT to a patient who is being maintained on lithium.[6] Additionally, the application of proper pharmacologic agents in conjunction with the treatment itself may facilitate a favorable response and avoid some unwanted adverse effects.[7] This chapter reviews some practical principles in the application of ECT which may facilitate safe and effective use of this potentially lifesaving treatment.

MECHANISMS OF ACTION OF ECT

In reviewing any therapeutic technique the two most fundamental concerns are safety and efficacy. Since most clinicians are uncomfortable with any technique whose mechanism of action is unknown, some anxiety occurs when ECT is considered. Older literature has suggested that the efficacy of ECT was dependent on the actual physical convulsion,[1] but modern techniques utilizing muscle relaxants and general anesthesia essentially avoid a physical convulsion yet may produce a highly beneficial result.[2] Furthermore, earlier thinking about ECT suggested that the beneficial effect was connected with the induction of memory loss and confusion, which somehow allowed for the patient's recovery. Again, with the application of newer techniques such as the administration of much smaller amounts of electrical energy to the nondominant hemisphere, a course of several treatments may be administered with little or no confusion or memory change but with a sizable therapeutic benefit.[1,2,9]

Although a variety of techniques of ECT have been associated with a therapeutic response, the only finding that appears absolutely necessary is the development of a generalized electrical seizure within the brain.[9] One thing that makes the response to ECT puzzling, as various mechanisms of action are considered, is the finding that although depression is the condition most responsive to ECT there may also be a favorable therapeutic response in manic patients and in some individuals with schizophrenia, wherein presumably different mechanisms of action must be invoked.[9]

There are many known neurotransmitters, and a larger number which are still either unknown or poorly understood. Most of the data thus far available regarding the effects of ECT on neurotransmitters are derived from animal studies. Effects on various transmitters appear contradictory at times, although this may help to explain what appear to be opposite results when ECT may benefit either depression or mania.[10,11] Some studies have suggested that following a series of electrically induced seizures in rats, there is increased turnover of norepinephrine and possibly a net increase in both brain level and synthesis of norepinephrine.[12] MHPG (3-methoxy 4-hydroxyphenyl-glycol) levels in the urine of depressed patients have been reported to increase following a series of ECT, presumably suggesting increases in norepinephrine turnover associated with improvement in mood.[11,12]

Brain levels and turnover of serotonin increase in animals following a series of electrically induced seizures.[11,12] Abnormally low CSF levels of the serotonin metabolite 5-hydroxyindolacetic acid (5-HIAA) may increase toward normal with ECT-induced remission in depression.[12] Electroconvulsive shocks administered to rats dramatically increase dopamine levels in the striatum, and electroconvulsive therapy has a beneficial effect in Parkinson's disease, suggesting that increased brain dopamine concentrations may occur with ECT.[13] Thus there is experimental evidence of enhancement of at least three neurotransmitters thought to be involved in the mechanism of depression by electroconvulsive therapy, yet there is not enough evidence to state with certainty that these mechanisms explain the beneficial effects of ECT. It is intriguing to postulate a more important role of dopamine deficiency states in some forms of depression to explain the therapeutic benefit of ECT in some patients who are unresponsive to conventional antidepressants. In humans electroconvulsive therapy has been found to activate the hypothalamic-pituitary-adrenal axis, resulting in the release of beta-endorphin.[14] There are conflicting data in the literature regarding changes in the serum levels of the catecholamine metabolites MHPG and HVA following ECT; on the other hand, most studies have confirmed ECT-induced increases of serum prolactin concentration proportional to seizure duration.[15,16]

In animal studies, ECT, like antidepressant drugs, has led to downregulation of both beta- and alpha-adrenergic receptors as well as Serotonin 5-HTz receptors.[12] There is evidence of a generalized release of acetylcholine throughout the brain during the course of ECT and of increases in spinal fluid acetylcholine and choline levels associated with the ECT.[12] Although it may be difficult to correlate increased acetylcholine levels with an improvement in mood in depressed patients, this finding is interesting since the administration of acetylcholine precursors to manic patients may improve the symptoms of mania.[12] Perhaps similar or related changes may account for some of the favorable observations of ECT in schizophrenia. The extracellular concentration of GABA is increased (though GABA synthesis is decreased) following ECT in animals.[12] The old idea of "brain scrambling" as a mechanism for ECT would seem to be far behind our sophisticated age of neurochemistry and psychopharmacology, yet more work is needed to correlate neurochemistry with observed therapeutic responses.[17]

INDICATIONS FOR ELECTROCONVULSIVE THERAPY

Although early studies suggested that ECT was as good as or better than pharmacotherapy in schizophrenia, virtually all current studies support the superiority of neuroleptics to ECT in schizophrenia.[1,10] Increased dopamine activity and increased density of receptor sites for this neurotransmitter suggest that the most specific intervention in schizophrenic psychosis would be the proper use of adequate dosages of dopamine-blocking agents such as haloperidol.[18] Not all schizophrenic patients respond to pharmacotherapy, and the limited response may at times need to be dealt with by careful clinical trial of a variety of neuroleptic agents. The possibility that ECT may be beneficial is worthy of consideration. The literature is far from definite in proving the therapeutic value of ECT in schizophrenia; therefore, this indication should be seen as questionable, except in circumstances where a patient remains psychotic and uncontrollable in spite of optimal pharmacotherapy.[5,9] If there is a response of schizophrenia to ECT, a larger number of treatments needs to be employed than in the treatment of depression. It appears that the depressive symptoms which occur in some schizophrenic patients are more likely to respond to ECT than the symptoms of the actual schizophrenic illness itself.[9]

With the advent of potent antipsychotic drugs and the widespread use of lithium carbonate, the necessity to employ ECT in the treatment of mania has diminished. One obvious risk of mania is that the patient will continue to expend great amounts of energy and will eventually suffer exhaustion. I have not encountered a situation where the judicious use of pharmacotherapy would not provide a considerable degree of control even to the most agitated manic individual. Nevertheless, the literature does support the potential value of ECT in controlling medication-refractory mania.[4]

Although a variety of other conditions have been treated with ECT,[9] the evidence is far from convincing that this treatment is truly specific or superior to other forms of treatment, except in the patient with refractory depression who has either been unresponsive to intensive pharmacotherapy or who presents an immediate risk of suicide.[3,19]

Electroconvulsive therapy should generally not be the initial treatment of choice in a depressed patient. There are, of course, some exceptions to the general rule. Severely depressed patients who have been unresponsive to full therapeutic doses of antidepressant medication administered over an adequate period of time and who present with serious suicidal intent, may often require immediate hospitalization and a course of ECT rather than a protracted period of pharmacotherapy, particularly if the risk of suicide seems imminent.[19] Furthermore, some severely depressed persons have had multiple trials of antidepressant medication and have been unable to tolerate this form of treatment. Many of those patients may be hospitalized and treated effectively by medication, with the added support and supervision provided in the inpatient setting. On the other hand, the continued presence of severe depression and suicidal ideation, along with a variety of drug side effects, may appropriately lead the physician to the administration of a course of ECT without unnecessary delay. In the severely depressed person who has made a previous suicide attempt and who continues to be preoccupied with a plan to end his life, a course of ECT may be rapidly beneficial and avoid the risks associated with the delay generally necessary to achieve an adequate pharmacologic response.[3]

TECHNIQUES IN THE CLINICAL ADMINISTRATION OF ECT

Techniques in the clinical administration of ECT have undergone a variety of advances since its first experimental application in 1938. A greater understanding of its mechanisms of action and clinical indications has improved the image of this form of treatment; simultaneously, its safety and efficacy have also improved. These advances have contributed to a more judicious application of this potent therapeutic technique. The use of ECT in situations where it is either not necessary or not likely to be beneficial, is hopefully, disappearing as our knowledge increases.

Electroconvulsive therapy was initially administered without the benefits of muscle relaxants or anesthesia. Thus patients who were awake underwent the frightening torture of experiencing their body writhing with convulsive movements. Unfortunately, this image continues to be portrayed in many lay publications and in the theater, as well as in the literature of individuals and organizations opposed to the therapeutic use of ECT. As I continue to train residents and nurses in the use of ECT, I am repeatedly told of their surprise to see that nothing happens to the patient except for the eventual lifting of the depression.

The use of ECT must begin with a thorough clinical evaluation of the patient, both psychiatrically and medically. Proper psychiatric indications must exist before this form of treatment is considered. Prior to proceeding, the patient should undergo a thorough physical examination and a series of laboratory studies. An ECG and chest x-ray are necessary in the ECT evaluation; it is also desirable to obtain x-rays of the spine, to rule out the presence of compression fractures or to document their presence so that their later appearance is not seen as a complication of the treatment. In my practice the thorough medical evaluation includes a complete blood count, an automated chemistry profile, and a urinalysis. A patient who has been receiving diuretics should have baseline electrolyte and creatinine determinations done. The automated blood chemistry profile, although not an absolute necessity, may point to some underlying medical condition that would either add to the understanding of the patient's depressive illness or perhaps complicate anesthesia. In the interest of optimal safety I prefer to obtain an EEG and CT scan of the brain. The EEG is useful since the presence of a previous seizure focus may produce an extended series of seizures in response to ECT; however, the presence of a prior seizure focus does not necessarily contraindicate ECT.[9] The primary contraindication to ECT is the presence of a brain tumor, since a space-occupying mass can cause herniation of the brain during the course of treatment.[9] Thus, obtaining a CT scan is an added safety measure. Patients with underlying organic brain dysfunction, particularly the elderly, are likely to have an increased confusional response to ECT; although the presence of this abnormality does not rule out treatment, it is useful to have the patient seen in consultation by a neurologist to clarify concerns regarding the proposed ECT. I generally prefer to have the patient seen in consultation by an internist once the appropriate laboratory tests have been completed and prior to instituting ECT. Although many physicians who utilize ECT do not employ an anesthesiologist to administer the anesthesia, I routinely utilize an anesthesiologist for this purpose. The presence of two physicians during the treatment adds further to the safety of the administration of ECT and provides more thorough backup if a complication should arise. The best means of dealing with complications is to avoid them by careful evaluation and screening of patients prior to treatment.

Electroconvulsive therapy should be done in an area that is large enough to accommodate the necessary equipment, including emergency equipment. The room must also provide adequate lighting and ventilation for the comfort of the patient and staff administering the treatment. The presence of other patients in the room should generally be avoided, as should the presence of staff members who are not directly involved in the treatment procedure.

Treatments are best administered during the early morning hours so that the patient is spared unnecessary waiting and anxiety. Patients should receive nothing by mouth from midnight until they are fully awake following the treatment. It is advisable to have staff periodically remind the patient of this requirement. It may also be useful to have someone with the patient in the morning until the procedure begins in order to reinforce the NPO status and to help allay fears and anxiety.

Since ECT is generally associated with vagal stimulation and a consequent bradycardia that may on rare occasions be associated with asystole, it has become standard clinical practice to administer an anticholinergic drug in an adequate vagolytic dose prior to anesthesia. This agent not only prevents bradycardia but also provides for a decrease in oral secretions, which could complicate anesthesia and proper ventilation of the patient. The standard anticholinergic drug utilized in preanesthetic medication, for a variety of surgical procedures as well as ECT, is atropine sulfate. If an inadequate dosage of atropine is given, there may be some initial parasympathomimetic effect with associated bradycardia.[20] Therefore, if atropine is employed, a relatively large dose, such as 1 mg given subcutaneously or intramuscularly, should be administered approximately 30 to 45 minutes prior to anesthesia. Atropine readily crosses the blood-brain barrier and exerts central as well as peripheral anticholinergic effects.[20] Unfortunately, the central manifestations of atropine effects are well known to psychiatrists, since this drug may produce a toxic delirium. The possibility of memory disturbance or confusion occurring during the course of ECT would therefore be enhanced if atropine is used as the anticholinergic agent. If an anticholinergic agent with a quarternary structure is utilized, this chemical structure prevents passage through the blood-brain barrier and thereby prevents the drug from affecting the CNS. Such a compound would therefore be unable to produce an anticholinergic delirium and would be potentially safer. I prefer to administer glycopyrrolate (Robinul), in a dose of 0.2 to 0.6 mg IM, 30 to 45 minutes prior to anesthesia.[20] This agent is a quarternary compound and does not cross the blood-brain barrier. It also does not produce a toxic delirium when given alone, and it appears not to enhance the potential for ECT-induced confusional states. It provides adequate peripheral cholinergic blockade, and with its extensive use I have not observed bradycardia in patients receiving this medication prior to

ECT. This agent also provides a satisfactory drying effect, thus avoiding excessive oral secretions, which can complicate the work of the anesthesiologist.[20]

Following IV administration of 1 mg/kg methohexital sodium (Brevital), a dose of 1 mg/kg succinylcholine chloride (Anectine) is given IV by the anesthesiologist, who then, for a brief period, hyperventilates the patient. The electrical stimulus is then administered, and the anesthesiologist continues to ventilate the patient until he is able to breathe spontaneously while awakening. Since standard ECT machines may administer an electric shock and produce a convulsion that is invisible by virtue of the anesthesia and muscle relaxation, it is useful to apply a blood pressure cuff to the arm and inflate it to 250 to 300 mmHg just before the succinylcholine administration. Using the cuff as a tourniquet will largely prevent paralysis of the musculature of the arm to which the tourniquet has been applied, so that the muscles of the arm can contract and graphically demonstrate that the patient indeed has had a seizure response to the electrical stimulation. The use of newer instruments such as the MECTA (Monitored ElectroConvulsive Therapy Apparatus) and the Thymatron, which provide simultaneous monitoring of both the ECG and the EEG, allows the electrical manifestations of a seizure to be observed so that visualization of its effects in the arm by the tourniquet technique is no longer essential.[21] It may still be of clinical value, however, for the clinician to observe the seizure by employing the tourniquet technique.

Once awake following the seizure, the patient should remain in bed in a quiet room with a staff member in attendance until fully alert and the posttreatment confusion has cleared. It is a good practice to orient the patient to time and date, the physical surroundings, and the fact that the treatment has been completed. The patient should be cautioned that dizziness may be present and that it is necessary to get up slowly because of potential weakness and residual confusion from the treatment and anesthesia. It may be necessary to provide physical support by a staff member as the patient begins to ambulate.

The patient should be breathing and swallowing satisfactorily before being given small quantities of clear liquids to drink. When up and about and able to tolerate small quantities of liquids, the patient may eat a limited quantity of food, assuming there is no nausea or swallowing difficulty. Subsequently, he may be encouraged to participate in the daily routine of the hospital. In the case of outpatient ECT, the patient may be observed for a period of time and then discharged home in the company of someone who will provide transportation, orientation, and support as required.

ECT INSTRUCTIONS

The technique of ECT has been refined through a variety of means, initially with the introduction of ECT administered under anesthesia with muscle relaxants. Other refinements have involved the development of more sophisticated instrumentation. Electroconvulsive therapy was initially administered by a simple device that could administer electrical energy in the form of a sine wave of 50 c/s with the ability to vary the voltage of the stimulus from 50 to 150 V. Standard ECT devices are quite similar to the original Cerletti apparatus, in that they produce a stimulus of constant voltage that can be varied at the discretion of the clinician. Since electrical resistance of the patient, and of the interface between the patient and the electrode, can vary, those devices which administer a constant voltage will provide considerable variation both in current and in total electrical energy administered. Older ECT devices are capable of administering up to several hundred joules. The form of the electrical stimulus is generally either a sine wave or a square wave that may be unidirectional or bidirectional.[1] With one standard older ECT machine (Elektra Laboratories) the voltage administered is generally set at between 100 and 300 V, in order to achieve a suitable seizure. Since the electrode interface impedance varies, the patient-electrode circuit acts as a voltage divider such that about one half of the voltage is lost at the electrode interface. Changes in this interface would obviously deliver varying amounts of electrical energy to the patient independent of the adjustment setting of the machine. This device also allows for a variation in the duration of administration of the electrical stimulus, generally between 0.5 and 1.5 seconds. The amount of electrical energy administered by a standard ECT device is comparable to the energy administered by commonly utilized heart defibrillators. If there is poor contact between the electrodes and the skin, electrical burns may occur.

The major advancement in ECT instrumentation was the development in 1973 of MECTA, which administers a reduced-energy, bipolar, square-wave pulse at constant current.[21] Anterograde and retrograde memory function have been found to be less impaired when lower-energy, brief-pulse, square-wave stimuli are employed.[22] Stimuli of these parameters produce seizures of equal length and equal therapeutic efficacy with less memory impairment than is encountered with sine-wave stimuli.[22]

Since the initial MECTA instrument was marketed, there have been several refinements in the basic design, with several different MECTA models being marketed since 1986. Another sophisticated ECT device, the Thymatron, was developed by a competing company and has been marketed since 1985. All of the MECTA models and the Thymatron deliver a constant-current (0.8 or 0.9 A) bipolar, square-wave stimulus. The maximum energy output of all of these devices is 100 J, although most often therapeutically satisfactory seizures can be induced at energy levels far below the maximum capability of the device. The maximum electrical charge generated by the Thymatron is 504 millicoulombs, while the maximum charge of the various MECTA units is 576 mC. Earlier MECTA models generally deliver a maximum energy level of only about 60 J, and occasional patients, particularly the elderly, who have higher seizure thresholds, fail to achieve seizure responses at the lower maximal energy levels. Though occasional claims are made that either the MECTA or the Thymatron is superior for seizure induction, these devices should be seen as comparable with respect to their production of electrical seizures. Both these devices deliver considerably less electrical energy and are safer than older units, such as the Elektra and the Medcraft.

All MECTA models and the Thymatron measure patient-electrode impedance and display these data on a meter or chart recorder. The MECTA will not deliver a stimulus unless the impedance value is satisfactory or the impedance override is used. The Thymatron does not require satisfaction of impedance parameters prior to delivering the stimulus. Because excessive patient-electrode impedance may allow for the occurrence of skin burns when the electrical stimulus is applied, inactivation of the stimulus circuitry of the MECTA by excessive impedance is an important safety factor.

MECTA manufactures two models, the JR-1 and the JR-2, which deliver ECT stimuli without having the capability of monitoring EEG and ECG. The MECTA SR-1 and SR-2 deliver ECT stimuli and simultaneously record EEG and ECG on built-in strip-chart recorders. The Thymatron does not record EEG, but utilizes a unique electronic system to present an auditory representation of the EEG through a loudspeaker. Changes in the audible sound generated allow the clinician to determine that a seizure has occurred. Claims have been made that this system of signaling a successful seizure is easier for the clinician to interpret than is a graphic EEG chart.[23] The Thymatron does not record the ECG, which I feel should generally be monitored for optimal safety of ECT. If this device is used, a standard ECG machine must also be employed, thus presenting a possible additional electrical hazard to the patient and canceling the financial advantage of the lower cost of the Thymatron.

The dose of electrical stimulus administered with the MECTA JR-1 and SR-1 requires the treating physician to adjust pulse frequency, pulse width, and stimulus duration. Dosage selection is easier with the MECTA JR-2 and SR-2, because these units require the adjustment of only a single energy level control, which varies the duration of the stimulus and, thereby, the dosage administered. The Thymatron also requires adjustment of only one control, labeled percent energy, which adjusts the stimulus duration in order to alter the electrical charge delivered to the patient.

The physician who administers ECT must decide which of the currently available devices is most suitable for his or her own use. Because of its simpler control panel, its requirement for satisfactory impedance, and its ability to provide a baseline recording of the ECG and EEG prior to and following seizure induction, I favor the MECTA SR-2.

Since the newer devices that deliver lower energy levels produce less memory impairment and confusion than do the older instruments, some clinicians have suggested the administration of two or more seizure-producing electrical stimuli during the same anesthesia session in order to achieve a greater therapeutic response more rapidly with fewer exposures to anesthesia. Except in emergency situations with severely suicidal patients, I favor the administration of only a single seizure during each treatment session.

In addition to advances in instrumentation, any consideration of ECT must take into account the role of variation in electrode placement. Most earlier work with ECT utilized the bilateral (bitemporal) placement of electrodes. This approach provides stimulation to both the dominant and nondominant hemispheres. Although it is highly effective, it may be associated with greater confusion and memory deficit than the use of the unilateral electrode placement, wherein one electrode is placed in the temporal region and the other on the forehead over the nondominant hemisphere.[9,24] There is controversy about differences in efficacy of these two electrode placements, with some claiming greater efficacy for the bitemporal electrode position as compared to the standard unilateral position.[9] The D'Elia electrode placement technique utilizes one electrode placed in the temporal region and another on the vertex of the skull over the nondominant hemisphere.[25] My experience, and that of others, suggests this placement is more effective than the standard unilateral technique, and usually comparable in efficacy to bilateral electrode placement.[22,24] The D'Elia position appears to produce less confusion and memory problems than bilateral ECT, with equal efficacy in most patients.[22,25]

The American Psychiatric Association Task Force on Electroconvulsive Therapy, which reviewed this field in depth several years ago, recognizes that each individual psychiatrist should decide whether to employ unilateral or bilateral treatment.[9] Members of the task force would generally favor unilateral ECT because of the potential of less memory disability. My clinical experience suggests that most severely depressed patients who require ECT will respond favorably to a course of six to eight treatments administered with the MECTA device, employing D'Elia electrode placement. I have, however, encountered some patients who do not respond to unilateral treatments by the D'Elia electrode technique. My standard practice is to initiate treatment with this technique and, if no response is observed after the third treatment, to change electrode placement to bilateral for the remaining series of treatments. I believe this approach will minimize the risk of a patient receiving a number of ineffective treatments and thereby having to undergo a larger total number of treatments and consequently a greater number of anesthesia sessions.

One of the most unfortunate aspects of ECT is the controversy that this technique has generated. This controversy centers primarily on the question of whether ECT produces persistent or even permanent brain damage. Those opposed to ECT obviously answer this question affirmatively, although the data do not support that position.[1,9,17] Most evaluations of patients who have been treated judiciously with short (6 to 12 treatment) courses of ECT have only temporary, minor, and reversible memory deficits.[9,17] Some patients who have had extensive ECT (more than 50 treatments) may develop long-lasting or permanent impairment in memory capacity or cognitive function.[17] A group of 231 psychiatric patients were evaluated with the Wechsler Adult Intelligence Scale and the Halstead-Reitan Neuropsychological Test Battery prior to and following ECT. Most of those patients received unilateral ECT, although 29% received bilateral treatment. Contrary to the popular belief of those who relate

ECT to brain damage, some improvement in these test parameters was seen in 96% of the measures, and statistically significant ($P < 0.05$) improvement was noted in 37.5% of measurements of cognition and memory, indicating generally improved functioning following ECT.[26]

PHARMACOTHERAPY DURING ECT

Patients who require ECT may be agitated or psychotic at the outset of treatment. Therefore some individuals will require antipsychotic medication prior to and during the course of ECT.[9] The choice of an antipsychotic drug to use in such individuals should take into account the actions of that drug on the autonomic nervous system and cardiovascular system.[27] The drug should be readily administered IM, so that oral medication can be avoided during the period the patient is NPO. In my experience haloperidol is clearly the antipsychotic drug of choice for patients receiving ECT; it can be conveniently and painlessly administered IM, has very little anticholinergic effect, and provokes very little hypotension.[27] The dose of haloperidol utilized before and during the course of ECT should be relatively low. I prefer to administer this drug in a dosage of between 2 and 10 mg daily during the course of ECT, as opposed to higher doses. Chlorpromazine is certainly less desirable, because of its ability to lower seizure threshold and produce hypotension and cholinergic antagonism. Likewise, thioridazine is not desirable because of its hypotensive and anticholinergic effects and the inability to administer it by the IM route. Clozapine, which lowers seizure threshold significantly and has potent hypotensive and anticholinergic activity, is best avoided during the course of electroconvulsive treatment, wherein it may increase seizure intensity or duration.

Although some investigators feel that tricyclic antidepressants should be avoided during the course of ECT, others, including myself, feel that tricyclics are generally safe during ECT. However, the more anticholinergic tricyclic antidepressants may enhance confusional problems and interact with other anticholinergic agents the patient may receive prior to ECT.[4] The hypotensive action of tricyclics is manifested primarily as postural change, although in an individual with hemodynamic instability it would be preferable to avoid these drugs during the course of ECT. The potential myocardial depressant and arrhythmogenic effects of tricyclics may also provide an added risk to the patient receiving anesthesia during ECT, particularly if there is associated cardiovascular disease. Some observations suggest that tricyclic antidepressants may enhance the response to ECT, but further work is needed to confirm this.

Since clomipramine lowers seizure threshold and may lead to more intense and prolonged seizures, this tricyclic should probably be used with caution or not at all during ECT. There is no evidence that SSRIs interact adversely with ECT; however, fluoxetine and paroxetine inhibit drug metabolism and may potentiate anesthetic agents.

Monoamine oxidase inhibitors should be avoided during ECT because of their ability to potentiate barbiturate anesthetics, enhance hypotensive responses to anesthesia, and potentiate the hypertensive response that is generally observed during the course of ECT.[27] There have been some isolated reports that MAOIs can enhance the speed of response to ECT, although other factors that have been mentioned would generally counsel against their use during ECT.[7]

Lithium carbonate should be discontinued several days prior to starting ECT. Several observations strongly support the ability of lithium to enhance and prolong memory deficits and confusional states which may occur during the course of ECT.[6,7] There is also evidence that lithium may increase the paralytic effect of succinylcholine, the muscle relaxant employed by most physicians during ECT.[28] This effect of lithium may make it more difficult for the patient to begin breathing spontaneously following metabolic breakdown of the administered muscle relaxant.

If antianxiety agents such as the benzodiazepines are necessary in the management of patients receiving ECT, it should be remembered that the durations of action and the half-lives of these agents are generally long and their sedative and respiratory depressant effects may be additive with any anesthesia agent administered.[27] Following completion of a course of ECT, the issue probably foremost in the minds of most patients and physicians is the likelihood of recurrence of the depressive illness. The risk of recurrence even after a highly successful response to ECT is great.[9] The prophylactic value of lithium carbonate and the various antidepressant drugs against recurrent depression has been well documented.[8,29] Following a course of ECT, either lithium or a suitable antidepressant should be administered to the patient over a prolonged period in order to prevent recurrence of the depressive illness which necessitated the ECT.[8,10,30] If we assume that only the more severe forms of depression are refractory to pharmacotherapy and therefore require ECT, then these patients are the ones most important to protect against a recurrence of their depressive illness. I find it difficult to defend the administration of ECT to a patient with refractory depression who is not provided with some program of maintenance pharmacotherapy following treatment in order to avoid recurrence.

REFERENCES

1. Abrams R: *Electroconvulsive therapy,* New York, Oxford University Press, ed 2. 1992.
2. Fink M: Electroconvulsive therapy. In Paykel ES (ed): *Handbook of affective disorders,* ed 2. New York, Guilford Press, 1992, 359-367.
3. Paul SM, Extein I, Calil HM, et al: Use of ECT with treatment resistant depressed patients at the N.I.M.H. *Am J Psychiatry* 1981;138:486-489.
4. Mukherjee S, Saxkeim HA, Schnur DB: Electroconvulsive therapy of acute manic episodes: a review of 50 years' experience. *Am J Psychiatry* 1994;151:169-176.
5. Milstein V, Small JG, Miller MJ, et al: Mechanism of action of ECT: schizophrenia and schizoaffective disorder. *Biol Psychiatry* 1990;27:1282-1292.
6. El-Mallakh RS: Complications of concurrent lithium and electroconvulsive therapy: a review of clinical material and theoretical considerations. *Biol Psychiatry* 1988;23:595-601.
7. Kellner CH (ed): ECT and drugs: concurrent administration. *Convulsive Ther* 1993;9:237-351.

8. Coppen AJ, Abou-Saleh MT, Miller P, et al: Lithium continuation therapy following electroconvulsive therapy. *Br J Psychiatry* 1981;139:284-287.

9. American Psychiatric Association Task Force on Electroconvulsive Therapy: *The practice of electroconvulsive therapy: recommendations for treatment, training, and privileging.* Washington DC, American Psychiatric Press, 1990.

10. NIMH Consensus Development Conference on Electroconvulsive Therapy. *JAMA* 1985;245: 2103-2108.

11. Modigh K: Long term effects of electroconvulsive shock therapy on synthesis, turnover, and uptake of brain monoamines. *Psychopharmacology* 1976;49:179-183.

12. Coffey CE (ed): *The clinical science of electroconvulsive therapy.* Washington DC, American Psychiatric Press, 1993.

13. McGarvey KA, Zis AP, Brown EE, et al: ECS-induced dopamine release: effects of electrode placement, anticonvulsant treatment, and stimulus intensity. *Biol Psychiatry* 1993;34:152-157.

14. Young EA, Grunhaus L, Haskett RF, et al: Heterogeneity in the beta-endorphin immunore-activity response to electroconvulsive therapy. *Arch Gen Psychiatry* 1991;48:534-539.

15. Devanand DP, Bowers MB, Hoffman FJ, et al: Acute and subacute effects of ECT on plasma HVA, MHPG, and prolactin. *Biol Psychiatry* 1989;26:408-412.

16. Rudorfer MV, Risby ED, Osman OT, et al: Hypothalamic-pituitary-adrenal axis and monoamine transmitter activity in depression: a pilot study of central and peripheral effects of ECT. *Biol Psychiatry* 1991;29:253-264.

17. Weiner RD: Does electroconvulsive therapy cause brain damage? *Behav Brain Sci* 1984;7:1-53.

18. Kane JM: The current status of neuroleptic therapy. *J Clin Psychiatry* 1989;50:322-328.

19. Mandel MR, Welch CA, Mieske M, et al: Prediction of response to ECT in tricyclic-intolerant or tricyclic-resistant depressed patients. *McLean Hosp J* 1977;2:203-209.

20. Swartz CM, Saheba NC: Comparison of atropine with glycopyrrolate for use in ECT. *Convulsive Ther* 1989;5:56-60.

21. Nilsen SM, Willis KW, Pettinati HM: Initial impression of two new brief-pulse electrocon-vulsive therapy machines. *Convulsive Ther* 1986;2:43-54.

22. Sackeim HA, Prudic J, Devanand DP, et al: Effects of stimulus intensity and electrode placement on the efficacy and cognitive effects of electroconvulsive therapy. *N Engl J Med* 1993;328: 839-846.

23. Swartz CM, Abrams R: An auditory representation of ECT-induced seizures. *Convulsive Ther* 1986;2:125-128.

24. Abrams R, Swartz CM, Vedak C: Antidepressant effects of high-dose right unilateral electroconvulsive therapy. *Arch Gen Psychiatry* 1991;48:746-748.

25. D'Elia G: Unilateral electroconvulsive therapy. *Acta Psychiatr Scand Suppl* 1970;215:5-98.

26. Malloy FW, Small IF, Miller MJ, et al: Changes in neuropsychological test performance after electroconvulsive therapy. *Biol Psychiatry* 1982;17:61-67.

27. Bernstein JG: Psychotropic drug prescribing. In Cassem NH (ed): *Massachusetts General Hospital Handbook of general hospital psychiatry,* ed 3, St Louis, Mosby, 1991, 527-569.

28. Packman PM, Meyer DA, Verdun RM: Hazards of succinylcholine administration during electrotherapy. *Arch Gen Psychiatry* 1978;35:1137-1141.

29. Quitkin F, Rifkin A, Kane J, et al: Prophylactic effect of lithium and imipramine in unipolar and bipolar II patients: a preliminary report. *Am J Psychiatry* 1978;135:570-572.

30. Sackeim H, Malitz S (eds): Electroconvulsive therapy: clinical and basic research issues. *Ann NY Acad Sci* 1986;462:1-410.

CHAPTER 8

Lithium and Other Mood-Stabilizing Drugs

OVERVIEW

Indications
1. Treatment of acute manic episodes in manic depressive illness — FDA approved.
2. Prophylaxis against recurrent mania in manic depressive illness — FDA approved.
3. Adjunct with TCA, SSRI, or MAOI in treatment of depression.
4. Alone as an antidepressant (?efficacy).
5. Treatment of impulse disorders and episodic violence
6. Treatment (with antipsychotic drug) of schizoaffective disorder
7. Treatment of emotionally unstable character disorder
8. Treatment of borderline syndrome
9. Treatment of schizophrenia (?)
10. Treatment of premenstrual syndrome; cyclic depression (?)

Patient Evaluation Prior to Lithium Therapy
1. Serum creatinine and/or BUN.
2. ECG (in patients over age 50, or with cardiac history)
3. Serum electrolytes if patient has been on low-salt diet or diuretics, or if clinically indicated (i.e. renal or cardiovascular disease).
4. Thyroid function tests: T_3, T_4, TSH.
5. White blood cell count and fasting blood sugar or 2-hour blood sugar may also be helpful.

Initiating Lithium Therapy and Monitoring Serum Lithium Concentration
1. Use lowest effective dosage: 300 mg 2 to 4 times daily, depending on age and body size.
2. Use concurrently with antipsychotic drugs such as haloperidol in treating acutely manic patients.
3. In acutely manic patients, lithium level ideally should be between 0.8 and 1.0 mEq/L.

Continued.

4. In maintenance of manic or depressed patients, lithium level should be 0.6 to 0.8 mEq/L. (Levels of 0.4 to 0.6 mEq/L may be adequate.)

5. In acutely ill hospitalized patients, lithium level is measured once or twice weekly—more often if there are concurrent medical problems.

6. In starting lithium therapy in less acutely ill outpatients, levels may be measured once weekly.

7. If diuretics are administered, determine electrolytes—especially potassium and serum creatinine at least once weekly initially and less often subsequently.

8. Lithium levels should always be measured taking into account the time interval since last dose, which should preferably be 12 ± 2 hours.

9. In the first month of lithium therapy, lithium levels should be obtained (using a reliable laboratory) once weekly.

10. During the next month or 2, lithium level every 2 weeks; gradually extend the time interval between levels to every 4 weeks.

11. After lithium level has been stable for 4 to 6 months, the frequency may be decreased so the level is measured every 6 and eventually every 8 weeks. In virtually all patients it should be measured at least every 2 or 3 months, as long as the patient is being maintained on lithium.

12. Lithium level increase in the presence of stable dosage and constant dose-to-level time interval may be the earliest sign of lithium-related change in renal function, requiring medical evaluation and creatinine clearance determination.

13. Carbamazepine and valproate are effective in controlling acute mania and in prophylaxis, alone or with lithium. However, C may produce leukopenia; V may produce hepatic dysfunction.

14. Carbamazepine and valproate are effective in refractory, dysphoric, or rapidly cycling patients, alone or with lithium.

15. Clonazepam has limited antimanic efficacy, primarily as an adjunct to lithium or other drugs.

16. Lorazepam may be useful in acute mania and may allow use of lower doses of neuroleptics.

Continued.

17. Clonidine is helpful in the treatment of some acutely manic patients. Hypotension may occur.
18. Verapamil and other calcium channel blockers are helpful, primarily adjunctively in some manic patients; may provoke or worsen depression.

Lithium is considered by most physicians to be a relatively new treatment in medicine. Its use in the treatment of affective illness was approved by the FDA in the United States in 1969. The clinical use of lithium had its origin in the first published report by Garrod in 1859, who considered it to be a safe and effective treatment for gout. In the late 1800s a variety of patent medicines containing lithium salts and a multitude of proprietary brands of "lithia water" were sold in the United States and elsewhere. The primary application of these preparations was in the treatment of gouty conditions and various other physical ailments.[1] It is interesting to note the labeling on a bottle of Buffalo Lithia Water: "This medication is safe and effective for the treatment of nervous disorders in all their forms." A multitude of lithium products—including mineral waters, salts, tablets, and even Lithia Beer—were sold for medicinal purposes in the late 1800s and early 1900s. The advertisement for Buffalo Lithia Water from *Harpers Monthly Magazine*, March 1888, the Lithia Beer label, and the products shown in Figure 8-1 illustrate the ubiquitousness of lithium at the turn of the century.

Initially, lithium preparations were considered safe and devoid of adverse effects. By the first decade of the 1900s reports of cardiac depression and dilatation associated with excessive and continued consumption of lithia tablets began to appear in the medical literature. In the same period, reports of mental depression, nausea, and giddiness significantly dampened the medical use of lithium preparations. In the late 1920s lithium bromide was considered a safe and effective sedative. Excessive use of these preparations was then recognized to be associated with toxicity that was attributed to the bromide ion, which also received credit for the sedative action of the lithium bromide preparations. In retrospect, it is apparent that in all likelihood the efficacy and the toxicity of these early sedative preparations were related to both the lithium ion and the bromide ion.[1]

HISTORY OF LITHIUM THERAPY IN PSYCHIATRY

John Cade, an Australian physician, employed lithium urate for his investigation of the toxicity of urea in guinea pigs, and found that the animals developed extreme lethargy while remaining fully conscious. Cade had been

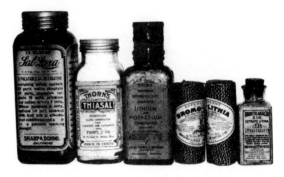

Fig. 8-1 Products used in the late 1800s and early 1900s for medicinal purposes.

involved in this work in relationship to his search for a toxin in the urine of manic patients. He then employed lithium salts experimentally, in an attempt to produce sedation in manic patients; he also used lithium preparations in epilepsy because of their apparent anticonvulsant action.[1] Prior to Cade's application of lithium in psychiatric patients, Henderson and Gillespie noted in their 1944 textbook of psychiatry that the waters taken from certain wells appeared to have special efficacy in the treatment of mental illness.[2] It was felt by Cade and subsequent workers that the therapeutic efficacy of those well waters was likely related to their lithium content.[1]

Cade's original report involved the use of lithium salts to treat ten patients suffering from mania, six diagnosed as having dementia praecox, and three who were called melancholic.[1] Although in the manic patients considerable improvement was noted paralleling lithium treatment, there was no fundamental improvement in the patients with dementia praecox except that three of them who were reported to be restless, noisy, and shouting nonsensical abuse did show some improvement. These three individuals may indeed have suffered from a manic illness rather than dementia praecox. The initial report failed to find a beneficial effect of lithium in patients suffering from chronic depressive psychoses. The initial clinical studies of lithium utilized lithium carbonate in a dose of 600 mg three times daily, gradually tapered down to 600 mg twice daily, and eventually to a maintenance dose of 600 mg once daily. Lithium citrate was used in doses of 1200 mg three times daily and likewise titrated downward to lower maintenance levels. Cade reported that adverse effects mainly involved the GI tract and nervous system.[1] The GI side effects reported were abdominal pain, anorexia, nausea, vomiting, and mild diarrhea. The neurologic side effects included giddiness, tremor, ataxia, slurred speech, myoclonic twitching, asthenia, and depression. Cade recommended immediate cessation of lithium if toxic effects appeared, and noted that the failure to withdraw the drug could be associated with a fatal outcome. It is interesting to note that Cade's initial studies did not involve monitoring of lithium blood levels, but rather utilized clinical

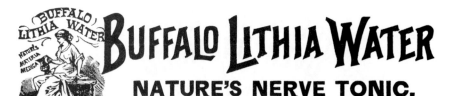

NATURE'S NERVE TONIC.
Nature's Specific for Bright's Disease.

A Powerful Nervous Tonic, it is a wonderful restorative in Nervous exhaustion, neuralgia, and affections generally of the nervous system. Both a remedy for and preventive of Mental and Physical Exhaustion from Overwork or Bright's Disease, Gout, Rheumatic Gout, Rheumatism, Acid Dyspepsia, Malarial Poisoning, &c. It is par excellence a remedy. Endorsed by medical men of the highest distinction.

Water in Cases of one dozen half gallon bottles, $5 per case, at the Springs.
THOS. F. GOODE, Proprietor, BUFFALO LITHIA SPRINGS, VA.

Reprinted from *Harpers Monthly Magazine*, March 1888.

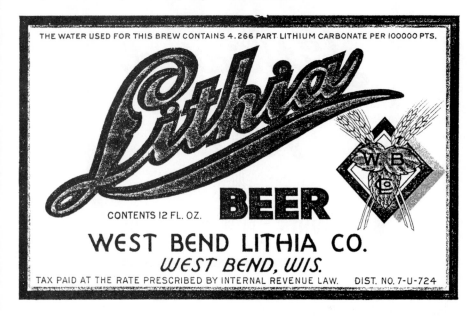

observations to adjust the dosage of lithium.[1] Unfortunately, the modern practitioner who has ready access to measuring serum lithium levels often forgets that clinical observation of the patient is at least of equal importance to the regular and careful monitoring of lithium levels.

It is as clear from Cade's original report in 1949 as it is today that lithium can be a safe and effective therapeutic agent in the treatment of psychiatric patients, particularly those with manic illness. Nevertheless, in many quarters, lithium continues to have a bad name and indeed is seen as a toxic or dangerous medication by psychiatrists, physicians in other specialties, and by laymen. One of the blackest chapters in our experience with lithium, and perhaps the origin of some of the negative feelings about the drug, particularly among internists,

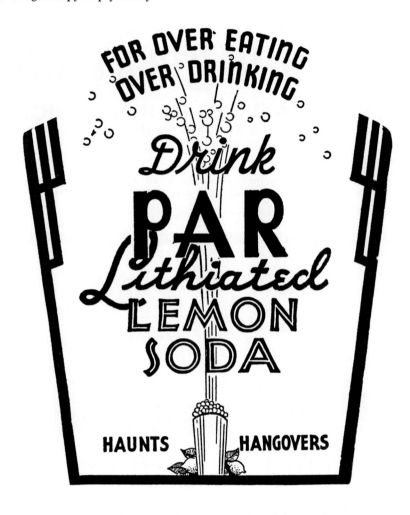

FOR OVER EATING OVER DRINKING

Drink

PAR

Lithiated

LEMON

SODA

HAUNTS HANGOVERS

is unrelated to the application of lithium in psychiatry. In the 1940s and early 1950s there were essentially no effective antihypertensive drugs. Therefore, the standard treatment of hypertension involved the use of a salt-restricted diet. Patients whose dietary intake of sodium was drastically reduced and who were unable to use sodium chloride to flavor their food were instructed to use a variety of salt substitutes. Lithium chloride was one of the most widely used salt substitute preparations.[3] Initially, it was felt to be a benign element, and since it was used to flavor food, no one considered the possibility of monitoring serum lithium levels or advising cautious use of this preparation. Furthermore, two other important factors were operative. It is now well-known that restriction of sodium intake causes the kidneys to increase retention of lithium.[3] Any physician prescribing lithium for the management of affective illness should warn his patients against consuming a salt-restricted diet.[4]

The other important factor that favored the development of toxicity in hypertensive patients using lithium as a salt substitute, was that, as we now know, many hypertensive patients tend to crave salt. Many hypertensive persons routinely salt their food prior to tasting it, in part because of habit and in part because of this craving. Therefore, the unfortunate salt-restricted hypertensive patient utilizing lithium as a salt substitute tended to use excessive quantities of this preparation, which enhanced toxicity. Physicians in medical practice in the days when lithium salts were used in this way will readily recall patients developing cardiac arrhythmias, obtundation, and a variety of neurologic complications. Fatalities associated with the use of lithium as a salt substitute were well-known in those early days. It seems very likely that much of the negative image associated with lithium is directly connected with these early complications, which in effect arose out of the absence of an understanding of the physiology of lithium and other electrolytes that existed at that time. The reality of this situation, and its potential for interfering with the therapeutic use of lithium in a manic patient whose internist recalls the early days of lithium, has repeatedly become apparent in my own clinical experience.

INDICATIONS FOR THE USE OF LITHIUM IN PSYCHIATRY

The use of lithium in the treatment of psychiatric patients, which began with the remarkable early work of Cade, spread to England and Denmark and subsequently throughout Europe. Eventually the tide of lithium reached the United States, which became the last country to authorize the therapeutic use of this valuable medication. At the present time, lithium carbonate is approved by the FDA for only two uses: in the treatment of manic episodes of manic-depressive illness and in the maintenance therapy of patients with a history of mania wherein it may prevent or diminish the intensity of subsequent manic episodes.[4] Despite these limited official applications of lithium, this simple element has been used throughout the world, and unofficially in the United States, in the treatment of a variety of other psychiatric illnesses. Many of these other uses of lithium remain controversial despite an expanding body of literature that supports broader therapeutic efficacy than the treatment and prophylaxis of mania.[4,6]

CLINICAL PRESENTATIONS OF MANIA

The acutely manic patient is relatively easy to recognize by the presence of an elevated, expansive, or irritable mood, and by associated findings which include (1) increased work, social, and sexual activity with or without physical restlessness; (2) increased talkativeness and pressure of speech; (3) flight of ideas and the feeling of racing thoughts; (4) inflated self-esteem and grandiosity; (5) decreased need for sleep; (6) easy distractibility; and (7) excessive participation in activities which may involve excessive danger or risk-taking, including the

---

DSM-IV CRITERIA

Box 8-1 Criteria for manic episode

A. A distinct period of abnormally and persistently elevated, expansive, or irritable mood, lasting at least 1 week (or any duration if hospitalization is necessary).

B. During the period of mood disturbance, three (or more) of the following symptoms have persisted (four if the mood is only irritable) and have been present to a significant degree:

(1) Inflated self-esteem or grandiosity

(2) Decreased need for sleep (e.g., feels rested after only 3 hours of sleep)

(3) More talkative than usual or pressure to keep talking

(4) Flight of ideas or subjective experience that thoughts are racing

(5) Distractibility (i.e., attention too easily drawn to unimportant or irrelevant external stimuli)

(6) Increase in goal-directed activity (either socially, at work or school, or sexually) or psychomotor agitation

(7) Excessive involvement in pleasurable activities that have a high potential for painful consequences (e.g., engaging in unrestrained buying sprees, sexual indiscretions, or foolish business investments)

C. The symptoms do not meet criteria for a Mixed Episode.

D. The mood disturbance is sufficiently severe to cause marked impairment in occupational functioning or in usual social activities or relationships with others, or to necessitate hospitalization to prevent harm to self or others, or there are psychotic features.

E. The symptoms are not due to the direct physiological effects of a substance (e.g., a drug of abuse, a medication, or other treatment) or a general medical condition (e.g., hyperthyroidism).

Note: Manic-like episodes that are clearly caused by somatic antidepressant treatment (e.g., medication, electroconvulsive therapy, light therapy) should not count toward a diagnosis of Bipolar I Disorder.

From American Psychiatric Association: *Diagnostic and statistical manual of mental disorders*, ed 4 [DSM-IV]. Washington DC, American Psychiatric Press, 1994.

---

tendency to get involved in fights, reckless driving, poor business judgments, sexual indiscretions, and spending sprees.[5] These findings, though not uniformly present in all manic patients, are consistent with the classical descriptions of mania and with those accepted by the DSM-IV, which are shown in Boxes 8-1 and 8-2.[2] Mania may present simply with restlessness or only some of these described findings. It is infrequently recognized by clinicians that manic patients may be extremely paranoid. Often the presence of agitated behavior, inappropriate verbalizations, and paranoid ideation is taken by the clinician to support a diagnosis of a schizophrenic illness. I have observed a number of persons suffering from manic illness and highly responsive to lithium, whose primary manifestation involved only pressure of speech and paranoid ideation.

The danger of an acute manic episode cannot be underestimated from the standpoint of its ability to interfere with or destroy family relationships, as well as the business and professional standing of the patient.[6] There is a high

DSM-IV CRITERIA
Box 8-2 Criteria for hypomanic episode

A. A distinct period of persistently elevated, expansive, or irritable mood, lasting throughout at least 4 days, that is clearly different from the usual nondepressed mood.
B. During the period of mood disturbance, three (or more) of the following symptoms have persisted (four if the mood is only irritable) and have been present to a significant degree:
   (1) Inflated self-esteem or grandiosity
   (2) Decreased need for sleep (e.g., feels rested after only 3 hours of sleep)
   (3) More talkative than usual or pressure to keep talking
   (4) Flight of ideas or subjective experience that thoughts are racing
   (5) Distractibility (i.e., attention too easily drawn to unimportant or irrelevant external stimuli)
   (6) Increase in goal-directed activity (either socially, at work or school, or sexually) or psychomotor agitation
   (7) Excessive involvement in pleasurable activities that have a high potential for painful consequences (e.g., the person engages in unrestrained buying sprees, sexual indiscretions, or foolish business investments)
C. The episode is associated with an unequivocal change in functioning that is uncharacteristic of the person when not symptomatic.
D. The disturbance in mood and the change in functioning are observable by others.
E. The episode is not severe enough to cause marked impairment in social or occupational functioning, or to necessitate hospitalization, and there are no psychotic features.
F. The symptoms are not due to the direct physiological effects of a substance (e.g., a drug of abuse, a medication, or other treatment) or a general medical condition (e.g., hyperthyroidism).
Note: Hypomanic-like episodes that are clearly caused by somatic antidepressant treatment (e.g., medication, electroconvulsive therapy, light therapy) should not count toward a diagnosis of Bipolar II Disorder.

From American Psychiatric Association: *Diagnostic and statistical manual of mental disorders*, ed 4 [DSM-IV]. Washington DC, American Psychiatric Press, 1994.

correlation between manic episodes and the tendency to consume excessive quantities of alcohol. The individual who suffers from repeated affective illness may simultaneously present with the problem of alcoholism. Most commonly, the first manic episode attacks the individual and his family by complete surprise, whether it originates gradually or suddenly. Likewise, most persons suffering their first episode will deny that anything is wrong and will rationalize the symptoms in a variety of ways. Many persons who suffer from this illness are extremely creative and intelligent, which further enhances their ability to deny illness. Most persons will become angry when approached by the physician attempting to prescribe treatment. There is no safe or effective nonsomatic treatment for mania.[6] Pharmacotherapy is almost always the preferable form of treatment, though ECT has been used effectively in the control of acute mania.[7]

Psychotherapy in the absence of medication is dangerous and ineffective. If the patient is kept in a totally safe environment and prevented from destroying family, business, and professional components of his life, the mania may eventually break, with or without psychotherapy. On the other hand, most affected individuals will have numerous contacts within society and many opportunities to irreparably damage their reputation. Awaiting the spontaneous disappearance of mania, with or without the use of psychotherapy, will be unduly costly and damaging to the patient.

Patients who are manic tend to sleep very little, and become involved in a variety of activities at a rapid and, at times, almost inhuman pace. Manic patients can suffer from exhaustion as a result of hyperactivity; and if there is underlying cardiovascular or pulmonary disease, or the presence of a metabolic disease such as diabetes, the individual may be more likely to suffer medical complications of his acute manic illness.[8] Many otherwise respectable people during the course of a manic episode, become involved in illegal or immoral activities which turn considerable negative attention toward themselves.[9] The person who has always been law-abiding, and suddenly becomes involved in fraudulent or otherwise illegal business or professional activities, should be seriously evaluated with the likelihood that he may be suffering from a manic illness.[9] The faithful spouse who begins to have a series of sexual liaisons is likewise a suspect for mania. The kind, responsible, and loving parent who suddenly becomes a child abuser may also be suffering from bipolar affective illness.

An individual may suffer one episode of mania and have no recurrences, and therefore would not need long-term medication maintenance. However, this situation is less frequent than the more common observation of a patient having repeated manic episodes throughout his life which may be interspersed with moderate to severe depression. There is clearly an inherited tendency to develop major affective illness; most patients will have biologic relatives who have suffered from episodes of mania or depression, or with problems of alcohol dependency, the latter appearing to be biologically and perhaps genetically connected with the propensity to develop affective illness.[9] A patient who has an acute manic episode, particularly in the presence of either a positive family history or a personal history of previous manic or depressive episodes, should be considered for long-term lithium maintenance.[4,9]

Manic episodes can occur at vastly different intervals in each patient and the frequency of manic episodes in a group of patients with bipolar affective illness will vary considerably. Some will suffer multiple manic episodes during the course of a year, while others may remain free of mania for periods of 10 or more years, even in the absence of lithium maintenance. Many of the latter individuals will intermittently experience mild to severe depressive episodes.[9] A given individual may have manic episodes at different times in his or her life with greater or lesser frequency. There is no age barrier to the development of manic symptoms. Manic illnesses have been reported in the literature in children as young as 4 years old,[10] and in adults in their 90s.[9] Manic symptoms associated with major affective illness are becoming recognized with increasing frequency in latency-age children and in adolescents.[11] Many of these children had previously been labeled as behavior problems and seen as "acting-out" teenagers. Some children who were previously labeled as attention deficit hyperactivity disorder (ADHD) are now being recognized as having major affective illnesses, responsive to lithium therapy.[10,12] I have observed the first episodes of symptoms consistent with mania appearing from age 11 to 80. As will be discussed later in this chapter, lithium therapy used with appropriate caution can be safe at either end of the age spectrum.

LITHIUM IN MANIA AND DEPRESSION

The efficacy of lithium carbonate in the treatment of acute mania has been well documented through a variety of controlled and uncontrolled clinical studies done over a period of many years.[4,13,14] In addition to the monitoring of blood levels and other parameters in patients taking lithium in the acute phase of manic illness, lithium requires a cooperative patient who will take daily oral medication, in contrast to neuroleptic drugs which can be given orally or IM intermittently as required. Perhaps the major disadvantage of lithium in the treatment of acute mania is that improvement is slow and gradual. It may require up to 3 weeks to adequately control manic symptoms if the administration of other medications is avoided. One excellent controlled study compared the efficacy of lithium carbonate, chlorpromazine, and haloperidol in the control of acute mania in hospitalized patients.[100] Lithium carbonate and haloperidol used alone produced significant improvement in manic symptoms without excessive sedation. Haloperidol had the most dramatic and rapid impact in controlling behavioral activity in the manic patients under study. Lithium produced a more even and gradual normalization of the study patients. Chlorpromazine, on the other hand, produced considerable sedation but did little to alter qualitatively the underlying manic symptoms.[14]

In addition to the documentation of safety and efficacy in acute mania, similar documentation exists supporting the use of lithium in the prophylaxis of recurrent mania.[4,6] Although specific techniques in the therapeutic use of lithium will be discussed later, it is important to note that there is some controversy as to the optimal therapeutic blood level and dosage regimen when lithium is employed either in the treatment of acute mania or its prophylaxis. The generally quoted therapeutic range for serum lithium levels is 0.6 to 1.2 mEq/L. Lithium blood levels should ideally be measured at approximately 12 hours (plus or minus 2 hours) after the last dose of lithium is administered.[4,6] Clinical observations must always accompany laboratory determination in adjusting the proper therapeutic and maintenance dose of the lithium ion. In addition to the well-documented prophylactic effect of lithium against recurrent mania, there is considerable evidence to support its highly beneficial effect in the prophylaxis of recurrent depression in patients suffering from bipolar illness. There is also evidence to support the prophylactic value of lithium against recurrent depression in patients who do not have a manic component to their major affective illness.[15,16] Careful regular use of adequate lithium dosage regimens in patients with bipolar illness is somewhat more effective in preventing the recurrence of mania than it is in preventing the recurrence of depression. In my experience and in that of other investigators, it can be estimated that between 30% and 40% of patients with bipolar illness being maintained on lithium will require an additional mood stabilizer or antidepressant for the treatment of a manic or depressive episode not adequately prevented by lithium maintenance.[6,17]

Lithium has been widely utilized in the treatment of depression, and many workers have supported a therapeutic as well as a prophylactic value of this ion in depression.[16,18] When used as the sole therapeutic agent in the treatment of depression, lithium appears to be less effective than conventional antidepressant drugs, though some patients do achieve an adequate therapeutic response without the need to add other antidepressants.[18] Perhaps one of the more interesting and clinically important applications of lithium in depression is its apparent ability to facilitate a therapeutic response to conventional antidepressant drug therapy in some patients.[19] One double-blind study found that lithium enhanced the antidepressant efficacy of imipramine, while there was less evidence to support a lithium enhancement of the antidepressant action of amitriptyline.[20] Other studies have found a synergistic effect of lithium when combined with tranylcypromine in refractory depressed patients.[21] I have seen many patients treated with a variety of SSRI or tricyclic antidepressant medications at adequate dosages who achieved a limited therapeutic benefit and dramatically improved within 3 days to 3 weeks after the addition of lithium carbonate. Likewise, I have seen a number of patients previously unresponsive to MAOIs who achieved a satisfactory therapeutic response when lithium was added to the regimen. Several of my patients who have experienced a partial therapeutic response to the combination of a tricyclic and an MAOI antidepressant subsequently experienced enhancement of the antidepressant response when lithium was added. An additional value of lithium in the treatment of depression is its potential for protecting an individual against the development of mania when treated with a conventional antidepressant drug in a standard or larger-than-standard therapeutic dose.[4] Lithium has some value in the prophylaxis of depression in patients with unipolar affective illness, though this effect is less dramatic than that seen with the prophylactic use of lithium in mania.[4,16]

LITHIUM IN OTHER PSYCHIATRIC DISORDERS

Lithium is not approved for the treatment of schizophrenia, and considerable controversy surrounds its use in this condition. Numerous studies have employed lithium alone or in combination with neuroleptics in the treatment of various subtypes of schizophrenia. One study found that six of 11 lithium-treated schizophrenic patients developed a toxic confusional organic brain syndrome.[22] A review of 24 published articles on lithium use in schizophrenia, most of which were uncontrolled studies, revealed some positive response in a third to a half of patients.[23] The same review found that there was a higher response rate in 22 publications on lithium treatment of schizoaffective disorder, and also some beneficial effect of lithium noted in nine reports on atypical or schizophreniform psychosis treated with lithium.[23] A somewhat more recent study has found a favorable response to lithium in schizophrenic patients judged to have a favorable prognosis.[24] A well-conducted study found lithium combined with haloperidol to be more effective than haloperidol alone in schizoaffective disorder.[25] I would not strongly recommend the use of lithium in schizophrenia except for its value in schizoaffective disorder, which most likely represents an affective illness with associated schizophrenic symptoms.

Schizoaffective disorder in accordance with the DSM-IV[5] presents as an uninterrupted period of illness with a Major Depressive Episode, a Manic Episode, or a Mixed Episode concurrently with symptoms meeting Criterion A for Schizophrenia. The latter criteria are as follows: (1) delusions, (2) hallucinations, (3) disorganized speech, (4) grossly disorganized or catatonic behavior, (5) negative symptoms (that is, affective flattening, alogia, or avolition). To make this diagnosis, there must have been delusions or hallucinations for at least 2 weeks in the absence of prominent mood symptoms, symptoms for the mood episode must be present for a substantial portion of the illness, and the disorder must not be related to drugs or a general medical condition. Furthermore, the mood symptoms must satisfy criteria for depression with depressed mood or for bipolar type with manic or mixed features.

Considerable variability exists in this syndrome, which is relatively common and responsive to pharmacotherapy. The therapeutic benefit of lithium carbonate alone has been demonstrated in schizoaffective illness.[4] Furthermore, there is considerable documentation to support the use of lithium carbonate in conjunction with low-dose high-potency neuroleptics such as haloperidol or trifluoperazine in the treatment of this syndrome.[4,25] I have treated many patients fitting the criteria of schizoaffective illness, both those showing signs consistent with the manic type and those showing evidence of the depressive type, with a variety of psychopharmacologic agents. In both forms, lithium appears to be beneficial, and the patients I have treated have generally done better with the addition of low-dose neuroleptics, particularly when the bipolar or manic type is present. Patients suffering from the depressed type tend to respond best to antidepressants if they are simultaneously receiving lithium and low-dose neuroleptics. Although I am sensitive to the concerns of many regarding polypharmacy, the judicious use of lithium in combination with a low-dose neuroleptic and an antidepressant in depressed patients with schizoaffective illness, may spell the difference between repeated hospitalizations and suicide attempts, and the patient's ability to remain functional and productive.

Emotionally unstable character disorder (EUCD), as defined by Rifkin, is a syndrome characterized by mood swings, both depressive and hypomanic, lasting from several hours to a few days and usually not precipitated by or reactive to environmental or interpersonal events. It is associated with one or more of the following activities: drug abuse, delinquent behavior, avoidance or inadequate performance at school or work, difficulty with authority, sexual promiscuity, and malingering.[26] The patients classified in this way by Rifkin were primarily women from their late teens into their early thirties. These patients bear many similarities to the more widely recognized group of patients labeled borderline personality disorder (BPD). The 21 hospitalized patients treated in a double-blind crossover design by Rifkin, wherein lithium was compared with placebo, demonstrated significantly more therapeutic efficacy with lithium than with placebo.[26] Unfortunately, these patients and those more commonly classified as BPD are often not willing to cooperate fully with a therapeutic trial of medication. Furthermore, both EUCD and BPD patients have a tendency to behave in a self-destructive manner, and present some increased risk of medication abuse and overdose.

Nevertheless, over many years I have used lithium to treat nearly 200 similar patients, both men and women, between 15 and 40 years of age. A sizable proportion of the patients I have seen with EUCD-BPD symptomatology have benefited from lithium. The benefit has been most marked in terms of a reduction in the frequency or severity of depressive symptoms and a decrease in impulsivity, as well as some decrease in antisocial behavior. Those individuals who would be considered more typically BPD compared with EUCD tended to have more severe and persistent affective symptoms, primarily depressive, and were more apt to make suicide threats or attempts. This latter group tended to do better if a low-dose high-potency neuroleptic was added to the lithium regimen; those borderlines with more significant affective features who were being treated with lithium tended to achieve a better therapeutic response when their depressive symptoms were treated by the addition of a TCA, SSRI, MAOI antidepressant. The published literature and my clinical experience suggest that it is often difficult to reliably differentiate patients labeled BPD classified as schizoaffective from those diagnosed as EUCD and those labeled BPD.[4,5,25,26] As these three groups of patients merge with one another, there appears to be an underlying affective component which may draw them together as a variant of major affective disorder. A therapeutic trial of lithium is clearly indicated, particularly if other agents have been unsuccessful and the patient's symptomatology is severe enough to significantly impair his ability to remain functional and productive.[27]

Lithium is particularly advantageous in these patients, since its blood level can be monitored, which may provide an added dimension of surveillance to reinforce proper use of the prescribed medication.[27] Furthermore, since lithium does not produce an enjoyable "high" or any desirable behavioral change of a recreational nature when excessive doses are employed, and since patients may be warned about the risks of excessive medication use, patients in this latter category may be less apt to abuse lithium than if the clinician attempts to treat them with benzodiazepines or antidepressant medication. Patients with impulse disorders and episodic violence or aggressive behavior may benefit from a therapeutic trial of lithium carbonate. It has been shown in some studies to reduce aggressive, impulsive, and violent behavior in patients of normal intelligence and in individuals suffering from mental retardation.[28-30]

The apparent connection between alcohol abuse and affective illness has already been mentioned. Indeed, prior to the modern era of psychopharmacology, *Par Lithiated Soda* claimed on its label to be helpful for excessive alcohol consumption. Some studies of lithium treatment in alcoholics have found that lithium decreases drinking and facilitates abstinence in depressed alcoholics. Others have found a beneficial effect of lithium on abstinence, independent of coexistent depression.[31] Some persons who are episodic alcohol abusers will develop hypomanic symptoms in response to moderate amounts of alcohol. Lithium has been shown to diminish the development of these responses, though not necessarily to affect the quantity of alcohol consumed.[32] Many persons who abuse a variety of drugs, including narcotics, sedatives, cocaine, and amphetamines, may indeed be suffering from an affective illness.[33] Empiric trial of lithium in selected patients with drug abuse problems who are motivated to participate in a treatment program may be associated with some stabilization of mood and a potential decrease in their substance abuse.[33,34]

Lithium has been used by a variety of investigators and clinicians in the treatment of premenstrual syndrome (PMS) associated with irritability, and mood shifts with either elation or depression.[4] Though lithium is not approved by the FDA for this use and should not be routine treatment for PMS, the positive results suggested in some published studies would support a therapeutic trial of this agent in women who experience PMS, particularly if associated with cyclic mood fluctuations.[35]

Although the indications which I have reviewed for the therapeutic application of lithium by no means include all of the conditions for which the drug has been tried, this is an attempt to present those clinical conditions in which lithium may be beneficial. The discussion of these potential indications for lithium is not meant to endorse its use beyond the treatment and prophylaxis of affective disorders. In treating a patient who has failed to respond to other regimens, where there is a potential of a beneficial response, a therapeutic trial of lithium should be considered.[35] A trial of lithium for an alternative indication should take place only if the patient is in good health and does not have any medical contraindications to lithium therapy. The patient should be told that lithium is being used for a nonapproved indication, and his permission to try the drug in this situation should be sought. It is appropriate to document in the patient's medical record that this discussion has taken place and that the patient has agreed to a trial of lithium. The clinician must ascertain that the patient will cooperate with the recommended therapeutic regimen, take the medication as prescribed, and present himself at appropriate intervals for lithium blood level determination. It is likewise important when lithium is utilized in one of these special situations to ask the patient to discontinue medication and notify the physician at the first sign of any significant adverse effect. The treatment of any patient with lithium carbonate should not proceed until the appropriate and necessary medical evaluation can be conducted.

PATIENT EVALUATION PRIOR TO LITHIUM THERAPY

Since lithium is an ion which is physiologically interchangeable with sodium and has a variety of physiologic and pathophysiologic actions in various organ systems, it is important to ascertain that the patient has no medical contraindications and has sufficient renal function to clear the ion adequately to prevent lithium intoxication.[4] If a patient is currently being treated by another physician for any other medical condition, the psychiatrist should talk with the other physicians managing the patient, to understand the overall medical condition and any other medications the patient may be receiving.[8] In a patient not receiving other medical care, the psychiatrist should take a medical history, including a review of systems, directly from the patient. I prefer to do a physical examination on the patient unless one has been done recently by another physician and I can obtain those data.

A serum creatinine and BUN determination should be done prior to starting lithium unless one has been done within the past month. If a patient is currently or has recently been on a low-salt diet or a diuretic regimen, or if there is any medical information to suggest the possibility of an electrolyte abnormality, serum electrolyte determinations should be done. Not uncommonly, patients taking diuretics under the care of other physicians may not have had serum electrolyte measurements done recently enough, although if electrolytes have been measured within a week before starting lithium, a repeat determination is generally unnecessary. Since lithium is not metabolized and is excreted unchanged by the kidney, an elevation in serum creatinine level would lead to increased lithium serum concentration and an increase of toxicity at conventional therapeutic doses. Hypokalemia, frequently induced by diuretic therapy, increases the risk of both cardiovascular and neurologic side effects of therapeutic serum lithium concentrations.[4] Patients being maintained on low-salt diets or diuretics will achieve greater-than-predicted serum lithium levels with conventional dosage and thereby stand a greater risk of lithium intoxication.[4,8]

Since lithium not uncommonly produces repolarization (ST and T wave) changes in the ECG at therapeutic dosages, a baseline ECG prior to starting the drug is useful, particularly since these changes may be misinterpreted as representing coronary insufficiency if they are found on a routine ECG during lithium treatment.[4,8] About 20% of patients taking lithium experience T wave flattening or inversion at therapeutic blood levels of lithium, although these changes are not indicative of underlying heart disease.[36] Conduction abnormalities and changes in sinus node function can occur at therapeutic as well as toxic levels of lithium.[37] Asymptomatic first-degree atrioventricular block has been reported in a young patient who was not lithium-toxic.[4] One study utilizing exercise testing and extended ambulatory monitoring of 12 patients receiving lithium therapy[37] found no adverse effect of lithium on cardiac function; furthermore, it was found that lithium does not aggravate exercise-associated ventricular arrhythmias. Isolated reports, however, have noted the appearance of atrial and ventricular arrhythmias in some patients receiving lithium and maintained at standard therapeutic blood levels.[4] In patients suffering from lithium intoxication, a variety of cardiovascular abnormalities may be seen, including arrhythmias, conduction disturbances, and hypotension.[37] The likelihood of these complications occurring would be enhanced by excessive serum lithium levels or by the presence of hypokalemia. Routine periodic monitoring of the ECG in patients receiving lithium is not clinically necessary, but if ECGs are done by the patient's internist during a periodic examination or because of the development of cardiovascular symptoms, it would be helpful for the psychiatrist to obtain copies.

Since lithium treatment may be associated with the development of euthyroid goiter, hypothyroidism with or without thyroid gland enlargement, or abnormalities in serum determinations of thyroid function,[4] it is useful to obtain baseline measurement of thyroid function (triiodothyronine [T_3], thyroxine [T_4], and thyroid-stimulating hormone [TSH]) prior to initiating lithium therapy. When administered at therapeutic levels, lithium may inhibit synthesis and release of T_3 and T_4 from the thyroid gland. This reduction in circulating thyroid hormones stimulates TSH secretion, leading to a compensatory stimulation of the thyroid gland in order to re-establish the euthyroid state.[4] During this compensatory process, a goiter may form or the patient may become clinically hypothyroid. Lithium has also been reported to decrease the rate of T_4 clearance from the blood, inhibit thyroglobulin synthesis, inhibit TSH-sensitive adenylcyclase, and inhibit iodine uptake into the gland with consequent inhibition of the formation of organic iodine.[38] In my experience the incidence of hypothyroidism or goiter formation in lithium-treated patients is exceedingly low. It is more common to find an increase in TSH on periodic follow-up thyroid function testing. If no other structural or functional thyroid changes are seen, this isolated finding does not require discontinuation of lithium or the administration of any specific treatment. The presence of hypothyroidism or of a goiter during lithium therapy would indicate the need for appropriate consultation and probably the simultaneous administration of thyroid replacement therapy along with continued lithium carbonate management.[4] In addition to the value of measuring thyroid hormone parameters prior to and at yearly intervals during lithium therapy, it is also clinically useful to palpate the thyroid gland before treatment and during the maintenance period.

Lithium administration is frequently associated with weight gain, which may be related to both fluid retention and to increased caloric intake.[39] Various studies have demonstrated either an increase or a decrease in glucose tolerance in lithium-treated patients, and there are no data to suggest that lithium is diabetogenic.[4] Furthermore, diabetes is not a contraindication to lithium therapy. On the other hand, it is useful to obtain a serum glucose determination prior to starting lithium therapy in diabetics as well as nondiabetics. This baseline information may be particularly useful in the event that some metabolic change occurs during lithium therapy. Furthermore, since many patients seen by the psychiatrist are receiving no other medical care, the opportunity to do selected laboratory tests may help to diagnose previously unsuspected medical illnesses such as diabetes.

Lithium frequently produces benign reversible leukocytosis, and WBC counts of 12,000 to 15,000/μL are not uncommonly seen during therapy. The increase in the WBC count is not indicative of any hematologic disease and does not require discontinuation of lithium.[4] The appearance of an elevated white cell count in a patient taking lithium, who is seen by a physician not aware of this association, may precipitate a series of medical evaluations which are not clinically necessary. It is generally useful to determine the white cell count before starting treatment, and to communicate with any physician managing a lithium-treated patient so that he will be aware of this association.

INITIATING LITHIUM THERAPY AND MONITORING LITHIUM CONCENTRATION

Once the clinician has established the need for lithium treatment and has completed the medical evaluation of the patient, treatment should be initiated utilizing the lowest dose necessary to achieve the desired therapeutic blood concentration.[4] In general, for the indications discussed previously, one should achieve a serum concentration of lithium of 0.6 to 0.9 mEq/L. Treatment at lower or higher serum lithium concentrations is appropriate in some patients who either have lithium side effects or fail to achieve adequate mood stabilization. As can be seen from Table 8-1, many of the adverse effects of lithium correlate with serum concentration. The technique used in the administration of lithium will differ somewhat in a patient being treated for an acute manic episode in the hospital, as opposed to the individual being started on the drug as an outpatient, for either mild manic symptoms or other clinical indications.

Since lithium is slow yet highly effective in controlling acute mania,[14] the therapeutic regimen of choice in dealing with an acute manic patient involves the simultaneous administration of appropriate neuroleptic drugs.[4,8] Haloperidol is a neuroleptic with the most rapid and dramatic antimanic action, and

Table 8-1   Adverse effects of lithium carbonate

Side effects (therapeutic serum concentration)	Impending toxicity (increased serum concentration)	Lithium toxicity (toxic serum concentration)
Polydipsia, polyuria	Nausea, vomiting	Cardiac arrhythmias
Nausea	Diarrhea	Impaired consciousness
Mild diarrhea	Coarse hand tremor	Muscle fasciculation
Fine hand tremor	Sleepiness	Hyperreflexia
Dizziness	Sluggishness	Nystagmus
Weight gain	Vertigo	Convulsions
Edema	Dysarthria	Coma
Hypothyroidism or goiter		Oliguria, anuria

therefore should be considered the neuroleptic of choice in acute manic psychosis.[14] Contrary to the alarmist publications which appeared some years ago calling attention to a presumed specific toxic interaction between lithium and thioridazine[39] and between lithium and haloperidol,[41] there is no good evidence that a specific toxic syndrome exists. Indeed, a review of 425 patients receiving a combination of lithium and haloperidol failed to confirm even one case with findings consistent with the initial report of four patients with a presumed toxic syndrome.[42] There is no question that the use of lithium can produce toxic reactions, particularly when excessive blood levels are employed, as in the report by Cohen and Cohen.[41] Furthermore, there are a variety of potential adverse effects associated with all of the neuroleptic drugs, including the potential development of the neuroleptic malignant syndrome discussed in chapter 9. Numerous publications fail to define a specific lithium-haloperidol toxic syndrome, and my own extensive clinical use of this combination has likewise failed to confirm the report of Cohen and Cohen. Although there are multiple case reports in the literature suggesting a toxic interaction between lithium and each of our currently available neuroleptic drugs,[4] a study of 60 manic patients given neuroleptics alone and 69 given neuroleptics and lithium together found no difference in frequency or severity of adverse effects.[43]

In the acutely manic patient, treatment should be initiated with haloperidol at a dose of 5 mg orally or IM with additional haloperidol or lorazepam administered as required to produce behavioral control and prevent the patient from harming himself or others. The dosage of lorazepam and haloperidol may be titrated upward during the initial course of treatment of the acute manic episode, until adequate behavioral improvement is noted and lithium has had time to become effective. The neuroleptic dosage is gradually titrated downward, and discontinued once the lithium effect is established. Instituting treatment with a neuroleptic such as haloperidol will not only produce a relatively prompt antimanic action in most patients, but it will also improve the safety of the patient while awaiting a therapeutic response to lithium. Lithium therapy can be started simultaneously with the neuroleptic. A variety of techniques for initiating lithium therapy have been recommended, with some physicians suggesting a more aggressive dosage regimen. My own preference is to avoid aggressive use of lithium. It is not likely to measurably increase the speed of the lithium response, and it is likely to increase the risk of unwanted side effects, including GI symptoms, confusion, and tremor.[4] Furthermore, the aggressive administration in acute manic illness may lead to an overshooting of the desired blood level so that lithium intoxication develops before the desired therapeutic response is achieved.

Although no particular formula can adequately govern an exact starting dose of lithium, and various techniques of administration of a test dose with subsequent lithium level determinations are often too cumbersome to employ in the patient who is agitated, I tend to recommend a graduated dosage schedule based on the patient's overall body size and age. Elderly patients are more likely than younger persons to develop a toxic confusional state when receiving lithium, and should generally be given a lower dose initially and throughout the course of treatment. In many elderly persons, particularly those with some organic brain dysfunction, it may be safer and more useful to maintain lithium levels in the range of 0.3 to 0.6 mEq/L rather than the conventional range of 0.6 to 0.9 mEq/L. Since the primary work of controlling mania in the first week is by an appropriate neuroleptic regimen, it seems less critical if the serum lithium level reaches a therapeutic range by the third day or by the end of the first week. In a patient who has had prior manic episodes and who has tolerated and required larger doses of lithium, it would be good clinical practice to follow the previous experience of the patient. With the first manic episode, it is reasonable to start lithium carbonate at a dose of 1200 mg daily in a patient who weighs 180 lb or more. In a person weighing between 120 and 180 lb, a dose of 900 mg daily is a reasonable starting point, while in the person weighing less than 120 lb, a starting dose of 600 mg daily is clinically appropriate. If the patient is elderly and has not had prior experience with lithium, the clinician may consider using a starting dose of one-half to three-quarters that used in a young, otherwise healthy, patient. The total daily lithium dose may be administered in divided doses or as a single daily dose at bedtime.

In the acutely manic patient it may be preferable to achieve a somewhat higher serum lithium concentration than one might wish to achieve during the maintenance phase. There is little evidence to suggest a significant advantage, however, in establishing serum levels above 1.2 mEq/L even in the acutely manic individual, though lithium levels in the 0.8 to 1.2 range may be more likely to be beneficial than levels in the 0.6 to 0.8 mEq/L range. With higher lithium levels, there is greater likelihood of unwanted side effects.[4]

Generally lithium has been administered to patients in two to four divided daily doses, with the rationale of providing a more stable serum concentration, with the potential that less peaks and troughs would minimize side effects such as tremor and maximize efficacy. Numerous studies have suggested potential benefits of less frequent, generally single daily doses of lithium. One such study found more sclerotic glomeruli, fibrosis and atrophic tubules in the kidneys of patients on a multiple dose schedule.[44] Several studies have found lower urine volumes in patients receiving lithium on a single daily dose schedule; one group examined 85 patients on single- or multiple-dose regimens being maintained in a lithium clinical and concluded that single daily doses were associated with significantly less polyuria.[45] It has been suggested that the once daily lithium dose regimen produces lower trough serum levels, allowing more time for renal distal tubular regeneration, which may have a protective effect and minimize the risk of lithium associated renal damage.[45] At the present time, there are still inadequate data to document whether or not once daily lithium dosing is as effective prophylactically as the multiple-dose regimens; furthermore, many of the studies have involved small numbers of patients and did not adequately control for total daily lithium doses, which were larger in some patients on multiple-dose regimens. Certainly it would be appropriate to cautiously convert patients who have persistent polyuria to once daily dosing as a means of trying to correct the polyuria.

The lithium side effect patients are most likely to experience is tremor of the hands and fingers. In starting a patient on a new medication, it is important to alert him or her of the unwanted effects which may occur. Likewise, it is important for the clinician to utilize whatever techniques he can to minimize the likelihood of developing side effects, since early side effects experienced with a particular medication may help to galvanize that patient against continued therapeutic use of that medication. Utilizing slow titration of lithium dosage as suggested, it is adequate to measure the serum lithium level once or twice weekly in the acutely manic patient. The most accurate determination of serum lithium level, and the measurement most likely to be comparable to data in the literature and least responsive to the postabsorptive peak of lithium, is the determination done approximately 12 hours after the prior lithium dose. If conditions dictate the need to measure lithium levels on a different time schedule from the 12-hour interval, the interval from dose to blood collection should be recorded so that it can be factored into any comparison of the series of lithium level determinations done on the patient.

AVAILABLE LITHIUM PREPARATIONS

Many lithium preparations are available for clinical use. Because of variations in manufacturing and in the inert ingredients present in any tablet or capsule, bioavailability variations are likely to be seen between brands. Changes from one brand to another may account for considerable variation in serum lithium levels. Therefore it is preferable to specify a particular brand of lithium and utilize it uniformly to increase the reliability of the correlation of blood level, therapeutic response, and dosage. It is also important to utilize a specific laboratory whenever possible, rather than having determinations done in a variety of laboratories whose results may be unpredictable.

Lithium carbonate manufactured under the trade name of Eskalith in both capsule and tablet form is a reliable preparation. Cibalith-S is a liquid preparation of lithium citrate which is clinically useful in patients who cannot take lithium in tablet or capsule form. Generally, within 1 to 2 hours following the administration of lithium in standard tablet, capsule, or liquid form, there is a peak in the blood level far exceeding the steady-state lithium serum concentration one seeks to maintain and monitor. There is evidence that in some patients the postabsorptive peak in the lithium level may contribute to transient worsening of side effects, particularly tremors of the hands and fingers, which may be minimized by the use of slow-release lithium tablets.[4]

Eskalith-CR and Lithobid are slow-release tablet formulations manufactured in special resin-based tablets which eliminate a considerable portion of the postabsorptive blood level peaks. Although these preparations are no more suitable than any other for employment with a single daily dose regimen, they do produce considerably less fluctuation in the serum level in the initial period following each administration, and therefore seem to be somewhat better tolerated by many patients. A small proportion of patients taking Eskalith-CR or Lithobid tablets (approximately 5% — 10%) complain of diarrhea, which they had not experienced with other preparations and which is not related to achievement of an excessive serum lithium concentration.[4] In such individuals, it is worth switching to another preparation, once the serum lithium level has been determined. If the change in preparation is associated with the disappearance of diarrhea, it is reasonable to continue treatment with the alternate form, except in those patients who experience a worsening of tremors, and who may require their lithium to be administered in smaller increments throughout the day or who may prefer to return to slow-release tablets and tolerate a certain amount of diarrhea. Once the manic symptoms are well controlled and a suitable serum lithium level is established, gradual titration and discontinuation of the coadministered neuroleptic should begin in most patients suffering from manic illness.

MONITORING LITHIUM THERAPY

During the first 4 weeks of lithium treatment serum levels should be monitored weekly — more frequently if higher doses are used, if there is an abnormality of renal function or serum electrolytes, or in the presence of cardiovascular disease or diuretic therapy. Lithium level determinations should be done every 2 weeks during the second month and once monthly thereafter. As the patient stabilizes over a number of months on lithium, serum determinations should generally be continued indefinitely every 4 to 6 weeks, although some patients who remain very stable and free of affective symptoms may eventually be adequately monitored by lithium levels every 2 to 3 months.

I am strongly opposed to maintaining patients on lithium with monitoring less often than every 2 to 3 months, for a variety of reasons. It is known that infrequently patients on lithium maintenance will develop abnormalities of renal structure or function; in these individuals often the first clue to renal impairment is the finding of gradually increasing serum lithium concentration, without changes in lithium dosage or time intervals between lithium dose and serum determination.[46] It would appear that more frequent serum lithium determinations may be one of the best early warning signs of lithium-related renal impairment, without the need for more complicated and costly laboratory procedures.[47] Furthermore, relatively frequent serum lithium level determinations may be useful in reinforcing patient compliance with long-term lithium maintenance. During the course of lithium therapy, alteration of the patient's diet for weight loss or sodium restriction or administration of diuretic therapy should lead to increased frequency of lithium, electrolytes, and creatinine monitoring. Likewise, the presence of vomiting, diarrhea, or fever is an additional indication for temporarily increasing the frequency of lithium level monitoring, as is any alteration in the prescribed dose of lithium.

Although the most dramatic response to lithium is in the acutely manic patient, lithium has an important role in the prophylaxis of mania and as an adjunct in the treatment of depression and other disorders.[4] Very often, patients whose indication for lithium is other than acute mania receive their treatment on an outpatient basis. One needs to make appropriate decisions about initiating lithium treatment, and provide adequate documentation in the patient's medical record. Also, pretreatment lithium evaluation must be done on the outpatient who is to receive therapy. A starting dosage regimen similar to the one previously described may be utilized, based on approximate body weight. Patients with schizoaffective disorder may be receiving low-dose neuroleptics, while patients with refractory depression may be receiving an antidepressant regimen to which lithium is added.

A patient on a salt-restricted diet should receive lithium only with cautious management and monitoring. Patients receiving diuretics as a part of their treatment for hypertension or congestive heart failure may be treated safely with lithium carbonate.[4] In a patient receiving a combined diuretic and lithium regimen, creatinine and electrolyte determinations need to be done on a regular basis. The frequency of monitoring is determined by the patient's clinical status, the potency of the diuretic regimen, and the use of supplemental potassium if indicated. The administration of digoxin or other digitalis preparations is not contraindicated with lithium therapy, although maintenance of normal serum potassium is essential to the safety of the therapeutic regimen.[4]

SIDE EFFECTS OF LITHIUM THERAPY

Because lithium is a simple ion whose traversal through the body is governed by the same physiologic mechanisms that govern sodium, it reaches all tissues.

Table 8-2 Medical complications of lithium therapy

Neurologic
   Tremors—may respond to dosage of slow-release lithium or β blockers
   Confusion, memory impairment, difficulty concentrating, slowed thought
   Seizures, EEG changes—primarily at toxic level
Cardiac
   ECG changes—usually minor ST-T wave changes
   Conduction disturbances; arrhythmia with toxic lithium levels
Renal
   Polyuria, polydipsia—may be benign; may respond to diuretics or to dosage adjustment
   Decreased urine-concentrating ability
   Decreased creatinine clearance
   Microscopic, structural renal dosage—severity and incidence uncertain
Metabolic
   Weight gain, fluid retention; changes in caloric intake
Thyroid
   Goiter with normal thyroid function tests—TSH elevated
   Hypothyroidism—without thyroid gland enlargement
   Skin rash; hair loss (rare)

Its prime site of action for the psychiatrist is obviously the central nervous system, which is likewise one of the major areas where adverse lithium effects are seen. Table 8-2 lists some of the common medical complications of lithium therapy.

Tremor which tends to be irregular in rhythm and amplitude affecting the fingers, and jerky movements with flexion and extension of the fingers, is commonly associated with lithium therapy.[48] The tremor tends to become more prominent with intentional movement, but remains present at rest. It varies in intensity and frequency, and may vary to some extent with the differences in serum lithium concentration and with upward fluctuation in the concentration that occurs following individual dosage administration. Table 8-3 compares lithium-induced tremors with other common tremors. Lithium tremors are somewhat less likely to occur early in treatment if the dosage is titrated upward slowly as opposed to a rapid-dosage regimen. Very often they disappear spontaneously as the dose is held constant after the first 2 or 3 weeks of lithium treatment. In some cases tremors will persist or worsen, even with relatively constant serum lithium concentration.[48] If the tremor appears at a concentration of 0.8 mEq/L or greater, perhaps the first approach to control the tremor is to reduce the dosage of lithium or advise the patient to take smaller doses several times throughout the day, rather than using a single or twice daily regimen.

As previously mentioned, the use of slow-release lithium preparations may, by reducing postabsorptive blood level peaks, reduce the severity of lithium tremor. If the tremor persists and is severe enough to cause inconvenience to the

Table 8-3 Differentiating tremors induced
by lithium from other common tremors

Lithium-related	Non lithium-related
1. Irregular amplitude and rhythm	*Anxiety tremor*
2. Jerking movements of fingers with flexion or extension; side thrusts may occur	1. Fine rapid rhythmic movements
	2. Usually no side-to-side movements
3. Present at rest; may worsen with intentional movement	
	Essential (familial) tremor
4. Rigidity on passive flexion generally absent	1. Long-standing, runs in families
	2. Smooth, wide range of movements
5. Usually confined to fingers; hands and wrists may become involved if severe	3. Propranolol diminishes or obliterates
6. Frequency and intensity vary throughout day and from day to day	*Parkinsonian tremor*
	1. Slow, rhythmic
7. Uncertain relationship to serum lithium concentration	2. Rotational and flexing movements prominent
8. May diminish with decreased lithium dosage, use of slow-release lithium preparations, or the administration of propranolol	3. Fingers, hand, and wrist tend to move as a unit

patient in his daily activities, specific pharmacologic intervention may be required. Propranolol, metoprolol, and nadolol, beta-adrenergic blocking agents which are effective in controlling familial or essential tremor, likewise are beneficial in reducing or eliminating lithium-induced tremor.[49,50] In my experience, many patients who are troubled by lithium-related tremor can recall other family members who have not taken lithium but who had persistent tremors. Lithium-induced tremors seem more likely to occur in patients who have a family history of essential tremor. In the treatment of lithium-induced tremor, the patient should be evaluated clinically for evidence of bronchospasm, congestive heart failure and other contraindications to β-blockers. The patient should then be started on propranolol at a dose of 10 mg 4 times daily. If after the initial week of therapy at this dose the tremor has not improved, the dose may be increased to 20 mg 3 to 4 times daily. Most patients with lithium-induced tremor are responsive to propranolol in a dose of 40 to 80 mg daily; occasionally, higher doses may be necessary, if the patient tolerates the medication satisfactorily without any adverse effect on heart rate and rhythm, blood pressure, or mood. Although the propranolol dose that is generally effective in lithium-related tremors is not likely to adversely affect mood, metoprolol 25 to 50 mg or nadolol 20 to 40 mg twice daily may be equally effective without risk of inducing depression.[49,50]

Many otherwise healthy persons suffering from affective illness will, when treated with lithium, complain of a variety of unwanted mental symptoms. Both normal volunteers and patients with affective illness who have undergone clinical evaluation and cognitive testing prior to and during the course of lithium administration have reported occasional difficulty concentrating or slowing of thought, as well as confusion and memory impairment. These findings are more apt to occur in the elderly or in people who have organic brain dysfunction. Usually, these changes in mentation are not severe in young healthy individuals with affective illness and do not limit the use of lithium therapy.[51] In situations where they compromise ability to function, the clinician would be well advised to consider a trial of a lower dose of lithium, even accepting a period wherein the serum lithium concentration might be maintained as low as 0.3 to 0.4 mEq/L.[52] I have seen a number of patients, including academically oriented students, who described changes in mentation associated with lithium but in whom lithium maintenance was necessary. In many of these individuals lithium levels of 0.3 to 0.4 mEq/L were better tolerated and adequately beneficial in protecting against the recurrence of mania. I have seen the same phenomena occur in the elderly, and at times have found it necessary to maintain lithium levels in the range that is generally not considered to be therapeutic in order to sidestep the changes in mentation. Again, in many of these situations there has been an improvement in the unwanted effect, and the beneficial effect has been maintained. Patients who become lithium intoxicated, either as a result of receiving an excessive dosage or as the result of an intentional overdose, will generally become confused and may suffer obtundation as well as impairments in mental acuity.

Lithium intoxication is often associated with the development of EEG abnormalities and seizures that may be grand mal in nature.[53] Seizures will occasionally occur in patients with convulsive disorders who are receiving therapeutic doses of lithium. A seizure disorder, if adequately controlled does not necessitate avoidance of lithium if it is otherwise clinically indicated.[54] In treating a patient who has taken an overdose of lithium, it is important to be aware of the risk of seizures and to provide proper medical management.[53]

A variety of cardiovascular effects may be seen in association with lithium. When this element is used at conventional therapeutic dosages the changes seen are usually minor ST-T wave abnormalities without associated cardiovascular symptoms.[36] Conduction disturbances may also be seen in association with therapeutic doses of lithium, but they are more likely seen at toxic levels.[37] A variety of ECG rhythm disturbances have been reported with lithium.[4] These are seen infrequently at therapeutic blood levels and tend to be more common in association with lithium intoxication.

LITHIUM AND THE KIDNEY

Somewhat over half of patients taking lithium will experience increased urination (polyuria) due to lithium antagonism of antidiuretic hormone (ADH), which normally acts to facilitate the reabsorption of free water in the distal renal tubule. These patients will excrete an excessive volume of dilute urine, and will experience increased thirst. This syndrome, known as nephrogenic diabetes insipidus (NDI), has generally been considered benign in most lithium-treated patients.[4] Most often judicious use of amiloride or thiazide diuretics will exert a paradoxical antidiuretic effect, with reduction in urine volume and thirst.[55]

There is now reason to question the benign nature of persistent polyuria and polydipsia in association with lithium therapy, although minor degrees of either symptoms should not be seen as alarming. In a 1977 report, 14 patients who had received lithium for periods ranging from 20 months to 15 years were referred for renal evaluation because of the presence of either acute lithium poisoning or lithium-induced nephrogenic diabetes insipidus (NDI).[46] All of these patients had reduced urine concentrating ability, decreased creatinine clearance, or both. The patients were observed to have gradually increasing serum lithium concentrations despite a stable or decreasing dosage of lithium. Renal biopsy specimens showed only insignificant acute lesions. However, in 13 patients, there was a pronounced degree of focal nephron atrophy, interstitial fibrosis, or both. There was no correlation between age or length of treatment and the degree of fibrosis. The authors of that initial report of lithium-related renal damage could not explain the origin of the pathologic process. They did speculate, however, that there may have been a relationship between the chronic renal changes observed and the fact that their patients had either experienced recurrent lithium intoxication or periods of persistent polyuria associated with NDI.[46] Other investigators studying small numbers of patients who developed evidence of renal functional impairment while receiving lithium have reported their findings, and clinicians have become concerned about the possibility of a lithium-associated renal functional impairment.[4]

Of the patients studied and reported in the literature who have had renal changes in association with therapeutic doses of lithium, only two have been reported to develop renal failure.[56] One study, which involved extensive noninvasive testing of renal function in 43 patients who had been taking lithium for 1 to 20 months, found a moderate but asymptomatic impairment in urine-concentrating ability.[57] The conclusion of this extensive clinical investigation on a series of patients, both men and women, aged 17 to 67 years, was that patients receiving lithium should be carefully evaluated and tested, and there is not enough evidence to justify avoidance of lithium therapy or discontinuation of lithium in patients who might otherwise benefit from its use.[57]

The awareness of some possible change in renal function during lithium treatment would support periodic evaluation of urine-concentrating ability. The simplest method to employ for this purpose is the measurement of urine osmolality following a 12-hour fast, during which time no fluids, food, or medication are taken.[47] Likewise, the periodic accurate determination of serum lithium levels at a fixed interval after a given dose of lithium is a useful means of detecting changes in renal function and lithium clearance. Although decreased creatinine clearance may occasionally be noted in association with lithium therapy, the routine use of creatinine clearance measurements during treatment is not necessary unless specific indications of renal disease or severe polyuria are present. Measurement of serum creatinine every 6 to 12 months during lithium maintenance may be useful, although in most patients who have been found to have renal structural or functional changes while taking lithium, serum creatinine determinations have generally been normal.[4]

According to a large controlled study by Vestergaard et al. morphologic kidney changes may be found in 10% to 20% of patients receiving long-term lithium therapy, which may be associated with impairment of water reabsorption.[58] Those investigators stated that the occurrence of morphologic changes is not indicative of a reduction in glomerular filtration rate (GFR) or the development of renal insufficiency.[58] A significant epidemologic study failed to find any elevated mortality due to nephrotoxicity among a large group of patients receiving chronic lithium maintenance treatment.[59] A series of 40 lithium-treated manic-depressive patients who each underwent two renal functional assessments 6 to 18 months apart showed no change in GFR.[60] That study concluded that with chronic lithium maintenance, most patients develop little renal-concentrating impairment while some show increasing polyuria during continuing lithium administration.[60]

Within the first year after the initial publication of findings in the 14 patients previously mentioned, I saw a number of patients who had been stable on lithium who discontinued the drug and subsequently experienced acute manic episodes necessitating hospitalization. One patient whom I have seen with significant renal functional impairment on lithium was an elderly woman of slight body build who was taking 600 mg lithium 3 times daily. This amount seemed excessive for her age and size. When I first saw her, she assured me that her lithium level had been maintained stable at 1.5 mEq/L; however, when I measured the lithium level on our initial visit, it was 2.8 mEq/L, and although my reduction in her dosage to 300 mg twice daily was associated with a subsequent decrease to 0.6 mEq/L, she subsequently developed further evidence of renal functional impairment which was marked by a gradual increase in her serum lithium concentration.

Although most of the earlier literature has taken a more benign view of the renal effects of lithium, increasing numbers of patients being maintained on lithium for longer periods signal the need for caution in arriving at conclusions regarding the effects of this ion on the kidney. Yet, excessive fear of lithium is not without risk — in that it is potentially lifesaving for patients with bipolar affective illness and can allow many to lead fully active, productive, and rewarding lives. The longest follow-up study of renal status in lithium-treated patients examined 27 individuals with a mean duration of over 19 years of lithium therapy.[61] In that group, no decline in glomerular filtration rate (GFR) was found; one patient had a serum creatinine of 3.2 mg/100 ml after 25 years of lithium, and another a creatinine of 2.26 mg/100 ml, with the finding of subacute tubulointerstitial nephritis on renal biopsy.[61] The first well-documented report of lithium-induced renal failure requiring dialysis appeared in the literature in 1990,[62] while the second was reported in 1993.[56] A series of 82 lithium-treated bipolar patients in an affective-disorders clinic found 3 (3.7%) to have serum creatinine levels greater than 2.0 mg/100 ml, all of whom began lithium with normal creatinine concentrations.[56] Clearly, as we continue to use lithium over longer courses of treatment of bipolar patients, there is a need to do anything possible to enhance its safety. Experimental administration of potassium supplementation to lithium-treated rats has been found to reduce adverse effects of this ion on growth as well as renal morphology and function.[63] Reduction of intracellular potassium may contribute to lithium-induced ST-T wave changes on the electrocardiogram, and it is known that hypokalemia increases the danger of lithium intoxication; yet there is not yet adequate documentation of a clinically beneficial effect of potassium supplementation during clinical treatment with lithium.[63] Nevertheless, it is important to provide adequate supplemental potassium if diuretics are administered with lithium and to consider a trial of conservative doses of oral potassium supplementation in some patients with lithium-induced polyuria, particularly if diuretic therapy does not adequately ameliorate this symptom.[63] It is too early and there are too few data to support the routine use of potassium in the hope of minimizing the risk of lithium-induced renal abnormalities. Amelioride, which is a potassium-saving diuretic in common use for lithium-induced NDI, has the added benefit of preventing lithium uptake into renal tubular cells; however, its potential benefit in protecting against adverse renal effects of lithium remains unknown.[63]

Perhaps the major guidelines regarding lithium and kidney damage are that the medication should not be prescribed unless there is reasonable clinical indication of its necessity and likelihood of providing a useful therapeutic benefit. Also, lithium and serum creatinine levels should be monitored carefully and on a regular basis, and appropriate consultations and investigations of renal function should be done in the presence of symptoms such as polyuria or if the serum lithium level increases while the patient is being maintained on a stable dose of lithium.

During the course of lithium treatment many patients will complain of edema of the ankle or lower leg. One early study of this phenomenon revealed the presence of normal renal, cardiovascular, and hepatic function and noted that the edema in some patients disappeared spontaneously while in others it responded favorably to spironolactone (50 mg twice daily), a specific aldosterone inhibitor, thus suggesting that tubular reabsorption of sodium had some role in the edema formation.[64] Patients who complain of edema may also respond favorably to intermittent administration of a diuretic such as hydrochlorothiazide in a dose of 50 mg daily or every other day. If hydrochlorothiazide is administered on a regular basis, it is important to monitor serum potassium and provide supplemental oral potassium chloride, as in any patient receiving a thiazide diuretic simultaneously with lithium.

METABOLIC EFFECTS OF LITHIUM

Although weight gain is common in patients taking lithium and may be due in part to fluid retention, there are variable changes in glucose metabolism which may be important in explaining this weight gain.[4] Patients taking lithium usually find it more difficult to successfully lose weight by dieting while taking lithium in comparison to previous experiences with dieting in the absence of lithium. Nevertheless, I have seen numerous patients who have lost significant amounts of weight (from 20 to 75 lb) while taking lithium and following a very restricted low-calorie diet. It is good practice to counsel patients that they must maintain adequate fluid and salt intake during the course of rapid weight loss and it is appropriate to measure serum lithium concentration more frequently during the course of any diet.

Lithium therapy may be associated with the development of goiter in the presence of normal thyroid function tests and a clinically euthyroid state. This is usually associated with an increased TSH level, and the enlargement of the thyroid gland is felt to be related to its attempt to maintain the euthyroid state in response to increased stimulation from the increased circulating level of TSH.[38] Hypothyroidism also may occur with lithium treatment, although neither the development of hypothyroidism nor the appearance of goiter indicates a need to change the dosage or discontinue the medication. The presence of either condition dictates the need for a proper medical evaluation. If the patient is clinically hypothyroid, the gland enlarged, or the TSH significantly elevated, thyroid hormone replacement therapy may be necessary in conjunction with lithium.[38]

Serum calcium has been found to be elevated in approximately 10% of patients receiving long term lithium therapy. Parathormone (PTH) levels are likewise not infrequently elevated during lithium therapy, although since PTH is not routinely monitored, the incidence of abnormalities is not known.[65,66] In a survey of a small series of chronic lithium maintained patients, I found approximately 10% to have mild hypercalcemia, while 3 of 6 patients had significantly elevated serum PTH. Although most patients with hypercalcemia or elevated PTH during lithium therapy simply have hyperactive parathyroid glands, some have been found to have parathyroid adenomas, which may well have preceeded lithium therapy. It would appear that lithium maintained patients with renal stones, or excessive tiredness, unrelated to depression or other pharmacotherapy, or who present with unexplained cognitive changes would be good candidates to screen for hypercalcemia and PTH elevation. Generally patients who have these laboratory findings during lithium therapy will revert to normocalcemia and normal PTH levels following lithium discontinuation, if this intervention is feasible.[65,66] The mechanism of hypercalcemia and PTH elevation during lithium therapy is that physiologically, PTH secretion is regulated by the concentration of calcium in the blood; lithium at therapeutic levels reduces parathyroid gland responsivity to calcium, thus PTH continues to be secreted at serum calcium levels which would normally turn off PTH production and release.[65,66]

DERMATOLOGIC ASPECTS OF LITHIUM

A variety of skin rashes may occur or worsen during the course of lithium therapy. Acne may appear for the first time or may worsen during the course of lithium administration.[4] Appropriate dermatologic consultation should be sought, and treatment instituted. In most cases acne can be satisfactorily treated, although in some cases its severity is such that a patient may refuse to continue lithium or the dermatologist may request a drug-free interval, in which case an alternative pharmacologic regimen to maintain mood stability may be required. Lithium has been reported to exacerbate psoriasis, and in some cases satisfactory treatment of the psoriasis requires the discontinuation of lithium.[4] Occasionally a maculopapular rash, with or without associated pruritus, may occur during the course of lithium treatment.[4] I have observed rashes of this type to disappear following discontinuation of lithium and not to reappear several weeks later when lithium therapy was reinstituted. Sometimes patients may continue lithium therapy and experience a disappearance of the rash during treatment with an antihistamine and the application of a topical steroid cream. One of the rare complications associated with lithium is thinning of hair and hair loss. Hair loss may be limited to the scalp or may affect other body hair as well.[4] Following discontinuation of lithium the hair usually returns to its normal pattern though some persons report only partial recovery. One middle-aged patient I observed lost hair from her scalp, arms, axillae, and pubic area. She subsequently discontinued lithium, and in the next 18 months noted regrowth of the hair that had been lost. She subsequently experienced an episode of depression, which had previously responded to lithium, since she was unable to tolerate any tricyclic antidepressant. Lithium therapy was then reinstituted, with an improvement in her mood, but the hair loss recurred. She subsequently discontinued lithium following stabilization of her mood over several months and has regained the hair. Since hair loss may result from hypothyroidism, thyroid function studies should be done when hair loss occurs during lithium therapy.[4]

LITHIUM AND THE DIGESTIVE SYSTEM

Many patients taking lithium carbonate will experience GI complaints, the most common being epigastric burning and persistent indigestion. I routinely advise patients to take lithium at mealtime or with a small snack. In most instances, lithium with food or milk will avoid associated epigastric distress; occasionally, however, an antacid preparation along with each dose of lithium is necessary to avoid GI distress. Mild diarrhea is occasionally associated with conventional therapeutic doses and blood levels of lithium carbonate but is more likely with excessive lithium concentration. Although anorexia occasionally occurs, it is less apt to occur at therapeutic dosage levels than in the presence of lithium toxicity.[4] Lithium toxicity is almost always associated with anorexia, nausea, and vomiting. One of the major risks of vomiting in a patient receiving lithium is that it will contribute to dehydration, which in turn is likely to further worsen the lithium toxicity.[4] Patients who develop nausea and vomiting as a component of a flulike syndrome during lithium therapy should be advised to discontinue lithium and maintain adequate fluid intake for a few days. Any patient who develops a febrile illness while taking lithium is likewise more apt to become dehydrated and may be more vulnerable to lithium intoxication.

Many patients taking psychotropic medication complain of excessive dental caries and increased periodontal disease. The ability of neuroleptics and tricyclic antidepressant drugs to decrease salivary secretion can be readily understood as a potential mechanism for decreasing the defense system against dental and oral inflammatory and carious conditions.[67] Although lithium is devoid of anticholinergic activity, it has been associated with a relatively high incidence of dental caries and periodontal disease; but the mechanism of this effect is not well understood. Any patient experiencing increased oral symptoms while taking lithium should be urged to thoroughly and gently brush his teeth and frequently rinse his mouth with warm salt water or other mild solutions. Evaluation and ongoing treatment by a periodontist may be necessary.

DETERMINATIONS OF LITHIUM LEVEL
DURING LITHIUM THERAPY

Laboratory determinations are a required part of proper lithium treatment during the acute phase of mania and during the course of maintenance.[4] The clinical value of lithium determinations is only as good as the accuracy of the laboratory and the standardization of the procedure in the laboratory and in the office where the patient is seen. Blood samples taken for lithium determination at unspecified intervals following previous doses of lithium may yield numbers, but those numbers are not necessarily meaningful data. That is to say, a lithium level of 0.8 would be considered therapeutic if it were determined 10 to 14 hours after the previous dose. The same level of 0.8 determined 2 hours after the previous dose would represent the contribution of that recent dose to the circulating lithium concentration, and would therefore not be meaningful in assessing the patient. The frequency of lithium level determination has been reviewed elsewhere in this chapter but needs to be reemphasized since the failure to determine serum lithium concentration on a regular basis may help reinforce the patient's irregularity in taking the medication. Also, the failure to determine lithium levels often enough may miss an opportunity to diagnose lithium-related renal dysfunction, which may become manifested in an excessive lithium concentration at a dose that previously provided a therapeutic concentration.[4] For optimal reliability, a laboratory that performs a reasonable volume of lithium determinations should be chosen. Ideally, that laboratory should be used for all patients whom the particular physician is maintaining on lithium, so that an unusual result appearing in one patient can be compared with other patients' results, in the event there is a defect in standardization in the laboratory on that particular day.

MONITORING SALIVARY LITHIUM CONCENTRATION

The necessity for careful standardized serum lithium level determinations throughout the course of lithium therapy cannot be overemphasized. In some patients, either because of their own reluctance to allow blood to be drawn on a frequent basis or because of the presence of small veins, regular measurement of serum lithium level is difficult or even impossible. Additionally, I have treated several patients who have spent extensive periods of time in localities that could not provide lithium serum determinations. The use of saliva samples to monitor lithium therapy has been employed by several investigators including myself.[68] A variety of formulas have been devised to correlate saliva lithium concentration and serum concentration.[69] Although the ratio of saliva to serum lithium concentration varies from individual to individual, it tends to be relatively constant in a given individual. In general, the saliva concentration as measured by standard lithium assay techniques will be approximately twice that found in serum. The preferred approach to utilizing lithium saliva determination is to measure serum and saliva lithium concentrations simultaneously on several occasions, calculate the ratio for the given individual, and apply that ratio in subsequent determinations of saliva lithium concentration in order to derive presumed serum concentrations. I have encountered some individuals whose saliva concentration of lithium was equal to their serum concentration. Thus far I have not seen individuals whose saliva concentration was lower than their serum concentration. At the other end of the spectrum, I have seen individuals whose saliva-serum ratio was as high as 3.0. If one wishes to start lithium in a patient and is unable to obtain blood samples for the measurement of lithium concentration, lithium therapy can be instituted and the saliva concentration can be measured and recorded. In the absence of any blood level determination to validate the saliva measurement, it would be appropriate to administer lithium in a dose that seems clinically appropriate, and adjust the dose as necessary to achieve initial saliva lithium concentrations in the range of 1.0 to 1.8 mEq/L. Assuming a ratio of 1:1, this yields a serum concentration in the range of 1.0 to 1.8 mEq/L, which, though somewhat high, is not in the range where significant toxicity can be anticipated. Assuming the more likely condition of a 2:1 ratio of saliva to serum, the serum level with the saliva in the range of 1.0 to 1.8 would be 0.5 to 0.9, which is within the range of lithium levels considered clinically effective.

MANAGEMENT OF LITHIUM INTOXICATION

When lithium toxicity is suspected, the drug should be immediately discontinued and blood samples should be sent to the laboratory for determination of serum lithium concentration, serum creatinine, and electrolytes. If the patient is obtunded, administration of additional medications should not be undertaken, with the exception of the cautious IM administration of trimethobenzamide (Tigan) to inhibit vomiting. The specific treatment of lithium intoxication requires that the patient be adequately hydrated. If vomiting is not severe and oral fluids can be tolerated, small quantities of water may be consumed. If the patient has persistent vomiting and is unable to tolerate fluids by mouth, IV fluids should be started immediately. The initial IV fluid that should be administered is normal saline solution, to which 40 to 80 mEq/L of potassium chloride has been added. Once IV fluid replacement therapy has been instituted and the serum determination of electrolytes, lithium, and creatinine is available, the rate and nature of fluid replacement can be adjusted accordingly.

It is important to monitor electrolytes and renal and cardiac function during lithium intoxication, and a baseline ECG should be done as quickly as possible.[4] The possibility of a cardiac arrhythmia occurring must be kept in mind.[37] The patient's myocardial contractility may be decreased during lithium intoxication, and antiarrhythmic drugs must be used cautiously to avoid a further decrease in myocardial contractility. The patient who is lithium toxic is likely to suffer a variety of CNS effects, including confusion and obtundation as well as seizures.[53] The changes in mental function may impair the patient's ability to give an accurate history of what has happened.

Pharmacologic agents may be necessary to manage seizures. Since hypoglycemic coma can mimic some of the findings seen in lithium intoxication, serum glucose level should be determined when initial laboratory studies are done prior to administering IV fluids. The patient who has had a toxic ingestion of lithium may simultaneously have taken a variety of other psychotropic or otherwise toxic compounds. Therefore blood and urine should be sent to the laboratory for a comprehensive toxic screen. Obviously, the management of a psychiatric patient who has suffered any kind of intoxication is dependent on the overall medical expertise of the physician in attendance, including the necessity for that physician to be able to provide lifesaving cardiopulmonary resuscitation if necessary.

ALTERNATIVE ANTIMANIC AND MOOD-STABILIZING DRUGS

When initially employed, lithium appeared to be universally effective in the treatment and prophylaxis of mania; with increasing experience, it appears that only 60% to 70% of bipolar patients respond optimally to this agent. The need for alternative antimanic and mood-stabilizing therapies has become more apparent with increasing recognition of the limitations of lithium, although it remains the primary agent in the treatment of bipolar affective disorders. Many patients do not tolerate lithium-induced side effects, or have medical contraindications to its use, and thus form one group for whom alternative agents are important. The other major indication for alternative drugs is those patients who continue to have manic or depressive episodes in spite of adequate and well-monitored lithium maintenance. Four conditions which are less likely to be lithium responsive are (1) Rapid Cycling bipolar disorder, (2) Dysphoric Mania, (3) Mixed States, and (4) Substance Abuse in bipolar disorder. In these conditions, lithium is often used in conjunction with one or more alternative agents; however, in many patients the alternative drug may be more effective or better tolerated than lithium, which can then be eliminated from the regimen. Some patients with refractory or recurrent depression may benefit from the combination of an antidepressant along with an alternative mood-stabilizing agent. The alternative antimanic or mood-stabilizing agents which have been most extensively studied and used clinically include carbamazepine, divalproex (valproate), clonazepam, clonidine, and the calcium-channel blockers — all of which are marketed in the United States for indications other than affective disorders. The extensive studies and clinical applications of these agents in affective disorders make it reasonable for physicians to prescribe them beyond their FDA-approved clinical indications, provided the physician understands their proper clinical applications and precautions, discusses their risks and benefits with the patient, and documents the reasons for their use in the medical record. Divalproex has recently received FDA approval for treatment and prophylaxis of mania.

Carbamazepine

Carbamazepine, which is structurally similar to tricyclic antidepressants, has been used clinically since the early 1960s, first in trigeminal neuralgia and subsequently as an anticonvulsant, particularly in temporal lobe epilepsy. The antimanic activity of carbamazepine (CBZ) was first discovered in the late 1960s at the NIMH and in studies in Japan.[70] Like other anticonvulsants, CBZ inhibits kindling and, similar to lithium and valproate, enhances activity of the inhibitory neurotransmitter γ-amino butyric acid (GABA).[6,70] Carbamazepine does not antagonize dopamine receptors or induce Parkinsonian side effects or tardive dyskinesia, which makes it safer than neuroleptics.[71]

One study found a moderate to excellent antimanic response in 10 of 17 patients who received carbamazepine as their sole psychopharmacologic intervention.[72] In a review of 11 open and six blind studies of the effect of carbamazepine in acute mania, 60% of 254 patients showed moderate to marked improvement with carbamazepine alone or combined with lithium or other medications.[73] A comparable response rate was found for carbamazepine as a prophylactic treatment in affective disorders among 240 patients included in this same review.[73] Carbamazepine was comparable to lithium when used as the sole agent in the treatment of acute mania in a series of 28 patients, half of whom received either treatment.[74]

Most studies, both controlled and uncontrolled, have confirmed the efficacy of carbamazepine in the treatment of acute mania and in prophylaxis of recurrence. Generally, it has been equal to lithium, but in some cases it has been effective when lithium failed.[75,76] I have seen numerous patients whose mania was resistant to lithium and neuroleptic regimens respond favorably to the addition of CBZ. Likewise, a number of my patients with recurrent affective episodes during conscientious lithium maintenance have been stabilized, with reduced frequency and/or severity of mood shifts, when either carbamazepine or divalproex (VPA) was added to the maintenance lithium. I have been less impressed with the ability of either CBZ or VPA to replace lithium in maintenance of bipolar patients. In severely ill acutely manic patients, neuroleptics in conjunction with lithium are, in my experience, more rapidly efficacious than CBZ or VPA alone or in combination with lithium.

In addition to its antimanic effect, carbamazepine has been shown to possess an antidepressant action when employed alone or in conjunction with other antidepressant drugs.[77,78,79] It decreases the severity of behavioral dyscontrol in patients with borderline personality disorder.[80] Two patients, however, were reported to develop melancholia during carbamazepine treatment of borderline personality disorder.[81] I have seen a number of patients with borderline personality disorder whose behavioral dyscontrol and affective symptoms showed a greater improvement with carbamazepine than with antidepressants, neuroleptics, or lithium. Nightmares, flashbacks, and intrusive recollections are reduced in intensity and frequency when carbamazepine is employed in the treatment of posttraumatic stress disorder.[82] When employed for psychiatric indications, carbamazepine is generally administered orally in a dose of 100 mg 3 times daily to 200 mg 4 times daily, although doses of up to 1600 mg daily, or occasionally higher, may be necessary in the control of acute mania.

Although plasma concentrations of carbamazepine correlate with its anticonvulsant effect, the relationship of blood level to antimanic activity is less clear.[4] Some patients do well at relatively low serum concentrations of the drug, whereas others require blood levels in excess of those commonly employed when the drug is used as an anticonvulsant. Nausea, anorexia, and occasional vomiting may be seen with CBZ, particularly if the drug is administered on an empty stomach or when relatively higher doses are employed. Sedation and drowsiness are other common side effects which may be minimized by using lower doses, or by administering the greater portion of the daily dose at bedtime. The sedative effect of carbamazepine may be useful in managing insomnia in some patients with affective disorders, particularly those receiving MAOI-type antidepressants. The most serious and, fortunately, rarest side effect of carbamazepine is the production of agranulocytosis.[4] Some patients may experience mild to moderate leukopenia, anemia, or thrombocytopenia. Complete blood counts (CBCs) with examinations of the blood smear should be done weekly during the first 1 to 2 months of therapy, and may be performed at progressively longer intervals during the course of treatment. Patients who have tolerated this drug without developing hematologic abnormalities, and who will be maintained on carbamazepine for prolonged periods of time, should generally have CBCs done at intervals of every 2 to 3 months during continuing treatment. The reduction in cellular elements of the blood may necessitate decreased dosage or discontinuation of carbamazepine. Some patients experience such dramatic benefit from this drug that, with careful periodic monitoring, mild leukopenia, anemia, or thrombocytopenia can be tolerated.

As discussed in chapter 12, coadministration of erythromycin and carbamazepine may produce carbamazepine toxicity with drowsiness, ataxia, and diplopia as a result of the ability of this antibiotic to inhibit carbamazepine metabolism. CBZ may also increase serum lithium concentration and decrease serum neuroleptic concentration. Neurotoxicity may occur when carbamazepine is combined with calcium-channel blockers or angiotensin-converting enzyme inhibitors.

Valproate

Valproic acid (VPA) and related compounds, including sodium valproate and divalproex, are anticonvulsants, used since the mid-1960s in the treatment and prophylaxis of mania.[83] VPA has been examined in controlled as well as open clinical studies for a wide variety of affective and anxiety disorders with generally positive results and a tolerable level of adverse effects.[84,85,86]

Unfortunately, most of the studies with sodium valproate have employed this drug in conjunction with lithium, neuroleptics, carbamazepine, or other drugs so that it is difficult to ascertain the specific contribution of valproate to the therapeutic response. In a review of six studies in which 144 patients were treated with sodium valproate, more than 50% of patients showed lasting improvement with this drug maintained over follow-up periods of 6 to 60 months.[87] Most of the patients reviewed, however, had received other drugs in addition to sodium valproate.[87] None of those studies reported serious adverse effects; however, patients did experience GI symptoms, mild alopecia, and lethargy occasionally. Transient mild thrombocytopenia and increased serum levels of transaminases, indicating mild hepatic dysfunction, were noted in a few patients.[87] A series of 36 patients treated with sodium valproate (750 to 3000 mg/day) for manic symptoms refractory to other pharmacotherapy found a moderate to marked response in 16 (44%) patients.[87]

The largest recent review of valproate in psychiatry examined uncontrolled studies in a total of 663 bipolar and schizoaffective patients and found that 63% had a moderate or marked response.[83] A similar response rate (62%) was found in 45 acutely manic bipolar patients who received valproate in published controlled studies.[83] Published studies indicate approximately equal efficacy of lithium, carbamazepine and valproate in the acute management of mania and its prophylaxis. Review of clinical experience and published studies indicate that VPA may be effective in some patients who do not respond to lithium or CBZ, just as CBZ or lithium will yield therapeutic benefit in some patients who are nonresponders to another mood-stabilizing drug. Although clear predictors of which agent to employ do not exist, it appears that rapid cycling and dysphoric or mixed states may be more likely to benefit from VPA or CBZ alone or in combination with each other or with lithium. There is no clear evidence of greater or differential efficacy between CBZ and VPA, although some investigators and clinicians favor one or the other as their first alternative to lithium. Some patients will better tolerate the side effects of one of these agents or be intolerant of another, which probably is one of the most important guidelines in choosing between them for a specific patient. Both CBZ and VPA treatment and maintenance require monitoring of CBC and liver function tests on a periodic basis, since alterations of hematologic parameters and hepatic function may occur. It is also important to periodically determine serum valproate levels, which for efficacy should generally be between 50 and 100 μg/ml, although some patients benefit from lower levels and acutely manic patients may require levels approximating 150 μg/ml for optimal efficacy.

Clonazepam

A double-blind crossover study comparing the anticonvulsant clonazepam with standard lithium treatment in 12 acutely manic patients found clonazepam to exert a clinically significant antimanic effect.[88] In that study, clonazepam-treated patients required lower daily doses of haloperidol and, with the exception of considerable drowsiness, experienced minimal adverse effects when receiving clonazepam doses of 2 to 16 mg/day.[88] A therapeutic trial of clonazepam at doses of 0.5 to 4 mg daily found a beneficial effect in an acutely manic and two schizoaffective patients.[89] Further studies of moderate to high-dose clonazepam have confirmed earlier experience indicating that this drug may have a useful antimanic effect.[90] I have seen a small number of manic patients, who were reluctant to receive neuroleptics during acute manic illness, in whom clonazepam proved to be a useful adjunct to lithium therapy in enhancing relatively early behavioral control. Clonazepam appears to be useful in acute mania, particularly in those situations where neuroleptic drugs cannot be employed, as in the case of a patient with Parkinson's disease in whom the movement disorder may be adversely affected by antipsychotic drug therapy. Clonazepam may also be useful as a maintenance drug in bipolar affective disorder in conjunction with lithium in patients who have previously required combined lithium-neuroleptic maintenance regimens.

Lorazepam

Lorazepam in doses of 3 to 20 mg daily was employed in lieu of neuroleptic drugs in conjunction with lithium carbonate in the treatment of acute manic agitation in four patients.[91] Its potential advantage compared with clonazepam is its shorter duration of action and the potential of administration by oral, IM, or IV routes. The primary adverse effect noted when using large doses of lorazepam is excessive sedation. If administered only for a few days, there is little risk of dependency or withdrawal. However, prolonged administration of this drug as an antimanic agent in high doses would carry with it a potential addictive risk. Alternatively, lorazepam may be employed to produce sedation and reduce agitation in conjunction with lower-than-usual neuroleptic doses in the management of acutely manic patients. Lorazepam may also minimize acute extrapyramidal side effects of high-potency antipsychotic drugs in the treatment of acute psychosis.

Clonidine

Clonidine, an antihypertensive drug, is being used for an increasingly wider array of psychiatric disorders. It is an alpha$_2$-adrenergic agonist whose most prevalent side effects are drowsiness and hypotension. A series of 24 newly hospitalized acutely manic patients were treated with 0.45 to 0.90 mg/day of clonidine for a period of 2 weeks.[92] A marked decrease in manic symptoms was observed in approximately half the patients after a 5- to 13-day period of treatment.[92] Some of the patients simultaneously received lithium carbonate. Patients that had previously had poor responses to neuroleptic drugs appeared to do better with clonidine than those who had previous favorable responses to antipsychotic drug therapy.[92] In another series of 24 patients treated with clonidine for acute mania, a better therapeutic response was achieved with lithium, which produced fewer side effects.[93] In the latter series, eight patients experienced hypotension and seven complained of depression while receiving clonidine.[93] The risk of depression occurring with clonidine therapy and the incompatibility of this drug with cyclic antidepressants has discouraged me from employing clonidine in the treatment of mania.

Calcium-channel blockers

Among alternative antimanic therapies, carbamazepine and valproate show clear efficacy, comparable to lithium, while clonazepam and the calcium-channel blockers have been less extensively studied and appear less efficacious. Acutely ill bipolar patients have increased intracellular calcium ion concentration in lymphocytes and platelets, which decreases with resolution of mania. Since lithium reduces platelet calcium ion concentration in manic patients, there is a theoretical basis for considering calcium-channel blockers (CCBs) as potential alternative antimanic agents.[94] A large number of nonblinded single-case reports and small uncontrolled studies which have appeared in the literature since the early 1980s have found the CCB verapamil to have antimanic activity. These reports are difficult to interpret in that many acutely ill patients also received other medications, including haloperidol, benzodiazepines, or lithium.[94] The dose of verapamil employed has varied widely but was most often between 160 and 320 mg/day. A few patients have received other CCBs, including diltiazem, nifedipine, and nimodipine.[94,95] CCBs have been used both in the treatment of acute mania and in the prophylaxis of mania, with efficacy being claimed for both uses.[96,97] The experience with verapamil in the treatment of depression has been mixed, with evidence of efficacy unconvincing,[98] furthermore I have seen at least eight patients who have become depressed during treatment with CCBs, including verapamil, diltiazem, and nifedipine.

An open clinical trial found a marked reduction in acute manic symptoms in six patients treated with 160 to 320 mg verapamil daily.[99] A double-blind crossover study found verapamil (320 mg/day) superior to clonidine in 20 manic patients who had been previously unresponsive to lithium.[100] Another study of 20 patients which used a double-blind randomized design found comparable efficacy between verapamil and lithium, although patients in the former group required more haloperidol and lorazepam than did the lithium patients.[96] In a 1-year maintenance study of 20 manic patients employing a double-blind crossover paradigm, verapamil was reported to be equal to lithium in efficacy.[97]

A study of verapamil in treatment-resistant mania yielded less favorable results, with eight of 14 patients studied showing no improvement of manic symptoms.[101] In that study, four patients experienced dysphoria with two of them switching into depression.[101] One patient experienced mild improvement and another had a clear positive response while receiving verapamil prophylactically for mania. Two patients with persistent pharmacologic hypomanias became euthymic while receiving verapamil.[101]

I have observed a stabilization of mood in a small number of hypomanic patients treated with verapamil or with nifedipine, and I have been consulted by at least six patients who became depressed while receiving calcium-channel blockers, including verapamil, diltiazem, and nifedipine. Although a causal relationship between the calcium-channel blocker and depression cannot be proven with certainty, in each case considerable mood improvement occurred following discontinuation of the calcium-channel blocker. In two of the patients, mild depression recurred following initiation of treatment with a calcium-channel blocker other than the agent the patient was taking at the time the depressed mood was noted. I have also seen two hypomanic patients who experienced mild depression when given a course of verapamil treatment for hypomania. The potential therapeutic value of calcium-channel blockers should be further explored, since these agents may offer useful therapeutic benefits to patients who do not respond adequately or experience intolerable side effects during conventional antimanic therapy or prophylaxis. In my experience, nifedipine appears less likely to produce depression than verapamil; therefore I am inclined to use nifedipine in a daily dose of 30 to 90 mg, most often along with lithium to enhance antimanic prophylaxis. Nifedipine also has the advantage of availability of a long-acting preparation for single daily dose usage. With any CCB it is important to monitor pulse and blood pressure as well as to obtain occasional electrocardiograms.

REFERENCES

1. Cade JFJ: Lithium salts in the treatment of psychotic excitement. *Med J Aust* 1949;2:349-352.
2. Henderson DK, Gillespie RD: *Textbook of psychiatry*, ed 6. Oxford, Oxford University Press, 1944, p 3.

3. Baldessarini RJ: Drugs and the treatment of psychiatric disorders. In Gilman AG, Rall TW, Nies AS, Taylor P (eds): *Goodman and Gilman's The pharmacological basis of therapeutics,* ed 8. New York, Pergamon Press, 1990, pp 383-435.

4. Jefferson JW, Griest JH, Ackerman DL, et al: *Lithium encyclopedia for clinical practice.* Washington DC, American Psychiatric Press, 1987.

5. American Psychiatric Association: *Diagnostic and statistical manual of mental disorders,* ed 4, [DSM-IV]. Washington DC, American Psychiatric Press, 1994.

6. Janicak PG, Davis JM, Preskorn SH, Ayd FJ: *Principles and practice of psychopharmacotherapy,* Baltimore, Williams & Wilkins, 1993.

7. Black DW, Winokur G, Nasrallah A: Treatment of mania: a naturalistic study of electroconvulsive therapy versus lithium in 438 patients. *J Clin Psychiatry* 1987;48:132-139.

8. Bernstein JG: Psychotropic drug prescribing. In Cassem NH (ed): *Massachusetts General Hospital Handbook of general hospital psychiatry,* ed 3. St Louis, Mosby, 1991, pp 527-569.

9. Akiskal HS: The clinical management of affective disorders. In Michels R, Cavenar JO, Brodie HKH, et al (eds): *Psychiatry.* Philadelphia, JB Lippincott, 1985, vol 1, ch 61, pp 1-27.

10. Rosenberg DR, Holttum J, Gershon S: *Textbook of Pharmacotherapy for child and adolescent psychiatric disorders,* New York, Brunner/Mazel, 1994.

11. McKnew DH, Cytryn L, Buchsbaum MS, et al: Lithium in children of lithium-responding parents. *Psychiatry Res* 1981;4:171-180.

12. Biederman J, Munir K, Knee D, et al: High rate of affective disorders in probands with attention deficit disorder and their relatives. *Am J Psychiatry* 1987;44:330-333.

13. Ortiz A, Dabbagh M, Gershon S: Lithium: clinical use, toxicology, and mode of action. In Bernstein JG (ed): *Clinical psychopharmacology,* ed 2. Boston, John Wright–PSG, 1984, pp 111-144.

14. Shopsin B, Gershon S, Thompson H, et al: Psychoactive drugs in mania. *Arch Gen Psychiatry* 1975;32:34-42.

15. Quitkin F, Rifkin A, Klein DF, et al: Prophylaxis in unipolar affective disorder. *Am J Psychiatry* 1976;133:1091-1092.

16. Goodwin FK, Murphy DL, Dunner DL, et al: Lithium response in unipolar versus bipolar depression. *Am J Psychiatry* 1972;129:44-47.

17. Chou JCY: Recent advances in treatment of acute mania. *J Clin Psychopharmacol* 1991;11:3-21.

18. Souza FGM, Goodwin GM: Lithium treatment and prophylaxis in unipolar depression: a meta-analysis. *Br J Psychiatry* 1991;158:666-675.

19. Nelson JC, Majore CM: Lithium augmentation in psychotic depression refractory to combined drug treatment. *Am J Psychiatry,* 1986;143:363-366.

20. Lingjaerde O, Edlund AH, Gormsen CA, et al: The effect of lithium carbonate in combination with tricyclic antidepressants in endogenous depression. *Acta Psychiatr Scand* 1974;50:233-242.

21. Price LH, Charney DS, Heninger GR: Efficacy of lithium-tranylcypromine treatment in refractory depression. *Am J Psychiatry* 1985;142:619-623.

22. Shopsin B, Kim SS, Gershon S: A controlled study of lithium vs chlorpromazine in acute schizophrenics. *Br J Psychiatry* 1971;119:435-440.

23. Delva NJ, Letemendia FJJ: Lithium treatment in schizophrenia and schizo-affective disorder. *Br J Psychiatry* 1982;141:387-400.

24. Garver DL, Hirschowitz J, Fleishman R, et al: Lithium response and psychoses: a double-blind, placebo-controlled study, *Psychiatr Res* 1984;12:57-68.

25. Biederman J, Lerner Y, Belmaker RH: Combination of lithium carbonate and haloperidol in schizo-affective disorder. *Arch Gen Psychiatry* 1979;36:327-333.

26. Rifkin A, Quitkin F, Carrillo C, et al: Lithium carbonate in emotionally unstable character disorder. *Arch Gen Psychiatry* 1972;27:519-523.

27. Kane JM, Quitkin FM, Rifkin A, et al: Lithium carbonate and imipramine in the prophylaxis of unipolar and bipolar II illness: a prospective placebo-controlled comparison. *Arch Gen Psychiatry* 1982;39:1065-1069.

28. Tardiff K: The current state of psychiatry in the treatment of violent patients. *Arch Gen Psychiatry* 1992;49:493-499.

29. Schiff HB, Sabin TD, Geller A, et al: Lithium in aggressive behavior. *Am J Psychiatry* 1982;139:1346-1348.
30. Tyrer SP, Walsh A, Edwards DE, et al: Factors associated with a good response to lithium in aggressive mentally handicapped subjects. *Prog Neuropsychopharmacol Biol Psychiatry,* 1984;8: 751-755.
31. Fawcett J, Clark DC, Aagesen CA, et al: A double-blind, placebo-controlled trial of lithium carbonate therapy in alcoholism. *Arch Gen Psychiatry* 1987;44:248-256.
32. Judd LL, Huey LY: Lithium antagonizes ethanol intoxication in alcoholics. *Am J Psychiatry* 1984;141:903-909.
33. Flamenbaum A, Cronson AJ, Weddige RL: Lithium in opiate abuse: a theoretical approach. *Compr Psychiatry* 1979;20:91-99.
34. Gawin FH, Kleber HD: Cocaine abuse treatment: Open pilot trial with desipramine and lithium carbonate. *Arch Gen Psychiatry* 1984;41:903-909.
35. Barklage NE, Jefferson JM: Alternative uses of lithium in psychiatry. *Psychosomatics* 1987;28:239-256.
36. Bucht G, Smipan L, Wahlin A, et al: ECG changes during lithium therapy: a prospective study. *Acta Med Scand* 1984;216:101-104.
37. Mitchell JE, MacKenzie TB: Cardiac effects of lithium therapy in man: a review. *J Clin Psychiatry* 1982;43:47-51.
38. Myers DH, Carter RA, Burns BH, et al: A prospective study of the effects of lithium on thyroid function and on the prevalence of antithyroid antibodies. *Psychol Med* 1985;15:55-61.
39. Bernstein JG: Induction of obesity by psychotropic drugs. In Wurtman RJ, Wurtman JJ (eds): Human obesity, *Ann N Y Acad Sci* 1987;499:203-215.
40. Spring GK: Neurotoxicity with combined use of lithium and thioridazine. *J Clin Psychiatry* 1979;40:135-138.
41. Cohen WJ, Cohen NH: Lithium carbonate, haloperidol, and irreversible brain damage. *JAMA* 1974;230:1283-1287.
42. Baastrup PC, Hollnagel P, Sorenson R, et al: Adverse reactions in treatment with lithium carbonate and haloperidol. *JAMA* 1976;236:2645-2646.
43. Goldney RD, Spence ND: Safety of the combination of lithium and neuroleptic drugs. *Am J Psychiatry* 1986;143:882-884.
44. Hetmar O, Brun C, Clemmesen L, et al: Lithium: long-term effects on the kidney. II, Structural changes. *J Psychiatr Res* 1987;21:279-288.
45. Bowen RC, Grof P, Grof E: Less frequent lithium administration and lower urine volume. *Am J Psychiatry* 1991;148:189-192.
46. Hestbech J, Hansen HE, Amdisen A, et al: Chronic renal lesions following long-term treatment with lithium. *Kidney Int* 1977;12:205-213.
47. Ramsey TA, Cox M: Lithium and the kidney: a review. *Am J Psychiatry* 1982;139:443-449.
48. Tyrer P, Lee I, Trotter C: Physiological characteristics of tremor after chronic lithium therapy. *Br J Psychiatry* 1981;139:59-64.
49. Zubenko GS, Cohen BM, Lipinski JF: Comparison of metoprolol and propranolol in the treatment of lithium tremor. *Psychiatr Res* 1984;11:163-164.
50. Kruse JM, Ereshefsky L, Scavone M: Treatment of lithium induced tremor with nadolol. *Clin Pharmacol* 1984;3:299-301.
51. Squire LR, Judd LL, Janowsky DS, et al: Effects of lithium carbonate on memory and other cognitive functions. *Am J Psychiatry* 1980;137:1042-1046.
52. Coppen A, Abou-Saleh M, Millen P, et al: Decreasing lithium dosage reduces morbidity and side-effects during prophylaxis. *J Affective Disord* 1983;5:353-362.
53. Sansone MEG, Ziegler DK: Lithium toxicity: a review of neurologic complications. *Clin Neuropharmacol* 1985;8:242-248.
54. Ghadirian AM, Lehmann HE: Neurological side effects of lithium: organic brain syndrome, seizures, extrapyramidal side effects and EEG changes. *Compr Psychiatry* 1980;21:327-335.

55. Batlle DC, von Riotte AB, Gaviria M, Grupp M: Amelioration of polyuria by amiloride in patients receiving long-term lithium therapy. *N Engl J Med* 1985;312:408-414.
56. Gitlin M: Lithium-induced renal insufficiency. *J Clin Psychopharmacol* 1993;13:276-279.
57. Gerner RH, Psarras J, Kirschenbaum MA: Results of clinical renal function tests in lithium patients. *Am J Psychiatry* 1980;137:834-837.
58. Vestergaard P, Shou M, Thomsen K: Monitoring of patients in prophylactic lithium treatment: an assessment based on recent kidney studies. *Br J Psychiatry* 1982;140:185-187.
59. Norton B, Whalley LJ: Mortality of a lithium-treated population. *Br J Psychiatry* 1984;145: 277-282.
60. DePaulo JR, Correa EI, Sapir DG: Renal function and lithium: a longitudinal study. *Am J Psychiatry* 1986;143:892-895.
61. Hetmar O, Povlsen UJ, Ladefoged J, Bolwig TG: Lithium: long-term effects on the kidney. A prospective follow-up study 10 years after kidney biopsy. *Br J Psychiatry* 1991;158:53-58.
62. von Knorring L, Wahlin A, Nystrom K, et al: Uraemia induced by long-term lithium treatment. *Lithium* 1990;1:251-253.
63. Jefferson JW: Potassium supplementation in lithium patients: a timely intervention or premature speculation? *J Clin Psychiatry* 1992;53:370-372.
64. Demers R, Heninger G: Pretibial edema and sodium retention during lithium carbonate treatment. *JAMA* 1970;214:1845-1848.
65. Potts JT: Diseases of the parathyroid gland and other hyper- and hypocalcemic disorders. In: Isselbacher KJ, Braunwald E, Wilson JD, et al (Eds) *Harrison's Principles of Internal Medicine*, ed 13, New York, McGraw-Hill, 1994, pp 2151-2171.
66. Mallette LE, Eichorn E: Effects of lithium carbonate on human calcium metabolism. *Arch Int Medicine* 1986;146:770-776.
67. Bassuk E, Schoonover S: Rampant dental caries in the treatment of depression. *J Clin Psychiatry* 1978;39:163-165.
68. Neu C, DiMascio A, Williams D: Saliva lithium levels: clinical applications. *Am J Psychiatry* 1975;132:66-68.
69. Othmer E, Powell B, Piziak B, et al: Prospective use of saliva determination to monitor lithium therapy. *J Clin Psychiatry* 1979;40:526-527.
70. Post RM, Uhde TW, Putnam FW, et al: Kindling and carbamazepine in affective illness. *J Nerv Ment Dis* 1982;170:717-731.
71. Post RM, Rubinow DR, Uhde TW, et al: Dopaminergic effects of carbamazepine. *Arch Gen Psychiatry* 1986;43:392-396.
72. Post RM, Uhde TW: Carbamazepine in bipolar illness. *Psychopharmacol Bull* 1985;21:10-17.
73. Post RM, Uhde TW, Joffe RT, et al: Anticonvulsant drugs in psychiatric illness: new treatment alternatives and theoretical implications. In Trimble MR (ed): *The psychopharmacology of epilepsy*. Chichester UK, Wiley, 1985, pp 141-171.
74. Lerer B, Moore N, Meyendorff E, et al: Carbamazepine versus lithium in mania: a double blind study. *J Clin Psychiatry* 1987;48:89-93.
75. Small JG, Klapper MH, Milstein V, et al: Carbamazepine compared with lithium in the treatment of mania. *Arch Gen Psychiatry* 1991;48:915-921.
76. Post RM, Leverich GS, Rosoff AS, et al: Carbamazepine prophylaxis in refractory affective disorders: a focus on long-term follow-up. *J Clin Psychopharmacology* 1990;10:318-327.
77. Post RM, Uhde TW, Roy-Byrne PP, et al: Antidepressant effects of carbamazepine. *Am J Psychiatry* 1986;143:29-34.
78. Stuppaeck CH, Barnas C, Schwitzer J, et al: Carbamazepine in the prophylaxis of major depression: a 5-year follow-up. *J Clin Psychiatry* 1994;55:146-150.
79. Cullen M, Mitchell P, Brodaty H, et al: Carbamazepine for treatment-resistant melancholia. *J Clin Psychiatry* 1991;52:472-476.
80. Gardner DL, Cowdry RW: Positive effects of carbamazepine on behavioral dyscontrol in borderline personality disorder. *J Clin Psychopharmacol* 1986;6:236-239.

81. Gardner DL, Cowdry RW: Development of melancholia during carbamazepine treatment in borderline personality disorder. *J Clin Psychopharmacol* 1986;6:236-239.

82. Davidson J: Drug therapy of post traumatic stress disorder. *Br J Psychiatry* 1992;160:309-314.

83. McElroy SL, Keck PE, Pope HG, et al: Valproate in the treatment of bipolar disorder: literature review and clinical guidelines. *J Clin Psychopharmacol* 1992 (suppl):12:42-52.

84. Bowden CL, Brugger AM, Swann AC, et al: Efficacy of divalproex vs lithium and placebo in the treatment of mania. *JAMA* 1994;271:918-924.

85. Deltito JA: The effect of valproate on bipolar spectrum temperamental disorders. *J Clin Psychiatry* 1993;54:300-304.

86. Jacobsen FM: Low-dose valproate: a new treatment for cyclothymia, mild rapid cycling disorders, and premenstrual syndrome. *J Clin Psychiatry* 1993;54:229-234.

87. McElroy SL, Keck PE, Pope HG Jr: Sodium valproate: its use in primary psychiatric disorders. *J Clin Psychopharmacol* 1987;7:16-24.

88. Chouinard G, Young SN, Annable L: Antimanic effects of clonazepam. *Biol Psychiatry* 1983;18:451-466.

89. Victor BS, Link NA, Binder RL, et al: Use of clonazepam in mania and schizoaffective disorders. *Am J Psychiatry* 1984;141:111-112.

90. Chouinard G: Antimanic effects of clonazepam. *Psychosomatics* 1985;26(suppl):7-12.

91. Midell JG, Lenox RH, Weiner S: Inpatient clinical trial of lorazepam for the management of manic agitation. *J Clin Psychopharmacol* 1985;5:109-113.

92. Hardy MC, Lecrubier Y, Widlocher D: Efficacy of clonidine in 24 patients with acute mania. *Am J Psychiatry* 1986;143:1450-1453.

93. Giannini AJ, Pascarzi GA, Loiselle RH, et al: Comparison of clonidine and lithium in the treatment of mania. *Am J Psychiatry* 1986;143:1608-1609.

94. Dubovsky SL: Calcium antagonists in manic-depressive illness. *Neuropsychobiology* 1993;27: 184-192.

95. Brunet G, Cerlich B, Robert P, et al: Open trial of a calcium antagonist, nimodipine, in acute mania. *Clin Neuropharmacol* 1990;13:224-228.

96. Garza-Trevino ES, Overall JE, Hollister LE: Verapamil versus lithium in acute mania. *Am J Psychiatry* 1992;149:121-122.

97. Giannini AJ, Taraszewski R, Loiselle RH: Verapamil and lithium in maintenance therapy of manic patients. *J Clin Pharmacol* 1987;27:980-982.

98. Hoschl C, Kozeny, J: Verapamil in affective disorders: a controlled, double-blind study. *Biol Psychiatry* 1989;25:128-140.

99. Brotman AW, Farhadi AM, Gelenberg AJ: Verapamil treatment of acute mania. *J Clin Psychiatry* 1986;47:136-138.

100. Giannini AJ, Loiselle RH, Price WA, et al: Comparison of antimanic efficacy of clonidine and verapamil. *J Clin Psychopharmacol* 1985;25:307-308.

101. Barton BM, Gitlin MJ: Verapamil in treatment-resistant mania: an open trial. *J Clin Psychopharmacol* 1987;7:101-103.

CHAPTER 9

Panic, Phobias, OCD, Eating Disorders, Seasonal Affective Disorder, Premenstrual Syndrome

OVERVIEW

1. In addition to depression and mania, a wide variety of conditions fit into a spectrum of affective disorders which merges into the spectrum of anxiety disorders.
2. These conditions share both symptom clusters and abnormalities of neurochemistry.
3. Patients with panic disorder, agoraphobia, OCD, anorexia, bulimia, SAD, and PMS have a higher prevalence of depressive disorders in first-degree biologic relatives than do unaffected matched control subjects.
4. Cyclic, SSRI, and MAOI antidepressants are effective in panic disorder, agoraphobia, OCD, eating disorders, and PMS.
5. SAD patients benefit from bright-light treatment, which inhibits melatonin release, and from fenfluramine and SSRIs, which enhance brain serotonin.
6. Although alprazolam in moderate- to high-dose regimens is effective for some patients with panic disorder and agoraphobia, withdrawal symptoms occur if this drug is suddenly discontinued, and seizures can occur with an abrupt switch from alprazolam to a TCA, which lowers seizure threshold.
7. MAOIs are often effective in patients with panic, agoraphobia, OCD, and bulimia who have not responded to TCAs or SSRIs. Postural hypotension is the most prevalent MAOI side effect.
8. Social phobia is an underrecognized condition, which can be treated with MAOIs, SSRIs, TCAs, benzodiazepines, or beta-blockers.
9. Obsessive-compulsive disorder, which if severe may be mistaken for a psychotic disturbance, is most effectively treated with SSRIs.
10. Clonazepam may be more effective than alprazolam in preventing panic attacks and is less likely to produce withdrawal symptoms following discontinuation.

With increasing frequency, we are recognizing a number of psychiatric conditions which may have, in the past, seemed to be distinct entities and which now appear to merge and be individualized expressions of related biochemical and physiologic disorders of brain function. Although many have attempted to see depression, panic, phobias, obsessive-compulsive disorder, anorexia, and bulimia as distinct entities related to unresolved psychological conflicts, this point of view is clearly no longer tenable. These diseases appear to be interrelated and may be different manifestations of similar pathogenic processes. Indeed, patients may, at times, present with an eating disorder, panic attacks, or agoraphobia and, at other times, show evidence of a major depressive disorder, or OCD.

Although the DSM-IV classifies panic, phobias, and obsessive-compulsive disorder as anxiety disorders, classifies SAD as a mood disorder, and separates the eating disorders from these groups, characteristics which they share in common suggest that they are different manifestations of a deficiency in brain serotonin. They may be thought of as belonging to a broad spectrum of mood disorders. Similarly the striking affective component of PMS would favor its placement in the mood disorder spectrum, also termed *affective spectrum disorders*.

Patients with atypical depression, who tend to have increased appetite and increased sleep, and who may be cheered up or let down by life events, also belong in the spectrum of mood disorders. We are beginning to recognize individuals who function normally throughout the year but who become depressed and experience increased appetite and hypersomnia during the fall and winter months, with spontaneous recovery in the spring. Patients with seasonal affective disorder (SAD) belong to this spectrum and can benefit from active, not psychodynamic, treatment. Women who experience depression, anger outbursts, anxiety, and fatigue in the week preceding their menstrual period have been seen by generations of physicians as undesirable and untreatable patients. These same women have often undergone a variety of psychotherapies and pharmacotherapies, with minimal benefit. Premenstrual syndrome (PMS) is a physiologically based disorder which may properly belong to the mood spectrum and may, hopefully, be responsive to judicious pharmacologic interventions. Obsessive thoughts and compulsive acts formerly were seen as components of obsessive-compulsive neurosis, another disorder presumed to be psychologically based. This condition may also belong to the affective spectrum and is responsive, often dramatically, to pharmacologic interventions which increase brain serotonin.

The evidence supporting a connection between these various conditions is gaining strength as new research unfolds. Many patients with histories of panic disorder, agoraphobia, and eating disorders will, in the course of their illnesses, experience clinically significant depressive episodes. Studies of family members of patients with panic disorder, agoraphobia, and eating disorders reveals a significantly higher incidence of depression in first-degree biological relatives than that found in unaffected control subjects or in the population at large.[1-3] Serotonin-selective reuptake inhibitors (SSRIs), tricyclic antidepressants (TCAs), and monoamine oxidase inhibitors (MAOIs) are effective in major depressive disorder and dysthymic disorder. These medications are also effective in the treatment of panic disorder, agoraphobia, and eating disorders. Antidepressants, particularly SSRIs, produce dramatic relief from obsessive thoughts and compulsive acts associated with obsessive-compulsive disorder. Indeed, many depressed patients do, at times, experience very uncomfortable obsessional thinking, which is relieved along with the depression when appropriate pharmacotherapy is undertaken. Many patients with obsessive-compulsive disorder, at some time during their lives, experience significant episodes of depression.

Abnormalities in neurotransmitters and their metabolites and in certain endocrine indicators, such as the dexamethasone suppression test, may appear in depressed patients and in those individuals suffering from panic, agoraphobia, and eating disorders.[1] Some PMS patients experience dramatic beneficial responses to SSRI antidepressants, lithium, or the centrally acting serotonergic compound fenfluramine. Subclinical hypothyroidism and abnormal responses to thyrotropin-releasing hormone (TRH) testing have been reported in some patients with PMS, similar to findings in some patients with major depressive disorder.[4,5] Patients with SAD often have rapid relief of their depression when exposed to bright light,[6] or SSRIs.

Family, biochemical, and pharmacologic studies all point to the existence of an affective spectrum made up of the above-described disorders and, in all likelihood, other disorders, which we will hopefully better understand in the future. The pharmacology of TCAs, SSRIs, MAOIs, antianxiety drugs, and lithium has been discussed earlier in this volume. This chapter focuses on some of the clinical characteristics and specific pharmacologic interventions applicable in the treatment of the affective spectrum disorders.

PANIC DISORDER

Patients with panic disorder experience discrete episodes of intense fear, discomfort, or anxiety, which may vary considerably in frequency and severity. During an attack, patients most commonly complain of shortness of breath,

---

DSM-IV CRITERIA

Box 9-1 Criteria for panic attack

Note: A Panic Attack is not a codable disorder. Code the specific diagnosis in which the Panic Attack occurs (e.g., 300.21 Panic Disorder With Agoraphobia).

A discrete period of intense fear or discomfort, in which four (or more) of the following symptoms developed abruptly and reached a peak within 10 minutes:
1. Palpitations, pounding heart, or accelerated heart rate
2. Sweating
3. Trembling or shaking
4. Sensations of shortness of breath or smothering
5. Feeling of choking
6. Chest pain or discomfort
7. Nausea or abdominal distress
8. Feeling dizzy, unsteady, lightheaded, or faint
9. Derealization (feelings of unreality) or depersonalization (being detached from oneself)
10. Fear of losing control or going crazy
11. Fear of dying
12. Paresthesias (numbness or tingling sensations)
13. Chills or hot flushes

From American Psychiatric Association: *Diagnostic and statistical manual of mental disorders*, ed 4 [DSM-IV]. Washington DC, American Psychiatric Press, 1994.

dizziness, palpitations, and sweating as noted in the DSM-IV criteria for panic disorder presented in Box 9-1.[7] During a panic attack, a patient may feel frightened of "going crazy" or losing control. Feelings of depersonalization or derealization are often part of the attack. The most important thing for the clinician to do is to recognize the occurrence of panic disorder and to define and describe it for the patient. The patient must be reassured that it is not his or her fault that the condition exists. The pharmacologic treatment alternatives should be discussed in detail, including potential adverse effects and favorable responses. Psychotherapy should not be recommended as a means of getting rid of the panic attacks, since it is more likely to provoke further recurrences and make the patient feel guilty that the attacks are continuing. In evaluating a patient with panic disorder, evidence of coexisting depression and family history of depression should be taken into account. Supportive psychotherapy may, along with pharmacotherapy, be beneficial, though open-ended or exploratory psychotherapeutic interventions may be painful and ineffective. Early in the assessment, the patient should be informed that though he may feel as if he were going to die or "go crazy" during a panic attack, this will not occur. Since experimental studies and clinical situations have demonstrated that caffeine can provoke panic attacks, it is important to advise patients to significantly decrease or discontinue their use of caffeine-containing beverages.[8]

Many popular articles have attributed a variety of physical and psychological symptoms to hypoglycemia, to the extent that this diagnosis has become somewhat of a fad. Many patients who present initially with complaints consistent with panic disorder will report that they had previously been diagnosed as having hypoglycemia or will suspect that their symptoms are due to low blood sugar rather than panic disorder. There is no evidence of an association between hypoglycemia and panic attacks other than the fact that administration of insulin experimentally may lower blood sugar and produce some of the symptoms of panic. In a study of 10 panic disorder patients given sodium lactate to provoke panic, none showed evidence of low blood sugar levels in association with anxiety symptoms.[9]

Studies of patients with panic anxiety and agoraphobia demonstrated an increased plasma level of the norepinephrine metabolite 3-methoxy-4-hydroxyphenylglycol (MHPG) in response to the administration of the alpha$_2$-adrenergic receptor antagonist yohimbine.[10] This suggests an increased sensitivity to augmented noradrenergic function in panic patients, and implies that impaired presynaptic noradrenergic regulation may exist in these patients.[10,11] As further confirmation of abnormal noradrenergic regulation in panic disorder, experimental administration of clonidine, an alpha$_2$-adrenergic receptor agonist, produces a greater decrease in plasma MHPG in panic patients than in normal controls.[11] The failure of the serotonin precursor tryptophan to produce greater elevation in serum prolactin levels in panic patients as compared with controls suggests that serotonin function may be normal in panic anxiety disorders, in spite of the presumed antipanic mechanism of alprazolam which some investigators link to a serotonergic effect.[12]

Various studies have found an association between the occurrence of mitral valve prolapse and panic disorder. Mitral valve prolapse may occur in up to 6% of normal women, while studies in patients with panic disorder have indicated an incidence of mitral valve prolapse ranging from 12% to 50%.[13] Some investigators have found that pharmacologic control of panic attack leads to echocardiographic or auscultatory normalization of mitral valve prolapse.[1] One study reported that 26% of women with panic disorder had an abnormality of thyroid function and that 17% of the patients studied showed evidence of thyroid microsomal antibodies.[14] The potential existence of abnormal thyroid function in some patients with major depressive disorder, PMS, and panic disorder is of interest and may lead to a better understanding of some of the common mechanisms that may underlie these conditions.

A subset of patients with atypical panic disorder with associated hostility, irritability, severe derealization, and social withdrawal has been described.[15] In these patients, though there was no clear evidence of temporal lobe epilepsy, there were temporal EEG abnormalities.[15] Some of these patients with atypical panic showed a therapeutic response to carbamazepine or alprazolam.[15]

Although sleep deprivation has been reported to have a beneficial effect in some depressed patients, panic attacks may be exacerbated following sleep deprivation as documented in a controlled study, wherein 40% of panic patients experienced an attack the day following sleep deprivation.[16]

Pharmacotherapy

Five classes of drugs have proven to be therapeutically effective in the management of panic attacks. Each has its advantages and disadvantages, and its range of side effects and characteristics, which may make a particular treatment more or less desirable for a specific patient. Benzodiazepines, including alprazolam and clonazepam, have the disadvantage of producing excessive drowsiness, tolerance, and physical dependence. Tricyclic and heterocyclic antidepressants exert antipanic effect, but may produce dry mouth, constipation, tachycardia, and postural hypotension. MAOIs require the avoidance of certain foods, beverages, and medications, which may, if consumed in conjunction with an MAOI provoke a hypertensive crisis. Furthermore, the MAOIs may produce significant dizziness and postural hypotension. The serotonin-selective re-uptake inhibitors (SSRIs) when used in low doses exert a potent antipanic effect with minimal side effects, but if higher doses are used may provoke or worsen panic; furthermore, it usually takes at least 2 weeks to begin to see a response.[20,21] Controlled clinical studies of each of these classes of drugs against placebo in patients with panic disorder indicate considerable benefit, with some variations in efficacy between drugs.[17-22]

In my experience, the MAOIs and SSRIs are often more effective and better tolerated than either tricyclics or benzodiazepines. Many patients treated with alprazolam or clonazepam experience excessive drowsiness prior to achieving adequate control of panic. Many people given tricyclics, such as imipramine, experience sinus tachycardia at the outset of treatment, making them feel that the drug is actually inducing panic symptoms. Beta-blockers reduce physiologic symptoms and are useful in some panic disorder patients who do not tolerate or benefit from more conventional antipanic agents.[22]

When the decision is made to treat a panic patient with a benzodiazepine, one may choose either alprazolam or clonazepam. Clonazepam has been used for a number of years as an anticonvulsant, and has more recently been employed in the treatment of anxiety disorders.[19,23] The side effects and risks of these drugs are discussed in detail in chapter 3. Rare instances of liver enzyme abnormalities have been reported during treatment with clonazepam, and therefore it may be useful to periodically perform liver function tests, particularly when higher doses or longer durations of administration are employed. There are a larger number of controlled studies indicating the efficacy of alprazolam in panic than there are for clonazepam.[24] Many studies, however, indicate that clonazepam is equal or superior to alprazolam in the treatment of panic disorder.[19,23]

Abrupt discontinuation of either drug after several weeks of treatment is to be avoided, since a withdrawal syndrome may occur. The longer half-life and slower clearance of clonazepam may produce a greater cumulative effect. However, this factor may also reduce the intensity and severity of withdrawal symptoms compared with alprazolam. In one study of 48 patients whose treatment regimen was changed from alprazolam to clonazepam, 39 patients (82%) preferred clonazepam because of decreased frequency of administration and lack of interdose anxiety.[25]

On a milligram-for-milligram basis, clonazepam is likely to be approximately twice as potent as alprazolam, and therefore can be administered in a smaller daily dose and taken on a once or twice daily basis as opposed to the regimen of 3 or 4 doses per day usually required with alprazolam. The average antipanic dose of alprazolam in young to middle-aged healthy persons is approximately 3 mg/day. However, some patients may require doses of up to 6 or 8 mg/day, and others may respond favorably to doses of only 1 to 2 mg/day. Generally, clonazepam exerts its antipanic effect at a daily dosage of approximately 1.5 mg, although some patients may require up to 3 times this dose whereas others will respond to a daily dose as low as 0.5 mg. With either alprazolam or clonazepam, a low dosage should be used initially with gradual upward titration as tolerated by the patient and as required to achieve symptom control. Alprazolam should be started at 0.25 mg 3 times a day with increases of 0.25 mg every 1 to 3 days. The rate of dosage adjustment must be governed by the continuing presence of symptoms and by the absence of excessive drowsiness or sedation. When initiating clonazepam, it is appropriate to start with 0.25 mg twice a day for the first 2 days, with dosage increments of 0.25 mg every day or two as tolerated. Since clonazepam may produce excessive drowsiness and may achieve control of panic anxiety with a single daily dose administered at bedtime, it is preferable to give the larger portion of the dose at bedtime and to increase the morning dose more slowly. A typical and effective clonazepam regimen may allow the patient to take 0.5 to 2.0 mg at bedtime, along with a morning dose of 0.25 to 0.5 mg. Since these benzodiazepines may produce drowsiness and impaired performance, patients whose dosage is being titrated should be advised against the operation of motor vehicles or machinery until a stable dosage is established at which the patient is free of significant impairment.

It is not advisable to utilize regimens combining two or more benzodiazepines. In those patients who, after receiving a benzodiazepine, do not achieve the desired therapeutic response it may be necessary to initiate another form of pharmacologic treatment, including a serotonin selective or tricyclic antidepressant or an MAOI. Since tricyclic antidepressants may lower seizure threshold and since seizures may occur in association with benzodiazepine withdrawal, it is important not to switch abruptly from alprazolam or clonazepam to a tricyclic, but rather to gradually titrate the benzodiazepine dosage downward as the tricyclic dosage is gradually titrated upward.[24] Although in some studies buspirone has been found to be comparable to benzodiazepines in generalized anxiety disorder, there is no evidence that buspirone is effective in the treatment of panic disorder.[27,28]

Several studies indicate the efficacy of the combined use of low-dose benzodiazepines and beta-adrenergic blocking agents such as propanolol.[22,29,30] There is evidence for noradrenergic hyperactivity in patients with panic disorder, and indeed, many of the physiologic manifestations of this condition may be related to excessive catecholamine activity. Thus the use of relatively low doses of propranolol, generally in the range of 10 to 20 mg 3 to 4 times daily may be a useful adjunct to a benzodiazepine in the management of panic disorder, particularly in those patients who do not tolerate or who are unwilling to take a tricyclic SSRI, or MAOI.[29,30]

Numerous studies have demonstrated therapeutic efficacy for imipramine in the treatment of panic disorder.[18] Several studies have also reported antipanic effects of other tricyclic and heterocyclic antidepressants, including amitriptyline, desipramine, and trazodone.[17,31] It has been suggested that trazodone may have specific antipanic activity due to its higher specificity as an inhibitor of serotonin reuptake.[31] When tricyclic or heterocyclic antidepressants are used in the management of panic disorder, initial doses should be 10 to 25 mg daily with slow increments as required to gain symptom control. Although conventional antidepressant doses may be required, starting with excessively high doses may provoke panic symptoms and lead the patient to premature discontinuation of the cyclic agent.

Clinical studies support the efficacy of MAOIs in panic anxiety.[17,18] Phenelzine and tranylcypromine are both effective in the management of panic.[18] When MAOIs are employed, it is extremely important to provide the patient with a printed sheet of dietary and medication instructions, such as that appearing in Appendix A. In addition to the printed instructions, patients should be carefully instructed by the physician regarding the dietary and medication restrictions and should be specifically told that MAOIs cannot be combined with SSRIs and cannot be taken until several weeks after stopping prior SSRI therapy. Since panic disorder is often difficult to control, patients may consult other physicians and have their medications changed; thus the SSRI interaction warning must be emphasized. Generally phenelzine is initiated at 15 mg twice daily with gradual dosage increase as tolerated and as required for symptom control up to 15 mg 4 times daily. When employing tranylcypromine, the initial dose should be 10 mg twice daily with gradual increase to 10 mg 4 times daily as tolerated and as necessary for efficacy. Blood pressure in sitting and standing positions should be monitored once weekly initially and less often later in treatment. Patients should be warned about the possible occurrence of dizziness with postural change and advised to increase salt and fluid intake should this side effect occur, as discussed in chapter 6.

The serotonin-selective reuptake inhibitors, when used in low doses, are often the most effective agents and easiest to use in the prophylaxis of recurrent panic attacks.[21,32] If an SSRI is initiated at too high a dose, panic attacks may be provoked or worsened, often leading to premature discontinuation of the drug trial. SSRIs, like MAOIs, and tricyclics generally must be given for at least 2 to 3 weeks and often require dosage adjustment before antipanic efficacy is seen. Since benzodiazepines generally produce an initial improvement in panic symptoms within a day or 2, it is often best to initiate treatment with a low dose of a benzodiazepine, such as 0.25 to 0.5 mg of clonazepam 1 to 3 times daily simultaneously with the SSRI. Generally in most patients, fluoxetine can be started at 5 mg daily and the dose not increased for at least the first 2 to 3 weeks, since conventional doses of 20 mg per day may increase panic symptoms. Fluoxetine, however, inhibits drug metabolism and will increase the effect of clonazepam, alprazolam, and most other benzodiazepines. I therefore prefer to initiate treatment and prophylaxis of panic disorder with sertraline, 25 mg daily in conjunction with the previously mentioned dose of clonazepam, since sertraline is often highly effective at this dose in panic disorder, with minimal potential to alter serum concentration or effect of coadministered benzodiazepines. If no response is seen after 2 to 3 weeks, the sertraline dose can be increased to 25 mg twice daily or 50 mg once daily. Fluvoxamine and other SSRIs have also been used successfully in the management of panic.[21] In obsessive-compulsive disorder and in depression, higher doses of SSRIs are commonly employed, and if one of these conditions coexists with panic the SSRI dosage may need to be titrated upward, although this may destabilize control of panic symptoms and may therefore necessitate continuing coadministration of the benzodiazepine. In many patients with panic disorder who do not also suffer concurrently from depression or OCD, treatment can continue with the SSRI while the benzodiazepine is gradually decreased and discontinued.

PHOBIAS

The two most common phobic disorders seen in adult psychiatry are agoraphobia, which may occur with or without panic attacks (Boxes 9-2 and 9-3), and social phobia. In agoraphobia there is a fear of being in places or situations from which escape may be difficult or embarrassing or in which help may not be readily available. Agoraphobic patients are often frightened to be away from their homes and may therefore remain at home, avoiding ordinary occupational and social interactions. Some agoraphobic patients arrange elaborate schemes so that they can go out of their homes with a companion. Many patients with agoraphobia will attempt to participate in normal life situations and endure intense anxiety in the process. The majority of severely agoraphobic patients, however, are unable to travel on public transportation and experience great difficulty standing in line, going to a theater, or shopping. Most agoraphobic individuals experience panic attacks, while some do not develop the full panic syndrome but experience somatic symptoms, including dizziness, loss of bladder control, chest pain, and shortness of breath. In some cases, even in the absence of a panic attack, agoraphobic patients may experience depersonalization or derealization.[7]

Agoraphobia

Agoraphobic patients with or without panic attacks may benefit from pharmacologic intervention. Some experience depression, and it is often difficult to differentiate between depressive symptoms that are secondary to the altered life-style of the agoraphobic individual and a primary depressive

Box 9-2 Diagnostic criteria for 300.01 panic disorder without agoraphobia

A. Both (1) and (2):
  (1) Recurrent unexpected Panic Attacks
  (2) At least one of the attacks has been followed by 1 month (or more) of one (or more) of the following:
      (a) Persistent concern about having additional attacks
      (b) Worry about the implications of the attack or its consequences (e.g., losing control, having a heart attack, "going crazy")
      (c) A significant change in behavior related to the attacks
B. Absence of Agoraphobia.
C. The Panic Attacks are not due to the direct physiologic effects of a substance (e.g., a drug of abuse, a medication) or a general medical condition (e.g., hyperthyroidism).
D. The Panic Attacks are not better accounted for by another mental disorder, such as Social Phobia (e.g., occurring on exposure to feared social situations), Specific Phobia (e.g., on exposure to a specific phobic situation), Obsessive-Compulsive Disorder (e.g., on exposure to dirt in someone with an obsession about contamination), Posttraumatic Stress Disorder (e.g., in response to stimuli associated with a severe stressor), or Separation Anxiety Disorder (e.g., in response to being away from home or close relatives).

From American Psychiatric Association: *Diagnostic and statistical manual of mental disorders,* ed 4 [DSM-IV]. Washington DC, American Psychiatric Press, 1994.

disorder. Because of similar pharmacologic responsiveness of panic disorder, agoraphobia, and depression, it is likely that there may be related underlying neurochemical processes in these disorders. In some cases behavioral therapy, including exposure techniques, are useful in agoraphobia, although behavioral therapy tends to be more effective when combined with pharmacologic intervention.[33] In most instances medical management of the agoraphobic patient will allow for fairly rapid recovery and return to more normal function, particularly when combined with at least some psychotherapeutic intervention, including supportive psychotherapy, cognitive therapy, and behavioral techniques.

Controlled clinical studies indicate the efficacy of alprazolam in agoraphobic patients.[18] In general, alprazolam needs to be used at relatively high dosages, generally between 3 and 6 mg/day, which carries with it the previously mentioned risk of excessive sedation and drug dependency. Several studies have found imipramine, alone or in combination with in vivo exposure techniques, to be highly beneficial in the treatment of agoraphobia.[3,34] Earlier studies suggested that agoraphobic patients and patients with panic disorder could be

---

Box 9-3 Diagnostic criteria for 300.21 panic disorder
with agoraphobia

A. Both (1) and (2):
   (1) Recurrent unexpected Panic Attacks
   (2) At least one of the attacks has been followed by 1 month (or more) of one (or
      more) of the following:
      (a) Persistent concern about having additional attacks
      (b) Worry about the implications of the attack or its consequences (e.g., losing
         control, having a heart attack, "going crazy")
      (c) A significant change in behavior related to the attacks
B. The presence of Agoraphobia.
C. The Panic Attacks are not due to the direct physiological effects of a substance
   (e.g., a drug of abuse, a medication) or a general medical condition (e.g., hyperthy-
   roidism).
D. The Panic Attacks are not better accounted for by another mental disorder, such as
   Social Phobia (e.g., occurring on exposure to feared social situations), Specific
   Phobia (e.g., on exposure to a specific phobic situation), Obsessive-Compulsive
   Disorder (e.g., on exposure to dirt in someone with an obsession about
   contamination), Posttraumatic Stress Disorder (e.g., in response to stimuli
   associated with a severe stressor), or Separation Anxiety Disorder (e.g., in response
   to being away from home or close relatives).

From American Psychiatric Association: *Diagnostic and statistical manual of mental disorders,* ed 4
[DSM-IV]. Washington DC, American Psychiatric Press, 1994.

---

responsive to rather low doses of tricyclic antidepressants, in the range of 10 to
75 mg/day, as opposed to the conventional antidepressant doses utilized.
However, some studies support the necessity of using conventional antidepressant doses of tricyclic drugs in the treatment of agoraphobic patients.[34] The
optimal dose of imipramine tends to be between 150 and 200 mg/day. Some
agoraphobic patients, like many panic patients, experience increased anxiety
when tricyclic therapy is initiated and may therefore need to start with a dose
as low as 10 mg daily, with gradual dosage increments as tolerated until a
therapeutic response is established. Amitriptyline, trazodone, and the more
strongly serotonergic TCA clomipramine, as well as the SSRIs (including
fluoxetine and fluvoxamine) have all been effective in agoraphobia, paralleling
their efficacy in panic disorder.[31,32,35]

MAOIs, particularly phenelzine, have been demonstrated to be dramatically
effective in the treatment of agoraphobia.[18,36] Indeed, many agoraphobic
patients who do not achieve optimal results with SSRIs or imipramine can
experience relief of their symptoms when phenelzine in conventional antidepressant doses is employed. There are two major disadvantages of MAOIs in

agoraphobic patients. Since it is necessary to alert patients to dietary and medication restrictions, some patients, finding this information frightening, will be reluctant to take these medications or may take them and, prior to their becoming effective, live in fear that they are about to have a hypertensive crisis. Another potential disadvantage of MAOIs is their ability to produce postural hypotension, which some patients may interpret either as evidence of continuing agoraphobic symptoms or as the occurrence of a hypertensive reaction.[37] If patients are adequately prepared and instructed, these drugs are often effective and may allow a patient who has been unable to leave home and use public transportation to be employed and return to a relatively normal life. Indeed, patients who are agoraphobic with or without panic attacks may benefit from MAOIs.

Social Phobia

Social phobia is a fairly common and at times disabling disorder, classified as an anxiety disorder in DSM IV although bearing some features in common with the affective spectrum disorders. Unfortunately, the diagnosis of social phobia is often missed by clinicians, who may instead make the diagnosis of generalized anxiety or of panic disorder (see Box 9-4).

Social phobia is a persistent fear of situations in which the individual is potentially exposed to the scrutiny of others. The social phobic patient is frightened that he or she may say or do something that will be humiliating or embarrassing. Such persons are often frightened of public speaking, unable to eat in restaurants, and even unable to urinate in a public lavatory.[1] Patients with social phobia may experience hand trembling when writing in the presence of others and may be embarrassed or unable to answer simple questions. They often avoid situations that require them to speak in public and may, as a result of their social phobia, severely curtail their social, personal, and professional lives.[1] Patients with social phobia often experience a variety of physiologic symptoms, similar to those seen in panic disorder during an attack. Performance anxiety prior to a public appearance, which actors and musicians may experience, may be a form of social phobia.

The pharmacologic interventions that have proved most effective in social phobia involve the use of benzodiazepines such as alprazolam or clonazepam, alone or in combination with beta-blocking drugs, or the use of SSRIs or MAOIs.[38,39,40,41] Social phobic symptoms may appear at any time, and the patient must have pharmacologic symptom control, endure the symptoms, or engage in avoidance behavior. It is preferable to establish an effective pharmacologic regimen and encourage the patient to function normally.

Benzodiazepines, when used in high doses, have the risk of excessive drowsiness and dependency; therefore their prolonged use may present some disadvantages. Many patients respond well to low doses of benzodiazepines, and do not require more intensive pharmacotherapy. In relatively mild social

DSM-IV CRITERIA

Box 9-4 Diagnostic criteria for 300.23 social phobia

A. A marked and persistent fear of one or more social or performance situations in which the person is exposed to unfamiliar people or to possible scrutiny by others. The individual fears that he or she will act in a way (or show anxiety symptoms) that will be humiliating or embarrassing. **Note:** In children, there must be evidence of the capacity for age-appropriate social relationships with familiar people and the anxiety must occur in peer settings, not just in interactions with adults.

B. Exposure to the feared social situation almost invariably provokes anxiety, which may take the form of a situationally bound or situationally predisposed Panic Attack. **Note:** In children, the anxiety may be expressed by crying, tantrums, freezing, or shrinking from social situations with unfamiliar people.

C. The person recognizes that the fear is excessive or unreasonable. **Note:** In children, this feature may be absent.

D. The feared social or performance situations are avoided or else are endured with intense anxiety or distress.

E. The avoidance, anxious anticipation, or distress in the feared social or performance situation(s) interferes significantly with the person's normal routine, occupational (academic) functioning, or social activities or relationships, or there is marked distress about having the phobia.

F. In individuals under age 18 years, the duration is at least 6 months.

G. The fear or avoidance is not due to the direct physiological effects of a substance (e.g., a drug of abuse, a medication) or a general medical condition and is not better accounted for by another mental disorder (e.g., Panic Disorder With or Without Agoraphobia, Separation Anxiety Disorder, Body Dysmorphic Disorder, A Pervasive Developmental Disorder, or Schizoid Personality Disorder).

H. If a general medical condition or another mental disorder is present, the fear in Criterion A is unrelated to it, e.g., the fear is not of Stuttering, trembling in Parkinson's disease, or exhibiting abnormal eating behavior in Anorexia Nervosa Or Bulimia Nervosa.

Specify if:
Generalized: if the fears include most social situations (also consider the additional diagnosis of Avoidant Personality Disorder).

From American Psychiatric Association: *Diagnostic and statistical manual of mental disorders*, ed 4 [DSM-IV]. Washington DC, American Psychiatric Press, 1994.

phobia, often the simplest initial pharmacologic intervention is clonazepam 0.25 to 0.5 mg once or twice daily, which may significantly improve symptoms, perhaps in part related to its serotonergic activity along with other benzodiazepine mechanisms. Some patients with social phobia will be responsive to beta-blocking drugs such as propranolol 10 to 20 mg 3 or 4 times daily, metoprolol 25 to 50 mg twice daily, or atenolol 50 to 100 mg once daily.[43,44] The use of beta-blocking drugs in conjunction with alprazolam or clonazepam generally allows for the administration of lower benzodiazepine dosage and the achievement of better control of phobic symptoms. Beta-adrenergic blocking drugs should not be prescribed by physicians who do not first take a careful medical history and then conduct physical examinations including blood pressure, pulse rate, heart sounds, and chest auscultation on a regular basis during treatment. A past history of congestive heart failure, bradyarrhythmias, or bronchial asthma is a contraindication to treatment with beta-adrenergic blocking drugs.

Several clinical studies have documented the therapeutic efficacy of tranylcypromine and phenelzine in the treatment of social phobia.[38,41,42,44] Imipramine has also been used with some success in the treatment of social phobia.[38] Studies which have compared the efficacy of phenelzine to that of imipramine or amitriptyline have found phenelzine to be superior.[43] Likewise, phenelzine is superior to atenolol in the treatment of social phobic symptoms.[41,44] When treating social phobia with MAOIs, these drugs should be used in conventional antidepressant dosage. Patients, of course, must be warned about dietary and medication restrictions and MAOIs should be started at one to two tablets daily with gradual upward titration. In a patient for whom MAOIs and beta-adrenergic blocking drugs are contraindicated, tricyclic antidepressants may be considered alone or in conjunction with a low dose of alprazolam. Buspirone, which has demonstrated efficacy in the treatment of generalized anxiety and which is largely free of sedating or dependency-producing effects, has not yet been documented to have significant efficacy in the treatment of social phobia.[27] Nevertheless, if other agents are ineffective or not tolerated, a trial of buspirone in a gradually titrated dosage of 15 to 30 mg/day may be considered in a patient suffering from social phobia.

The serotonin-selective reuptake inhibitors, clearly proven effective in depression, obsessive compulsive disorder, and panic disorder, have been used to a limited extent in social phobia with encouraging results.[35,40] Major advantages of the SSRIs include the absence of hypotensive and anticholinergic side effects, since many social phobic patients complain of feeling dizzy and experience "fogginess" when given tricyclics. If SSRIs are initiated at ordinary doses, anxiety symptoms may be worsened; therefore, as in the case of panic disorder, starting doses for fluoxetine should be 5 mg daily and for sertraline 25 mg daily. I favor the latter drug since in the event of an unfavorable response the effect will end much sooner than that of fluoxetine, which has the added disadvantage of increasing serum concentration, and the effect of benzodiazepines which may be coadministered. Unfortunately, SSRIs generally must be given for at least 2 or 3 weeks before a response begins; thus the patient may be most appropriately treated initially by the concurrent administration of clonazepam or a similar drug. It still appears that phenelzine is more effective in social phobia than are the SSRIs; however the latter drugs are easier to administer, do not require dietary or medication restrictions, and may be more easily accepted by patients who are reluctant to receive pharmacotherapy.

Obsessive-Compulsive Disorder

Formerly thought to be relatively uncommon, obsessive-compulsive disorder (OCD) is becoming recognized with increasing frequency. Classified in DSM IV as an anxiety disorder, it bears many similarities to mood disorders and very likely can be seen as a component of the affective spectrum (see Box 9-5). Furthermore, within OCD there are many variations on the theme with some patients having only recurrent and persistent thoughts, impulses, or images, termed *obsessions*, and others driven to perform repetitive behaviors such as washing or checking or mental acts such as counting or praying, termed *compulsions*. Patients may experience primarily obsessions or compulsions or both, a critical point being the feeling that these thoughts or actions are uncontrollable. Depressed patients often experience obsessional thinking, and patients who have OCD often become depressed. The occurrence of depression in a patient with OCD generally worsens obsessive and compulsive symptoms. Patients with OCD are more likely to have a family history of a major depressive or bipolar disorder.[45] As we become more familiar with obsessive-compulsive disorder, it is becoming apparent that this is a family or spectrum of disorders which includes body dysmorphic disorder (BDD), trichotillomania, hypochondriasis, Tourette's syndrome, and very likely anorexia nervosa and a number of other conditions with compulsive and impulsive features including pathologic gambling and depersonalization disorder.[45] At times the severity of OCD-related symptoms is so intense as to suggest a psychotic disorder. Generally studies utilizing pharmacologic probes and various pharmacotherapies strongly suggest that a disturbance of central serotonergic function plays an etiologic role in this group of disorders.[45] Indeed, the most promising pharmacotherapies for OCD-related disorders include clomipramine and the various SSRIs, along with MAOIs and clonazepam, both of which also enhance central serotonin activity.[46] The occurence of certain abnormal behaviors in animals suggests the potentially ubiquitous nature of a serotonin deficit syndrome, similar to obsessive-compulsive disorder. In dogs, where the phenomenon of acral lick may cause the animal to macerate the foot "compulsively" and in birds, where partial denudation may occur through "compulsive" feather picking, the therapeutic benefit of clomipramine and SSRIs such as fluoxetine has been demonstrated.[47,48]

Obsessions represent recurrent and persistent ideas, thoughts, impulses, or images which are experienced generally as intrusive and senseless. Frequently the individual attempts to ignore or suppress such thoughts or to neutralize them with some other thought or action.[1] Compulsions are repetitive, purposeful, and intentional behaviors performed in response to an obsession or in accordance with certain rules the patient has established. Compulsive acts are designed to neutralize or prevent discomfort or to avoid some dreaded situation or event. Obsessions and compulsions cause distress, are time consuming, and may significantly interfere with the person's normal level of occupational and social function.[1]

DSM-IV CRITERIA

Box 9-5 Diagnostic criteria for 300.3 obsessive-compulsive disorder

A. Either obsessions or compulsions:

Obsessions as defined by (1), (2), (3), and (4):

(1) Recurrent and persistent thoughts, impulses, or images that are experienced, at some time during the disturbance, as intrusive and inappropriate and that cause marked anxiety or distress

(2) The thoughts, impulses, or images are not simply excessive worries about real-life problems

(3) The person attempts to ignore or suppress such thoughts, impulses, or images, or to neutralize them with some other thought or action

(4) The person recognizes that the obsessional thoughts, impulses, or images are a product of his or her own mind (not imposed from without as in thought insertion)

Compulsions as defined by (1) and (2):

(1) Repetitive behaviors (e.g., hand washing, ordering, checking) or mental acts (e.g., praying, counting, repeating words silently) that the person feels driven to perform in response to an obsession, or according to rules that must be applied rigidly

(2) The behaviors or mental acts are aimed at preventing or reducing distress or preventing some dreaded event or situation; however, these behaviors or mental acts either are not connected in a realistic way with what they are designed to neutralize or prevent or are clearly excessive

B. At some point during the course of the disorder, the person has recognized that the obsessions or compulsions are excessive or unreasonable. **Note:** This does not apply to children.

C. The obsessions or compulsions cause marked distress, are time consuming (take more than 1 hour a day), or significantly interfere with the person's normal routine, occupational (or academic) functioning, or usual social activites or relationships.

D. If another Axis I disorder is present, the content of the obsessions or compulsions is not restricted to it (e.g., preoccupation with food in the presence of an Eating Disorder; hair pulling in the presence of Trichotillomania; concern with appearance in the presence of Body Dysmorphic Disorder; preoccupation with drugs in the presence of a Substance Use Disorder; preoccupation with having a serious illness in the presence of Hypochondriasis; preoccupation with sexual urges or fantasies in the presence of a Paraphilia; or guilty ruminations in the presence of Major Depressive Disorder).

E. The disturbance is not due to the direct physiological effects of a substance (e.g., a drug of abuse, a medication) or a general medical condition.

Specify if:

With Poor Insight: if, for most of the time during the current episode, the person does not recognize that the obsessions and compulsions are excessive or unreasonable.

From American Psychiatric Association: *Diagnostic and statistical manual of mental disorders*, ed 4 [DSM-IV]. Washington DC, American Psychiatric Press, 1994.

Prior to the advent of clomipramine and the SSRIs, tricyclic antidepressants and MAOIs were the most widely used agents in treating obsessive compulsive disorder. Numerous controlled and uncontrolled clinical studies have documented the efficacy of TCAs and MAOIs in OCD, however more recent work has clearly shown the superiority of clomipramine and SSRIs to these drugs.[46] Although occasional benefits have been seen with alprazolam in OCD, clonazepam which is a more serotonergic benzodiazepine is more effective and appears to exert an anti-obsessional effect beyond simple reduction of anxiety.[49] Although clonidine has been used at times for OCD, there is no convincing evidence of its efficacy.[49] Lithium has been used in the treatment of OCD and as an adjunct to enhance other anti-obsessional drugs; although occasionally beneficial clinically, controlled studies fail to document its value in OCD.[50] Some patients' obsessional thoughts are so intense that they may be mistaken for hallucinations, furthermore there is the possibility of co-morbidity of OCD with a psychotic disorder, in these situations, failure to respond adequately to an SSRI or clomipramine suggests the possibility of achieving further benefit by the addition of a neuroleptic, though the latter should be employed cautiously.[51,52]

Clomipramine is the most serotonergic of currently marketed tricyclics, and has been well documented as a potent anti-obsessional drug, it does however produce typical tricyclic side effects and is therefore not well tolerated by many patients.[46,49] The ordinary dosage of clomipramine ranges between 100 and 200 mg daily, most or all of which may be given at bedtime; some OCD patients will respond favorably to significantly lower or higher doses. Because of sedation, anticholinergic or hypotensive side effects, some patients with OCD are unable to tolerate large enough doses of clomipramine to adequately control symptoms. Clomipramine is clearly more effective than other tricyclics in most people with OCD.

The serotonin selective reuptake inhibitors are being used with increasing frequency not only in depression and panic disorder but are rapidly becoming the drugs of choice in the management of OCD. Although only fluoxetine and fluvoxamine are specifically approved in the treatment of OCD, sertraline, paroxetine, and venlafaxine also have significant anti-obsessional effects and may have some advantages as discussed in chapter 5. Although fluvoxamine is the most recently approved SSRI for use in OCD in the United States, it is the SSRI which has been most extensively studied and employed for this condition world-wide. Experience with fluvoxamine in depression and OCD abroad suggests that it will be an important and useful addition to our pharmacologic armamentarium, particularly in the management of severe OCD, which is not infrequently resistant to pharmacotherapy.[46,50,51] In OCD, fluvoxamine in daily doses of 200 to 300 mg are generally employed with favorable therapeutic responses and a tolerable level of side effects, which resemble those of other SSRIs. As discussed in chapter 5, fluvoxamine has a half-life of 15 hours with no active metabolites, and although it may inhibit metabolism of co-administered drugs as does fluoxetine, its shorter half-life reduces its impact on drug metabolism and interactions.

Since clonazepam is an effective and commonly used adjunct in the management of OCD, the lesser potential of sertraline and venlafaxine to interact with benzodiazepines may be advantageous. The long half-life of fluoxetine may be advantageous in establishing and maintaining a stable serum concentration and pharmacologic activity, yet this drug can significantly increase the serum concentration of clomipramine and other tricyclics, which could increase the risk of clomipramine toxicity including seizures. Many patients with severe OCD require high doses of anti-obsessional medications and not uncommonly combined regimens are employed; therefore if fluoxetine and clomipramine are administered simultaneously, it is important to monitor clomipramine serum concentrations, since the latter drug can lower seizure threshold and provoke convulsions as well as cardiac arrhythmias, particularly at high serum concentrations.

In spite of the considerable efficacy of clomipramine and SSRIs in OCD, some patients fail to respond adequately and may require adjunctive agents including clonazepam and neuroleptics. I have seen a number of patients whose OCD failed to respond to tricyclics, clomipramine, or an SSRI who eventually responded best to a monoamine oxidase inhibitor; it must be emphasized again that an adequate period after discontinuing clomipramine or an SSRI must elapse prior to starting an MAOI. Furthermore, if an MAOI treated patient needs to be treated subsequently with clomipramine or an SSRI, they must remain off the MAOI for 2 weeks prior to initiating the alternative medication.

In addition to more typical OCD, many variants and partial symptom forms of OCD have been recognized. Serotonergic drugs have been shown to be effective in compulsive nail biting (onychophagia) which may occur as an isolated symptom or as a component of OCD.[53] Likewise, these anti-obsessional drugs are effective in trichotillomania,[54] religious scrupulosity,[55] and pathologic jealousy.[56]

EATING DISORDERS

Anorexia nervosa and bulimia nervosa are classified in the DMS-IV[1] as eating disorders, yet a broad clinical and biologic examination of these conditions suggests association with obsessive-compulsive disorder, in that there is a distorted view of body image along with compulsive behavior including dieting, bingeing, and purging.[45] Furthermore, the well-known association of these conditions with depressive symptoms and family histories suggests their membership in the spectrum of affective disorders. Family studies of patients with anorexia or bulimia reveal a higher-than-expected incidence of depression and affective illness.[3,57,58] In one study of 82 female outpatients with anorexia nervosa or bulimia, research diagnostic criteria for major depressive disorder were met by 55.6% of the anorexic patients and by 23.6% of the bulimic patients.[58] In that study, a modified Hamilton Depression Rating Scale found that 40.7% of the anorexics and 23.6% of the bulimics had scores in the moderately or severely depressed range.[58] Abnormal neurochemical markers, such as altered MHPG excretion, may occur in anorexia nervosa and bulimia as well as in some depressed patients.[58] Patients with bulimia often respond favorably to treatment with TCAs, SSRIs, and MAOIs.[59,60,61] The therapeutic response of eating disorders to antidepressant drug treatment, along with the numerous population studies that have found a high incidence of affective illness and substance abuse in families of patients with eating disorders, is supportive of the placement of these conditions within the affective spectrum, although the exact nature of this interaction remains to be better defined.[3]

Many studies support an association between brain serotonin and appetite, behavior, and food preference.[62,63,64,65] Decreased serotonin neurotransmission increases carbohydrate craving and may be an important mechanism of bingeing, which is seen in bulimia.[62] Increased CNS serotonergic activity may decrease carbohydrate craving and bingeing behavior.[67]

In anorexia nervosa there is refusal to maintain body weight above a minimal normal level for age and height. Anorexic patients have an intense fear of gaining weight and see themselves as fat, even when they are emaciated. Female anorexics generally develop amenorrhea.[65] Clinical studies indicate that amitriptyline may be effective in allowing anorexic patients to gain weight and stabilize, avoiding recurrent patterns of weight loss.[68] An open study of fluoxetine found that 29 of 31 patients with anorexia nervosa maintained their weight at or above 85% average with restrictor anorexics responding better than bulimic or purging-type anorexics.[66] Cyproheptadine, a serotonin receptor antagonist, has also been used to control anorexic behavior and facilitate weight maintenance.[68] It is not helpful in bulimia and may, presumably as a result of its serotonin antagonist activity, increase bingeing.

Patients with bulimia have recurrent episodes of binge eating, which involves the consumption of a large amount of food in a relatively short time.[7] During eating binges, bulimic patients feel a lack of control over their eating behavior.[7] The DSM-IV criteria for bulimia include a minimum of two binge-eating episodes a week, overconcern with body shape and weight, and the regular use of self-induced vomiting, laxatives, diuretics, strict dieting, or vigorous exercise in an attempt to prevent weight gain in spite of the continuing binge eating.[7]

Controlled clinical studies indicate that various TCAs, including amitriptyline, desipramine, and imipramine, may be effective in the treatment of bulimia and the control of binge eating in this disorder.[59,69,70] Fluoxetine given in a daily dose of 60 mg decreased the frequency of weekly binge eating and vomiting episodes in a placebo-controlled outpatient study of 387 bulimic women.[61] MAOIs, including phenelzine and tranylcypromine, also are effective in controlling bulimia.[60] Among the MAOIs, phenelzine has been subjected to the most extensive double-blind placebo-controlled studies.[60] Although amitriptyline has been reported to control binge eating in bulimic patients, it is the tricyclic antidepressant most likely to stimulate carbohydrate hunger and cause weight gain in depressed, nonbulimic patients. For this reason, tricyclics such as desipramine and imipramine, which are less likely to stimulate appetite and weight gain, may be preferable in the treatment of bulimic patients.

Other tricyclic and heterocyclic antidepressants have occasionally been used in the treatment of bulimia, but there is less extensive documentation for the efficacy of these compounds. Since bulimic patients are obsessed with their eating behavior and weight, it is likely that phenelzine and SSRIs may have particular efficacy not only in controlling the binge-eating behavior but also in controlling the obsessional thinking about food, eating, and bingeing. In my experience, tricyclics have been less effective in bulimia than SSRIs or MAOIs; my preference has been to use either sertraline or tranylcypromine. Venlafaxine should also be considered and eventually studied formally in eating disorders, because of its dual serotonergic and noradrenergic activity.

SEASONAL AFFECTIVE DISORDER

Seasonal affective disorder (SAD) was first described in 1984 by Rosenthal's group at the National Institute of Mental Health (NIMH). This syndrome is characterized by recurring cycles of fall and winter depression and spring-summer hypomania or euthymia.[71,72] Typically, the depressions occur in October or November, persist throughout the winter months, and begin to disappear in March or April. The recovery period is often characterized by mild hypomanic symptoms.[72,73] Characteristically, the depression itself is associated with hypersomnia, rather than insomnia, and increased hunger with specific craving for carbohydrates, rather than diminished appetite, which is typical of major depressive disorders. During the depressive phase of SAD, patients complain of anergia, fatigue, and weight gain. Though present in both men and women, the incidence is greater in women and most often begins early in adult life, although childhood SAD has been described.[6,72]

In the course of SAD, depression may be quite severe and may be associated with suicidal ideation, although in most cases SAD patients experience less severe depressive symptoms. The hormone melatonin, manufactured in the pineal gland, is thought to have a role in SAD. Animals and people exposed to prolonged periods of darkness generally manufacture and release larger quantities of melatonin, a serotonin-derived indole molecule.[6] Exposure of animals and humans to extended periods of bright light suppresses melatonin secretion. Preliminary evidence suggests that patients suffering from SAD may indeed have elevated serum concentrations of melatonin during their depressive periods.[6]

Patients with SAD generally experience a prompt remission of their depressive symptoms when traveling during the fall and winter months to regions of the world that have longer periods of bright sunlight each day.[71] It has become established that the administration of bright light therapy to depressed SAD patients will generally bring about marked relief of the depression, diminution in carbohydrate craving, and an improved sense of well-being within 48 hours. The initial studies of SAD involved administration of 3 hours of bright light twice daily, in the early morning and early evening. Light was administered by having patients sit approximately 3 ft from a fixture containing eight Vitalite full-spectrum fluorescent light bulbs.[71,72] The brightness of the light administered by that technique was rated at 2500 lux. Subsequent studies have utilized various light intensities and varying periods of administration. There is evidence to support the antidepressant efficacy of as little as 1 hour of phototherapy per day throughout the fall and winter months. Although earlier studies of light therapy focused on a circadian phase-delay hypothesis, more recent work indicates that depressive symptoms are improved by either morning or evening bright light therapy.[74] Some patients experience hypomania as they recover from SAD depression with light therapy. It is presumed that the administration of phototherapy suppresses melatonin release and its antidepressant effect may involve serotonin, which is a precursor for the synthesis of melatonin in the pineal gland.[6]

Preliminary studies indicate that some SAD patients achieve partial relief of their depression when treated with the beta-adrenergic antagonist atenolol in a dose of 50 to 100 mg nightly at bedtime.[76] Beta-adrenergic blocking drugs, like bright light, inhibit the synthesis and release of melatonin.[76] Double-blind controlled studies have found that D-fenfluramine, which stimulates release and inhibits reuptake of serotonin, alleviates both depressed mood and carbohydrate craving associated with SAD.[77] Bright light therapy, which improves mood and decreases carbohydrate craving, appears to be more effective than beta-adrenergic blocking agents; however, data do not yet exist to compare the efficacy of light therapy to that of D-fenfluramine. Since D-fenfluramine is an investigational drug currently not available in the United States, the related compound DL-fenfluramine (Pondimin) may be useful for the pharmacologic treatment of SAD. The most common side effects of DL-fenfluramine are drowsiness and dizziness, which can usually be minimized by starting at a dose of 10 mg twice daily and gradually titrating the dosage upward to 20 mg (one tablet) 3 times daily.[78] Following a period of DL-fenfluramine administration, the dosage should be gradually tapered and then discontinued, rather than stopped abruptly. There have been isolated reports in the literature of depression occurring following abrupt discontinuation of DL-fenfluramine.[78] The cause of these depressive episodes is unclear; however, since the drug exerts an antidepressant action, the withdrawal depressions that have been reported may be the result of discontinuation of what had been an effective antidepressant medication. The SSRIs, including fluoxetine and sertraline, have been effective in my clinical experience and in limited clinical studies in the management of depressed mood and carbohydrate craving associated with SAD. Bupropion has also been shown to be beneficial in winter depression associated with SAD.[75]

PREMENSTRUAL SYNDROME

The DSM-IV includes research criteria for premenstrual dysphoric disorder (PDD), although neither this condition nor the more commonly described premenstrual syndrome (PMS) is considered an official diagnostic category. The research criteria presented in Box 9-6 are typically similar in severity, though not in duration, to those of a major depressive disorder. The DSM-IV differentiates premenstrual dysphoric disorder from PMS by requiring the symptoms to significantly interfere with work, school, and social activities and relationships to meet the criteria for PDD.

The presence of depressed mood and affective lability and the common familial association with other persons suffering from major affective disorder suggest that PDD and PMS belong in the affective spectrum. The presence of low energy and a tendency to sleep excessively, along with increased appetite and, most commonly, carbohydrate cravings, suggests an association between PDD/PMS and atypical depression, which is described in chapter 6. One uncontrolled study found that 51 (94%) of 54 patients with PMS had laboratory evidence of thyroid dysfunction. An exaggerated response of thyroid-stimulating hormone (TSH) to an administered test dose of thyrotropin-releasing hormone (TRH) was found in 35 PMS patients.[4] That study reported a favorable therapeutic response to the administration of L-thyroxine in a dose of 100 μg/day.[4] Another investigation found a greater variability in TSH response to TRH among PMS patients than among controls. In that study, three patients exhibited a blunted TSH response while four had an augmented response.[5] On the basis of preliminary evidence, it may be appropriate in evaluating a PMS patient to request triiodothyronine (T_3), thyroxine (T_4), and TSH measurements and to consider the possibility of thyroid antibody and TRH testing.

Experimental attempts to shorten the luteal phase and induce menses with the progesterone antagonist mifepristone in 14 women with PMS failed to alter the timing or severity of PMS symptoms.[79] That study concluded that endocrine events during the late luteal phase do not directly generate the symptoms of PMS. Some patients with PMS benefit from the administration of medroxyprogesterone (Provera) in a dose of 2.5 to 10 mg daily, beginning approximately 10 days prior to menses and stopping when menstruation occurs. Clinical studies have reported variable results, and it is unlikely that the majority of patients will respond to progesterone; yet in some patients symptomatic relief may occur with minimal side effects.[80] Some patients with PMS benefit from cyclic administration of estrogen and progesterone; however, these hormones should be prescribed by a gynecologist, internist, or family physician who will conduct appropriate breast and pelvic examinations and periodic Papanicolaou smears while monitoring hormone treatment.[80,81]

DSM-IV CRITERIA

Box 9-6 Research criteria for premenstrual dysphoric disorder

A. In most menstrual cycles during the past year, five (or more) of the following symptoms were present for most of the time during the last week of the luteal phase, began to remit within a few days after the onset of the follicular phase, and were absent in the week postmenses, with at least one of the symptoms being either (1), (2), (3), or (4):
  (1) Markedly depressed mood, feelings of hopelessness, or self-deprecating thoughts
  (2) Marked anxiety, tension, feelings of being "keyed up," or "on edge"
  (3) Marked affective lability (e.g., feeling suddenly sad or tearful or increased sensitivity to rejection)
  (4) Persistent and marked anger or irritability or increased interpersonal conflicts
  (5) Decreased interest in usual activities (e.g., work, school, friends, hobbies)
  (6) Subjective sense of difficulty in concentrating
  (7) Lethargy, easy fatigability, or marked lack of energy
  (8) Marked change in appetite, overeating, or specific food cravings
  (9) Hypersomnia or insomnia
  (10) A subjective sense of being overwhelmed or out of control
  (11) Other physical symptoms, such as breast tenderness or swelling, headaches, joint or muscle pain, a sensation of "bloating," weight gain
  Note: In menstruating females, the luteal phase corresponds to the period between ovulation and the onset of menses, and the follicular phase begins with menses. In nonmenstruating females (e.g., those who have had a hysterectomy) the timing of luteal and follicular phases may require measurement of circulating reproductive hormones.
B. The disturbance markedly interferes with work or school or with usual social activities and relationships with others (e.g., avoidance of social activities, decreased productivity and efficiency at work or school).
C. The disturbance is not merely an exacerbation of the symptoms of another disorder, such as Major Depressive Disorder, Panic Disorder, Dysthymic Disorder, or a Personality Disorder (although it may be superimposed on any of these disorders).
D. Criteria A, B, and C must be confirmed by prospective daily ratings during at least two consecutive symptomatic cycles. (The diagnosis may be made provisionally prior to this confirmation.)

From American Psychiatric Association: *Diagnostic and statistical manual of mental disorders*, ed 4 [DSM-IV]. Washington DC, American Psychiatric Press, 1994.

Numerous psychotropic drugs have been used, with variable and inconsistent effects, including alprazolam, TCAs, MAOIs, and lithium.[82] Some PMS patients benefit from each of these agents, yet no large-scale or well-controlled study supports their efficacy. Alprazolam in a double-blind placebo-controlled study failed to significantly reduce PMS symptoms.[83] Studies at MIT with the investigational serotonergic agent D-fenfluramine have shown significant beneficial effects of this drug on carbohydrate craving and depressed mood in patients with PMS. Clinically I have seen beneficial effects of DL-fenfluramine (Pondimin) on these parameters of PMS at a dose of 10 to 20 mg 3 times daily. I have also seen occasional favorable responses to tranylcypromine and to lithium, although the potential for weight gain with the latter makes it less than optimal in PMS. The most promising therapeutic agents in PMS are the serotonin selective reuptake inhibitors, and I have often seen dramatic responses to either fluoxetine or sertraline. Nine of 10 subjects receiving fluoxetine in a double-blind controlled study had significant reductions in PMS-associated symptoms.[84] Other open studies of fluoxetine in PMS, including individual case reports, have found that continuous intermittent or even single-dose administration of this serotonergic agent can alleviate PMS symptoms, suggesting that SSRIs at this time be considered the optimal available pharmacologic intervention in PMS and PDD, both of which can be both unpleasant and incapacitating. In a preliminary nonblinded study, nefazodone, which is a serotonin-reuptake inhibitor with serotonin (5-HT$_2$) antagonist activity, was shown to reduce symptoms in PMS patients with and without coexisting major depression.[85]

REFERENCES

1. Ballenger JC: Biological aspects of panic disorder. *Am J Psychiatry* 1986;143:516-518.
2. Breier A, Charney DS, Heninger GR: The diagnostic validity of anxiety disorders and their relationships to depressive illness. *Am J Psychiatry* 1985;142:787-797.
3. Swift WJ, Andrews D, Barklage NE: The relationship between affective disorder and eating disorders: a review of the literature. *Am J Psychiatry* 1986;143:290-299.
4. Brayshaw ND, Brayshaw DD: Thyroid hypofunction in premenstrual syndrome. *N Engl J Med* 1986;315:1486-1487.
5. Roy-Burne PP, Robinow DR, Hoban C, et al: TSH and prolactin responses to TRH in patients with premenstrual syndrome. *Am J Psychiatry* 1987;144:480-484.
6. Rosenthal NE, Genhard M, Jacobsen FM, et al: Disturbances of appetite and weight regulation in seasonal affective disorders. *Ann NY Acad Sci* 1987;499:216-230.
7. American Psychiatric Association: *Diagnostic and statistical manual of mental disorders, ed 4 [DSM-IV].* Washington DC, American Psychiatric Press, 1994.
8. Charney DS, Heninger GR, Jatlow PI: Increased anxiogenic effects of caffeine in panic disorders. *Arch Gen Psychiatry* 1985;42:233-243.
9. Gorman JM, Martinez JM, Liebowits MR, et al: Hypoglycemia and panic attacks. *Am J Psychiatry* 1984;141:101-102.
10. Charney DS, Heninger GR, Breier A: Noradrenergic function in panic anxiety. *Arch Gen Psychiatry* 1984;41:751-763.
11. Charney DS, Heninger GR: Abnormal regulation of noradrenergic function in panic anxiety. *Arch Gen Psychiatry* 1984;41:751-763.
12. Charney DS, Heninger GR: Serotonin function in panic disorders. *Arch Gen Psychiatry* 1986;43:1042-1054.
13. Liberthson R, Sheehan DV, King ME, et al: The prevalence of mitral valve prolapse in patients with panic disorders. *Am J Psychiatry* 1986;143:511-515.
14. Matvzas W, Al-Sadir J, Uhlenthuth EH, et al: Mitral valve prolapse and thyroid abnormalities in patients with panic attacks. *Am J Psychiatry* 1987;144:493-496.
15. Edlund MJ, Swann AC, Clothier J: Patients with panic attacks and abnormal EEG results. *Am J Psychiatry* 1987;144:508-509.

16. Roy-Byrne PP, Uhde TW, Post RM: Effects of one night's sleep deprivation on mood and behavior in panic disorder. *Arch Gen Psychiatry* 1986;43:895-899.
17. Ballenger JC: Pharmacotherapy of the panic disorders. *J Clin Psychiatry* 1986;47 (suppl 6):27-32.
18. Klerman GL: Treatments for panic disorder. *J Clin Psychiatry* 1992;53(3 suppl) :14-19.
19. Pollack MH, Otto MW, Tesar GE, et al: Long-term outcome after acute treatment with alprazolam or clonazepam for panic disorder. *J Clin Psychopharmacol* 1993;13:257-263.
20. Tiffon L, Coplan JD, Papp LA, et al: Augmentation strategies with tricyclic or fluoxetine treatment in seven partially responsive panic disorder patients. *J Clin Psychiatry* 1994;55:66-69.
21. Black DW, Wesner R, Bowers W, et al: A comparison of fluvoxamine, cognitive therapy, and placebo in the treatment of panic disorder. *Arch Gen Psychiatry* 1993;50:44-50.
22. Ravaris CL, Friedman MJ, Hauri PJ, et al: A controlled study of alprazolam and propranolol in panic-disordered and agoraphobic outpatients. *J Clin Psychopharmacol* 1991;11:344-350.
23. Beauclair L, Fontaine R, Annable L, et al: Clonazepam in the treatment of panic disorder: a double-blind, placebo-controlled, trial investigating the correlation between clonazepam concentrations in plasma and clinical response. *J Clin Psychopharmacol* 1994;14:111-118.
24. Jonas JM, Cohon MS: A comparison of the safety and efficacy of alprazolam versus other agents in the treatment of anxiety, panic, and depression: a review of the literature. *J Clin Psychiatry* 1993;54 (10 suppl):25-45.
25. Herman JB, Rosenbaum JF, Brotman AW: The alprazolam to clonazepam switch for the treatment of panic disorder. *J Clin Psychopharmacol* 1987;7:175-178.
26. Fyer AS, Liebowitz MR, Gorman JM, et al: Discontinuation of alprazolam treatment in panic patients. *Am J Psychiatry* 1987;144:303-308.
27. Olajide D, Lader M: A comparison of buspirone, diazepam, and placebo in patients with chronic anxiety states. *J Clin Psychopharmacol* 1987;7:148-152.
28. Schweizer E, Rickels K: Buspirone in the treatment of panic disorder: a controlled pilot comparison with clorazepate. [Letter]. *J Clin Psychopharmacol* 1988;8:303.
29. Shehi M, Paterson WM: Treatment of panic attacks with alprazolam and propranolol. *Am J Psychiatry* 1984;141:900-901.
30. Noyes R, Anderson DJ, Clancy J, et al: Diazepam and propranolol in panic disorders and agoraphobia. *Arch Gen Psychiatry* 1984;41:287-292.
31. Mavissakalian M, Perel J, Bowler K, et al: Trazodone in the treatment of panic disorder and agoraphobia with panic attacks, *Am J Psychiatry* 1987;144:785-787.
32. Solyom L, Solyom C, Ledwidge B: Fluoxetine in panic disorder. *Can J Psychiatry* 1991;36:378-380.
33. Mavissakalian M, Michelson L: Two-year follow-up of exposure and imipramine treatment of agoraphobia. *Am J Psychiatry* 1986;143:1106-1112.
34. Mavissakalian M, Perel J: Imipramine in the treatment of agoraphobia: dose response relationships. *Am J Psychiatry* 1985;142:1032-1036.
35. DenBoer JA, Westenberg HGM, Kamerbeek WDJ, et al: Effect of serotonin uptake inhibitors in anxiety disorders: a double-blind comparison of clomipramine and fluvoxamine. *Int Clin Psychopharmacol* 1987;2:21-32.
36. Phol R, Berchou R, Rainey JM: Tricyclic antidepressants and monoamine oxidase inhibitors in the treatment of agoraphobia. *J Clin Psychopharmacol* 1982;2:399-407.
37. Kronig MH, Roose SP, Walsh BT, et al: Blood pressure effect of phenelzine. *J Clin Psychopharmacol* 1983;3:307-310.
38. Liebowitz MR, Gorman JM, Fyer AJ, et al: Social phobia. *Arch Gen Psychiatry* 1985;42:729-736.
39. Davidson JRT, Potts N, Richichi E, et al: Treatment of social phobia with clonazepam and placebo. *J Clin Psychopharmacol* 1993;13:423-428.
40. Sternbach H: Fluoxetine treatment of social phobia. [Letter]. *J Clin Psychopharmacol* 1990;10:230-231.
41. Gelernter CS, Uhde TW, Cimbolic P, et al: Cognitive-behavioral and pharmacological treatments of social phobia. *Arch Gen Psychiatry* 1991;48:938-945.

42. Versiani M, Mundim FD, Nardi AE, Liebowitz MR: Tranylcypromine in social phobia. *J Clin Psychopharmacol* 1988;8:279-283.
43. Liebowitz MR, Campeas R, Levin A, et al: Pharmacotherapy of social phobia. *Psychosomatics* 1987;28:305-308.
44. Liebowitz MR, Schneier F, Campeas R, et al: Phenelzine vs atenolol in social phobia: a placebo-controlled comparison. *Arch Gen Psychiatry* 1992;49:290-300.
45. Hollander E(ed): *Obsessive compulsive related disorders.* Washington DC, American Psychiatric Press, 1993.
46. Jenike MA: Pharmacologic treatment of obsessive compulsive disorders. *Psychiatr Clin North Am* 1992;15(4):895-919.
47. Rapoport JL: Treatment of behavioral disorders in animals. [Letter]. *Am J Psychiatry* 1990;147:1249.
48. Grindlinger HM: Compulsive feather picking in birds. [Letter]. *Arch Gen Psychiatry* 1991;48:857.
49. Hewlett WA, Vinogradov S, Agras WS: Clomipramine, clonazepam, and clonidine treatment of obsessive-compulsive disorder. *J Clin Psychopharmacol* 1992;12:420-430.
50. McDougle CJ, Price LH, Goodman WK, et al: A controlled trial of lithium augmentation in fluvoxamine-refractory obsessive-compulsive disorder: lack of efficacy. *J Clin Psychopharmacol* 1991;11:175-184.
51. McDougle CJ, Goodman WK, Price LH, et al: Neuroleptic addiction in fluvoxamine-refractory obsessive-compulsive disorder. *Am J Psychiatry* 1990;147:652-654.
52. Zohar J, Kaplan Z, Benjamin J: Clomipramine treatment of obsessive compulsive symptom atology in schizophrenic patients. *J Clin Psychiatry* 1993;54:385-388.
53. Leonard HL, Lenane MC, Swedo SE, et al: A double-blind comparison of clomipramine and desipramine treatment of severe onychophagia (nail biting). *Arch Gen Psychiatry* 1991;48: 821-827.
54. Pollard CA, Ibe IO, Krojanker DN, et al: Clomipramine treatment of trichotillomania: a follow-up report of four cases. *J Clin Psychiatry* 1991;52:128-130.
55. Fallon BA, Liebowitz MR, Hollander E, et al: The pharmacotherapy of moral or religious scrupulosity. *J Clin Psychiatry* 1990;51:517-521.
56. Lane RD: Successful fluoxetine treatment of pathologic jealousy. *J Clin Psychiatry* 1990;51: 345-346.
57. Rivinus TM, Biederman J, Herzog DB, et al: Anorexia nervosa and affective disorders: a controlled family history study. *Am J Psychiatry* 1984;141:1414-1418.
58. Herzog DB: Are anorexic and bulimic patients depressed? *Am J Psychiatry* 1984;141:1594-1597.
59. Mitchell JE, Groat R: A placebo-controlled double blind trial of amitriptyline in bulimia. *J Clin Psychopharmacol* 1984;4:186-193.
60. Walsh BT, Gladis M, Roose SP, et al: Phenelzine vs placebo in 50 patients with bulimia. *Arch Gen Psychiatry* 1988;45:471-475.
61. Fluoxetine Bulimia Nervosa Collaborative Study Group: Fluoxetine in the treatment of bulimia nervosa. *Arch Gen Psychiatry* 1992;49:139-147.
62. Garattini S, Mennini T, Samanin R: From fenfluramine racemate to D-fenfluramine: specificity and potency of the effect on the serotoninergic system and food intake. *Ann NY Acad Sci* 1987;499:156-166.
63. Kaye WH, Ebert MH, Gwirtsman HE, et al: Differences in brain serotonergic metabolism between nonbulimic and bulimic patients with anorexia nervosa. *Am J Psychiatry* 1984;141: 1598-1601.49B. Blouin AG,
64. Blouin JH, Perez EL, et al: Treatment of bulimia with fenfluramine and desipramine. *J Clin Psychopharmacol* 1988;8:261-269.
65. Kaye WH, Weltzin T, Hsu LKG: Anorexia nervosa. in Hollander E (ed): *Obsessive compulsive related disorders.* Washington DC, American Psychiatric Press, 49-70.

66. Kaye WH, Weltzin TE, Hsu LKG, et al: An open trial of fluoxetine in patients with anorexia nervosa. *J Clin Psychiatry* 1991;52:464-471.
67. Wurtman JJ: Disorders of food intake. *Ann NY Acad Sci* 1987;499:197-202.
68. Halami KA, Eckert E, LaDut J, et al: Anorexia nervosa: treatment efficacy of cyproheptadine and amitriptyline. *Arch Gen Psychiatry* 1986;43:177-181.
69. Hughes PL, Wells LA, Cunningham CJ, et al: Treating bulimia with desipramine. *Arch Gen Psychiatry* 1986;43:182-186.
70. Pope HG Jr, Hudson JI, Jonas JM, et al: Bulimia treated with imipramine: a placebo-controlled, double blind study. *Am J Psychiatry* 1983;140:554-558.
71. Rosenthal NE, Sack DA, Gillin JC, et al: Seasonal affective disorder: a description of the syndrome and preliminary findings with light therapy. *Arch Gen Psychiatry* 1984;41:72-80.
72. Weht TA, Jacobsen FM, Sack DA, et al: Phototherapy of seasonal affective disorders. *Arch Gen Psychiatry* 1986;43:870-875.
73. Rosenthal NE, Sack DA, Carpenter CJ, et al: Antidepressant effect of light in seasonal affective disorder. *Am J Psychiatry* 1985;142:163-170.
74. Wirz-Justice A, Graw P, Krauchi K, et al: Light therapy in seasonal affective disorder is independent of time of day or circadian phase. *Arch Gen Psychiatry* 1993;50:929-937.
75. Dilsaver SC, Qamar AB, Del Medico VJ: The efficacy of bupropion in winter depression: results of an open trial. *J Clin Psychiatry* 1992;53:252-255.
76. Parry BL, Rosenthal NE, Tamarkin L, et al: Treatment of a patient with seasonal premenstrual syndrome. *Am J Psychiatry* 1987;144:762-766.
77. O'Rourke D, Wurtman J, Brezinski A, et al: Treatment of seasonal affective disorder with D-fenfluramine. *Ann NY Acad Sci* 1987;499:329-330.
78. Bernstein JG: Induction of obesity by psychotropic drugs. *Ann NY Acad Sci* 1987;499:203-215.
79. Schmidt PJ, Nieman LK, Grover GN, et al: Lack of effect of induced menses on symptoms in women with premenstrual syndrome. *N Engl J Med* 1991;324:1174-1179.
80. Freeman EW, Sondheimer SJ, Rickels K, et al: PMS treatment approaches and progesterone therapy. *Psychosomatics* 1985;26:811-816.
81. Oppenheim G: Estrogen in the treatment of depression: neuropharmacological mechanisms. *Biol Psychiatry* 1983;18:721-725.
82. Harrison WM, Rabkin JG, Endicott J: Psychiatric evaluation of premenstrual changes. *Psychosomatics* 1985;26:789-799.
83. Schmidt PJ, Grover GN, Rubinow DR: Alprazolam in the treatment of premenstrual syndrome. *Arch Gen Psychiatry* 1993;50:467-473.
84. Stone AB, Pearlstein TB, Brown WA: Fluoxetine in the treatment of late luteal phase dysphoric disorder. *J Clin Psychiatry* 1991;52:290-293.
85. Freeman EW, Rickels K, Sondheimer SJ, et al: Nefazodone in the treatment of premenstrual syndrome: a preliminary study. *J Clin Psychopharmacol* 1994;14:180-186.

CHAPTER 10

Medical Complications
of Psychotropic Drugs

OVERVIEW

Idiosyncratic Drug Reactions — Not Predictable
1. *Allergic reactions:* leukopenia and skin rashes may occur with any drug, cholestatic jaundice occasionally occurs with chlorpromazine.
2. *Agranulocytosis and leukopenia* can be fatal; most serious potential complication of clozapine (CZ). WBC must be done weekly throughout CZ therapy; drug stopped and patient evaluated before resuming if WBC below 3000 and granulocytes below 1500. CZ must be stopped and probably not restarted if WBC is less than 2000 with granulocyte count 1000 or below. Patient needs protective isolation, hematologic evaluation, and treatment for infectious complications.

Adverse Reactions — Related to Known Pharmacology
1. *Central nervous system depression:* sedatives (barbiturates, benzodiazepines, etc); excessive drowsiness may occur with psychotropic drugs alone or in combination with nonpsychotropic agents.
   Management: Discontinue the drug and reinstitute at a lower dosage.
2. *Anticholinergic effects* can involve CNS (confusion, toxic delirium) or peripheral (blurred vision, dry mouth, tachycardia, constipation, urinary retention, decreased sweating). Most common with cyclic antidepressants and neuroleptics. Reversed by physostigmine.
   Management: Discontinue the drug and treat with a similar agent possessing less anticholinergic activity. High-potency neuroleptics (risperidone, haloperidol) are least anticholinergic; thioridazine, chlorpromazine, and clozapine are most anticholinergic. Of the antidepressants, amitriptyline and imipramine are most anticholinergic; desipramine, trazodone, bupropion, maprotiline, and amoxapine least. The SSRIs and MAOIs lack anticholinergic activity.

Continued.

3. *Adrenergic blockade* of alpha-receptors by low-potency neuroleptics such as clozapine, chlorpromazine, mesoridazine, and thioridazine accounts for their prominent hypotensive action. High-potency antipsychotic agents, particularly haloperidol, have little hypotensive action.

4. *Adrenergic stimulation* produced by antidepressants is partially responsible for their arrhythmogenic potential.

5. *Myocardial depression* and decreased membrane excitability may occur, particularly with tricyclic drugs and phenothiazines (particularly thioridazine and chlorpromazine). These effects can be manifested by antiarrhythmic action of tricyclics and by additive interaction of these drugs with conventional antiarrhythmic agents. Decreased myocardial contractility may lead to or worsen congestive heart failure. Cardiac rhythm and conduction abnormalities may also occur.

6. *Electrocardiographic changes* produced, particularly by thioridazine and to a lesser extent by chlorpromazine and some tricyclic antidepressants, may resemble changes seen in ischemic coronary heart disease, specifically ST segment depression, decreased T wave amplitude, or inverted or biphasic T waves.

7. *Postural hypotension* is among the more common adverse effects of tricyclic antidepressants, MAOI antidepressants, and low-potency antipsychotic drugs.

8. *Hypertensive reactions,* which may be mild or severe enough to produce a cerebrovascular accident, can occur in MAOI-treated patients who eat large quantities of tyramine-rich foods or take stimulants or vasoconstrictors.

Continued.

9. *Neuroleptic malignant syndrome* (NMS) (potentially fatal) occurs with muscular rigidity and akinesia, often with catatonic appearance. There is hyperthermia (temperature from 101° to 106° F), and consciousness is altered — the patient may be alert and show "dazed mutism" and stupor, or may be comatose. There is profound autonomic dysfunction with labile blood pressure, profuse diaphoresis, sialorrhea, incontinence, dysphagia, and dyskinesia. Treatment requires discontinuation of all neuroleptic drugs, maintenance of adequate hydration by oral or IV route, correction of electrolyte abnormalities, symptomatic management of fever, and specific management of complications including pneumonia and pulmonary emboli. If medication is required to control behavior, use small doses of short-acting benzodiazepine (e.g., lorazepam). Antiparkinsonian drugs are not specific to reverse NMS; however, cautious use of benztropine may be helpful. Bromocriptine or dantrolene may be beneficial in severe cases of NMS.

10. *Serotonin syndrome* (potentially fatal) can occur when MAOI-treated patient is given meperidine, clomipramine, or any of the SSRIs.

11. *Convulsions* can occur with clozapine, chlorpromazine, bupropion, clomipramine, and maprotiline, particularly when given in higher doses or to patients susceptible to seizures. Tricyclics may also lower seizure threshold; SSRIs and high-potency neuroleptics are unlikely to provoke convulsions.

12. *Appetite* is increased and there is often weight gain with neuroleptics, cyclic and MAOI antidepressants, and lithium. Bupropion and SSRIs are unlikely to increase appetite; may decrease appetite, carbohydrate craving, and weight.

13. *Sexual dysfunction:* decreased ability to achieve and maintain erection; impaired orgasmic function in men and women is most likely to occur with SSRIs and MAOIs, but also with cyclic antidepressants and neuroleptics.

Continued.

14. *Skin pigmentation* may occur with phenothiazines, especially chlorpromazine. This also produces increased sensitivity to sunlight and greater risk of sunburn, even with limited sun exposure.
15. *Retinal pigmentation* may occur with phenothiazines, especially thioridazine and chlorpromazine. The risk of retinal damage with thioridazine is so great that long-term administration at doses exceeding 400 mg/day should generally be avoided, and doses exceeding 800 mg/day should never be prescribed.

Every known drug possesses a spectrum of activity affecting multiple organ systems. By convention we classify drugs into different therapeutic groups depending primarily on which organ system is most affected by the drug and on the pathologic state most likely to benefit from its action.[1] The primary therapeutic action of a given pharmacologic agent is considered the wanted effect, while actions on other organ systems are considered unwanted or adverse effects. For practical purposes adverse drug actions may be divided into two major groups, those that are unpredictable and those that are predictable. The unpredictable effects are called idiosyncratic and are not generally based on the known pharmacology of the drug.[1] These effects include allergic reactions that bear some relationship to the chemical structure of the compound but are not predictable in their occurrence, except in an individual who has had a previous reaction to the same compound or one closely related chemically. These reactions tend to be relatively rare. The only possible means of avoiding them is the clinician's awareness that the patient has had a prior idiosyncratic allergic reaction to the compound. If a patient does experience an idiosyncratic drug reaction, the offending agent should be discontinued promptly. If there is continuing need for treatment, the clinician should select a drug from the same therapeutic group which is as chemically different as possible from the compound that produced the initial adverse reaction.

It is important to differentiate idiosyncratic or unpredictable drug reactions from those which are predictable based on the known pharmacology of the drug, such as anticholinergic actions associated with tricyclic antidepressants or extrapyramidal reactions to neuroleptic drugs, which are pharmacologically based adverse drug reactions and not idiosyncratic or allergic reactions. Most patients are not aware of the difference between these two types of major drug reactions. They may urge the physician not to administer a particular therapeutic agent they believe they are allergic to, although in reality they may have had a pharmacologically produced adverse response such as an extrapyramidal reaction. Awareness by the physician that such a reaction has occurred is useful in guiding him or her in the proper choice of, in this case, a neuroleptic drug with less extrapyramidal effect, or the possibility of combining an antiparkinsonian agent with the prescribed neuroleptic. Unfortunately, patients' medical records are often labeled with a variety of drug allergies that are not drug allergies at all, but predictable pharmacologically based adverse drug effects.

IDIOSYNCRATIC DRUG REACTIONS

Any patient may develop an allergic rash covering the trunk and extremities in response to any psychotropic or nonpsychotropic medication. If an allergic rash does appear, prompt discontinuation of the offending agent, symptomatic treatment of the rash and associated itching, and subsequent prescription of a chemically distinct and therapeutically appropriate alternative medication is the management of choice. Although hair loss is rare with psychotropic drugs, clinicians should be aware that it can occur in response to lithium therapy, with or without an associated skin rash. Many patients who develop skin rashes or hair loss in response to lithium can have the medication discontinued and then restarted several months later without recurrence of either the skin rash or hair loss.

Hepatic Dysfunction

Another infrequent, and uncommon, idiosyncratic drug reaction to psychotropic drugs is the development of cholestatic jaundice, which may occur with tricyclic antidepressants and phenothiazines. The agent most likely to be associated with cholestatic jaundice is chlorpromazine; this reaction occurs in approximately 1% of patients, typically within the first few months of therapy.[2] Patients developing this reaction tend to have a prodrome, including fever, chills, nausea, abdominal pain, and malaise, followed in several days by pruritus and jaundice. A prior history of liver disease does not appear to increase the likelihood of chlorpromazine-induced cholestatic jaundice. Serum alkaline phosphatase and conjugated bilirubin are typically elevated, though transaminase levels are not strikingly elevated as they would be in the presence of hepatocellular jaundice. This condition may be purely an allergic reaction, although some investigators have suggested that chlorpromazine exerts a direct toxic effect on bile secretory mechanisms of the liver.[2,3] Cholestatic jaundice induced by chlorpromazine is generally self-limited and has a good prognosis, though the drug should be discontinued immediately and the patient should be treated with a chemically dissimilar antipsychotic drug such as haloperidol. Routine monitoring of liver function tests during the initial course of chlorpromazine or other phenothiazine therapy is not generally necessary, and has a very low yield in detecting presymptomatic cases of cholestasis. In the presence of liver disease or recent hepatitis, chlorpromazine should be avoided and haloperidol, which has rarely been associated with hepatic dysfunction, should generally be employed.[3] Mild, usually benign, elevations of alkaline phosphatase and transaminases may occur during treatment with cyclic antidepressants and generally do not necessitate drug discontinuation, although periodic liver function tests are indicated.[13] Bilirubin, alkaline phosphatase, and SGOT should be monitored every week or two initially, then every month or two during carbamazepine or valproate therapy. Hepatotoxicity infrequently occurs with phenelzine, valproate, and carbamazepine and calls for drug discontinuation and periodic monitoring of liver function tests.[1]

Hematologic Abnormalities

Leukopenia and agranulocytosis are rare complications of psychotropic drug therapy.[5,6] Leukopenia is generally not a dangerous adverse effect, and in most instances the WBC count returns to normal within a short interval after discontinuing the offending agent. Agranulocytosis is much more serious and has been associated with a mortality rate of 20% to 50%, even after discontinuation of the offending medication and appropriate supportive treatment.[4,5,7] One comprehensive study of WBC abnormalities in psychiatric patients involved careful monitoring of over 11,000 consecutive admissions over a 15-year period in a university hospital setting. Of these, approximately 6000 were receiving psychotropic medication, mostly phenothiazines. White blood cell counts below 3700 were recorded in 1100 patients.[5] In 84 patients whose data were adequate for study, 30 had received no medication and 54 were receiving psychotropic medication; 41 patients were receiving phenothiazines while 13 were receiving other psychotropic drugs alone or in combination with phenothiazines. Only a few patients in the study had agranulocytosis. They had been receiving chlorpromazine, but after drug discontinuation and appropriate supportive therapy they recovered fully. That study indicated that there was no benefit obtained from periodic WBC monitoring in providing for early detection of leukopenic reactions to psychotropic drugs.[5] Agranulocytosis is a very rare complication of tricyclic antidepressants.[4] Leukopenia, anemia, and thrombocytopenia occur occasionally with carbamazepine therapy although agranulocytosis is rare.[8] Studies have evaluated the possible beneficial effects of periodic monitoring of patients receiving maintenance neuroleptics or other psychotropic agents.[9] Periodic laboratory monitoring is an essential feature of patient management when clozapine, carbamazepine, and valproate are prescribed; otherwise, routine laboratory tests are not likely to yield significant abnormalities with other psychotropic agents. Eosinophilia is an unusual side effect of neuroleptics and tricyclics which will most often disappear when the medication is changed to a chemically different drug. This finding may at times occur independently of other allergic manifestations, or in association with a rash or other allergic signs or symptoms.[6] Complete blood counts (CBCs) should be done periodically during carbamazepine therapy.[8]

The risk of leukopenia and agranulocytosis with clozapine exceeds that with all other psychotropic drugs and is significant enough that the distribution of this drug to patients in the United States mandates that they have weekly white blood cell counts done and reported to the pharmacy and physician. Leukopenia is generally a benign condition, with white counts between 2500 and 4000 and absolute neutrophil counts exceeding 500.[10] The risk of infection is not increased if there are adequate granulocyte precursors in bone marrow. The condition is to be distinguished from agranulocytosis — characterized by a sudden loss of white cells, paralysis of the defenses against infection, chills, fever, sepsis, and the likelihood of death.[10] In either case, at the first sign of a precipitous drop in the WBC or the occurrence of a WBC below 3000 and a granulocyte count of less than 1500, clozapine must be immediately discontinued and appropriate hematologic assessment done. If the WBC has fallen to 2000 or less with granulocytes less than 1000, clozapine should be stopped, and protective isolation, hematologic assessment, and appropriate evaluation and treatment for concurrent infection initiated. Although the mechanism of clozapine-induced agranulocytosis is uncertain, evidence supports the generation of a toxic metabolite which attacks bone marrow stem cells, presumably by an immunologic mechanism, rendering them incapable of proliferation and maturation to form polymorphonuclear leukocytes, which are essential in host defenses against infection.[7] As of December 31, 1989, there had been 149 cases of agranulocytosis reported worldwide associated with clozapine, 32% of which were fatal. Few such deaths have occurred since careful WBC monitoring was instituted in 1977. Utilizing weekly WBC monitoring, there were 68 cases of agranulocytosis with only one fatality in the United States as of January 1, 1991. A disproportionate share of the agranulocytosis cases have occurred in patients of Finnish or Jewish origin, for reasons which remain unknown.[7] Clearly, weekly monitoring of the WBC in clozapine-treated patients adds to the cost and inconvenience of this form of therapy, but of greater significance is the fact that this drug is uniquely beneficial for some patients and early detection of WBC reduction can generally avoid serious hematologic complications by immediate clozapine discontinuation and appropriate monitoring and supportive patient care.

Predictable Adverse Reactions

Having discussed *unpredictable* adverse reactions to drugs, I will now turn my attention to those adverse reactions which are *predictable* based on the pharmacology and structure-activity relationships of the various medications used in psychiatric practice. In prescribing psychotropic drugs it is important to have a thorough understanding of their pharmacologic properties in addition to a knowledge of their therapeutic action. Furthermore, it is important to know something about the chemical structures of the variety of drugs that we call psychotropic. A general awareness of the structural similarities and differences between drugs within therapeutic classes allows the physician to predict, to some extent, a particular patient's response to a new medication, having knowledge of his responses to other medications in the past.[11] This prediction, based on pharmacologic profile and structure-activity relationships, not only allows us to make some choices as to which therapeutic agent to employ, particularly in a patient with extensive previous experience with psychotropic drugs, but also allows us to be aware of which adverse drug effects to anticipate. For the most part, the acute medical complications occurring with psychotropic drug therapy may be anticipated by a thorough knowledge of these drugs, and an awareness that the adverse effects seen clinically tend most often to be directly related to their pharmacology.[12]

This chapter concentrates on those pharmacologically determined adverse drug reactions which may be minimized or avoided by an awareness of the pharmacologic properties of psychotropic drugs, and by consequent judicious selection of one psychotropic agent or another. I will concentrate on medical reactions which occur frequently enough to be seen by most clinicians prescribing these medications — specifically, reactions that present either significant discomfort to patients or the potential of serious or fatal outcome. Some of the medical problems associated with psychotropic drugs occur in previously healthy persons; however, patients who are medically ill or elderly are likely to be particularly vulnerable to unwanted drug effects because of the action of the disease process or the aging process on physiologic systems. Furthermore, patients suffering from medical illnesses and elderly persons are likely to be taking a variety of medications in addition to psychotropic drugs. There is considerable potential for interaction between nonpsychotropic and psychotropic medications. I point out those medical problems which may predispose an individual to specific adverse drug reactions, and highlight some of the more important drug interactions involving psychotropic and nonpsychotropic medications. A detailed discussion of the medical complications of lithium is presented in chapter 8, and management of the adverse effects of MAOIs is discussed in chapter 6.

CENTRAL NERVOUS SYSTEM DEPRESSION

The majority of antipsychotic drugs and tricyclic antidepressants produce some degree of sedation or drowsiness. With tricyclic antidepressants, drowsiness appears to parallel their antihistaminic activity and may also correlate with their anticholinergic potency.[12] Amitriptyline and trazodone are most sedating, while desipramine, amoxapine, and protriptyline are least sedating. Doxepin and maprotiline are somewhat less sedating than amitriptyline, while imipramine produces a lesser degree of sedation. Among the antipsychotic drugs, clozapine, chlorpromazine, mesoridazine, and thioridazine are most sedating, while the piperazine phenothiazines such as trifluoperazine are much lower in sedative effect. Haloperidol has limited sedative effect in lower doses, while at higher dosage moderate degrees of sedation occur.[12] Despite the sedative effects of these psychotropic agents, they do not produce significant CNS depressant action such as that produced by barbiturates or alcohol.[11] Excessive doses of the benzodiazepines may produce considerable CNS depression as well as persistent respiratory depression. In the elderly or the medical patient even very small amounts of drugs such as diazepam may produce excessive sedation along with the potential of respiratory depression.[12] Perhaps the most dangerous medical complication of antianxiety agents such as the benzodiazepines is the potential of these drugs to induce addiction; after abrupt withdrawal of moderate doses of drugs such as diazepam, one may encounter a withdrawal syndrome including delirium, seizures, and fever. A person who becomes dependent on sedatives of the benzodiazepine type should be hospitalized and undergo a pentobarbital tolerance test to determine whether addiction does indeed exist, in which case detoxification needs to be done utilizing gradually diminishing doses of phenobarbital.[12] Failure to diagnose the existence of sedative addiction, and consequent failure to slowly detoxify the patient, may be fatal.

In considering unwanted CNS depression induced by psychotropic drugs, one must also be aware that lithium toxicity can cause confusion, obtundation, delirium, and seizures.[14] The generally accepted range of therapeutic blood levels for lithium is 0.6 to 1.2 mEq/L; serious toxicity, with accompanying CNS depression, tends to occur at serum lithium levels above 2.0 mEq/L. It is essential to be aware that some people are more sensitive to lithium than others, and signs of CNS toxicity from lithium as well as the presence of cardiac arrhythmias may occur in some individuals at lithium levels of 1.0 mEq/L or lower. Bupropion and all currently available serotonin-selective reuptake inhibitors have no direct CNS depressant activity, although they may each occasionally produce some tiredness or drowsiness.[6] Fluoxetine, fluvoxamine, and paroxetine inhibit cytochrome P-450, with resultant potentiation and prolongation of any coadministered drug which is metabolized through this enzyme system. Therefore if one of these SSRIs is administered along with a benzodiazepine, barbiturate, or cyclic antidepressant, the sedative or central nervous system depressant effect of the coadministered drug will be increased.[6] Bupropion, fluoxetine, sertraline, and venlafaxine are devoid of affinity for cholinergic receptors and anticholinergic side effects.[6] Paroxetine and fluvoxamine have very weak cholinergic receptor affinity and produce only minimal anticholinergic side effects.[6]

ANTICHOLINERGIC EFFECTS

Essentially all of the antiparkinsonian drugs, such as benztropine and trihexiphenidyl, are strongly anticholinergic. Both cyclic antidepressants and antipsychotic agents have considerable potential to produce cholinergic blockade. Among antidepressants, amitriptyline is the most anticholinergic, imipramine, trimipramine, and doxepin are intermediate, and trazodone, amoxapine, maprotiline, and desipramine are least anticholinergic.[12] Among neuroleptic drugs, clozapine and thioridazine are most anticholinergic, followed by mesoridazine and chlorpromazine.[12] Loxapine, trifluoperazine, and thiothixine are less anticholinergic, and haloperidol is the least anticholinergic of the antipsychotic drugs.[12] Drugs from each of these groups will produce additive effects with one another in terms of cholinergic blockade. Anticholinergic effects are manifested peripherally by dry mouth, blurred vision, tachycardia, decreased or increased sweating, constipation, and urinary retention. Additionally, and of great importance, each of these drugs may produce CNS manifestations of cholinergic blockade, including confusion, halting or stuttering speech,[15] disorientation, delirium, hallucinations, and the worsening of existing psychotic symptoms.[12] One of the most important and confusing areas where these symptoms arise clinically is in a patient who becomes more psychotic or confused following a small dose of a strongly anticholinergic antipsychotic agent such as thioridazine or clozapine. If such a situation arises and is not promptly recognized, the clinician may administer a larger dose of the initial therapeutic agent and see an even more pronounced worsening of symptoms. Elderly persons, or those with even minor degrees of organic brain dysfunction, are particularly vulnerable to anticholinergic complications of psychotropic drugs.

In a patient who becomes confused, disoriented, or psychotic following the use of a neuroleptic or cyclic antidepressant drug, it may be of great help to perform a physostigmine test. Physostigmine is a cholinesterase inhibitor that increases brain acetylcholine levels and thus counteracts cholinergic blocking drugs. Physostigmine causes increased salivation, sweating, bradycardia, and abdominal cramps with associated desire to urinate and defecate. Additionally, in the presence of a confusional state or delirium induced by cholinergic blockade, these symptoms may clear dramatically 15 to 20 minutes following physostigmine administration.[12,16] The preferred technique for the physostigmine test is to dilute 1 mg physostigmine to a total volume of 10 mL with normal saline. This solution may then be injected slowly IV over a period of three to five minutes. Prior to administering physostigmine it is advisable to obtain baseline blood pressure and pulse measurements, and to have these repeated at frequent intervals following the injection. Patients with cardiac disease present increased risk of adverse reactions to physostigmine and may develop profound bradycardia or transient sinus arrest. Likewise, individuals with pulmonary disease, particularly those with bronchial asthma, may develop bronchospasm following physostigmine injection. Healthy persons given physostigmine slowly are not likely to have serious adverse reactions. In an individual who fails to show any response to the initial 1 mg dose, the injection may be safely repeated 30 to 40 minutes later. The effect of physostigmine lasts only ½ to 1 hour, and once the diagnosis is established there is no justification for repeated administration. Having established the diagnosis of an anticholinergic-induced toxic state, it is preferable to withhold further medication until the offending agent is metabolically cleared. If it is necessary to medicate such a patient to control agitation or belligerent behavior, lorazepam may be administered orally or parenterally. The advantage of this drug is that it is short-acting and has no significant anticholinergic effect. Although benzodiazepines are not strongly anticholinergic, acute confusional states produced by diazepam and other members of this group often clear dramatically in response to IV-administered physostigmine.[17] Patients with narrow-angle glaucoma should receive low-anticholinergic antidepressants and have intraocular pressure measured before and periodically during treatment.[18]

ADRENERGIC EFFECTS

Tricyclic antidepressants have multiple pharmacologic actions, including inhibition of nerve reuptake of norepinephrine. This latter effect may explain the ability of these drugs to precipitate psychotic symptoms in some patients.[11,12] Furthermore, this mechanism, coupled with their anticholinergic effect, may explain their ability to induce or worsen cardiac arrhythmias such as atrial and ventricular premature beats.[4,19,20] The ability of tricyclics to block norepinephrine reuptake is responsible for their ability to block the hypotensive action of antihypertensive drugs such as guanethidine and clonidine.[4,11,20]

Monoamine oxidase inhibitors commonly produce postural hypotension. If tyramine-rich foods such as fermented cheeses, red wine, and tap beer are taken along with MAOIs, serious hypertensive reactions may occur. Furthermore, the use of phenylethylamine-containing drugs such as stimulants and decongestants along with MAOIs may produce hypertensive crises.[12,19]

The antipsychotic drugs produce varying degrees of alpha-adrenergic blockade. This causes peripheral vasodilatation, a fall in total peripheral resistance, and a consequent reduction in blood pressure.[3,12] Hypotensive reactions to antipsychotic drugs may be profound in individuals who are particularly sensitive to these drugs or in those who have received excessive dosage. Of the neuroleptic drugs, chlorpromazine, clozapine, thioridazine, and mesoridazine are most likely to produce hypotensive reactions.[3,12] Haloperidol, trifluoperazine, and fluphenazine have the least alpha-adrenergic blocking action and are consequently least likely to produce hypotensive reactions.[3,12] Combinations of two or more antipsychotic drugs enhance the potential for hypotension to occur. There appears to be a significant risk for hypotension in patients given haloperidol IM followed by IM chlorpromazine.[12] It is preferable to use only one antipsychotic agent at a time, and gradually increase the dosage or administer repeated doses until the desired response is achieved, as opposed to using combinations of drugs or repeatedly switching from one drug to another.

CARDIOVASCULAR SIDE EFFECTS

A variety of unwanted cardiovascular effects of psychotropic agents have been described and explained on the basis of anticholinergic, positive adrenergic, and adrenergic blocking mechanisms. Postural hypotension occurs commonly in patients receiving MAOIs as a result of reduced sympathetic tone in small arteries and arterioles of the peripheral vasculature.[3,12,21] In some cases reduction of the MAOI dosage will allow the patient to continue to achieve the therapeutic effect of the agent and minimize postural symptoms. In other patients reduction of the dosage to the level at which postural symptoms disappear is associated with a disappearance of the antidepressant or antiphobic action of the drugs.[21] Increased dietary salt intake, salt tablets (1 g 2 to 3 times daily), triiodothyronine (25 μg/day), thyroxine (100 to 200 μg/day), or in some cases fludrocortisone (0.1 to 0.2 mg/day) are often helpful in reducing or eliminating MAOI-induced postural hypotension.[12] Methylphenidate (5 to 10 mg, 1 to 3 times daily) may also counteract the postural hypotension of MAOIs; however, there is then a possible risk of hypertensive reactions.[22]

Although cyclic antidepressants are less likely to produce postural hypotension than are MAOIs, this is a common side effect of these drugs.[19,23] Hypotension is related to a direct vasodilator effect of these compounds on the peripheral vasculature. Although amoxapine, maprotiline, and nortriptyline are less likely to produce postural hypotension than other cyclic agents are, this effect also occurs with these compounds.[12,20] Postural hypotension produced by cyclic antidepressants may benefit from dosage reduction, use of a different antidepressant, administration of several smaller divided doses throughout the day, or administration of thyroid hormones.

Based in part on their actions upon the autonomic nervous system, the tricyclic antidepressants may produce cardiac arrhythmias. The use of antidepressants with less anticholinergic activity may yield less arrhythmic complications, and administration of smaller doses divided throughout the day may increase safety.[12] Amoxapine, maprotiline, and trazodone can also affect cardiac rate, rhythm, and conduction. Indeed, there have been reports of serious ventricular arrhythmias with trazodone in spite of the earlier suggestion that it might be free of cardiac toxicity. Extensive clinical use and research studies indicate that bupropion and the SSRIs fluoxetine, fluvoxamine, paroxetine, sertraline, and venlafaxine lack clinically significant cardiac or vascular adverse effects. These agents are devoid of alpha-adrenergic antagonism and do not produce postural hypotension. They are also without electrophysiologic activity and do not alter cardiac rate, conduction, or contractility.[6,23] Furthermore, they lack quinidinelike activity and are not likely to be arrhythmogenic or antiarrhythmic.[23] Electrocardiographic changes are not seen with bupropion or SSRIs. The inhibition of cyclic antidepressant metabolism by the above-mentioned SSRIs, however, may increase the risk of cardiac toxicity of the cyclic antidepressants if combined antidepressant regimens are utilized or if a patient being treated with a cytochrome P–450 inhibiting SSRI takes an overdose of a tricyclic antidepressant. Table 10-1 illustrates some of the cardiovascular effects which may occur with psychotropic drugs.

Tricyclic antidepressants, such as amytriptyline and imipramine, and related compounds, including thioridazine, exert a quinidinelike effect which may be

Table 10-1 Cardiovascular effects of psychotropic drugs

Drug	Anticholinergic effect	Supine BP	Postural hypotension	Heart rate	Rhythm	ECG	Cardiac conduction	Myocardial contractility
Cyclic antidepressants	Low to high	Minimal effects	Mild to moderate	Increased	Arrhythmogenic or antiarrhythmic	ST-T wave changes	Prolonged	High doses may decrease
Monoamine oxidase inhibitors	None	Decreased	Moderate to marked	Unchanged or decreased	No effect	No effect	No effect	No effect
High-potency antipsychotics	Low	Minimal effect	Mild	Unchanged or slight increase	No effect	Haloperidol—no effect	Haloperidol—no effect	No effect
Low-potency antipsychotics	High	Decreased	Moderate to marked	Increased	Arrhythmogenic or antiarrhythmic	ST-T wave changes	ST-T wave changes	High doses may decrease
Lithium	None	No effect	None	No effect	May be arrhythmogenic	ST-T wave changes may occur	Rarely prolonged	No effect at therapeutic level
SSRIs	None*	No effect	None	No effect	No effect	No effect	No effect	No effect
Bupropion	None	No effect	None	No effect	No effect	No effect	No effect	No effect

*Fluvoxamine and paroxetine have mild anticholinergic effects.

manifested clinically by reducing the frequency of atrial or ventricular premature beats.[24,25] This quinidinelike action is more likely to be manifested after several weeks of therapy, while patients in the first several days of therapy are more apt to experience the arrhythmogenic action of these compounds. One important aspect of the quinidinelike effect of cyclic antidepressants and thioridazine is that it will add to similar pharmacologic actions of conventional antiarrhythmic drugs, such as quinidine and procainamide, when they are administered simultaneously. Thus, in prescribing thioridazine or cyclic antidepressants for a patient receiving an antiarrhythmic drug, or in starting an antiarrhythmic agent in a patient being treated with one of these psychotropic agents, it is useful to monitor the plasma concentration of both therapeutic agents. Periodic ECGs should be obtained to ascertain that a suitable therapeutic effect is occurring without undue adverse effects on cardiac conduction or automaticity, since the electrophysiologic properties of some psychotropic drugs may produce ventricular tachyarrhythmias.[26] In addition to their electrical effects on the heart,[27] the tricyclic antidepressants may produce myocardial depression and decreased cardiac output when used in conventional therapeutic dosage.[28,29] These effects appear to account for the ability of tricyclic drugs to produce congestive heart failure or to worsen already existing congestive heart failure. Patients with myocardial disease who are to be treated with tricyclic antidepressants need periodic physical examinations. ECG monitoring, and cautious dosage titration. Peripheral edema occasionally occurs in patients treated with cyclic drugs, particularly amitriptyline, imipramine, and trazodone. This may well be a manifestation of developing congestive heart failure or, as some have proposed, the result of increased capillary permeability induced by these drugs.[4,12,30]

Tricyclic antidepressants have long been known to produce dosage-related ECG changes, including prolongation of the PR interval, widening of the QRS complex, and nonspecific ST and T wave changes.[27,31,32] These changes do not indicate myocardial damage produced by these drugs; they may occur without clinical symptoms or they may exist in association with alterations in myocardial function, heart block, or tachyarrhythmias, even in patients with a previously normal cardiovascular history.[28,31] Both ECG and clinical abnormalities of cardiovascular function are more likely to occur in patients taking overdoses of tricyclic compounds.[33] One study of 66 patients who had no evidence of cardiovascular disease found significant increases in heart rate and PR interval in patients treated with a variety of antidepressants.[34] That study also observed prolongation of QT and QRS intervals though those changes were not statistically significant. Statistically significant flattening of T waves was also observed. These changes were all reversible following discontinuation of the antidepressant, and after 13 months of antidepressant therapy in a subgroup of the patients, it was found that, except for heart rate, the ECG abnormalities reverted to normal. That study also noted that antidepressants were associated with a prolongation of the pre-ejection time and shortening of the left ventricular ejection time, indicating a decrease in myocardial contractility.[34] In that study—which included patients receiving trimipramine, amitriptyline, maprotiline, mianserin, and imipramine—no differences in ECG effects were noted between the various antidepressants administered. Nortriptyline appears to have less effect on cardiac conduction than other cyclic antidepressants that have been studied.[20,31] Patients with preexisting bundle-branch block are more likely to develop second-degree atrioventricular block with cyclic drugs.[32] There have been reports in the literature indicating the occurrence of sudden death in a relatively small number of patients receiving tricyclic antidepressants.[35] This is most likely related to sudden cardiac arrhythmias, such as ventricular tachycardia degenerating to ventricular fibrillation as well as disturbances in cardiac conduction. Again, these complications of tricyclic antidepressants are likely to be seen more often in a patient taking an overdose, or in an individual with underlying coronary heart disease, which would predispose him to cardiac rhythm disturbances. Careful hemodynamic and ECG monitoring may be necessary because of the risk of an additive interaction when an antiarrhythmic agent is coadministered.[33]

Hypotensive reactions to antipsychotic drugs are largely based on their ability to produce alpha-adrenergic blockade. Chlorpromazine, clozapine, thioridazine, and mesoridazine are most likely to produce significant hypotension either in the recumbent patient, or, to an even greater extent, in association with postural change.[12] These hypotensive effects are more pronounced when the antipsychotic agent is administered IM. Trifluoperazine, loxapine, and molindone have relatively less hypotensive action, while haloperidol appears to be the least hypotensive antipsychotic agent available.[12,36] The risk of dizziness, falling, and hip fracture in elderly psychiatric patients has been well studied.[37] It is particularly likely to occur in patients receiving low-potency antipsychotic agents alone or in combination with other blood pressure-lowering drugs, including antidepressants and antihypertensive agents.[37-39]

Electrocardiographic abnormalities have long been associated with phenothiazines.[39,40] The ECG changes produced by antipsychotic drugs are not necessarily indicative of their ability to produce myocardial disease, and tend to be reversible after discontinuation of the drug.[39,40] There is some conflict in the literature as to whether they are dosage-dependent or may occur at any dose of a specific therapeutic agent. There is evidence to support a strong association between the administration of thioridazine and abnormalities of the ECG, even in patients receiving fairly low doses of this compound.[40] One study reported that 27 (90%) of a group of 30 patients receiving less than 300 mg thioridazine per day had ECG changes.[41] The ECG changes most frequently associated with phenothiazines are repolarization changes, resembling those produced by quinidine and similar to the changes observed in association with myocardial ischemia.[27,39,41] These changes include depression, widening, notching, inversion, and flattening of the T wave, the presence of U waves, and prolongation of QT intervals.[41] In a study of patients receiving thioridazine in doses of 150 to 400 mg/day, only 32% of patients had normal ECGs while 44% had low voltage T waves and 23% had T wave widening. In patients receiving thioridazine 150 to 900 mg/day, the incidence of abnormalities in ECGs was 70%.

Similar ECG abnormalities have been noted in patients receiving clozapine, chlorpromazine, trifluoperazine, mesoridazine, fluphenazine, and pimozide.[3,27,43,44] The presence of first-degree atrioventricular block with conduction delay, nonconducted premature atrial beats, and atrial flutter with varying degrees of block have also been reported in patients receiving thioridazine.[3,27] Phenothiazine therapy, particularly thioridazine, is also likely to be associated with ST segment flattening or depression.[3,11,41] Recurrent unifocal and multifocal ventricular premature beats, ventricular tachycardia, and ventricular fibrillation have also been described in healthy persons receiving phenothiazine. In one study patients receiving combined oral and IM fluphenazine had a 91% incidence of abnormal ECGs.[27] In patients with previous histories of cardiovascular disease and in those without evidence of heart disease, haloperidol has repeatedly been demonstrated to be the antipsychotic agent least likely to produce ECG change or abnormalities in cardiac function.[36] Studies with varying dosages of haloperidol have not shown evidence of ECG abnormalities or clinically detectable changes in cardiac function.[36,43]

NEUROLEPTIC MALIGNANT SYNDROME

An infrequent complication of antipsychotic drug therapy, the neuroleptic malignant syndrome (NMS), characterized by muscular rigidity, hyperthermia, altered consciousness, and autonomic dysfunction, has been recognized since 1960.[45] It was first described in the French literature, which may be more than coincidental, as French clinicians tend more often than others to utilize a combination of multiple neuroleptic drugs simultaneously in the treatment of a given patient. There is some evidence to suggest that the combination of multiple neuroleptics may increase the risk of adverse effects and perhaps the risk of the development of this syndrome.[46] Since NMS is very serious and potentially fatal, it is of utmost importance that the clinician be able to recognize the syndrome, diagnose it early, discontinue neuroleptic medication, and institute supportive therapy as quickly as possible.[46]

A review of 500 neuroleptic-treated patients in a large psychiatric hospital during a 1-year period found that seven patients (1.4%) had experienced definite or probable NMS.[47] One patient experienced two episodes of NMS. In that series NMS developed with a wide variety of neuroleptic drugs, including chlorpromazine, thioridazine, fluphenazine, haloperidol, perphenazine, trifluoperazine, and clozapine. Data presented by that study confirm other studies and case reports which indicate that all neuroleptics present a risk of NMS, including both high- and low-potency drugs.[45-48] Although earlier reports suggested a higher risk of NMS developing in patients treated with long-acting injectable neuroleptics, and some investigators have suggested that low-potency neuroleptics were unlikely to produce NMS, which they attribute to high-potency drugs, there are no data to support these conclusions.[45] There does, however, appear to be a somewhat greater risk of NMS in patients receiving high doses of high-potency neuroleptic drugs, particularly when given by IM injection or with very rapid dose titration.[48,49] I have observed NMS in patients receiving a wide variety of high-potency and low-potency antipsychotic drugs and have seen this syndrome in patients receiving modest doses of medication. Although I have treated a large number of acutely psychotic patients with moderate to high doses of haloperidol administered orally, utilizing gradual dosage titration, I have not seen an inordinately high incidence of NMS with this therapeutic approach.

Though published reports generally indicate an incidence of 0.5% to 2.0% for the occurrence of NMS in neuroleptic-treated patients, most reports have found an incidence of less than 1.0%. Virtually all authors agree that patients who are medically ill, and those with neurologic disorders, dehydration, and exhaustion are more likely to suffer from NMS. Although earlier reports indicated that young males were at higher risk of developing the syndrome, there is no evidence that young or old age is a particular risk factor, in spite of the fact that males are indeed more often affected.[50] A wide spectrum of severity and symptoms exists in the different studies.[50] Although the earlier literature indicated a fatal outcome in 20% to 30% of patients, with better recognition and treatment, mortality is now in the 10% to 12% range.[51] Some evidence exists in support of the idea that patients with nonschizophrenic disorders are more likely than those with schizophrenia to have NMS.[47] Many patients with NMS have undergone multiple previous courses of neuroleptic therapy without developing the syndrome, and some have developed NMS following their first exposure to antipsychotic medication. Many who have experienced NMS have, following their recovery, been re-exposed to the same or a different neuroleptic without recurrence of NMS.[45,52]

The clinical signs and symptoms of NMS resemble those of malignant hyperthermia, which occurs secondary to inhalational anesthetic agents, and may also resemble the clinical manifestations of lethal catatonia, a condition described more than 100 years before neuroleptic agents were available.[53] Lethal catatonia may present with catatonic hyperactivity or stupor, along with high fever, altered consciousness, and autonomic lability with diaphoresis, tachycardia, and labile blood pressure.[53] It is likely that malignant hyperthermia, lethal catatonia, NMS, and the serotonin syndrome share common physiologic mechanisms involving disordered dopaminergic neurotransmission and an imbalance between dopaminergic, cholinergic and serotonergic functions. Each of these conditions has a significant potential for a fatal outcome. Table 10-2 differentiates some important features of NMS and the serotonin syndrome.

In NMS there is muscular rigidity ("lead pipe rigidity"), akinesia, and catatonia. Patients are febrile and may have temperatures up to 106° F, although

Table 10-2 Comparison of neuroleptic
malignant and serotonin syndromes

	Neuroleptic malignant (NMS)	Serotonin syndrome
Mental status	Dazed mutism	Confusion, disorientation, mania
Hyperthermia	Mild to marked	Mild to marked
Autonomic dysfunction	+	+
Tachycardia	+	+
Labile BP	+	+
Diaphoresis	+	+
Tremor	+	+
Incontinence	+	0
Sialorrhea	+	0
Dyspnea	+	0
Shivering	0	+
Restlessness	0	+
Extrapyramidal effects	+	0
Myoclonus	0	+
Hyperreflexia	0	+
Ataxia	0	+
Leukocytosis	+	0
CPK elevation	+	0
Muscular rigidity	+	0

many have low-grade hyperthermia with temperatures between 101° and 102° F. The state of consciousness is altered and may progress from alertness, through dazed mutism, and on to stupor and finally coma. There is profound dysfunction of the autonomic nervous system, with pronounced tachycardia, labile blood pressure or hypertension, profuse diaphoresis, dyspnea, sialorrhea, and incontinence. Patients with NMS often have dysphagia, which makes them vulnerable to the development of aspiration pneumonia. Dyskinesia is often a component of the spectrum of movement disorders seen in NMS.

Patients with NMS are subject to a variety of potentially dangerous complications—including dehydration with electrolyte imbalance, aspiration pneumonia, and pulmonary emboli—as a result of remaining immobile in bed.[45-48] Symptoms often begin abruptly and progress rapidly over the first 24 to 72 hours, and death may occur within 3 to 30 days from the onset of symptoms.[45] No specific laboratory test is diagnostic, although leukocytosis ranging from 15,000 to 30,000 is a common finding. Creatine phosphokinase (CPK) is elevated in most cases, though it may range only from a slightly abnormal value up to 15,000 units or higher.[45,47] Many factors, including IM injection and increased muscle tension, can produce mild to moderate CPK elevation which is not specific for NMS. The absence of CPK elevation or leukocytosis does not rule out the diagnosis of NMS. The EEG usually shows evidence of diffuse metabolic encephalopathy.[45]

Neuroleptic malignant syndrome has been reported to occur initially after 1 day to several months of antipsychotic drug exposure.[47] Many patients who have developed NMS were concurrently receiving lithium in combination with antipsychotic chemotherapy.[45] It is likely that the use of high doses of high-potency neuroleptic agents in conjunction with relatively high serum lithium levels may increase the risk of this syndrome.[45] Patients with preexisting brain dysfunction appear more likely to develop NMS when exposed to neuroleptics.[45,48] The symptoms of NMS generally persist for 5 to 10 days after discontinuation of the neuroleptics. Symptoms may be more intense and persist for longer periods of time following prolonged, high-dose, or depot neuroleptic administration.[45] The most common causes of fatality in NMS include respiratory or renal failure and severe cardiovascular disturbances.[45,48]

Early diagnosis and discontinuation of neuroleptic drugs is the most effective means to limit the severity, duration, and risk of complications of NMS. A high index of suspicion for the development of this syndrome must be in the mind of every clinician who prescribes antipsychotic medication. The syndrome may vary in severity from mild temperature elevation and muscle rigidity to the full-blown syndrome characterized by a febrile, rigid, catatonic-appearing patient, lying motionless in bed, staring off into space with beads of sweat on the forehead and chest and streams of saliva issuing from the mouth. In the event that the physician is overly suspicious and discontinues neuroleptic medication in an otherwise healthy catatonic patient, the worst that can occur is a delay in that patient's recovery from the psychotic process. In the event that an NMS patient is misdiagnosed as catatonic and is given increasing doses of neuroleptic medication, there may be a fatal outcome. It is better clinical practice to be overly vigilant, discontinue medication early, and observe the patient than to continue aggressive treatment in the presence of suggestive signs and symptoms.

Supportive medical care is more important than aggressive pharmacotherapy in the management of NMS. Since patients with this syndrome have difficulty swallowing and may suffer aspiration pneumonia, and since they are also likely to experience dehydration and electrolyte imbalance, proper fluid and electrolyte therapy needs to be instituted immediately following discontinuation of neuroleptic drugs. Fluids should be administered IV with careful attention to laboratory determinations and correction of any electrolyte disturbance. Nothing should be given by mouth until the clinician is certain that dysphagia is no longer present and that the gag reflex is present and the patient alert enough to take fluids by mouth. Blood pressure, pulse, temperature, and respiratory rate and depth should be monitored carefully. The patient should have periodic physical examinations, including chest auscultation, and laboratory determinations, including sputum and urine cultures where indicated, to detect the presence of infection. Chest physical therapy and attempts to ambulate the patient may also facilitate recovery. Antiembolism stockings and a footboard in bed may help to avoid the occurrence of thrombophlebitis, which may contribute to pulmonary embolization.

Most patients who are diagnosed early, have neuroleptic medication discontinued, and receive appropriate supportive medical care recover promptly and without complications. Patients with more severe NMS or who are diagnosed later in their course may benefit from a variety of pharmacologic interventions. Since NMS appears, at least in part, to be due to dopamine antagonism by neuroleptic drugs, the dopamine agonist bromocriptine has been used in treating a number of patients with this syndrome.[54] In one series of patients who received bromocriptine (7.5 to 45 mg/day in three divided oral doses), all five experienced significant improvement within 24 to 72 hours.[54]

Amantadine has also been used successfully in NMS. Since muscular rigidity and excessive salivation are important components of NMS, some patients will benefit from oral or IM administration of benztropine. This anticholinergic antiparkinsonian drug may increase autonomic instability, so that, if there is not a favorable response to the first or second dose, its administration should be discontinued and the patient treated with either bromocriptine or dantrolene or a combination of these two agents. Dantrolene inhibits muscular spasticity and has been employed as a standard therapeutic agent in the treatment of malignant hyperthermia. There have been several case reports of successful treatment of NMS utilizing dantrolene alone or in combination with bromocriptine.[55,56] Dantrolene may be administered either IV or orally and is usually given as an initial IV dose of 1 mg/kg, followed by 50 to 100 mg 4 times daily orally. If sedation is required at any point during the course of NMS, agents without dopamine-blocking activity should be employed, such as low doses of lorazepam, which may be administered parenterally as well as orally. Large doses of sedatives should be avoided because of the potential risk of respiratory depression.

Following the patient's recovery from NMS the clinician is often faced with the problem of how to treat the psychosis. The risk of recurrence with subsequent neuroleptic treatment is quite variable. From 15% to 30% of patients who initially developed NMS have experienced a recurrence with subsequent neuroleptization.[46,52] If a patient requires continuing neuroleptic therapy, a different agent should be administered, although some investigators suggest that the same drug can be readministered without risk of recurrence. If NMS occurred with a low-potency agent, it may be preferable to use very small, cautiously monitored, doses of high-potency agents. If the syndrome initially appeared during treatment with a high-potency agent, cautious use of low-potency antipsychotic drugs would be preferable if further neuroleptic therapy is required. A patient who develops NMS during treatment with depot neuroleptic medication should probably not be rechallenged with further depot neuroleptic therapy. Whenever possible, following recovery from NMS, alternative drugs which are not dopamine antagonists should be considered. In many patients, carbamazepine or valproate can be used for acute and maintenance treatment of the psychotic disorder. Patients whose psychotic illness may have been consistent with mania should be considered for treatment and prophylaxis with lithium, valproate, or carbamazepine. Nevertheless, many patients who develop NMS may have a continuing psychotic disturbance requiring antipsychotic chemotherapy. In these instances, antipsychotic drugs are not contraindicated, though they should be utilized with caution, adequate consultation with colleagues, full disclosure to the patient and family members, and well-defined notes in the patient's clinical record.

Lithium-Neuroleptic Syndromes

A number of years ago, a syndrome was described consisting of leukocytosis, fever, and neurologic symptoms with lethargy, tremulousness, confusion, and extrapyramidal as well as cerebellar dysfunction. There were initially four cases reported, and the authors attributed to them a specific toxic interaction between haloperidol and lithium.[57] Subsequent review of this report and of the rather extensive clinical experience with the combination of lithium and haloperidol strongly suggests that this combination of medications is safe and is not the cause of a specific toxic syndrome. One extensive review of a series of 425 patients treated with haloperidol and lithium in combination failed to reveal a single case of the presumed lithium-haloperidol syndrome.[58] My extensive use of this combination as the preferred therapeutic approach to treatment of acutely manic patients has failed to reveal the occurrence of this syndrome as described by Cohen and Cohen.[57] Several investigators reviewing the initial report of four cases suggested the possibility that this cluster of patients within a single institution in a short time span was consistent with a viral encephalomyelitis rather than with a specific toxic syndrome. The similarity between this syndrome and NMS should be considered, particularly since a similar syndrome has been reported with thioridazine and lithium.[59] In the patients reported by Cohen and Cohen[57] lithium levels were above the generally accepted therapeutic range of 0.6 to 1.2 mEq/L, and the contribution of lithium toxicity to the signs and symptoms noted by these authors cannot be denied.

Serotonin Syndrome

The use of more strongly serotonergic antidepressants and the generally ill-fated attempts to combine these drugs with the serotonin precursor L-tryptophan or with MAOI antidepressants have produced the serotonin syndrome, a potentially fatal complication of psychopharmacologic treatment.[60] There are mental status changes with confusion, disorientation, and in some cases manic or hypomanic symptoms. Serotonin syndrome (SS) is characterized by a variety of autonomic, hypothalamic regulatory and neuromuscular signs and symptoms resembling those seen in neuroleptic malignant syndrome, from which it must be differentiated, as shown in Table 10-2.

Muscular rigidity, dyspnea, sialorrhea, high fever, leukocytosis, and CPK elevation are typical of most cases of NMS and generally not prominent in serotonin syndrome. Patients with the latter usually have prominent shivering, myoclonus, hyperreflexia, and ataxia which help differentiate the serotonin syndrome from NMS. One of the more problematic aspects of SS is that the most widely used SSRI, fluoxetine, and its active metabolite have long half-lives, generally requiring 5 or more weeks to be cleared from the patient after their discontinuation; thus the syndrome may occur quite late when an MAOI is given to a patient who was formerly receiving an SSRI. At the first suspicion of serotonin syndrome, all serotonergic drugs including SSRIs, meperidine, and MAOIs must be stopped. Careful patient monitoring, medical consultation, and supportive medical care must be initiated. Seizures may complicate SS, and appropriate anticonvulsant medication may need to be instituted. Serotonin $5-HT_2$ antagonists have not been found to be effective interventions. However, $5-HT_1$ antagonists or nonspecific serotonin antagonists such as methysergide or cyproheptadine may be beneficial.[60] Additionally, clonazepam is useful for myoclonus and nifedipine is appropriate for management of hypertension.[60] Although chlorpromazine has been recommended by some for sedation, the autonomic lability generally present would most often make lorazepam a safer sedative in patients with SS. If significant hyperthermia is present, optimal clinical management may require the use of a cooling blanket.[60]

EEG and Convulsive Effects of Psychotropic Drugs

It is well known that a variety of psychotropic drugs may affect the EEG. Chlorpromazine and most other phenothiazines are capable of lowering seizure threshold and thereby increasing the risk of epileptic patients having seizures while being treated with this and related medications.[61] Thioridazine, a piperidine phenothiazine, appears to have the least ability to lower seizure threshold; likewise, haloperidol has a very limited effect on the EEG and minimal ability to lower seizure threshold, thus making these two agents perhaps the safest antipsychotic agents to use in patients with convulsive disorders.[12] Clozapine has the greatest risk of provoking convulsions among neuroleptic drugs, an effect which is clearly dose dependent. There is a 1% to 2% risk at doses up to 300 mg daily, with a 3% to 4% risk at doses of 300 to 600 mg daily, increasing to a 5% risk at daily doses of 600 to 900 mg.[44] Patients with a previous head injury or convulsive disorder should be treated cautiously with clozapine, and EEG should be done before and during treatment, with higher doses being avoided. If seizures occur in a clozapine-treated patient, the dosage should be reduced, anticonvulsants added or clozapine therapy discontinued.

Tricyclic antidepressants likewise are capable of lowering the seizure threshold and increasing the risk of seizures occurring in patients with epilepsy during the course of antidepressant therapy.[12,61] There is no evidence that any of the cyclic antidepressants is free of the risk of lowering seizure threshold or provoking convulsions, though these agents can be used with cautious monitoring in patients with convulsive disorders. Clomipramine is the tricyclic with the greatest risk of provoking convulsions, again on a dose-related continuum. With stable maintenance at moderate doses, its seizure rate appears to approximate 0.7% or less. With higher doses or rapid dosage increase the risk of seizures may approach 1% with clomipramine. It is preferable not to use this agent in patients with prior head injury or convulsive disorders, particularly since the SSRIs, which are generally free of epileptogenic effect, are in most cases similarly effective in depression and obsessive-compulsive disorder.[6] Maprotiline carries a significantly greater risk of seizures than do most other antidepressants, and generally lacks outstanding therapeutic advantages, so that its use is generally not appropriate in patients with convulsive disorders.[62] Bupropion in doses of 450 mg/day has a seizure risk of 0.44%, which is somewhat higher than the figure generally quoted for tricyclics, which approximates 0.2% to 0.3%.[63] Lower doses of bupropion would carry a lower risk, and higher doses a higher seizure risk. Generally bupropion is contraindicated in patients with prior head injury, bulimia, or convulsive disorder, who have been found to be at increased risk with respect to seizure occurrence.[63] As stated elsewhere, lithium carbonate, particularly in toxic serum concentrations, is capable of lowering seizure threshold and inducing seizures, which is one of the manifestations of lithium intoxication.[14]

ENDOCRINE, METABOLIC AND APPETITE EFFECTS

Neuroleptic drugs increase the secretion of prolactin in humans. This mechanism is important in the potential production of galactorrhea and gynecomastia with the phenothiazines. Although haloperidol is the most potent dopamine antagonist used clinically, and should theoretically have the greatest effect on prolactin levels, it appears to have less likelihood of producing galactorrhea than some of the less potent antipsychotic agents such as chlorpromazine and thioridazine.[61] So far there is no evidence to suggest that the antipsychotic agents increase the risk of carcinoma of the breast, despite their actions on prolactin.[11] Amantadine has been found to be effective in the treatment of neuroendocrine side effects of neuroleptics such as gynecomastia, galactorrhea, breast tenderness, decreased libido, and amenorrhea, which are mediated by excess prolactin release.[64] Chlorpromazine tends to decrease the secretion of adrenocorticosteroids as a result of diminished release of corticotropin.[11] Chlorpromazine may impair glucose tolerance and insulin release in some prediabetic patients.[11]

Appetite increase, carbohydrate craving, and weight gain are common side effects of most psychotropic drugs.[65] Chlorpromazine, thioridazine, and clozapine are prominent in their ability to increase appetite, carbohydrate craving, and weight. Molindone is least likely to stimulate appetite and weight gain, while piperazine phenothiazines are more likely to do so than are molindone or haloperidol.[65] Risperidone, which is a relatively weak dopamine antagonist with considerable serotonin 5-HT$_2$ receptor antagonist activity, appears to significantly increase appetite and carbohydrate craving. Considerable evidence suggests that serotonin antagonism by psychotropic drugs contributes to carbohydrate craving, increased appetite, and weight gain.[65]

Tricyclic antidepressants, most notably amitriptyline and imipramine, increase carbohydrate craving, appetite, and body weight; indeed a weight gain of 30 pounds is not uncommon during the first year of treatment.[65] Desipramine, amoxapine, and trazodone are less likely than other cyclic antidepressants to facilitate weight gain.[65] Among MAOIs, phenelzine not uncommonly increases appetite and weight while tranylcypromine often has no effect or may actually facilitate weight loss.

The SSRIs, presumably by increasing central serotonergic activity may decrease carbohydrate craving and with high doses actually facilitate weight loss.[65] In general, the conventional antidepressant doses of SSRIs have little ability to increase or decrease hunger, carbohydrate craving, or body weight.[65] Patients who have gained weight on other antidepressant regimens are good candidates for treatment with SSRIs or bupropion, since these agents generally facilitate weight loss rather than weight gain. At ordinary therapeutic dosage, bupropion is the antidepressant most likely to decrease appetite and facilitate weight loss when employed in conjunction with an appropriate reduced-calorie and reduced-fat diet.

SEXUAL DYSFUNCTION

Phenothiazines and other neuroleptics decrease libido and interfere with erection and ejaculation in men and likewise may inhibit orgasm in women.[66] Less potent neuroleptics with more prominent autonomic side effects, particularly thioridazine, appear more likely to inhibit sexual function than moderate doses of high-potency agents such as haloperidol.[66] In the absence of lithium intoxication, lithium generally has little or no effect on sexual function except that it may reduce the heightened sexual response associated with mania or hypomania.

Tricyclic antidepressants generally do not impair libido, though they occasionally, in a dose-dependent fashion, decrease erectile and ejaculatory function and impair orgasm intensity in women. Monoamine oxidase inhibitors often diminish orgasmic function in both men and women, reducing the firmness of erections and the ability to ejaculate in male patients without altering libido significantly in men or women.[67]

The serotonin-selective reuptake inhibitors occasionally decrease libido somewhat; however, their most prominent sexual side effects are reduced excitement, decreased ability to achieve erection and ejaculation, and inhibition of orgasm in women.[68] Although these effects are dose dependent, many people, including those who have otherwise been fully functional sexually, experience pronounced inhibition of sexual excitement and orgasmic function even at very low doses. I have encountered a number of men and women in their 30s, 40s, and 50s who have been unable to function sexually with sertraline doses as low as 12.5 mg daily, or fluoxetine at 5 mg daily, or clomipramine at 25 mg daily. The sexual side effects of clomipramine more closely resemble those of the SSRIs than of the TCAs. In most patients with antidepressant-induced sexual dysfunction, considerable improvement can be achieved with dosage reduction. In some patients it is necessary to change therapy to an alternate antidepressant. Trazodone rarely can induce persistent, painful erections known as priapism, yet this drug can be safely employed in many men who have erectile dysfunction either alone as an antidepressant or in smaller doses along with SSRIs to treat SSRI-induced erectile difficulty. Although many authors have suggested cyproheptadine, a serotonin antagonist, as a treatment for SSRI-induced sexual dysfunction, I do not recommend this approach since the serotonin antagonist may also inhibit the antidepressant efficacy of the SSRI. Yohimbine has been used successfully in many men with erectile dysfunction due to a variety of antidepressant drugs. Although not uniformly effective, the side effects, which are most often limited to increased anxiety, make this therapeutic approach worth trying; cholinergic agents such as bethanechol are most often ineffective.[69]

TERATOGENIC EFFECTS

There has been continuing concern about the teratogenic potential of psychotropic drugs, as these agents are sometimes administered to pregnant women for major psychiatric illnesses such as depression or acute psychosis. The teratogenic potential of psychotropic drugs is discussed in detail in chapter 14.

SKIN AND EYE COMPLICATIONS

Most phenothiazines increase sensitivity of the skin to sunlight and may therefore cause severe sunburn with only limited brief exposure to the sun. This photosensitization is far more common with chlorpromazine than with other phenothiazines. Since metabolites of this drug persist for many months after its administration has been discontinued, the photosensitivity may continue long after the drug has been discontinued. Patients receiving chlorpromazine or other phenothiazines should use carefully applied sunscreens prior to any sun exposure. Photosensitization does not occur with haloperidol or other nonphenothiazine neuroleptic drugs. Many believe that tricyclic antidepressants can produce photosensitivity reactions. There is no clear evidence that this is true although these agents may at times produce a patchy erythematous skin rash.[6]

High-dosage phenothiazine treatment may give rise to pigmentary changes in the skin or conjunctiva. These changes are most likely to occur with chlorpromazine, particularly when administered in high doses. Phenothiazine-induced skin changes generally begin with a tan or brownish coloration, progressing to slate-gray, metallic blue, or purple discoloration of exposed skin surfaces.[6] Biopsy of the involved skin reveals pigmentary granules similar in appearance to melanin. Long-term high-dose chlorpromazine administration produces whitish-brown granular deposits in the anterior subcapsular area of the eye or in the anterior cortex of the lens. These changes may also involve the endothelium and be associated with corneal opacities and in some cases brownish discoloration of the conjunctiva. Avoidance of long-term, high-dose administration of chlorpromazine is the best way to avoid these pigmentary changes.[6] Thioridazine may produce pigmentary retinopathy, although in most instances this complication does not occur in daily dosages of less than 800 mg.[6] Since questions have arisen regarding these retinal changes occurring in association with smaller doses of thioridazine, I do not recommend long-term maintenance at dosages exceeding 400 mg/day. The loss of visual acuity in association with phenothiazine-induced changes in the lens or retina has been reported, although this effect appears to be quite rare. There is no evidence that tricyclic antidepressants produce corneal, lenticular, or retinal changes.[6] Blurred vision and excessive sensitivity to light are due to pupillary dilatation and relaxation of muscles of accommodation produced by the anticholinergic effects of these drugs. Patients with open-angle glaucoma may generally be treated with various psychotropic agents without the fear of worsening this condition, although periodic tonometry may be a useful means of following the patient. Individuals with narrow-angle glaucoma should be treated with caution when tricyclic drugs or neuroleptics must be administered. These patients should receive medications possessing the least possible anticholinergic potency, and antiparkinsonian drugs should generally be avoided. Periodic tonometry in patients with narrow-angle glaucoma being treated with psychotropic medication is of greater necessity than in individuals with open-angle glaucoma.[6,18] Tinnitus is a rare side effect that has been reported with cyclic antidepressants which may also occur with MAOIs. Frequently tinnitus disappears spontaneously or with dosage reduction.[70]

MANAGEMENT OF ANTICHOLINERGIC SIDE EFFECTS

Patients being treated with tricyclic and heterocyclic antidepressants, antipsychotic drugs, and antiparkinsonian agents are likely to have a variety of peripheral manifestations of cholinergic blockade, particularly if two or more of these agents are administered simultaneously. Dry mouth associated with these agents will often be improved somewhat by encouraging the patient to suck on hard candy or chew gum, particularly one of the commercially available sour chewing gums such as Gatorade. When these simple remedies are ineffective patients will often have a more significant improvement in salivary flow if they wash their mouth several times daily with a 1% solution of pilocarpine, a cholinergic stimulant, or if they gradually dissolve in the mouth a tablet containing 5 or 10 mg of bethanechol chloride. Orally administered bethanechol may also be useful in reducing the blurred vision related to anticholinergic effects on the eye. It may also benefit constipation and urinary retention which occur secondary to cholinergic blockade by psychotropic agents.[71] If bethanechol is administered orally in tablet form for these GI and genitourinary complaints, it may be necessary to administer a dose of 10 to 25 mg 3 or 4 times daily. Occasionally, patients who have acute urinary retention while on anticholinergic medication may require the IM or subcutaneous injection of 5 to 10 mg of bethanechol chloride.[71]

Urinary retention associated with anticholinergic drugs tends to increase the risk of lower urinary tract infection. The persistence of this symptom should lead the clinician to obtain periodic urinalysis and urine culture in the presence of urinary tract dysfunction and to prescribe appropriate antibacterial treatment if the need arises. Since constipation is often a prominent side effect of psychotropic medications producing cholinergic blockade, it is useful to maintain adequate hydration of the bowel contents by the regular administration of a stool softener such as docusate (Colace) or the daily administration of a bulk laxative such as psyllium hydrophilic mucilloid (Konsyl or Metamucil). In addition patients receiving strongly anticholinergic drugs may require the intermittent use of a laxative such as casanthranol (Peristim) or a similar peristaltic stimulant. Psychotic individuals who lose interest in normal bodily functions may become so severely constipated when treated with psychotropic agents as to develop fecal impaction. This may require manual disimpaction if an adequate laxative regimen is not regularly and appropriately maintained.

MANAGEMENT OF INTOXICATION DUE TO OVERDOSE

It is well known that barbiturates produce a CNS depressant effect when taken in excessive dosage, and they may yield a fatal outcome when taken with suicidal intent.[1] On the other hand, overdoses of benzodiazepines have generally been found to be quite benign with respect to the potential of a fatal outcome.[11] Relatively few patients take a single agent if they are seriously interested in committing suicide. The most common agent to be combined with any drug overdose is alcohol. If alcohol is taken in conjunction with a benzodiazepine drug, even though the doses of either one may not be massive, there may indeed be a fatal outcome. When a patient has taken an overdose of alcohol, barbiturates, or a benzodiazepine, he must receive appropriate hydration and supportive therapy, including maintenance of adequate respiratory function, in order to survive until the offending agent has been satisfactorily metabolized.[1] The antipsychotic drugs are among the safest when taken in excessive dosage, in that when taken alone the likelihood of a fatal reaction occurring is quite small.[72] Since antipsychotic agents are likely to be combined with alcohol or other drugs, the risk of a fatal reaction of a combined intoxication will be greater than with the antipsychotic alone. Based on animal data, the therapeutic index is lowest for thioridazine.[26] Chlorpromazine is less toxic, with a therapeutic index of 200, while the potent antipsychotic agents have been found to have therapeutic indices in excess of 1000. Patients have survived chlorpromazine dosages up to 10,000 mg, while there have been no documented deaths due to haloperidol taken alone.[11] Patients taking overdoses of neuroleptic drugs will exhibit symptoms comparable to those seen when the drugs are given in therapeutic doses, except that they will be more prominent. Those antipsychotics that produce prominent hypotensive effects are likely to produce profound hypotension when an overdose is taken. Compounds such as chlorpromazine, which lowers the seizure threshold, may provoke the appearance of convulsions when an overdose has been taken.[11] Urinary retention and paralytic ileus are likely complications of a large dose of any agent with prominent anticholinergic activity.

Unfortunately, depressed patients are those who are most likely to make serious suicide attempts, and the agents used to treat such persons present the greatest risk of serious or even fatal intoxication.[33,73] If a large dose of a tricyclic antidepressant is taken, the blood level is likely to remain elevated for several days, and the patient is likely to have symptoms of intoxication for a long period of time.[33,73] Patients taking large tricyclic overdoses probably should have continuous cardiac monitoring for five to seven days following the overdose. These patients are likely to show persistent QRS prolongation, ST segment and T wave changes, and tachyarrhythmias.[33] The EEG is likely to be diffusely abnormal and may show focal seizure activity, as seizures may occur following an overdose of tricyclic drugs.[11] Abnormal neurologic signs, including choreiform movements, athetosis, and myoclonus, may occur and persist for several days following the tricyclic overdose.[73] If a patient has not been taking a tricyclic drug regularly but suddenly takes a large overdose, it is possible to find relatively low plasma tricyclic concentrations because of avid tissue binding of the drug. Tricyclics are fairly rapidly excreted by the kidneys, and neither dialysis nor forced diuresis are particularly helpful in managing tricyclic intoxication.[73] If a patient is seen shortly after the overdose, the oral administration of several grams of activated charcoal may be of value, since it may bind that portion of the drug remaining in the GI tract, thereby reducing its absorption and systemic toxicity.[11] Patients suffering from tricyclic overdoses may need intubation and respiratory support. They may also require the cautious administration of antiarrhythmic agents, though the potential for an addictive drug interaction with a tricyclic must be borne in mind.[33] Since these patients may develop seizures, the potential need for appropriate anticonvulsant therapy such as amobarbital or diazepam must be considered. Caution should be exerted in deciding to administer physostigmine to a patient who has taken an overdose of cyclic antidepressants since in the event of a major degree of myocardial depression, a physostigmine-induced bradyarrhythmia may produce further cardiac decompensation.[11]

Hypertensive reactions to MAOIs have been discussed in chapter 6, and it is important for the physician who uses these drugs to be aware of the management of these reactions. Very often a patient taking an ordinary therapeutic dose of MAOIs who has a hypertensive reaction in response to a tyramine-rich food or a phenylethylamine-derived drug product will simply need to lie quietly in a darkened room until the reaction passes spontaneously. In some situations, the cautious administration of propranolol alone or in combination with phentolamine or trimethaphan may be necessary to lower the patient's blood pressure.[1,12,38] Patients taking an overdose of an MAOI may develop agitation, hallucinations, hyperreflexia, fever, or convulsions.[61] The reactions of an MAOI overdose may not occur immediately, but may take several hours to develop and may persist for several days.[11,61] Maintenance of adequate fluid and electrolyte balance and conservative management of fever are essential. A patient should be hospitalized for several days following an MAOI overdose, and the fewest possible medications should be administered. The cautious use of diazepam or amobarbital may be of value in controlling seizures, and in controlling agitation, without evoking significant autonomic effects. I have encountered only one patient who has intentionally overdosed on an MAOI, and this patient survived after having a seizure and a moderate temperature elevation. I have not encountered patients who have intentionally taken substances which would produce a hypertensive crisis while taking MAOIs.

Patients taking lithium carbonate may develop toxic effects when the serum concentration becomes elevated either through unintentional means or by means of an intentional overdose. Patients developing lithium toxicity are apt to be confused, disoriented, or frankly obtunded.[14] Lithium toxicity is often associated with nausea, vomiting, and diarrhea, and if it has occurred through a gradual process, the patient is apt to be quite dehydrated when initially seen.[14] More severe forms of intoxication with lithium are associated with ataxia, coma, and convulsions. Patients who are lithium-intoxicated will almost always show tremors of the fingers, hands, arms, and legs. These patients are apt to be hyperreflexic and dysarthric, and may show focal neurologic signs. Cardiac arrhythmias, hypotension, and albuminuria are also likely to be seen with lithium intoxication. Treatment of lithium intoxication is supportive, and it is critical to maintain salt and water balance providing adequate hydration for the patient who is apt to become increasingly dehydrated.[14] Lithium excretion can be accelerated in the presence of adequate renal function by osmotic diuresis and the IV administration of sodium bicarbonate solution. In cases of severe lithium poisoning dialysis may be a necessary part of the clinical management.[14] Since gradually acquired lithium intoxication is associated with considerable intracellular lithium concentration, there may be a rather slow recovery, even when the serum concentration of lithium is rapidly lowered by hemodialysis.[14]

As mentioned repeatedly in this book, SSRIs, such as fluoxetine, fluvoxamine, and paroxetine, inhibit drug metabolism; therefore they will increase the likelihood of a fatal outcome of a tricyclic overdose.

REFERENCES

1. Gilman AG, Rall TW, Nies AS, Taylor P (eds): *Goodman and Gilman's The pharmacological basis of therapeutics,* ed 8. New York, Pergamon Press, 1990.
2. Jones JK, Van de Carr SW, Zimmerman H, et al: Hepatotoxicity associated with phenothiazines. *Psychopharmacol Bull* 1983;19:24-27.
3. Levinson DF, Simpson GM: Antipsychotic drug side effects. In Hales RE, Frances AJ (eds): *APA annual review.* Washington DC, American Psychiatric Press, 1987, vol 6, pp 704-723.
4. Blackwell B: Side effects of antidepressant drugs. In Hales RE, Frances AJ (eds): *APA annual review.* Washington DC, American Psychiatric Press, 1987, vol 6, pp 724-745.
5. Litvak R, Kaebling R: Agranulocytosis, leukopenia, and psychotropic drugs. *Arch Gen Psychiatry* 1971;24:265-267.
6. Kane JM, Lieberman JA (eds): *Adverse effects of psychotropic drugs.* New York, Guilford Press, 1992.
7. Pisciotta AV: A brief review of drug-induced agranulocytosis. *J Clin Psychiatr Monogr* 1990;8:22-29.
8. Joffe RT, Post RM, Roy-Byrne PP, et al: Hematologic effects of carbamazepine in patients with affective illness. *Am J Psychiatry* 1985;142:1196-1199.
9. Donlon PT: Medical screening of patients on maintenance neuroleptics. *Psychosomatics* 1977;18:51-54.
10. Pisciotta AV: Hematologic reactions associated with psychotropic drugs. In Kane JM, Lieberman JA (eds): *Adverse effects of psychotropic drugs.* New York, Guilford Press, 1992, pp 376-394.
11. Baldessarini RJ: Drugs and the treatment of psychiatric disorders. In Gilman AG, Rall TW, Nies AS, Taylor P (eds): *Goodman and Gilman's The pharmacological basis of therapeutics,* ed 8. New York, Pergamon Press, 1990, pp 383-435.
12. Bernstein JG: Psychotropic drug prescribing. In Cassen NH (ed): *Massachusetts General Hospital Handbook of general hospital psychiatry,* ed 3. St Louis, Mosby, 1991, pp 527-569.
13. Richelson E: Antidepressants and brain neurochemistry. *Mayo Clinic Proc* 1990;65:1227-1236.
14. Jefferson JW, Greist JH, Ackerman DS, et al: *Lithium encyclopedia in clinical practice,* ed 2. Washington DC, American Psychiatric Press, 1987.
15. Schatzberg AF, Cole JO, Blumer DP: Speech blockage: a tricyclic side effect. *Am J Psychiatry* 1978;135:600-601.
16. Granacher RP, Baldessarini RJ: Physostigmine. *Arch Gen Psychiatry* 1975;32:375-380.
17. Bourke DL: Physostigmine effectiveness as an antagonist of respiratory depression and psychomotor effects caused by morphine or diazepam. *Anesthesiology* 1984;61:523-528.
18. Lieberman E, Stoudemire A: Use of tricyclic antidepressants in patients with glaucoma. *Psychosomatics* 1987;28:145-148.
19. Goldman LS, Alexander RC, Luchins DJ: Monoamine oxidase inhibitors and tricyclic antidepressants: comparison of their cardiovascular effects. *J Clin Psychiatry* 1986;47:225-229.
20. Glassman AH, Preud'homme XA: Review of the cardiovascular effects of heterocyclic antidepressants. *J Clin Psychiatry* 1993;54(2 suppl):16-22.
21. O'Brien S, McKeon P, O'Regan M, et al: Blood pressure effects of tranylcypromine when prescribed singly and in combination with amitriptyline. *J Clin Psychopharmacol* 1992;12:104-109.
22. Feighner JP, Herbstein J, Damlouji N: Combined MAOI, TCA, and direct stimulant therapy of treatment-resistant depression. *J Clin Psychiatry* 1985;46:206-209.
23. Roose SP, Dalack GW: Treating the depressed patient with cardiovascular problems. *J Clin Psychiatry* 1992;53(9 suppl):25-31.
24. Connolly SJ, Mitchell LB, Swerdlow CP, et al: Clinical efficacy and electrophysiology of imipramine for ventricular tachycardia. *Am J Cardiol* 1984;53:516-521.
25. Yoon MS, Han J, Dersham GH, et al: Effects of thioridazine on ventricular electrophysiologic properties. *Am J Cardiol* 1979;43:1155-1158.

26. Khan MM, Lopan KR, McComb JM, et al: Management of recurrent ventricular tachyarrhythmias associated with Q-T prolongation. *Am J Cardiol* 1981;47:1301-1308.

27. Fowler NO, McCall D, Chou T, et al: Electrocardiographic changes and cardiac arrhythmias in patients receiving psychotropic drugs. *Am J Cardiol* 1976;37:223-230.

28. Jefferson JW: A review of the cardiovascular effects and toxicity of tricyclic antidepressants. *Psychosom Med* 1975;37:160-179.

29. Young RC, Alexopoulos GS, Shamoian CA, et al: Heart failure associated with high plasma 10-hydroxynortriptyline levels. *Am J Psychiatry* 1984;141:432-433.

30. Barrnett J, Frances A, Kocsis J: Peripheral edema associated with trazodone: A report of ten cases. *J Clin Psychopharmacol* 1985;5:161-164.

31. Georgotas A, McCue RE, Friedman E, et al: Electrocardiographic effects of nortriptyline, phenelzine and placebo under optimal treatment conditions. *Am J Psychiatry* 1987;144:798-801.

32. Roose SP, Glassman AH, Giardina EGV, et al: Tricyclic antidepressants in depressed patients with cardiac conduction disease. *Arch Gen Psychiatry* 1987;44:273-275.

33. Bailey DN, Van Dyke C, Langou RA, et al: Tricyclic antidepressants: Plasma levels and clinical findings in overdose. *Am J Psychiatry* 1978;135:1325-1328.

34. Burckhardt D, Rader E, Mullen V, et al: Cardiovascular effects of tricyclic and tetracyclic antidepressants. *JAMA* 1978;239:213-216.

35. Swett CP Jr, Shader RI: Cardiac effects and sudden death in hospitalized psychiatric patients. *Dis Nerv Syst* 1977;38:69-72.

36. Tesar GE, Murray GB, Cassem NH: Use of high-dose intravenous haloperidol in the treatment of agitated cardiac patients. *J Clin Psychopharmacol* 1985;5:344-347.

37. Ray WA, Griffin MR, Schaffner W, et al: Psychotropic drug use and the risk of hip fracture. *N Engl J Med* 1987;316:363-369.

38. Bernstein JG: Drug interactions. In Cassem NH (ed): *Massachusetts General Hospital Handbook of general hospital psychiatry*, ed 3. St Louis, Mosby, 1991, pp 571-610.

39. Risch SC, Groom GP, Janowsky DS: The effects of psychotropic drugs on the cardiovascular system. *J Clin Psychiatry* 1982;43:16-31.

40. Axelsson R, Aspenstrom G: Electrocardiographic changes and serum concentrations in thioridazine-treated patients. *J Clin Psychiatry* 1982;43:332-335.

41. Banchey MH, Lee JH, Amin R, et al: High and low potency neuroleptics in elderly psychiatric patients. *JAMA* 1978;239:1860-1862.

42. Huston JR, Bell GE: The effect of thioridazine hydrochloride and chlorpromazine on the electrocardiogram. *JAMA* 1966;198:16-20.

43. Fulop G, Phillips RA, Shapiro AK: ECG changes during haloperidol and pimoxide treatment of Tourette's disorder. *Am J Psychiatry* 1987;144:673-675.

44. Safferman A, Lieberman JA, Kane JM, et al: Update on the clinical efficacy and side effects of clozapine. *Schizophr Bull* 1991;17:247-261.

45. Caroff SN: The neuroleptic malignant syndrome. *J Clin Psychiatry* 1980;41:79-83.

46. Pearlman CA: Neuroleptic malignant syndrome: a review of the literature. *J Clin Psychopharmacol* 1986;6:257-273.

47. Pope HG Jr, Keck PE Jr, McElroy SL: Frequency and presentation of neuroleptic malignant syndrome in a large psychiatric hospital. *Am J Psychiatry* 1986;143:1227-1233.

48. Shalev A, Munitz H: The neuroleptic malignant syndrome: Agent and host interaction. *Acta Psychiatric Scand* 1986;73:337-347.

49. Keck PE, Pope HG, Cohen BM, et al: Risk factors for neuroleptic malignant syndrome. *Arch Gen Psychiatry* 1989;46:914-918.

50. Gurrera RJ, Chang SS, Romero JA: A comparison of diagnostic criteria for neuroleptic malignant syndrome. *J Clin Psychiatry* 1992;53:56-62.

51. Shalev A, Hermesh H, Munitz H: Mortality from neuroleptic malignant syndrome. *J Clin Psychiatry* 1989;50:18-25.

52. Rosebush PI, Stewart TD, Gelenberg AJ: Twenty neuroleptic rechallenges after neuroleptic malignant syndrome in 15 patients. *J Clin Psychiatry* 1989;50:295-298.
53. Mann SC, Caroff SN, Bleier HR, et al: Lethal catatonia. *Am J Psychiatry* 1986;143:1374-1381.
54. Dhib-Jalbut S, Hesselbrock R, Mouradian MM, et al: Bromocriptine treatment of neuroleptic malignant syndrome. *J Clin Psychiatry* 1987;48:69-73.
55. Rosenberg MR, Green M: Neuroleptic malignant syndrome: review of response to therapy. *Arch Intern Med* 1989;149:1927-1931.
56. Gratz SS, Levinson DF, Simpson GM: Treatment and management of neuroleptic malignant syndromes. *Prog Neuropsychopharmacol Biol Psychiatry* 1992;16:425-443.
57. Cohen WJ, Cohen NH: Lithium carbonate, haloperidol, and irreversible brain damage. *JAMA* 1974;230:1283-1287.
58. Baastrup PC, Hollnagel P, Sorenson R, et al: Adverse reactions in treatment with lithium carbonate and haloperidol. *JAMA* 1976;236:2645-2646.
59. Spring GH: Neurotoxicity with combined use of lithium and thioridazine. *J Clin Psychiatry* 1979;40:135-138.
60. Sternbach H: The serotonin syndrome. *Am J Psychiatry* 1991;148:705-713.
61. Rosenstein DL, Nelson JC, Jacobs SC: Seizures associated with antidepressants: a review. *J Clin Psychiatry* 1993;54:289-299.
62. Dessain EC, Schatzberg AF, Woods BT, et al: Maprotiline treatment in depression: a perspective on seizures. *Arch Gen Psychiatry* 1986;43:86-90.
63. Davidson JRT: Seizure risk during antidepressant therapy. *J Clin Psychiatr Monogr* 1993;11:50-54.
64. Correa N, Opler LA, Kay SR, et al: Amantadine in the treatment of neuroendocrine side effects of neuroleptics. *J Clin Psychopharmacol* 1987;7:91-95.
65. Bernstein JG: Induction of obesity by psychotropic drugs. *Ann NY Acad Sci* 1987;499:203-215.
66. Kotin J, Wilbert DE, Verburg D, et al: Thioridazine and sexual dysfunction. *Am J Psychiatry* 1976;133:82-85.
67. Segraves RT: Treatment-emergent sexual dysfunction in affective disorder: a review and management strategies. *J Clin Psychiatr Monogr* 1993;11(1):57-60.
68. Zajecka J, Fawcett J, Schaff M, et al: The role of serotonin in sexual dysfunction: fluoxetine-associated orgasm dysfunction. *J Clin Psychiatry* 1991;52:66-68.
69. Hollander E, McCarley A: Yohimbine treatment of sexual side effects induced by serotonin reuptake blockers. *J Clin Psychiatry* 1992;53:207-209.
70. Tandon R, Grunhaus L, Greden JF: Imipramine and tinnitus. *J Clin Psychiatry* 1987;48:109-111.
71. Pollack MH, Rosenbaum JF: Management of antidepressant-induced side effects. *J Clin Psychiatry* 1987;43:3-8.
72. Allen MD, Greenblatt DJ, Noel BJ: Overdosage with antipsychotic agents. *Am J Psychiatry* 1980;137:234-236.
73. Nicotra MB, Rivera M, Paol JL, et al: Tricyclic antidepressant overdose: clinical and pharmacological observations. *Clin Toxicol* 1981;18:599-613.

CHAPTER 11

Movement Disorders and Neurologic Aspects of Psychotropic Drugs

OVERVIEW

1. Acute dystonic reactions are common when starting antipsychotic chemotherapy — diphenhydramine (Benadryl) 50 mg IV provides most rapid and safe relief within minutes. Alternatively, diphenhydramine may be given IM or benztropine may be given IV or IM (1 to 2 mg).

2. Parkinsonism is common in the first few weeks of antipsychotic chemotherapy. There may be stiffness, reduced arm movement when walking, tremors, and sialorrhea. Prophylactic administration of an antiparkinsonian drug in low dosage 2 to 4 times daily may reduce the incidence and severity of extrapyramidal symptoms (EPS). They should not be used prophylactically in elderly patients or those with dementia. More potent antipsychotic agents with less anticholinergic activity are more likely to produce acute extrapyramidal effects. There is no evidence that neuroleptics with lower potential for producing acute EPS are less likely to produce tardive dyskinesia, with the exception of clozapine.

3. Akathisia, the most common acute EPS, responds best to treatment with antiparkinsonian drugs (e.g., trihexyphenidyl 6 to 10 mg/day), β-blockers (e.g., propranolol 10-20 mg tid), or Lorazepam (2 to 4 mg/day).

4. Akinesia, which may be mistaken for schizophrenic withdrawal or depression, should be treated with antiparkinsonian drugs.

5. When psychotic symptoms improve, antipsychotic dosage should be reduced, which will decrease EPS and other side effects and minimize the need for antiparkinsonian medication.

Continued.

6. Most antiparkinsonian medications exert their beneficial effect by blocking acetylcholine, and may thereby induce a toxic delirium.
7. Tricyclic antidepressants reduce neuroleptic-induced EPS; when these two classes of medication are administered simultaneously, antiparkinsonian drugs are usually unnecessary.
8. Most patients on long-term antipsychotic chemotherapy do not need long-term antiparkinsonian drugs.
9. Antipsychotic drugs should never be discontinued abruptly, since this may produce withdrawal dyskinesia, which looks exactly like tardive dyskinesia clinically but will gradually disappear with slow dosage reduction and eventual discontinuation of antipsychotic drug therapy.
10. Patients receiving fluphenazine or haloperidol decanoate may require antiparkinsonian medication for 3 to 5 days starting on the second or third day after each injection as the neuroleptic blood level is approaching its peak concentration.
11. Typical neuroleptic drugs produce tardive dyskinesia (TD) in approximately 20% of patients receiving prolonged treatment. Lower doses or short-term administration may reduce the risk. TD will often diminish and disappear after a prolonged neuroleptic-free interval. Clozapine, clonidine, cholinergic drugs, GABA-ergic drugs, valproate, and vitamin E may be useful treatment for TD.
12. Movement disorders due to abnormal neurotransmission: Torsion dystonia, which may be mistaken for a conversion reaction, should be treated with high-dose trihexyphenidyl, carbamazepine, and baclofen. Parkinson's disease patients are often depressed, commonly develop dementia, and not infrequently become acutely psychotic in response to levodopa and other therapies. Tourette syndrome with motor tics and OCD symptoms is treated with neuroleptics and often SSRIs.

Increasing use of psychotropic medications has alerted us to the occurrence of movement disorders, such as EPS, as side effects and TD as a long-term complication of neuroleptics, as well as the utility of these drugs to treat neurologic conditions. Modern psychiatrists should be aware that many abnormalities of movement were known to exist in psychiatric patients long before any of the presently used psychotropic medications were available. The 1907 *Textbook of Psychiatry* by Kraepelin described choreiform ataxia, which, among other abnormal movements, included the occurrence of "chorea of the mouth" long before the use of neuroleptic medications.[1] The English edition of Eugen Bleuler's *Textbook of Psychiatry*, published in 1924, noted that "tremors very frequently accompany the psychoses."[2] Bleuler also described choreiform and athetoid movements in psychiatric patients. Under the category of infectious deliria, Bleuler described chorea minor psychosis, wherein there was irritability, lability of affect, fatigue, and a decline of the tenacity of attention in association with choreic movements. He also noted that, "unfortunately, hysterical epidemics in schools, manifesting themselves in abnormal movements and similar things are also still called chorea." Patients who suffered from abnormal movements in association with psychotic illnesses a half-century ago, obviously had these symptoms in the absence of antipsychotic therapy.

Dystonia was originally described in 1911 as a condition involving fluctuating hypertonia and hypotonia of muscle groups, giving rise to abnormalities in locomotion and other skeletal muscle movements.[3] Most psychiatrists think of dystonia simply as an adverse effect of neuroleptic drugs; in patients with no prior history of neuroleptic drug treatment, this condition is frequently misdiagnosed as a hysterical conversion reaction.[4] Failure to recognize the distinct syndrome of torsion dystonia may lead the psychiatrist to a vain search for the causative pharmacologic agent or, more seriously, lead the patient into an extended course of unnecessary and ineffective psychotherapeutic intervention for a presumed conversion reaction.[4]

In a pharmacologically oriented age of medicine, physicians often forget that Parkinson's disease was initially described as "shaking palsy" in 1817.[5] Furthermore, parkinsonism, which is associated with a progressive muscular rigidity, abnormality of posture and gait, as well as arrhythmic tremors, may be associated with emotional lability, obsessive-compulsive personality features, and depressive reactions, even in the absence of any prior psychotropic drug therapy.[5] Multiple sclerosis is a progressive demyelinating disease that may be associated with paranoid ideation and mood lability, with associated depressive or hypomanic reactions. Patients with this condition may suffer emotional instability that may seriously disturb interpersonal relationships; they may also have impaired control of laughter and crying resulting from bilateral upper motor neuron lesions.[5] Huntington's disease is a genetically based degenerative disease of the central nervous system first described in 1872. In addition to having persistent chorea and other abnormal movements, these patients are often irritable, obstinate, and moody. They may lack motivation to function and they may be at times agitated and assaultive. Patients with Huntington's disease may experience euphoria or depression.[5]

In view of the effect of psychotropic drugs, particularly the neuroleptics, on a variety of neurotransmitters and their receptor sites in the brain, it is not surprising that movement disorders occur with the use of these drugs, which have a significant effect on basal ganglia function.[6] Furthermore, a variety of movement disorders including Huntington's disease,[7] parkinsonism,[8] and torsion dystonia,[3] may either improve or worsen in response to drugs that modify neurotransmitter function in the brain. Box 11-1 presents a lexicon of drug-related movement disorders.

EVALUATION AND MANAGEMENT OF DRUG-INDUCED MOVEMENT DISORDERS

Shortly after the introduction of neuroleptic drugs in the treatment of psychotic illness, a high incidence of acute extrapyramidal, or parkinsonian, reactions became recognized. Since antiparkinsonian drugs such as trihexyphenidyl and benztropine had been used previously for the treatment of spontaneously occuring parkinsonism, these drugs were used with the expectation that they would reduce the frequency or severity of unwanted extrapyramidal reactions.[10] Two studies conducted in the early 1970s of hospitalized chronic schizophrenic patients found that antiparkinsonian medication could be discontinued while a patient was maintained on neuroleptic therapy, without the development of major or persistent extrapyramidal symptoms.[11,12]

As a result of some of the early studies indicating the lack of necessity for antiparkinsonian medication, it became accepted as bad medical practice to routinely administer these drugs to patients receiving neuroleptics. I modified my own clinical practice and began to avoid combining antiparkinsonian

Box 11-1 A lexicon of drug-related movement disorders

A variety of abnormal movements may occur during psychotropic drug treatment or following discontinuation of such treatment. These abnormal movements which are more often associated with neuroleptic drugs than other psychotropics, result from the ability of these agents to affect neurotransmission at dopamine- and acetylcholine-mediated synapses. In the basal ganglia, movement abnormalities may result from blockade of receptor sites, supersensitivity of these receptor sites, or the actions of other modifying neurotransmitters such as γ-aminobutyric acid (GABA) and various neuropeptides. Abnormal movements are often responsive to a variety of treatment approaches — including dosage adjustment, discontinuation of the offending agent, or the addition of a suitable antiparkinsonian, muscle relaxant, β-blocker, or alpha$_2$-agonist compound.

Akathisia: Motor restlessness accompanied by the subjective sense of inner restlessness, impatience, nervousness, and a vague feeling of discomfort that is worsened by physical inactivity. These patients often fidget, pace, rock forward and backward when sitting, or continuously shift their weight from side to side when standing.

Akinesia: Decreased motor movements often associated with weakness, decreased spontaneous movements, and paresthesias. Akinetic patients tend to have a rigid posture and walk with a shorter stride and diminished spontaneous swings of the arms. These patients appear apathetic, have difficulty initiating usual activities including speech, and may have their movement disorder interpreted as indicative of depression or a withdrawn schizophrenic illness.

Athetosis: Slow, writhing, purposeless movements.

Catatonia: Patient is withdrawn, isolated, and mute, and may show bizarre posture rigidity or immobility, and waxy flexibility. NMS, a complication of neuroleptic drugs, must be differentiated from catatonia — a symptom of schizophrenic illness — which will benefit from discontinuation of medication rather than increased dosage.

Chorea: Rapid, jerky, quasipurposeful nonrhythmic movements.

Dyskinesia: Arrhythmic involuntary spasms of groups of muscles giving rise to a variety of abnormal movements.

Myoclonus: Abrupt, sudden, jerky movements.

Tardive dyskinesia (TD): May occur following prolonged administration of any neuroleptic drug. TD consists of slow, sometimes stereotyped, involuntary movements of the nose, tongue, mouth, face, and, at times, extremities or other parts of the body. The movements are writhing, purposeless, and may or may not be continuous. Mouth movements including sucking, licking, lip pursing, tongue movements, and chewing are the most frequently recognized manifestations of TD. Antiparkinsonian drugs should not be used to treat this disorder.

Withdrawal dyskinesia: Withdrawal dyskinesia, which is generally associated with the same type of involuntary movements as those seen in TD, may occur following the abrupt discontinuation of any neuroleptic drug, after either brief or long-term treatment. Not infrequently, withdrawal dyskinesia is incorrectly diagnosed as tardive dyskinesia.

Respiratory dyskinesia: May be manifested as an irregular respiratory rate, shortness of breath, and chest discomfort. This is a rare syndrome that may occur in association with drug-induced TD.

Continued.

Dystonia: An abnormality in muscle tone associated with persistent abnormal position of one or more extremities or of the face, neck, or trunk. Dystonia may take the form of an overextended or overflexed posture of the hand, inversion of the foot, pulling of the head to one side, or retraction of the head with or without associated twisting of the back. Acute dystonic reactions to neuroleptic drugs most often manifest themselves by rapid and sustained retroflexion of the neck, which may occur in association with abnormal movements of the tongue, difficulty speaking or swallowing, and occulogyric movements. Rarely, dystonic reactions may affect laryngeal or pharyngeal muscles and be associated with gagging or respiratory distress.

Tardive dystonia: A complication of long-term neuroleptics.

Parkinsonism: Muscular rigidity, poverty and slowness of voluntary movement, tremor at rest (pill-rolling, 4/sec), stooped posture, festinating gait, and lack of facial expression often associated with drooling and excessive saliva production. This syndrome may occur spontaneously, due to lesions of the CNS, or may occur during treatment with neuroleptic drugs.

Rabbit syndrome: Fine, rapid tremor of the lips (neuroleptic-induced).

Rigidity: Increased muscle tone with continuous passive resistance to movement, lack of facial expression, and micrography are manifestations of muscular rigidity associated with parkinsonism.

Tremor: Rhythmic alternating movements of opposing muscle groups, most often manifested in the fingers. Anxiety produces fine tremors associated with rapid rhythmic movements. Essential tremor is smooth in character, shows a wide range of movements, is usually long-standing, and has a tendency to run in families. Parkinsonian tremor is slow, rhythmic, and often associated with rotational and flexing movements affecting the fingers, hands, and wrists, which tend to move as a unit. Lithium-induced tremor is irregular in rhythm and amplitude. There are jerky movements with flexion and extension of fingers, but usually the hand and wrist are not involved until the condition is far advanced. Lithium-induced tremors are present at rest and tend to become more prominent with intentional movements; they usually fluctuate in intensity and frequency from day to day and there is generally no associated rigidity on passive flexion.

medication with antipsychotic drugs in light of these findings and the suggestion from another group of investigators that the coadministration of antiparkinsonian agents reduced blood levels of chlorpromazine in patients receiving combined treatment.[13] I then noted with increasing frequency a variety of extrapyramidal symptoms, most notably akathisia, akinesia, and dystonic reactions in patients receiving neuroleptics alone. I subsequently returned to my previous pattern of using antiparkinsonian medication routinely along with antipsychotic medication in the first 3 to 4 weeks of neuroleptic therapy, and found a decrease in the number of extrapyramidal reactions.

It is important to recognize that elderly patients and those with organic brain dysfunction are most likely to experience complications when anticholinergic-type antiparkinsonian medication is added to their regimens, and that these patients are the ones most likely to experience confusion, delirium, and changes in mentation in association with these potent anticholinergic agents.[14] In my experience the use of antiparkinsonian agents along with neuroleptics may reduce the frequency or severity of extrapyramidal reactions and thereby reduce the patient's exposure to a potentially frightening symptom. Some patients will need long-term administration of antiparkinsonian medication, in low dosage as long as they are maintained on neuroleptics. There are now double-blind controlled clinical studies that indicate the usefulness of these medications in conjunction with neuroleptic treatment.[15] In one study, wherein procyclidine was withdrawn from patients receiving antipsychotic medication, 54% of those removed from an active drug and placed on placebo experienced a variety of extrapyramidal side effects, while these effects were not seen in any of the patients whose antiparkinsonian regimen was continued.[16]

In addition to studies demonstrating the beneficial effect of antiparkinsonian medications in preventing drug-induced akinesia and akathisia,[15,16] prophylactic use of these agents has been shown to diminish or avoid drug-induced dystonic reactions.[17,18] A double-blind study of 39 hospitalized patients beginning treatment with high-potency neuroleptics (thiothixene, haloperidol, fluphenazine, or trifluoperazine) were randomly given either benztropine 2 mg or placebo twice daily.[17] Of 17 placebo-treated patients, eight (47%) experienced acute dystonic reactions, while none of the 22 benztropine-treated patients had dystonic reactions.[17] A retrospective study found that 15 of 16 haloperidol-treated young adults who did not receive benztropine experienced acute dystonic reactions while none of the patients who received comparable haloperidol doses along with 1 to 2 mg of benztropine daily had dystonic reactions.[18] Another study not employing antiparkinsonian medication found a lower incidence of acute extrapyramidal reactions when haloperidol was given IV rather than orally.[19]

As the symptoms of acute psychosis diminish in response to neuroleptic therapy, patients will often experience an increase in the incidence and severity of a variety of side effects, including sedation and extrapyramidal reactions. Once clinical improvement is noted, antipsychotic medication must be gradually tapered so that the patient is not exposed unnecessarily to excessive doses of medication and so that there will be a diminution in the sedative and extrapyramidal side effects.[20] The gradual dosage reduction of neuroleptics will generally reduce the need for continuous administration of antiparkinsonian medication. Dosage reduction of neuroleptic therapy may cause withdrawal dyskinesia, wherein a disorder resembling tardive dyskinesia can occur when neuroleptic drugs are tapered rapidly or discontinued suddenly.[21] Sudden dosage reduction or neuroleptic discontinuation can produce nausea, vomiting, diarrhea, abdominal pain, and a variety of autonomic symptoms and abnormal movements.[22] Table 11-1 presents guidelines for dosage range and suggested use of medications in managing movement disorders.

Table 11-1   Drugs in movement disorders

Drugs	Mechanism of action	Dosage range (daily)	Indications and comments
Benztropine (Cogentin)	Anticholinergic	0.5-6.0 mg (PO, IM, IV)	Parkinsonism, acute dystonic reactions
Biperidin (Akineton)	Anticholinergic	2-6 mg (PO, IM, IV)	Parkinsonism, acute dystonic reactions
Cycrimine (Pagitane)	Anticholinergic	2.5-20 mg PO	Parkinsonism
Diphenhydramine (Benadryl)	Anticholinergic, antihistaminic	25-50 mg IV, IM	Specific for acute dystonic reactions; parkinsonism, especially in elderly
Ethopropazine (Parsidol)	Anticholinergic	20-100 mg PO / 20-200 mg PO	Parkinsonism (nonneuroleptic phenothiazine derivative)
Procyclidine (Kemadrin)	Anticholinergic	2-220 mg PO	Parkinsonism
Trihexyphenidyl (Artane)	Anticholinergic, antihistaminic	2-10 mg PO (tablets, liquid)	Parkinsonism, akathisia (sustained-release capsules stabilize blood level) (20-60 mg/day in torsion dystonia)
Amantadine (Symmetrel)	Dopaminergic stimulant	50-300 mg (capsules, liquid)	Parkinsonism, tardive dyskinesia; useful in elderly; may be psychotogenic
Levodopa (Larodopa)	Increases central dopamine	0.1-8.0 g	Non–drug-induced parkinsonism, tardive dyskinesia
Carbidopa and levodopa (Sinemet)	Increases central dopamine; peripheral inhibition of dopa decarboxylase allows response to lower dopa dose	10-100/day to 25-250 4 times/day (dosage titration)	Non–drug-induced parkinsonism, tardive dyskinesia
Baclofen (Lioresal)	Increases GABA, substance P centrally	15-60 mg	Antispastic, tardive dyskinesia, torsion dystonia
Carbamazepine (Tegretol)	Uncertain	100-800 mg	Torsion dystonia, ?tardive dyskinesia
Clonidine (Catapres)	Central alpha$_2$-adrenergic agonist	0.1-0.6 mg	Tardive dyskinesia, ?antipsychotic Tourette syndrome, akathisia

Continued.

Table 11-1 Drugs in movement disorders — cont'd.

Drugs	Mechanism of action	Dosage range (daily)	Indications and comments
Clozapine (Clozaril)	Atypical/neuroleptic	25-400 mg	Tardive dyskinesia
Choline	Increases brain acetylcholine	2-8 g	Tardive dyskinesia, Alzheimer's disease,
Lecithin	Increases brain acetylcholine	10-40 g	?antimanic
Propranolol (Inderal)	Beta-adrenergic antagonist	30-160 mg	Inhibits lithium-induced tremors, akathisia; ?benefit in tardive dyskinesia
Valproate	Increases GABA	1-2 g	Tardive dyskinesia
Nifedipine	Calcium-channel blocker	30-60 g	Tardive dyskinesia

GABA = γ-aminobutyric acid.

TRIHEXYPHENIDYL

Akathisia

Although not the most dramatic-appearing of the movement disorders associated with the neuroleptic drugs, akathisia is among the most prevalent.[27] It is, unfortunately, often not recognized by clinicians, who are more apt to make a diagnosis of anxiety and prescribe non-specific treatment with a benzodiazepine.[27] In a survey of 3775 patients receiving phenothiazines, 39% developed extrapyramidal reactions, approximately half of whom, or 21% of the total treated patients, experienced akathisia.[28] Other investigators have found that akathisia may occur in 50% or more of neuroleptic-treated patients. This side effect does not appear immediately and generally increases in incidence as therapy is prolonged and as tissue levels of the drug accumulate. There is no predilection for either sex or any particular age group. Patients experience restlessness, vague feelings of discomfort, jitteriness, and nervousness.[27] Akathisia is more uncomfortable when the patient is at rest, and may lead him to pace, fidget, tap his feet, rock forward and backward when sitting, or shift his weight from side to side when standing. Akathisia has been described as "restless legs" or the "need to keep moving." In the early days of neuroleptic chemotherapy the increased motor activity of medicated patients was at times described as an activating effect of a drug that was considered to be favorable. Although akathisia will improve somewhat in response to a reduction of neuroleptic dosage, it will almost always persist, producing continued discomfort until appropriate medication is administered.

Several pharmacologic approaches have proven effective in the management of akathisia. Benzodiazepines, such as diazepam and lorazepam, are often useful but nonspecific treatments for various movement disorders. Amantadine in a daily dose of 100 to 300 mg may be helpful in controlling drug-induced parkinsonism and akathisia.[29] Since, unlike other antiparkinsonian drugs, amantadine lacks anticholinergic activity, it is less likely to produce memory impairment and confusion.[30] Amantadine, however, is a dopaminergic compound which can exacerbate psychotic symptoms.[31] Anticholinergic-type antiparkinsonian drugs are the agents which have been most extensively used over the longest period of time in the management of drug-induced parkinsonism and akathisia.[15] Akathisia tends to be more resistant to treatment with antiparkinsonian drugs than is the parkinsonian syndrome, which consists of tremor, rigidity, micrographia, and decreased fine motor coordination. In the management of akathisia, trihexyphenidyl, which has both antihistaminic and anticholinergic activity, appears to be more effective than benztropine or other antiparkinsonian medications. However, trihexyphenidyl generally must be administered in a larger dose of 2 mg 4 times/day. When used in the treatment of akathisia, the dose employed is often larger than needed in drug-induced parkinsonism.

Several studies have found the β-blocker propranolol to be effective in the treatment of neuroleptic-induced akathisia.[32,33,34] Propranolol is also effective in the management of tremor induced by lithium and by tricyclic antidepressants but is ineffective in the management of parkinsonism and tardive dyskinesia.[32] In one study, where raters were blind to the treatment being administered, propranolol in daily doses of 20 to 30 mg was more effective in controlling neuroleptic-induced akathisia than was lorazepam in a daily dose of 2 mg. Propranolol may be administered in a dose of 10 to 20 mg 3 to 4 times daily in the treatment of drug-induced akathisia. Propranolol is a nonselective beta$_1$- and beta$_2$-antagonist with both central and peripheral effects and has been shown to be more effective in the treatment of akathisia than nadolol or metoprolol, which have little or no central beta-blocking activity.[35] Clonidine, an adrenergic agonist, suppresses noradrenergic activity by activating presynaptic, inhibitory alpha$_2$-autoreceptors. Clonidine in a dose of 0.05 to 0.20 mg twice daily has been shown to reduce akathisia and anxiety during neuroleptic treatment.[36] Sedation and hypotension are the most prominently observed side effects of clonidine and may limit the patient's ability to tolerate an effective dosage regimen. Clonidine has also been found to be effective in the treatment of "restless legs," which may occur as part of the akathisia syndrome or as a separate and distinct entity either secondary to or independent of drug therapy.[37] In addition to the potential risk of hypotension and sedation during clonidine treatment, the psychiatrist should be aware of the ability of cyclic antidepressants to antagonize the actions of this drug. Patients who have severe akathisia, unresponsive to antiparkinsonian medications or who have bronchial asthma, which contraindicates the use of beta-adrenergic blocking drugs, should be considered for a therapeutic trial of clonidine or lorazepam.

Although akathisia has been primarily seen as a side effect of neuroleptics, it has also been occasionally reported with tricyclic and heterocyclic antidepressants. The serotonin-selective reuptake inhibitors, particularly paroxetine and fluoxetine, are being increasingly recognized as a potential source of iatrogenic movement disorders, including primarily akathisia but also to a limited extent dystonic reactions.[23,24,25] Evidence suggests that SSRIs can inhibit dopaminergic neurotransmission, most likely by enhanced serotonergic activity inhibiting the synthesis and release of striatal dopamine.[26] This effect is in most instances seen only with higher doses of SSRIs, and the occurrence

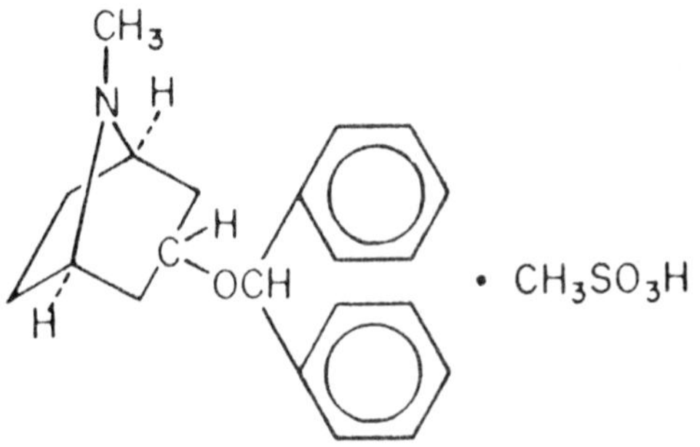

CH$_3$

N   H

C—H

C—OCH

H

· CH$_3$SO$_3$H

BENZTROPINE

of akathisia during fluoxetine treatment was one explanation offered for the occurrence of suicidal ideation during treatment with this antidepressant.[24] Multiple small series of case reports of akathisia with fluoxetine have appeared, and there have been a few cases of apparent drug-induced dystonia in the literature.[23,24,25] I have seen several patients with akathisia during treatment with fluoxetine and other SSRIs, which has resolved with dosage reduction or discontinuation; furthermore, lorazepam and propranolol have also been helpful in several patients. Several patients I have treated with SSRIs have complained of painful muscle spasms or myoclonus which responded favorably to dosage reduction, discontinuation of SSRI, or the addition of small doses of clonazepam. When neuroleptics are combined with SSRIs, there is often an increase in extrapyramidal side effects, particularly akathisia, which is a direct result of either inhibited dopamine transmission by the SSRI or, in the case of some drugs such as fluoxetine and paroxetine, inhibition of neuroleptic metabolism, with consequent increased neuroleptic serum concentration.

Akinesia

Akinesia is a disturbance of extrapyramidal function produced by neuroleptics and manifested by a lessening of spontaneous movements, paucity of gestures, diminished conversation, and apathy.[38] Patients with akinesia often confuse the clinician and may be diagnosed as suffering from depression or a chronic withdrawn schizophrenic state.[15,27] Since an absence of movement characterizes akinesia, rather than the appearance of more dramatic abnormal movements, it is not surprising that it has been easy to deny the necessity of antiparkinsonian medication for this syndrome, which is often not clearly recognized as a movement disorder.[15,27] The pattern of walking reveals a shorter stride, rigid posture, and diminution or absence of spontaneous arm swings.[38] Although there are no good data on the incidence of akinesia, in my experience it is quite prevalent. In one study of a small number of patients four of the five who experienced akinesia were receiving fluphenazine decanoate.[16] There is no evidence that any neuroleptic is free of the ability to produce akinesia, nor is there evidence that a particular neuroleptic is more apt to do so. Akinesia may appear in the absence of any other signs of extrapyramidal disturbance.[15,38] If akinesia is misdiagnosed as depression, the patient may be treated with antidepressant medication unnecessarily, and though he may benefit from such treatment, the benefit is likely to be more related to the anticholinergic effect of the antidepressant than to other pharmacologic actions of the drug. Furthermore, these patients may experience an antidepressant-induced worsening of their psychotic symptoms. The preferred therapeutic approach to akinesia should have two stages. The first stage is to reduce neuroleptics to the lowest dose that is effective for the patient, trying to avoid the risk of too rapid reduction or the administration of dosages that are insufficient to maintain the patient relatively free of psychotic symptoms.[15] Since neuroleptics remain in the body for a long time following prolonged treatment, there is apt not to be a rapid improvement in the paucity of motor activity following dosage reduction. The second phase of treatment, after dosage adjustment, is the addition of an antiparkinsonian medication such as trihexyphenidyl, benztropine, or procyclidine. The dose of antiparkinsonian medication should be started relatively low. However, since these medications have short durations of action, it is preferable to administer them in two to four doses divided throughout the day.[16,20]

Catatonia

Although catatonic behavior has been recognized for many years prior to the availability of neuroleptic drugs as a symptom seen in some forms of schizophrenia, it must also be recognized as a rare complication of neuroleptic treatment. This syndrome is characterized by isolation, withdrawal, and mutism, as well as motor abnormalities including bizarre posture, rigidity, immobility, and waxy flexibility.[39] The catatonic patient is fertile ground for a variety of medical complications including dehydration, hyperthermia, pulmonary emboli, and pneumonia.[40] Catatonia should be considered as a possible complication of neuroleptic therapy, and may represent a variant of the neuroleptic malignant syndrome discussed in chapter 10.[41] The patient who develops catatonia in response to medication should have neuroleptic drugs discontinued for a period of one to several days to allow for tissue concentration to decline as he is being appropriately monitored and observed.[39] It is of utmost importance to maintain appropriate fluid and electrolyte balance in such patients by the administration of IV fluids if clinically necessary.[41] Vital signs, including temperature, must be monitored to detect the appearance of an infectious complication. Catatonic patients may need antiembolism stockings and chest physical therapy, as well as any practical attempt at ambulation to reduce possible medical complications from lying in bed for a prolonged period of time. Any difficulty in swallowing associated with this syndrome must also be noted and managed by the clinician so that aspiration and consequent pneumonia are avoided. When catatonia does appear the clinician is often tempted to increase the dose of neuroleptic drugs in the belief that this is a manifestation of the psychotic disturbance. However, the possibility that this is a neurologic complication of the medication must be seriously considered. It must be recognized that the risk of temporarily discontinuing neuroleptic therapy may be less than the risk of escalating the dosage upward.[40]

Dyskinesia

Dyskinesia implies abnormal motor activity of basal ganglia origin. Although the cyclic antidepressants as a group are strongly anticholinergic and are generally free of significant ability to block dopamine, it would not appear that these compounds could produce abnormal movements. Since many patients receiving antidepressants may also have received neuroleptics, it is difficult to determine if antidepressants alone can produce abnormal movements. The anticholinergic effects of these drugs may in fact exert an antiparkinsonian action, so that patients receiving combined neuroleptic and cyclic drug therapy most often do not require the concomitant administration of antiparkinsonian medication. There have been sporadic reports in the literature associating tricyclic antidepressants with dyskinetic movements. Two patients reported to develop dyskinesia in association with amitriptyline were also receiving perphenazine, a neuroleptic.

As discussed in chapter 5, amoxapine and trazodone are atypical antidepressants with weak dopamine-blocking activity. Parkinsonian side effects and akathesia can occur infrequently when these drugs are employed at relatively high dose. Dyskinesias, which have been reported in a small number of amoxapine-treated patients, have in almost all cases disappeared after drug discontinuation. These dyskinesias appear to have been more consistent with withdrawal dyskinesia than tardive dyskinesia.

Patients who have been treated with neuroleptic drugs and have the medication abruptly discontinued may experience a variety of withdrawal symptoms, including nausea, vomiting, diarrhea, excessive perspiration, restlessness, insomnia, rhinorrhea, headache, increased appetite, and giddiness.[22] In addition, patients whose neuroleptic dosage is abruptly reduced or discontinued may experience abnormal movement of the extremities, neck, face, and mouth. These abnormal movements are indistinguishable from those observed in patients developing tardive dyskinesia during long-term administration of neuroleptic drugs.[21,22] Dyskinesia associated with the withdrawal of these drugs is related to increased dopaminergic and cholinergic activity and changes in the dopamine-acetylcholine balance within the basal ganglia.[21] The administration of antiparkinsonian medication is generally of no more value in the treatment of withdrawal dyskinesia than in the treatment of tardive dyskinesia. The treatment of choice for withdrawal dyskinesia is to reinstitute neuroleptic treatment at a dosage approximating the previously maintained dosage and then to very gradually reduce it over a period of several weeks while observing the patient for signs of dyskinesia. The neuroleptic tapering procedure may require 1 to 3 months to safely remove the drug without the reappearance of withdrawal symptoms. In those patients who have reappearance of dyskinesia, even following a very gradual drug-withdrawal schedule, it may be necessary to continue observation over a period of months without drug therapy before the dyskinesia symptoms gradually disappear.[21]

Tardive Dyskinesia

Tardive dyskinesia (TD) is a potential complication of long-term neuroleptic drug therapy related to the ability of these drugs to block a variety of receptor sites including dopamine sites.[38] This pharmacologic action of neuroleptics is essential for their therapeutic benefit and at the same time yields the complication of TD. There is no evidence that any effective neuroleptic drug with the possible exception of clozapine, is free of the liability of producing this complication.[43,44,45] Studies have failed to demonstrate that any typical neuroleptic drug is more apt to produce TD or that any is less likely to produce this unwanted complication.[43,45] The suggestion in some pharmaceutical advertising that a particular neuroleptic, by virtue of its lesser ability to produce acute extrapyramidal effects, is more benign from the standpoint of production of tardive dyskinesia is unsupported by scientific evidence.[45]

Animal experimentation has been fundamental to our attempts to understand the neurochemistry and pharmacology of TD although animal data cannot always be extrapolated and applied to the clinical situation. In the laboratory, carefully regulated dosage and experimental conditions allows neuroleptic drugs that have relative selectivity for different types of dopamine receptors to produce differential behavioral and motor responses.[46] Since the clinical situation cannot be controlled as easily as that in the laboratory, and since currently available drugs have only relative selectivity for different types of dopamine receptors, we cannot yet effectively antagonize limbic dopamine receptors while sparing those of the striatum. The lesser ability of thioridazine to produce supersensitivity of the dopamine receptor in animal models does not confer on this drug a freedom from the development of TD.[38]

The atypical neuroleptic drugs, including clozapine and risperidone, are relatively weaker dopamine antagonists than typical neuroleptics and, in addition, are potent antagonists of serotonin 5-HT$_2$ receptors.[47,48,49] Although it was initially thought that the relatively greater affinity of clozapine for limbic versus striatal dopamine receptors accounted for its decreased extrapyramidal side effects, it may well be that the ratio of serotonin to dopamine antagonism accounts for this characteristic.[48] Most clinical and research evidence indicates that clozapine has minimal likelihood of inducing acute extrapyramidal effects, akathisia, and dystonia.[48] Although most publications indicate the lack of TD as a complication of clozapine, one older and one recent report suggest that this complication, though rare can occur with clozapine.[50,51] Risperidone, which is chemically unrelated to clozapine, likewise is a potent 5-HT$_2$ and a weak dopamine antagonist which appears to have a lower risk of extrapyramidal side effects at conventional doses than typical neuroleptics.[49] Higher doses of risperidone, however, produce extrapyramidal side effects, and akathisia is more likely with this drug than with clozapine in some patients. Both risperidone and clozapine have been shown to reduce abnormal movements of tardive dyskinesia and tardive dystonia.[49,52] A review of clozapine studies in patients with TD found that this drug produced improvement in 43% of patients with this devastating movement disorder.[52] Clozapine, unfortunately, produces prominent sedation, hypotension and anticholinergic side effects along with the risk of leukopenia and the rare potential of agranulocytosis. Risperidone is essentially free of major autonomic side effects and has no adverse hematologic effects. At the present time evidence is inadequate to support or deny a low long-term risk of tardive dyskinesia with risperidone, although if it proves relatively benign in this respect, this agent may well earn a preeminent position in the management of psychotic disorders.

In spite of clinical experience and research studies over the past three decades, the mechanisms of TD are not yet fully understood. The most commonly accepted theory for the pathogenesis of TD is based on the assumption that chronic blockade of postsynaptic receptors results in denervation supersensitivity of the striatal tracts of the basal ganglia. This hypersensitivity is thought to induce the hyperdyskinetic manifestations of TD.[55] Although this explanation sounds complicated enough, it is far from the full story. There is evidence of noradrenergic hyperactivity, GABA-ergic underactivity, decreased cholinergic activity, and a variety of other neurotransmitter abnormalities in TD.[38,56] It is also likely that abnormalities of serotonergic and peptidergic transmission play a role in the pathogenesis of this complex disorder.

Estimates of the prevalence of TD range from 0.5% to 68% of neuroleptic-treated patients.[50,53,54] A review of 44 epidemiologic studies indicated that tardive dyskinesia may occur in 24% to 56% of patients receiving long-term neuroleptic therapy.[44] A study of 398 adult outpatients treated with neuroleptics for 3 months to 33 years found a 5-year risk for the development of tardive dyskinesia of 20%, which is in agreement with many previous studies.[45] That investigation also confirmed previously reported findings that, although the greatest risk of TD is in the first 5 years of neuroleptic treatment, new persistent cases continue to occur later with continued neuroleptic exposure.[45] It was also found in that study that type of neuroleptic used and coadministration of other medications, including lithium, antidepressants, antiparkinsonian drugs, and benzodiazepines, did not alter the risk of development of TD.[45] Psychiatric diagnosis also failed to alter the risk of TD occurrence, contrasting with other studies which had suggested that patients with affective illnesses were at greater risk for TD occurrence.[53,57] One of the important confirmatory findings was that total dose of neuroleptic and duration of exposure were positively correlated with risk of developing TD, thus again supporting the practice of minimizing dosage and duration of neuroleptic exposure as much as clinically possible to reduce the risk of TD.[45] Another study, of 362 chronic psychiatric outpatients who were free of TD at the outset and were maintained on neuroleptic medication, found a 32% risk of TD after 5 years of neuroleptic exposure, 57% after 15 years of exposure, and 68% after 25 years of neuroleptic treatment.[53] Although many earlier studies suggested a greater risk of TD in females, most data now support an approximately equal prevalence in males and females, although studies continue to indicate that TD is more likely to occur in the elderly.[53] Tardive dystonia, which in the past has been combined with tardive dyskinesia, is emerging as a separate entity characterized by abnormally sustained posturing associated with neuroleptic treatment.[58] Tardive dystonia is about twice as common in men as in women and tends to occur at an earlier age, with approximately two thirds of affected individuals being under age 50; furthermore, it is associated generally with a shorter neuroleptic exposure than is TD.[58] Anticholinergics, which often worsen TD, may benefit tardive dystonia, which is also likely to be improved by neuroleptic treatment, particularly with atypical agents such as clozapine and risperidone. Tardive dystonia appears to be more common in patients with affective disorders, in contradistinction to TD, although the latter was in the past thought to be more prevalent in affectively ill individuals.[45,58]

Some studies have suggested that drug holidays, wherein neuroleptic chemotherapy is interupted for 1 or 2 days each week, may reduce the risk of TD; other investigators have suggested that drug holidays may actually increase the risk.[43] It has been suggested that the continual administration of antiparkinsonian medication along with neuroleptics may increase the risk of the development of TD. There is no evidence to support this contention.[45] There is increasing evidence, however, that the presence of severe and persistent akathisia may be a risk factor for the development of TD.[59,60] It is unknown whether adequate control of akathisia by the administration of antiparkinsonian drugs, beta-adrenergic blocking drugs, or clonidine could potentially reduce the risk of tardive dyskinesia. Once tardive dyskinesia is present, antiparkinsonian drugs worsen abnormal movements, although beta-adrenergic blocking drugs and clonidine may have some beneficial effect.[50]

The classical clinical appearance of TD involves abnormal movements of the mouth, the presence of persistent chewing motions, peculiar movement of the tongue — often termed "fly catcher's tongue" — as well as sucking, licking, lip pursing, and blowing. The movements of TD are choreiform, coordinated, involuntary, stereotyped, and rhythmic, and continue as long as they are not disturbed by other events.[38,44,61] Patients with TD may also have choreiform movements and rapid unpredictable, often dramatic, thrusts of the extremities or neck. Respiratory dyskinesias occur rarely in association with TD and may be manifested by an irregular respiratory rate, shortness of breath, and chest discomfort.[62-64] Respirations are often somewhat faster and more irregular in patients with TD, although dyspnea and chest discomfort are usually not seen in patients who have TD.[63] Patients who have abnormal mouth movements in association with TD most often will salivate excessively and may drool continuously. Although some have suggested that patients with TD are not disturbed by their movements, this is unlikely; furthermore, family members complain of the unsightliness as well as the abnormal sounds and excessive salivation. Patients with TD may grunt or make strange sounds, thus calling further attention to their unfortunate plight.[43]

Treatment of tardive dyskinesia

Tardive dyskinesia was originally seen as a permanent and untreatable neurologic complication of antipsychotic medication. Early approaches to treatment generally involved the administration of large doses of high-potency antipsychotic drugs to suppress abnormal movements.[38] Because of the likelihood of prolonging and worsening TD, this treatment approach should not be employed except as an emergency measure in the management of severe dyskinesias with associated respiratory distress.[62] Whenever possible, the first treatment approach should be to discontinue antipsychotic medication.[38] There is significant potential for partial recovery from TD after several months free of neuroleptic therapy. One study of 12 schizophrenic patients and 21 nonschizophrenic patients with TD found equal improvement in abnormal movements in both groups beginning 7 months after discontinuation of neuroleptics.[65] That study estimated that if a patient can be kept off neuroleptic medication for 18 months there is an 87.2% probability of a 50% reduction in abnormal movements.[65] In those patients who can be removed from antipsychotic drug therapy, treatment with alternative agents, including lithium, carbamazepine, valproate, clonidine, and clonazepam, may be useful in managing the psychotic illness and may, perhaps, facilitate recovery from the dyskinesia. Many patients cannot be maintained free of neuroleptic therapy and, despite the dyskinesia, need continuing administration of these drugs. There is evidence that the severity of TD may reach a plateau and not worsen despite continuing conservative dosage management with antipsychotic medication. One 5-year follow-up study of 85 schizophrenic patients found that the long-term trend was for the dyskinesia to plateau after reaching mild intensity, with further extension or worsening of the movement disorder occurring in a minority of patients.[66]

Some clinicians favor discontinuing high-potency neuroleptics and administering thioridazine, which produces less acute extrapyramidal side effects. The disadvantage of this approach is that thioridazine, which is a relatively weak dopamine antagonist and strong cholinergic antagonist, will actually worsen dyskinetic movements. The administration of anticholinergic-type antiparkinsonian drugs to patients with mild dyskinesia will often worsen the dyskinesia. Other centrally acting anticholinergic drugs, including thioridazine, may produce a similar result. If neuroleptics cannot be discontinued, because of continuing psychosis, the patient's dosage should be reduced to the lowest effective level or the regimen changed to clozapine or risperidone. Although anticholinergic-type antiparkinsonian drugs should not be administered, amantadine, which is a dopamine receptor agonist, may be administered in a dose of 100 mg 2 to 3 times daily with significant potential of improving abnormal movements.[67] Amantadine, however, can exacerbate psychotic symptoms.[31]

Levodopa has been reported to worsen, have no effect, or improve TD.[50] Use of low doses of levodopa is likely to produce a transient worsening of TD followed by gradual improvement in up to 60% of patients.[50] I have treated TD patients successfully with low doses of this compound, generally beginning at 100 mg daily with gradual dosage increase over a period of several weeks to a maximum of 2 g daily. It would generally be more appropriate, however, to use levodopa in conjunction with carbidopa (Sinemet) in an initial dose of one-half tablet (10 / 100 mg) twice daily with gradual dosage increase by one-half tablet every 3 to 7 days. Since both amantadine and levodopa enhance dopaminergic activity, increased psychotic symptoms may result from this therapeutic approach. Furthermore, if neuroleptic drugs are administered simultaneously, the potential therapeutic activity of the dopaminergic substance is likely to be diminished.

The atypical neuroleptic drugs, including clozapine and risperidone, antagonize serotonin $5-HT_2$ receptors to a greater extent than dopamine sites, which may explain their decreased extrapyramidal side effects. These agents have also been found to be more effective than other neuroleptics in suppressing tardive dyskinesia.[49,67,68] There is considerable experience and investigative evidence to support clozapine as the most promising agent in the treatment of tardive dyskinesia at this time.[68] Since the majority of patients being maintained on long-term neuroleptics will have an exacerbation of psychotic symptoms when neuroleptic therapy is withdrawn in an attempt to control TD, the most practical therapeutic technique is to initiate clozapine therapy. When this approach is not clinically feasible, a trial of risperidone, which is generally better tolerated, without the need for hematologic monitoring, is likely to reduce symptoms of tardive dyskinesia as well as those of tardive dystonia and maintain antipsychotic efficacy.

Tiapride, a selective dopamine D_2-receptor antagonist, has also been found to produce significant beneficial effects in patients with TD.[69] Preliminary studies suggest that clonidine in a daily dose of 0.3 to 0.7 mg can produce marked improvement in TD and reduce concurrent psychotic symptoms.[70] Unfortunately, a subsequent double-blind crossover study of clonidine and placebo did not find a statistically significant therapeutic effect of this drug in the management of TD.[55] Nevertheless, on the basis of clinical observations and sporadic reports in the literature, clonidine is an agent that should be considered for a therapeutic trial in a patient with persistent tardive dyskinesia.[67]

γ-Aminobutyric acid (GABA) has an inhibitory effect on nigrostriatal dopaminergic activity. There is evidence that brain GABA activity is diminished in patients with TD and preliminary studies have found some beneficial effects when the GABA agonist baclofen is administered to TD patients.[71] This drug is available commercially and may be worth a therapeutic trial in TD starting at a dose of 5 mg tid with gradual increase to a maximum of 20 mg tid. Sodium valproate also possesses GABA agonist activity and may have a beneficial effect in TD.[50] An investigational GABA analogue, γ-vinyl GABA, has been used with some success in TD.[50] More potent GABA analogues are being studied investigationally and may eventually prove useful in the management of TD. Benzodiazepines, including diazepam and clonazepam, which effect GABA neurotransmission, are occasionally useful in the management of TD.[50]

There is experimental evidence that brain cholinergic activity is diminished in TD and this hypothesis has been tested by the IV administration of the cholinesterase inhibitor physostigmine.[72] When administered IV, physostigmine has been shown to diminish abnormal movements of TD.[72] Limited experience has also found transient reduction of abnormal movements following IV administered arecoline, a direct-acting cholinergic agonist.[50] Limited work with orally administered physostigmine and arecoline has found limited transient improvement in abnormal movements. Numerous studies have utilized the acetylcholine precursors, choline and lecithin, administered orally to TD patients. Preliminary experience suggested a favorable response, although subsequent studies have been unable to find a significant or prolonged beneficial effect of cholinergic precursors in TD.[50,73] In selected cases of TD, however, it still may be useful to employ highly purified lecithin (PHOS-chol capsules) along with orally administered physostigmine in the management of severe and persistent TD.

Some investigators have found that ordinary therapeutic doses of lithium carbonate may reduce abnormal movements in TD.[50] Likewise, occasional beneficial results are seen in TD with the oral administration of the dopamine-depleting drug reserpine.[50] Reserpine has also occasionally been found to be useful in the treatment of rabbit syndrome, which is a late-occurring neuroleptic-induced disorder characterized by rapid fine rhythmic movements of the lips that mimic the chewing movements of a rabbit.[74] Reserpine, however, does have the disadvantage of potentially producing severe depressive symptoms and must also be used with caution since it may produce significant hypotension and facilitate peptic ulceration. Since no agent is uniformly effective in TD, many agents are tried, and occasionally some benefit is seen. The calcium channel blocker nifedipine and the serotonin antagonist buspirone are sometimes effective.[75,76] One of the more novel approaches to the treatment of TD has been the use of vitamin E. One 12-week study using 1200 IU of vitamin E daily and another 36-week study using 1600 IU daily have shown significant reductions in AIMS scores and TD manifestations with this treatment, which produced essentially no side effects.[77,78]

Dystonic Reactions

Dystonic reactions, characterized by acute torsion spasms primarily affecting the neck muscles, jaw, and tongue, occur fairly commonly when potent neuroleptic drugs are initially administered. They are very rarely associated with dystonic spasms of the larynx and pharynx, and on those occasions acute dystonic reactions may be associated with difficulty speaking, swallowing, or breathing.[79] The vast majority of acute dystonic reactions are simply manifested by a tightness in the jaw, with associated retroflexion and twisting of the neck, but without associated difficulty in breathing and swallowing.[17,38] Among the high-potency neuroleptic agents there is no evidence that any one is more or less likely to produce acute dystonic reactions. The most immediate and dramatic treatment for acute dystonic reactions is the IV administration of 50 mg diphenhydramine.[20,80] If the dystonic reaction is severe, the patient is likely to be very frightened; therefore, the most effective and rapid therapeutic response possible utilizing IV administered diphenhydramine is to be recommended. Benztropine in a dose of 1 to 2 mg IV or IM may also be highly effective, and if an IV injection cannot be immediately given, diphenhydramine could alternatively be administered by the IM route.[20,80] Patients who have had dystonic reactions during prior courses of antipsychotic chemotherapy are likely to have a recurrence of these reactions during the initial phases of subsequent courses of chemotherapy. A patient not uncommonly will have several acute dystonic reactions if an initial reaction has occurred. Therefore, following the initial dystonic reaction it is preferable to begin the patient on a course of prophylactic medication or to increase the dose of prophylactic antiparkinsonian medication if the patient has been receiving such treatment prior to the acute dystonic reaction.[80] Benztropine in a dose of 1 to 2 mg orally 3 to 4 times daily, or diphenhydramine in an oral dose of 50 mg 3 to 4 times daily, may provide effective prophylaxis against recurrent dystonic reactions. Trihexyphenidyl appears to be less effective in preventing dystonic reactions than benztropine, although it is more efficacious in the treatment of persistent akathisia. Oculogyric movements occasionally accompany an acute dystonic reaction and likewise respond favorably to either benztropine or diphenhydramine.[38,80] Once the patient is established on a regular antipsychotic and antiparkinsonian regimen, recurrent acute dystonic reactions are unlikely to occur.[80]

Parkinsonian Reactions

Less dramatic than the acutely occurring dystonic reactions, or the potentially late-occurring dyskinetic reactions to neuroleptic drugs, is the appearance of an extrapyramidal syndrome in the form of parkinsonism, probably the most common neurologic sequela of neuroleptic treatment. The patient gradually develops parkinsonian signs — marked by a flattening of facial expression, muscular rigidity, and a reduction and slowing of voluntary

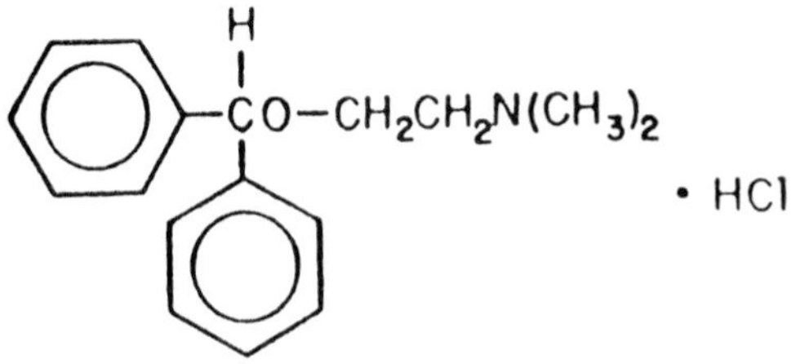

$$\text{(structure)} \quad \overset{H}{\underset{|}{C}}O-CH_2CH_2N(CH_3)_2 \quad \cdot \; HCl$$

DIPHENHYDRAMINE

movement. Patients with parkinsonism often have a stooped posture, a festinating gait (in which small steps are taken) and a reduction in accessory movements of the arms. Patients with this syndrome will often salivate and drool excessively and will generally show a coarse "pill-rolling" tremor of the thumb and fingers at rest.[5] These parkinsonian reactions to neuroleptics are not likely to occur in the first few days of treatment, but occur with increasing frequency as treatment is continued.[16,38] They are less severe in patients receiving simultaneously administered antiparkinsonian medication. In association with the parkinsonian manifestations, the patient may experience akathisia or restlessness, and at times akinesia or a reduction in total movement. Use of the lowest effective dose of neuroleptic medication, once the acute symptoms of psychosis have diminished, is the best approach to limiting the severity and persistence of parkinsonian reactions. In most situations, except in the elderly or in the patient with organic brain dysfunction, the simultaneous administration of benztropine in a dose of 0.5 to 1.0 mg, or trihexyphenidyl in a dose of 2 mg 2 to 4 times daily, is likely to produce significant improvement in parkinsonian reactions to antipsychotic chemotherapy.[9,38] These medications diminish both the muscular rigidity and the tremor of drug-induced parkinsonism. Since their anticholinergic effect may enhance confusion or may produce a delirium in the elderly, these drugs should generally be avoided in older patients or those with organic brain dysfunction.[20] In such individuals the use of diphenhydramine in a dose of 10 to 25 mg 2 to 4 times daily may be useful and produce fewer unwanted effects.[80] Alternatively, the use of amantadine in a dose of 50 to 100 mg 2 to 3 times daily may be useful in controlling drug-induced extrapyramidal symptoms.[29]

Tremor

Although tremors may occur in patients receiving SSRIs and tricyclic antidepressants, these drugs do not produce parkinsonism and antiparkinsonian medication is more likely to produce anticholinergic effects than it is to improve tremor. Paroxetine appears more likely to produce tremor than are other SSRIs. Patients who experience tremors with SSRI or tricyclic antidepressants may benefit from propranolol, in a dose of 10 to 20 mg 3 to 4 times daily.[35] Tremors not infrequently occur in patients treated with lithium carbonate. Lithium-associated tremors are not reduced by antiparkinsonian medication, but may improve or disappear in response to dosage adjustment or the coadministration of propranolol.[81] Propranolol, which is more effective than other β-blockers in the treatment of lithium-induced tremor, is also useful in the treatment of familial or essential tremor.[82]

NON–DRUG-INDUCED MOVEMENT DISORDERS
Parkinson's Disease

Although the psychiatrist most frequently encounters parkinsonism as a drug-induced side effect, this condition was recognized many years before the advent of neuroleptic drugs.[5] Parkinson's disease is most frequently treated with cholinergic antagonists and dopamine agonists.[8] Patients with this disorder may have a flattened affect and appear depressed.[83] Some Parkinson patients who are depressed will experience relief of depression when treated with antiparkinsonian medication. Many patients with Parkinson's disease have a true depressive disorder due to their neurochemical deficit.[83] Decreased synthesis of dopamine and related neurotransmitters in the brain contribute not only to the biochemical defect which produces a movement disorder but a profound effect on affect and mood.[83] Significant improvement of depressive symptoms may be achieved by the use of SSRI or cyclic antidepressants in conjunction with antiparkinsonian therapy.[83] The selective inhibitor of MAO-B selegiline (deprenyl) is beneficial in the treatment of depression as well as the movement disorder components of Parkinson's disease.[84] Unfortunately, one of the most devastating aspects of Parkinson's disease is the development of dementia, which closely resembles Alzheimer's dementia and which may be worsened by antiparkinsonian medication.[83,85]

Although the dopamine precursor levodopa has produced dramatic therapeutic results in the management of Parkinson's disease, this drug has many limitations, including the potential to produce dyskinesias, "on-off" phenomena and an eventual diminution in therapeutic activity.[83,85] Levodopa can produce a drug-induced psychosis that may resemble acute mania clinically and which is frequently associated with grandiosity and hypersexuality.[85] Anticholinergic-type antiparkinsonian drugs may produce a toxic delirium, even in the absence of dementia.[83,85] Treatment of confusional states or psychosis in a Parkinson patient must take into account the possibility that a dementia is developing. The first step in management is to adjust the dosage of antiparkinsonian medications. Often hypersexuality and psychotic symptoms related to levodopa can be minimized or eliminated by dosage reduction. Confusional states can frequently be controlled by reducing or eliminating anticholinergic-type drugs. In the event that psychotic symptoms persist in spite of medication adjustment, low doses of high-potency antipsychotic drugs, such as risperidone 0.25 to 0.5 mg 1 to 4 times daily, may be useful.

Generally, low doses of high-potency agents are preferable to higher doses of low-potency agents since the latter may further confound the picture by adding to the anticholinergic toxicity of antiparkinsonian therapy. It must be recognized that the administration of any antipsychotic medication will inhibit the therapeutic benefits of levodopa and may transiently worsen the movement disorder. When depression occurs in a patient that is being treated with anticholinergic-type antiparkinsonian drugs, it is preferable to use SSRIs or cyclic antidepressants with lower anticholinergic potency in order to avoid an additive drug interaction. Nonselective MAOIs should not be used as antidepressants in levodopa-treated patients with Parkinson's disease. Lithium may be a useful drug in the management of affective disorders in patients with Parkinson's disease and there is no contraindication to using lithium in conjunction with any of the conventional antiparkinsonian therapies.

Multiple Sclerosis

Since patients suffering from multiple sclerosis (MS) may become paranoid, depressed, or hypomanic, they often come to the attention of psychiatrists prior to the diagnosis of their MS or later, as the clinical course of their illness waxes or wanes.[5,86] Psychiatrists should have a high index of suspicion for neurologic disease, as psychiatric manifestations may precede other manifestations of neurologic illnesses such as MS. Some patients with MS experience rapidly fluctuating mood and require treatment with lithium carbonate to control or prevent manic symptoms.[5] Depression in the course of MS may require antidepressant drug therapy, and the occurrence of paranoid ideation or psychotic symptoms may require the use of antipsychotic medications.[86] There is no evidence that any particular psychotropic medication needs to be avoided in patients with MS. Since neuroleptic drugs may produce movement disorders, their dosage should be started relatively low and titration should follow a more gradual course in a patient with MS. Since the clinical course of MS is so variable and its impact on the physiology of the nervous system is so profound, it is not surprising that this illness may present initially as a psychiatric condition, wherein the primary care physician believes the patient is hysterical; furthermore, depression is becoming increasingly recognized as a possible initial presenting complaint in patients with multiple sclerosis.[5,86]

Huntington's Disease

Huntington's disease is a genetically transmitted degenerative disease of the CNS.[7] In addition to choreiform movements and a variety of disturbances of the neuromuscular system, patients with Huntington's disease may have psychiatric symptoms including irritability, obstinance, moodiness, and lack of initiative.[5] These patients may be destructive or assaultive and may have difficulties in interpersonal relationships. As the condition progresses, these patients often become severely depressed. Dopamine levels in the corpus striatum are normal in patients with Huntington's whereas they are low in patients with Parkinson's disease.[7] Levodopa exacerbates, while dopamine antagonists alleviate, the choreic movements of Huntington's disease.[5,7] In the caudate nucleus of the brain in a choreic patient there is a decrease in synthesizing enzymes for GABA as well as acetylcholine-synthesizing enzymes.[7] There is a decrease in muscarinic cholinergic as well as serotonin receptor binding in the caudate nucleus. Sodium valproate, which increases brain GABA levels, has not been effective in controlling involuntary movements in patients with Huntington's disease. The potent cholinergic agonist arecoline has also failed to improve chorea, and has produced an exacerbation in patients with Huntington's disease.[87] With increasing availability of substances that affect neurotransmitter function in the brain, it is hoped that more effective therapeutic agents will be found for controlling the abnormal movements of Huntington's disease. Neuroleptics such as haloperidol[7] have some beneficial effect and may be of value in managing psychotic symptoms in these patients. Because of the previously noted disturbance in acetylcholine synthesis, it seems prudent to treat depressed patients with this condition with those antidepressants having lower anticholinergic potential.

Torsion Dystonia

Patients with no prior exposure to neuroleptic drugs may develop dystonic symptoms which at first may appear intermittently and then gradually worsen, become persistent, and affect multiple muscle groups of the extremities, trunk, and neck. Although some patients sporadically develop generalized dystonia, the condition more commonly occurs in persons of Ashkenazic Jewish background, where it is inherited as an autosomal dominant trait with low penetrance. This form of dystonia has been known in the past as dystonia muscularum deformans, and is now termed torsion dystonia.[3] Its initial presentation is most often a mild abnormality of gait, or spasticity and difficulty with fine motor coordination in the hands. Early in the course of dystonia the patient may experience abnormal muscle tone in one of the extremities, more often the foot or leg, which may make the psychiatrist think of this as a conversion reaction and therefore recommend psychotherapy. In one survey of 84 patients with torsion dystonia, 37 (44%) had originally been misdiagnosed with a psychiatric illness, most often hysterical conversion reaction.[4]

There is no evidence of a structural anatomical lesion in torsion dystonia, and there is no uniformly effective treatment available. Thalamic surgery has been used successfully in a number of patients but is generally associated with the need for repeated operation and the production of considerable speech disturbance.[3] The ability of psychotropic drugs that modify sensitivity of CNS receptor sites to improve or worsen symptoms in torsion dystonia suggests that this condition is related to an abnormality in neurotransmission. Biochemical studies have found a marked decrease in norepinephrine in the hypothalamus, mamillary body, subthalamic nucleus, and locus ceruleus as well as reduced serotonin in the dorsal raphe nucleus and decreased dopamine in the nucleus accumbens in dystonia.[88] During the course of the illness there is considerable variation in the severity of symptoms and in the response to medications. The variability observed during the course of a day or during a number of months may make the psychiatrist believe that this is an illness of psychiatric origin, or that psycho-therapy is actually producing a beneficial effect.[4] Haloperidol in relatively low doses will improve the abnormal movements and posturing in some patients, suggesting the possibility of a dopamine-related dysfunction.[3] Trihexyphenidyl, in doses far in excess of those ordinarily used in parkinsonism (20-100 mg daily), may gradually produce significant improvement in the dystonic patient's ability to walk and perform voluntary muscle acts.[89] Carbamazepine also has some ability to decrease dystonic movements, particularly thrusting of the limbs, which occurs frequently in torsion dystonia.[89]

Patients with this condition often have painful spasms of the muscles of the extremities, which may respond dramatically at times to the administration of baclofen in doses of 15 to 60 mg daily.[90] This agent appears to act partly through enhancement of GABA activity. Baclofen is also useful in the treatment of tardive dyskinesia, multiple sclerosis and cerebral palsy, where there is spasticity of skeletal muscles.[6] Baclofen may be beneficial for the management of anxiety in some patients without the risk of drug dependency.[14] One interesting pharmacologic aspect of torsion dystonia is the ability of these patients, often children, to tolerate massive doses of the potent anticholinergic agent trihexyphenidyl, without the development of confusion, delirium, or other abnormal behavioral states.[3] This suggests the likelihood of an abnormality in cholinergic transmission in dystonia, and also serves as an opportunity for clinicians to recognize that in varying clinical conditions a favorable drug response may require doses that are far in excess of the range we ordinarily consider usual therapeutic doses. This further suggests that receptor sites potentially have a tremendous variation in their sensitivity and affinity for various agonists and antagonists under different conditions.

Tourette's Syndrome

Another neurologic condition, which often comes to the attention of the psychiatrist, is Tourette's syndrome. These patients generally present with a variety of motor tics and compulsive involuntary utterance of noises, words, or foul language. Although psychotherapy will not alter the course of this condition, a variety of pharmacologic interventions, including haloperidol, pimozide, clonidine, and in some cases clonazepam may be beneficial. This condition is discussed in detail in chapter 15.

Myoclonus, Neurotoxicity, and Seizures

Myoclonus, which consists of abrupt, irregular muscle contractions and sudden jerky movements, may be a side effect of a variety of psychotropic drugs. Myoclonic jerks may occur in patients receiving cyclic antidepressants, SSRIs, or MAOIs. These phenomena tend to be dose-related and are discussed in detail in chapters 5 and 6. Neurotoxicity, including clouded consciousness, seizures, and EEG abnormalities, can occur during lithium therapy and during the combined use of lithium and neuroleptic drugs, as discussed in chapter 8. Seizures may occur at ordinary therapeutic doses of tricyclic and heterocyclic antidepressants and are frequent consequences of the overdose of these drugs. The presence of an underlying convulsive disorder increases the risk of inducing seizures during treatment with cyclic antidepressants and some neuroleptic drugs, particularly clozapine and chlorpromazine. Maprotiline, clomipramine, and bupropion are the antidepressants most likely to provoke seizures and should generally be avoided in patients with convulsive disorders. Drug-induced lowering of convulsive threshold and seizure induction are discussed in chapters 4, 5, and 10.

REFERENCES

1. Ross-Diefendorf A: *Clinical psychiatry* (adapted from Kraepelin's *Lehrbuch der Psychiatrie*). New York, Macmillan, 1907.
2. Bleuler E: *Textbook of psychiatry* (A.A. Brill, translator and editor). New York, Macmillan, 1924.
3. Fahn S: Generalized dystonia: concept and treatment. *Clin Neuropharmacol* 1986;9 (suppl 2):S37-S48.
4. Lesser RP, Fahn S: Dystonia: a disorder often misdiagnosed as a conversion reaction. *Am J Psychiatry* 1978;135:349-352.
5. Hopkins A: *Clinical neurology: a modern approach*. New York, Oxford University Press, 1993.
6. Jeste, DV, Wyatt RJ: *Understanding and treating tardive dyskinesia*. New York, Guilford Press, 1982.
7. Martin JB, Gusella JF: Huntington's disease: pathogenesis and management. *N Engl J Med* 1986;315:1267-1276.
8. LeWitt PA: New perspectives in the treatment of parkinson's disease. *Clin Neuropharmacol* 1986;9(suppl 1):S37-S46.
9. Kruse W: Treatment of drug induced extrapyramidal symptoms. *Dis Nerv Syst* 1960;21:79-81.
10. Freyhan FA: Psychomotility and parkinsonism in treatment with neuroleptic drugs. *Arch Neurol* 1957;78:465-472.
11. Orlov P, Kasparian G, DiMascio A, et al: Withdrawal of antiparkinson drugs. *Arch Gen Psychiatry* 1971;25:410-412.
12. Klett CJ, Caffey E Jr: Evaluating the long term need for antiparkinson drugs. *Arch Gen Psychiatry* 1971;25:410-412.
13. Rivera-Aalimlin L, Nasrallah H, Strauss J, et al: Clinical response and plasma levels: effects of dose, dosage schedules and drug interactions on plasma chlorpromazine levels. *Am J Psychiatry* 1976;133:636-642.
14. Bernstein JG: Drug Interactions. In Cassem NH (ed): *Massachusetts General Hospital Handbook of General hospital psychiatry*, ed 3. St Louis, Mosby, 1991, pp 571-610.
15. Rifkin A, Quitkin F, Kane J, et al: Are prophylactic antiparkinsonian drugs necessary? *Arch Gen Psychiatry* 1978;35:483-489.
16. Rifkin A, Quitkin F, Klein DF: Akinesia. *Arch Gen Psychiatry* 1975;32:672-674.
17. Winslow RS, Stillner V, Coons DJ, et al: Prevention of acute dystonic reactions in patients beginning high-potency neuroleptics. *Am J Psychiatry* 1986;143:706-710.

18. Boyer WF, Bakalar NH, Lake CR: Anticholinergic prophylaxis of acute haloperidol-induced acute dystonic reactions. *J Clin Psychopharmacol* 1987;7:164-166.
19. Menza MA, Murray GB, Holmes VF, et al: Decreased extrapyramidal symptoms with intravenous haloperidol. *J Clin Psychiatry* 1987;48:278-280.
20. Bernstein JG: Psychotropic drug prescribing. In Cassem NH (ed): *Massachusetts General Hospital Handbook of general hospital psychiatry,* ed 3. St Louis, Mosby, 1991, 527-569.
21. Gardos G, Cole CO, Tarsy D: Withdrawal syndromes associated with antipsychotic drugs. *Am J Psychiatry* 1978;135:1321-1324.
22. Mitchell JR: Discontinuation of antipsychotic drug therapy. *Psychosomatics* 1981;22:241-247.
23. Lipinski JF, Mallya G, Zimmerman P, et al: Fluoxetine-induced akathisia: clinical and theoretical implications. *J Clin Psychiatry* 1989;50:339-342.
24. Rothschild AJ, Locke CA: Reexposure to fluoxetine after serious suicide attempts by three patients: the role of akathisia. *J Clin Psychiatry* 1991;52:491-493.
25. Baldessarini RJ, Marsh E: Fluoxetine and side effects (letter). *Arch Gen Psychiatry* 1990;47: 191-192.
26. Black B, Uhde TW: Acute dystonia and fluoxetine. [Letter.] *J Clin Psychiatry* 1992;53:327.
27. Weiden PJ, Mann JJ, Haas G: Clinical non-recognition of neuroleptic-induced movement disorders: a cautionary study. *Am J Psychiatry* 1987, 144:1148-1153.
28. Ayd FJ Jr: A survey of drug induced extrapyramidal disorders. *JAMA* 1961:175;1054-1060.
29. Fann WE, Lake CR: Amantadine versus trihexyphenidyl in the treatment of neuroleptic-induced parkinsonism. *Am J Psychiatry* 1976;133:940-943.
30. McEvoy JP, McCue M, Spring B, et al: Effects of amantadine and trihexyphenidyl on memory in elderly normal volunteers. *Am J Psychiatry* 1987;144:573-577.
31. Nestelbaum Z, Siris SG, Rifkin A, et al: Exacerbation of schizophrenia associated with amantadine. *Am J Psychiatry* 1986;143:1170-1171.
32. Lipinski JF, Zubenko GS, Cohen BM, et al: Propranolol in the treatment of neuroleptic-induced akathisia. *Am J Psychiatry* 1984;141:412-415.
33. Adler L, Angrist B, Peselow E, et al: Efficacy of propranolol in neuroleptic-induced akathisia. *J Clin Psychopharmacol* 1985;5:164-166.
34. Adler LA, Peselow E, Rosenthal M, et al: A controlled comparison of the effects of propranolol, benztropine, and placebo on akathisia: an interim analysis. *Psychopharmacol Bull* 1993;29: 283-286.
35. Comaty JE: Propranolol treatment of neuroleptic-induced akathisia. *Psychiatr Ann* 1987;17: 150-155.
36. Adler LA, Angrist B, Peselow E, et al: Clonidine in neuroleptic-induced akathisia. *Am J Psychiatry* 1987;144:235-236.
37. Handwerker JF Jr, Palmer RF: Clonidine in the treatment of "restless legs" syndrome. *N Engl J Med* 1985;313:1228-1229.
38. Jeste DV, Grebb JA, Wyatt RJ: Psychiatric aspects of movement disorders and demyelinating diseases. In Hales RE, Frances AJ (eds): *APA annual review,* Washington DC, American Psychiatric Press, 1985, vol 4, pp 159-189.
39. Gelenberg AJ, Mandel MR: Catatonic reactions to high potency neuroleptic drugs. *Arch Gen Psychiatry* 1977;34:947-950.
40. Brenner I, Rheuban WJ: The catatonic dilemma. *Am J Psychiatry* 1978;135:1242-1243.
41. Caroff SN: The neuroleptic malignant syndrome. *J Clin Psychiatry* 1980;41:79-83.
42. Fann WE, Sullivan JL, Richman BW: Dyskinesias associated with tricyclic antidepressants. *Br J Psychiatry* 1976;128:490-493.
43. Ananth J: Tardive dyskinesia: myths and realities. *Psychosomatics* 1980;21 389-396.
44. Tepper SJ, Haas JF: Prevalence of tardive dyskinesia. *J Clin Psychiatry* 1979;40:508-516.
45. Morgenstern H, Glazer WM: Identifying risk factors for tardive dyskinesia among long-term outpatients maintained with neuroleptic medications. *Arch Gen Psychiatry* 1993;50:723-733.
46. Klawans HL, Carvey P, Tanner CM, et al: The pathophysiology of tardive dyskinesia. *J Clin Psychiatry* 1985;46 (4, sec 2):38-41.

47. Small JG, Milstein V, Marhenke JD, et al: Treatment outcome with tardive dyskinesia, neuroleptic sensitivity, and treatment-resistant psychosis. *J Clin Psychiatry* 1987;48:263-267.

48. Safferman A, Lieberman JA, Kane JM, et al: Update on the clinical efficacy and side effects of clozapine. *Schizophr Bull* 1991;17:247-261.

49. Marder SR, Meibach RC: Risperidone in the treatment of schizophrenia. *Am J Psychiatry* 1994;151:825-835.

50. Tanner CM, Klawans HL: Tardive dyskinesia: prevention and treatment. *Clin Neuropharmacol* 1986;9(suppl 2):576-585.

51. Dave M: Clozapine-related tardive dyskinesia. *Biol Psychiatry* 1994;35:886-887.

52. Lieberman JA, Saltz BL, Johns CA, et al: The effects of clozapine on tardive dyskinesia. *Br J Psychiatry* 1991;158:503-510.

53. Glazer WM, Morgenstern H, Doucette JT: Predicting the long-term risk of tardive dyskinesia in outpatients maintained on neuroleptic medications. *J Clin Psychiatry* 1993;54:133-139.

54. Gardos G, Casey DE, Cole C, et al: Ten-year outcome of tardive dyskinesia. *Am J Psychiatry* 1994;151:836-841.

55. Browne J, Solver H, Marin R, et al: The use of clonidine in the treatment of neuroleptic-induced tardive dyskinesia. *J Clin Psychopharmacol* 1986;6:88-92.

56. Thaker GV, Tamminga CA, Alphs LD, et al: Brain γ aminobutyric acid abnormality in tardive dyskinesia. *Arch Gen Psychiatry* 1987;44:522-529.

57. Mukherjee S, Rosen AM, Caracci G, et al: Persistent tardive dyskinesia in bipolar patients. *Arch Gen Psychiatry* 1986;43:342-346.

58. Wojcik JD, Falk WE, Fink JS, et al: A review of 32 cases of tardive dystonia. *Am J Psychiatry* 1991;148:1055-1059.

59. Munetz MR, Corners CL: Distinguishing akathisia and tardive dyskinesia: a review of the literature. *J Clin Psychopharmacol* 1983;3:343-350.

60. Barnes TRE, Braude WM: Akathisia variants and tardive dyskinesia. *Arch Gen Psychiatry* 1985;42:874-878.

61. Gardos G, Cole CO, Salomon M, et al: Clinical forms of severe tardive dyskinesia. *Am J Psychiatry* 1987;144:895-902.

62. Chiang E, Pitts WM, Rodriguez-Garcia M: Respiratory dyskinesia: review and case reports. *J Clin Psychiatry* 1985;46:232-234.

63. Weiner WJ, Goetz CG, Nausieda PA, et al: Respiratory dyskinesias: extrapyramidal dysfunction and dyspnea. *Ann Intern Med* 1978;88:327-331.

64. Jackson IV, Volavka J, James B, et al: The respiratory component of tardive dyskinesia. *Biol Psychiatry* 1980;15:485-487.

65. Glazer WM, Moore DC, Schooler NR, et al: Tardive dyskinesia: a discontinuation study. *Arch Gen Psychiatry* 1984;41:623-627.

66. Gardos G, Cole CO, Perenyi A, et al: Five-year follow-up study of tardive dyskinesia. *Adv Biochem Psychopharmacol* 1985;40:37-42.

67. Jeste DV, Lohr JB, Clark K, et al: Pharmacological treatments of tardive dyskinesia in the 1980s. *J Clin Psychopharmacol* 1988;8:38S-48S.

68. Lieberman JA: Neuroleptic-induced movement disorders and experience with clozapine in tardive dyskinesia. *J Clin Psychiatr Monogr* 1990;8:3-8.

69. Perenyi A, Arato M, Bagdy G, et al: Tiapride in the treatment of tardive dyskinesia: a clinical and biochemical study. *J Clin Psychiatry* 1985;46:229-231.

70. Freedman R, Bell J, Kirch D: Clonidine therapy for coexisting psychosis and tardive dyskinesia. *Am J Psychiatry* 1980;137:629-630.

71. Stewart RM, Rollins J, Beckham B, et al: Baclofen in tardive dyskinesia patients maintained on neuroleptics. *Clin Neuropharmacol* 1982;5:365-373.

72. Weis KJ, Ciraulo DA, Shader RI: Physostigmine test in rabbit syndrome and tardive dyskinesia. *Am J Psychiatry* 1980;137:627-628.

73. Jackson IV, Nuttal EA, Ibe IO, et al: Treatment of tardive dyskinesia with lecithin. *Am J Psychiatry* 1979;136:1458-1460.

74. Yassa R, Lal S: Prevalence of the rabbit syndrome, *Am J Psychiatry* 1986;143:656-657.
75. Stedman TJ, Whiteford HA, Eyles D, et al: Effects of nifedipine on psychosis and tardive dyskinesia in schizophrenic patients. *J Clin Psychopharmacol* 1991;11:43-47.
76. Moss LE, Neppe VM, Drevets WC: Buspirone in the treatment of tardive dyskinesia. *J Clin Psychopharmacol* 1993;13:204-209.
77. Dabiri LM, Pasta D, Darby JK, et al: Effectiveness of vitamin E for treatment of long-term tardive dyskinesia. *Am J Psychiatry* 1994;151:925-926.
78. Adler LA, Peselow E, Duncan E, et al: Vitamin E in tardive dyskinesia: time course of effect after placebo substitution. *Psychopharmacol Bull* 1993;29:371-374.
79. Flaherty JA, Lahmeyer HW: Laryngeal-pharyngeal dystonia as a possible cause of asphyxia with haloperidol treatment. *Am J Psychiatry* 1978;135:1414-1415.
80. McGreer PL, Boulding JE, Gibson WS, et al: Drug induced extrapyramidal pyramidal reactions. *JAMA* 1961;177:665-670.
81. Lapierre YD: Control of lithium tremor with propranolol. *Can Med Assoc J* 1976;114:619-624.
82. Findley LJ: The pharmacological management of essential tremor. *Clin Neuropharmacol* 1986;9(suppl 2):561-575.
83. Harvey NS: Psychiatric disorders in parkinsonism. I. *Psychosomatics* 1986;27:91-103.
84. Yu PH, Boulton AA: Clinical pharmacology of MAO-B inhibitors. In Kennedy SH (ed): *Clinical advances in monoamine oxidase inhibitor therapies.* Washington DC, American Psychiatric Press, 1994, 61-82.
85. Harvey NS: Psychiatric disorders in parkinsonism. II. *Psychosomatics* 1986;27:175-184.
86. Goodstein RK, Ferrell RB: Multiple sclerosis presenting as depressive illness. *Dis Nerv Syst* 1977;38:127-131.
87. Nutt JG, Robin A, Chase TN: Treatment of Huntington's disease with a cholinergic agonist. *Neurology* 1978;28:1061-1064.
88. Hornykiewicz O, Kish SJ, Becker LE, et al: Brain neurotransmitters in dystonia musculorum deformans. *N Engl J Med* 1986;315:347-353.
89. Greene P, Fahn S: Treatment of torsion dystonia. In Johnson RT (ed): *Current therapy in neurologic disease,* Philadelphia, Decker, 1990, pp 267-270.
90. Greene P: Baclofen in the treatment of dystonia. *Clin Neuropharmacol* 1992;15(4):276-288.

CHAPTER 12

Drug Interactions

OVERVIEW

1. One drug may alter absorption, metabolism, or excretion of another.
2. Drugs may have additive or inhibitory interactions at the receptor site.
3. Idiosyncratic interactions are those wherein one drug enhances or antagonizes the action of another through a mechanism that is not discernible.
4. Two or more psychotropic drugs from different therapeutic groups may increase the sedative, hypotensive, or anticholinergic effects of one another. These effects can also be increased by nonpsychotropic drugs.
5. Psychotropic drugs may prevent therapeutic effects of some nonpsychotropic drugs (eg, TCAs block hypotensive effects of guanadrel, guanethidine, and clonidine).
6. One drug may inhibit metabolism and increase serum concentration of another (eg, methylphenidate, neuroleptics, and serotonin-selective reuptake inhibitors can increase serum concentration, therapeutic effects or toxic effects of TCAs).
7. The most dangerous, potentially fatal, interaction of psychotropic drugs is the serotonin syndrome which occurs when an MAOI is taken along with an SSRI or meperidine.
8. ACE inhibitors (eg, captopril) may produce profound hypotension when coadministered with chlorpromazine.
9. Diuretics, dehydration, and hypokalemia can increase the risk of lithium toxicity.
10. Calcium channel blockers, ACE inhibitors, and carbamazepine administered with lithium can provoke lithium neurotoxicity.

Continued.

11. Erythromycin and calcium channel blockers can inhibit metabolism of carbamazepine and provoke carbamazepine neurotoxicity.
12. A detailed medication history before prescribing psychotropic drugs is essential, as is periodic review of all prescribed and nonprescribed medications the patient is taking.

Before prescribing any psychotropic medication, the physician must take a detailed medication history. This history must include information about favorable and adverse effects of psychotropic and nonpsychotropic medications the patient has taken in the past. It is essential to determine all medications the patient is currently receiving, including prescription drugs, over-the-counter remedies, and illicit drugs. Before any medication is prescribed, the clinician must consider potential interactions with other drugs. Since many psychotropic medications can produce adverse pharmacologic effects and since medications used to treat nonpsychiatric illnesses may yield behavioral complications, the psychiatrist must be familiar with a wide variety of unwanted drug reactions.[1]

Many patients require long-term maintenance on psychotropic drugs and, during the course of treatment, may develop unrelated illnesses for which medications are prescribed by other physicians. It is important to remind patients periodically during follow-up that they should notify the psychiatrist regarding the addition or subtraction of medications by other physicians whom they may consult. The initiation or discontinuation of a diuretic in a lithium-treated patient may significantly affect a previously stable serum lithium concentration.[1] Administration of erythromycin for treatment of a bacterial infection may provoke ataxia and diplopia in a patient who has previously been stabilized on carbamazepine.[1] Prescribing propranolol or captopril to a patient previously stabilized on chlorpromazine may produce hypotension.[1] Prescription of cimetidine to a patient who has been receiving a long-acting benzodiazepine or a tricyclic antidepressant (TCA) may cause an adverse reaction.[1] Many SSRIs, including fluoxetine, fluvoxamine, and paroxetine, are potent inhibitors of cytochrome P-450, as is cimetidine and will therefore increase serum concentration and potential toxic effects of TCAs, benzodiazepines, and carbamazepine. Although many interactions between psychotropic and nonpsychotropic drugs have relatively minor consequences, an increasing number of potentially serious interactions are being recognized. Unfortunately, some drug interactions, such as that of SSRIs or meperidine with monoamine oxidase inhibitors (MAOIs), can be fatal.[1] Many patients, when providing a medication history, do not consider over-the-counter remedies to be medication and will omit this information unless it is specifically requested by the physician. Since many over-the-counter drugs contain decongestants, antihistamines, and drugs with anticholinergic activity, the potential for these remedies to interact with psychotropic drugs is great and can be dangerous.

This chapter discusses mechanisms of drug interactions, cites specific drug interactions, and discusses the clinical management of drug interactions. Since new drugs are constantly being developed and marketed, the astute clinician will often have an opportunity to observe firsthand a new drug-drug interaction not yet reported in the literature. When a drug interaction appears to have occurred, the first step of management is to discontinue the suspected agent, even if the apparent interaction has not been documented in the medical literature.

MECHANISMS OF DRUG-DRUG INTERACTIONS

The three general mechanisms of drug-drug interactions include pharmacokinetic, pharmacologic, and idiosyncratic interactions.[2]

Pharmacokinetic Interactions

Pharmacokinetic interactions include those interactions involving drug absorption, wherein one drug may enhance or impair GI absorption of another. For example, drugs that reduce GI motility may slow the transit time of another drug, allowing it to be present in the GI tract for a longer period of time, and thereby enhancing systemic absorption of the second drug. Drugs may speed GI motility to the extent that there is decreased absorption of another therapeutic agent. Administration of cholestyramine resin or a gel antacid with phenothiazines, TCAs, or other psychotropic drugs leads to formation of an insoluble complex with resultant impaired absorption and therapeutic effect.[3] The cholesterol-lowering agent colestipol (Colestid) and psyllium-containing bulk laxatives will adsorb lithium, anticonvulsants, and most psychotropic drugs, significantly reducing their serum concentrations and therapeutic effects.

Another pharmacokinetic interaction involves the binding of a drug to plasma proteins, with the resultant availability of a lower concentration of free drug. If another drug is administered that displaces the first drug from plasma protein binding sites, the concentration and pharmacologic action of the first drug, now freed from binding sites, is increased. A common example of this is the displacement of warfarin from plasma protein binding sites by the coadministration of chloral hydrate.[3] In addition to protein binding, lipid solubility and binding are extremely important in that all psychotropic medications, with the exception of lithium carbonate, are highly lipid-soluble. As the fat-to-lean body mass ratio increases in an elderly patient, increased plasma concentrations are encountered with a variety of lipid-soluble psychotropic medications.[4]

Interactions at the site of biotransformation are another form of pharmacokinetic drug interactions. For example, barbiturates induce a variety of hepatic microsomal enzymes, thus enhancing the rate of metabolic degradation of many drugs, including TCAs and phenytoin. Inhibition of drug-metabolizing enzymes by one drug may increase plasma concentration and pharmacologic action of another drug. Inhibition of cytochrome P-450 IID6, which is central to oxidative metabolism of many psychotropic and nonpsychotropic drugs by fluoxetine, fluvoxamine, and paroxetine, is the most commonly encountered example of a metabolic interaction which is likely to produce clinically significant alterations in serum drug concentration as well as potentially dangerous adverse effects. MAOIs not only inhibit the activity of monoamine oxidase, enhancing the effects of a variety of sympathomimetic amines, but also impair metabolic degradation of unrelated drugs, including sedatives and narcotics, thereby increasing their pharmacologic effects.[3,4]

Finally, pharmacokinetic drug interactions at the site of drug elimination may enhance or impair the pharmacologic action of a variety of medicinal substances. Alkalinization of the urine by the administration of sodium bicarbonate, for instance, may hasten the excretion of long-acting barbiturates such as phenobarbital; this interaction may thus be useful in the treatment of phenobarbital overdoses. However, the same interaction may prevent the desired pharmacologic effect of phenobarbital in a patient with a seizure disorder.[3] Acidification of the urine by ascorbic acid or ammonium chloride increases the rate of excretion of amphetamines and phencyclidine hydrochloride (PCP). Thus the administration of acidifying agents may be an important therapeutic technique in the treatment of PCP or amphetamine intoxication.

Pharmacologic Interactions

Pharmacologic interactions occur when two simultaneously administered drugs act similarly on the same receptor site or antagonize the action of each other at the receptor site. At times, a desired therapeutic effect can be achieved by administering two drugs that act similarly at the same receptor site. Two drugs acting at the same receptor site in a similar fashion may, however, produce an unwanted additive drug interaction, as in the case of a patient developing an anticholinergic delirium when receiving a combination of neuroleptic, tricyclic antidepressant, and antiparkinsonian medication. Two drugs, each with important and desired therapeutic effects, may antagonize the action of each other, thus preventing a desired therapeutic response. The classical example of this kind of drug interaction occurs when a hypertensive patient on a regimen of guanethidine receives amitriptyline or another tricyclic antidepressant and thereby loses the antihypertensive effect of guanethidine. Tricyclic antidepressants block nerve reuptake mechanisms, which are necessary to achieve the antihypertensive action of guanethidine, clonidine, guanadrel, bethanidine, debrisoquine, and related drugs.

Idiosyncratic Reactions

Another form of drug-drug interaction is the idiosyncratic phenomenon wherein we do not understand the mechanism of interaction leading to either a diminished therapeutic response of one or the other drug or the occurrence of a toxic or adverse effect of one drug when administered in the presence of another. One form of idiosyncratic reaction involves allergic reactions to drugs wherein the patient has been sensitized by the prior administration of a similar medication so that immunologically mediated reaction occurs.[2,4] Although in the idiosyncratic category, allergic reactions are, by definition, largely unpredictable, familiarity with chemical structural similarities between various therapeutic agents may allow the clinician to avoid allergic reactions when the patient has previously experienced an allergic reaction to a chemically related substance.[4] The infrequent occurrence of elevated serum lithium concentration or lithium intoxication when this agent is combined with fluoxetine is an example of a nonallergic idiosyncratic drug interaction. As we gain better understanding of the mechanism of action and adverse effects of medications, hopefully we will encounter fewer idiosyncratic drug interactions. As we understand mechanisms better, we may be able to avoid combined therapeutic application of substances that have previously been demonstrated to interact with each other in an adverse fashion.

• • •

Having reviewed some mechanisms of common drug interactions, we now focus on specific interactions between various psychotropic drugs and medications administered for nonpsychiatric illness. The role of coexisting medical and neurologic disorders in the occurrence of adverse drug reactions, as well as the psychiatric complications of nonpsychotropic medications, is also discussed. Those reactions under discussion have been well documented in published literature and are common enough that the average clinician should be prepared to recognize them.

SEDATIVES

A wide variety of chemical compounds including barbiturates, benzodiazepines, antihistamines, meprobamate, glutethimide, ethchlorvynol, chloral hydrate, and ethanol, are used to treat anxiety and insomnia. Sedatives are also known as minor tranquilizers or antianxiety drugs.

All sedatives, with the exception of antihistamines, have the capability of producing a dose-related CNS depressant effect. Administration of excessive doses or their use in combination with each other or with other centrally acting drugs may produce CNS depression and respiratory depression. Patients suffering from chronic obstructive pulmonary disease are more likely to suffer prolonged respiratory depression. With the exception of the antihistamines, they are capable of inducing tolerance, physical dependence, and addiction when administered over a prolonged period of time. Patients suddenly withdrawn from any of these drugs following long-term use may suffer a withdrawal syndrome marked by seizures, delirium, high fever, and even death. Patients who have become dependent on any of the sedative drugs require careful gradual detoxification under medical supervision. Although benzodiazepines have relatively minor anticholinergic action, confusional states and prolonged sedation resulting from their use may be reversed by the cautious IV administration of physostigmine.[5]

Barbiturates, particularly phenobarbital, are potent enzyme inducers and may enhance metabolic degradation of a variety of drugs including phenytoin and anticoagulants, reducing their therapeutic effects.[3,6]

Benzodiazepines, which were initially believed to be relatively free of drug interactions, have been found to interact with a variety of therapeutic agents. Cimetidine inhibits benzodiazepine metabolism, producing increased and prolonged effects, particularly of longer-acting benzodiazepines such as chlordiazepoxide and diazepam.[7,8] Likewise, disulfiram, which decreases benzodiazepine metabolism, may enhance and prolong the pharmacologic action of these compounds.[8] When diazepam is administered along with neuromuscular blocking drugs such as gallamine or succinylcholine, prolonged neuromuscular blockade and paralysis result.[9]

Fluoxetine, like cimetidine, is a potent inhibitor of the drug metabolizing enzyme, cytochrome P-450 IID6 and through this mechanism will increase serum concentration, as well as duration and extent of pharmacologic activity of all benzodiazepines except lorazepam and oxazepam, which are not metabolized by this enzyme system.[10,11] The half life of fluoxetine and its active metabolite is 7 to 9 days, further increasing its impact on drug metabolism.[11] Fluvoxamine and paroxetine also inhibit benzodiazepine metabolism through this mechanism, but like cimetidine have much shorter half-lives than fluoxetine.[10]

Chloral hydrate, which displaces a variety of drugs from plasma protein binding sites may, by this mechanism, increase the anticoagulant effects of warfarin and related compounds, and may also interact with the diuretic furosemide to produce diaphoresis and a hypertensive reaction.[12]

Hydroxyzine, a sedating antihistamine without CNS depressant or addictive effect, has been reported to interact with phenothiazines, particularly thioridazine, tricyclic antidepressants, and lithium to increase the risk of cardiac arrhythmias.[13]

Estrogenic hormones appear to inhibit metabolic degradation of benzodiazepines and may thereby increase their plasma concentration and pharmacologic action.[8] The antituberculous drug isoniazid inhibits a variety of enzymes and may thereby increase the effect of coadministered benzodiazepines.[8] Rifampin, another antituberculous drug, is an enzyme inducer and may decrease the pharmacologic effect of benzodiazepines by enhancing their metabolism.[8]

Likewise, tobacco smoking may decrease benzodiazepine activity by enzyme induction.[8] For reasons which are at this time unclear, administration of benzodiazepines along with digoxin may increase the half-life of the latter drug.[8]

Oral contraceptives have been reported to decrease the effects of oral lorazepam, oxazepam, and temazepam, perhaps by altering their glucuronidation.[9] Metabolism of triazolobenzodiazepives, such as triazolam and alprazolam, appears to be inhibited by oral contraceptives.[9] Toxicity and serum concentration of triazolam and midazolam are increased by erythromycin, which appears to inhibit their metabolism.[9] Although benzodiazepines have commonly been used together with clozapine without adverse effects, a rare phenomenon of circulatory collapse and respiratory arrest has occurred with this combination.[14] This appears similar to but more severe than the phenomenon of deep sedation with shallow respiration and hypotension which is occasionally seen when benzodiazepines are combined with other low-potency neuroleptics. Table 12-1 demonstrates some of the currently recognized interactions between sedatives and other drugs.

ANTIPSYCHOTIC DRUGS

Antipsychotic or neuroleptic drugs include seven chemically distinct groups of therapeutic agents: phenothiazine, thioxanthene, butyrophenone, dihydroindolone, dibenzoxazepine, dibenzodiazepine, and benzisoxazole. These drugs alleviate hallucinations, delusions, disordered thinking, and other major manifestations of psychotic illness, as a result of their ability to block dopamine and/or $5\text{-}HT_2$ receptors in the brain. The various antipsychotic drugs differ from one another in their potency and selectivity with respect to dopamine and $5\text{-}HT_2$ receptor blockade. They also differ from one another in respect to their side effects. Chlorpromazine, clozapine, mesoridazine, and thioridazine are most sedating whereas haloperidol, risperidone, loxapine, molindone, and the piperazine phenothiazines such as trifluoperazine are much less sedating. If a highly sedating antipsychotic agent is used in combination with a barbiturate or benzodiazepine, the patient may experience excessive somnolence and an additive drug interaction. The patient may become difficult to arouse or may experience respiratory depression, particularly if there is underlying chronic obstructive pulmonary disease or if the patient is elderly.[4,6]

Chlorpromazine, clozapine, mesoridazine, and thioridazine are potent alpha-adrenergic blocking agents and may produce considerable hypotension. If these drugs are combined with coronary, cerebral, or peripheral vasodilators or with antihypertensive drugs, more profound hypotension may be encountered.[1,4] Likewise, the combination of the previously mentioned phenothiazines with an MAOI antidepressant can produce hypotension that may be difficult to reverse since the MAOI may increase the risk of any pressor agent administered and the phenothiazine will reduce the response when a pressor agent is administered.[4,6] Hypotension resulting from these drug interactions is best

Table 12-1 Drug interactions: sedatives

Drug	Interacts with	Effects	Mechanism
Benzodiazepines (except lorazepam, oxazepam)	Fluoxetine, fluvoxamine, paroxetine	Increased benzodiazepine effect	SSRIs inhibit cytochrome P-450 drug-metabolizing enzymes
Benzodiazepines	Clozapine	Circulatory collapse, respiratory arrest	Additive effect, mechanism unknown
Benzodiazepines (except oxazepam, lorazepam)	Cimetidine	Increased benzodiazepine effect	Decreased benzodiazepine metabolism
Benzodiazepines	Disulfiram	Increased benzodiazepine effect	Decreased benzodiazepine metabolism
Benzodiazepines	Antacids	Decreased benzodiazepine effect	Impaired GI absorption
Benzodiazepines	Isoniazid	Increased benzodiazepine effect	Enzyme inhibition
Benzodiazepines	Estrogens	Increased benzodiazepine effect	Enzyme inhibition
Benzodiazepines	Tobacco smoking	Decreased benzodiazepine effect	Enzyme induction
Benzodiazepines	Rifampin	Decreased benzodiazepine effect	Enzyme induction
Benzodiazepines	Digoxin	Increased digoxin half-life	Unknown
Barbiturates	Phenytoin	Decreased phenytoin effects	Enzyme induction
Barbiturates	Anticoagulants (warfarin, dicumarol)	Decreased anticoagulant effect	Enzyme induction
Barbiturates	β-Blockers	Decreased β-blocker plasma level	Enzyme induction
Barbiturates	Tricyclic antidepressants	Decreased antidepressant effect	Decreased tricyclic antidepressant serum concentration
Chloral hydrate	Anticoagulants (warfarin, dicumarol)	Increased warfarin effect	Trichloroacetic acid displaces warfarin from plasma protein
Chloral hydrate	Furosemide	Diaphoresis, hot flashes, hypertension	Uncertain

Continued.

Table 12-1 Drug interactions: sedatives — cont'd.

Drug	Interacts with	Effects	Mechanism
Diazepam	Gallamine, succinylcholine	Prolonged neuromuscular blockade	Uncertain
Ethanol	CNS depressants	CNS depression	Additive effect
Hydroxyzine	Phenothiazines, tricyclic antidepressants, lithium carbonate	Cardiac toxicity	Increased effect on cardiac repolarization
Phenytoin	Anticoagulants	Phenytoin toxicity	Decreased phenytoin metabolism
Triazolam	Erythromycin	Increased triazolam plasma level	Metabolism of triazolam inhibited

treated by keeping the patient in a recumbent position and administering fluids intravenously, with careful patient monitoring to avoid congestive heart failure, which may result from excessive fluid replacement. If pressor agents must be administered, phenylephrine is the safest to employ, but it must be used cautiously because of the need to balance reduced sensitivity to the drug as a result of phenothiazines versus the increased sensitivity to the drug resulting from monoamine oxidase inhibition. Epinephrine should be avoided because it may, as a result of its β-adrenergic stimulant effect, induce further hypotension. The use of indirect-acting agents, such as metaraminol, which release catecholamines from the adrenal medulla, may be associated with unwanted hypertensive and arrhythmic effects.[15]

Haloperidol has the least α-adrenergic blocking effect and is least likely among antipsychotic drugs to induce hypotension.[16] The potential of an additive interaction with vasodilators or antihypertensive drugs is less with haloperidol than with the previously mentioned phenothiazines. Haloperidol and the piperazine phenothiazines such as trifluoperazine are safer if used in conjunction with MAOIs than are the lower-potency more hypotensive neuroleptics. When used alone, haloperidol is much less likely than other neuroleptics to induce unwanted hypotensive effects. When phenothiazines are used in combination with a variety of anesthetics such as halothane, enflurane, and isoflurane, there is considerable possibility of a profound hypotensive reaction; therefore, this drug combination should be avoided.[17] Phenothiazines may produce an additive drug interaction with succinylcholine resulting in prolonged neuromuscular blockade in association with anesthesia employing this muscle relaxant.[3,17]

Numerous drugs prescribed by psychiatrists exert a pronounced anticholinergic effect. Most antiparkinsonian medications exert their therapeutic action as a result of cholinergic blockade. Tricyclic and heterocyclic antidepressants have potent anticholinergic activity. Among antipsychotic drugs, clozapine, thioridazine, and mesoridazine can cause pronounced cholinergic blockade. Chlorpromazine is also strongly anticholinergic while the piperazine phenothiazines including trifluoperazine and the butyrophenone compound haloperidol exert much less anticholinergic action. Clinicians are generally aware that anticholinergic drugs produce blurred vision, dry mouth, tachycardia, constipation, and urinary retention. Anticholinergic agents may also have a central effect including the production of stuttering speech and impaired memory and concentration.[4] Since patients receiving neuroleptic drugs frequently are also taking antiparkinsonian medication, and, tricyclic antidepressants as well, it is possible that the patient will experience excessive cholinergic blockade as a result of the interaction of these psychotropic drugs.

Patients receiving neuroleptic drugs in combination with tricyclic antidepressants should generally not be given an antiparkinsonian medication. The latter will generally be unnecessary for controlling extrapyramidal side effects and will certainly add to the potential for an adverse central or peripheral anticholinergic syndrome. Clinicians must realize that patients often take nonprescription medications in addition to those which have been prescribed. Many over-the-counter cold remedies, tranquilizers, and sleeping medications contain potent anticholinergic agents and antihistamines. It is not inconceivable that a patient may therefore be taking at any given time three to five separate medications with anticholinergic activity, thus heightening the risk of an anticholinergic delirium or of peripheral manifestations of cholinergic blockade including tachycardia and dysrhythmias. Similar toxic anticholinergic syndromes are commonly seen in patients who have taken an overdose of a variety of prescribed and over-the-counter medications. Physostigmine is a cholinesterase inhibitor that may be used as a diagnostic test to assess anticholinergic toxicity.[4]

Neuroleptic drugs, by virtue of their ability to block dopamine receptor sites, commonly induce a variety of extrapyramidal effects including stiffness, tremors, increased salivation, and a parkinsonian gait with small steps and reduced accessory movements. The high-potency antipsychotic agents such as piperazine phenothiazines and haloperidol are more likely to produce acute extrapyramidal effects than are the lower-potency agents such as chlorpromazine clozapine and thioridazine. The simultaneous administration of antiparkinsonian medications including trihexyphenidyl or benztropine is useful to reduce or avoid these unwanted extrapyramidal effects of antipsychotic medications. Patients who have Parkinson's Disease are likely to have the symptoms of their movement disorder worsened by the administration of neuroleptic drugs, although such medications may be essential if the patient has a concurrent psychotic illness. In a patient with Parkinson's Disease, it may be worthwhile to initiate antipsychotic drug treatment with a lower-potency agent such as chlorpromazine, clozapine, or thioridazine rather than a higher-potency dopamine blocker.

Patients receiving levodopa for Parkinson's Disease may have the beneficial effect of that medication rather quickly reversed if neuroleptic medication is prescribed.[9] Despite its beneficial effects, levodopa itself may produce psychotic symptoms. In a Parkinson patient who requires antipsychotic chemotherapy, it may be best to utilize anticholinergic antiparkinsonian medications alone or in combination with amantadine to control symptoms of the movement disorder rather than continue the administration of levodopa in conjunction with antipsychotic chemotherapy. A levodopa-treated Parkinson patient who develops psychotic symptoms may best be treated by terminating levodopa therapy, and observing for evidence of behavioral improvement before initiating antipsychotic drugs unless the situation is urgent. In such patients temporary administration of lorazepam may control agitation while awaiting clearance of a potential toxic levodopa reaction.

Although it is well known that tricyclic antidepressants may inhibit the antihypertensive effects of guanadrel, guanethidine, clonidine, and related drugs, neuroleptics such as chlorpromazine also block nerve reuptake mechanisms and may antagonize the therapeutic action of these antihypertensive medications.[9] Another interaction involving nueroleptics and antihypertensives is the occurrence of a transient dementia in patients receiving haloperidol in combination with methyldopa.[18] This interaction appears to result from the ability of the antipsychotic drug to block dopamine receptor sites and the antihypertensive drug to reduce neurotransmitter synthesis.[18] The ability of methyldopa to reduce catecholaminergic neurotransmitter synthesis appears to explain its ability to induce severe depression when used in the treatment of hypertension.[19] This finding is certainly reminiscent of reports nearly 40 years ago that reserpine administered for the treatment of hypertension could cause profound depression and suicidal behavior.[20]

Since phenothiazines may exert prominent α-adenergic blockade, their administration in conjunction with epinephrine may result in a reversal of the pressor action of epinephrine with the occurrence of a hypotensive reaction due to unopposed β-adenergic stimulation induced by epinephrine.[4,15] Tricyclic antidepressants have long been associated with disturbances of cardiac rhythm.[21] Some phenothiazines, most notably thioridazine and chlorpromazine, have been associated with the occurrence of cardiac arrhythmias.[22] An important and potentially dangerous drug interaction may occur when thioridazine is administered simultaneously with quinidine, resulting in depressed myocardial function and dysrhythmias, presumably due to the fact that both drugs exert similar electrophysiologic effects on the myocardium.[17] It is likely that other antiarrhythmics and other phenothiazines may interact in a similar fashion based on our knowledge of their electrophysiologic effects. Significant ECG effects and interactions with cardiac drugs have not been reported for haloperidol even though the latter drug has been used in a number of studies in rather high dosage in patients following acute myocardial infarction or open heart surgery.[16]

Colestid, cholestyramine, psyllium, activated charcoal, and antacids all decrease GI absorption, serum concentration, and therapeutic effects of phenothiazines.[9] The common practice of mixing liquid preparations of phenothiazines with various beverages such as fruit juices to increase palatability presents considerable risk since many juices and other beverages when mixed with liquid phenothiazines result in the formation of an insoluble precipitant whose GI absorption appears to be poor, resulting in the possibility of therapeutically inadequate serum drug concentrations.[6] Liquid preparations of haloperidol are compatible with beverages, do not form insoluble precipitates, and are readily absorbed from the GI tract. Cigarette smoking has been reported to decrease the antipsychotic action of chlorpromazine, due to increased chlorpromazine metabolism.[9]

Clozapine is the neuroleptic which has the greatest ability to lower seizure threshold and to cause seizures, particularly at doses exceeding 300 mg per day.[23] Among other neuroleptics, chlorpromazine presents the most significant convulsive risk.[24] Any neuroleptic taken in overdose can produce seizures; furthermore, increased serum concentration of neuroleptics which may occur when fluoxetine is coadministered may cause seizures.[9,24,25] Thioridazine and haloperidol are least likely to provoke seizures in normal persons and in those with convulsive disorders. Chlorpromazine and clozapine should generally be avoided in patients who have convulsive disorders. Patients receiving any neuroleptic drug in combination with an anticonvulsant should have periodic monitoring of the latter to be certain that pharmacotherapy is adequate and thereby reduce the risk of seizures.

Decreased antipsychotic action has been reported in patients receiving neuroleptics along with carbamazepine, dichloralphenazone, griseofulvin, and rifampin, presumably due to increased metabolic degradation of the neuroleptic.[9] Although the mechanism is unknown, phenylbutazone administered along with neuroleptics may produce marked drowsiness and sedation.[8] Increased CNS toxicity has been reported when lithium is combined with neuroleptic drugs; however, this is generally seen only when high doses of either or both drugs are administered.[9] When both drugs are administered cautiously and the patient is carefully monitored, there does not appear to be undue risk from this commonly utilized medication combination.

Simultaneous administration of chlorpromazine and propranolol has been shown to cause a significant increase in plasma concentrations of both drugs, along with increased pharmacologic action.[26] Two studies have demonstrated a three- to fivefold increase in plasma thioridazine concentration when this drug is administered along with propranolol.[27,28] In one of these studies, coadministration of propranolol and haloperidol failed to alter plasma concentrations of haloperidol.[28] The implication is that when propranolol is administered along with a neuroleptic to control agitated or violent behavior, it would be safer to utilize haloperidol than thioridazine.

SSRIs are known to produce tremors; and extrapyramidal symptoms, including dystonic reactions, have occasionally been reported. Furthermore, several of these drugs, including fluoxetine, fluvoxamine, and paroxetine, impair metabolism of many drugs including neuroleptics. Therefore it is not surprising that there have been several reports in the literature of increased extrapyramidal side effects when neuroleptics are combined with SSRIs.[29,30]

Low-potency, more hypotensive phenothiazines, such as chlorpromazine, clozapine, mesoridazine, and thioridazine, should not be administered with ACE inhibitors. The multitude of currently marketed ACE inhibitors include benazepril, captopril, enalapril, fasinopril, lisinopril, quinapril, and ramipril. Profound, symptomatic hypotension was reported in a patient simultaneously receiving chlorpromazine and captopril.[31] The sympathomimetic amine phenylpropanolamine has been reported to produce ventricular arrhythmias when administered along with thioridazine.[8] Interactions between antipsychotic drugs and other commonly used medications are shown in Table 12-2.

Table 12-2 Drug interactions: antipsychotics

Drug	Interacts with	Effect	Mechanism
Neuroleptics	Levodopa	Decreased levodopa effect	Dopamine blockade
Neuroleptics	Lithium	Increased CNS toxicity	Synergism
Neuroleptics	Phenytoin	Phenytoin toxicity	Synergism
Neuroleptics	Phenylbutazone	Increased drowsiness	Unknown
Neuroleptics	Carbamazepine, dichloralphenazone, griseofulvin, rifampin	Decreased neuroleptic effect	Increased metabolism
Neuroleptics	All SSRIs	Increased EPS	Serotonergic mediated reduction of DA release
Neuroleptics	Fluoxetine, fluvoxamine, paroxetine	Increased neuroleptic serum level and effects	SSRI inhibition of cytochrome P-450–mediated drug metabolism
Phenothiazines (especially clozapine, chlorpromazine, thioridazine, mesoridazine)	Antihypertensive drugs and coronary vasodilators	Hypotension	Peripheral vasodilation
Phenothiazines	Epinephrine	Hypotension, vasodilation	α-Adrenergic blockade and β-adrenergic stimulation
Phenothiazines	Monoamine oxidase inhibitors	Hypotension	α-Adrenergic blockade and direct vasodilation
Phenothiazines	Anesthetics: enflurane, isoflurane, halothane	Hypotension	Potentiation of vasodilation, myocardial depression

Continued.

Table 12-2 Drug interactions: antipsychotics—cont'd.

Drug	Interacts with	Effect	Mechanism
Phenothiazines	Opiates, sedatives, hypnotics, barbiturates, benzodiazepines, antihistamines	Prolonged somnolence, respiratory depression	Additive CNS depression and hypotension
Phenothiazines	Succinylcholine	Prolonged neuromuscular blockade	Phenothiazines decrease levels of cholinesterase
Phenothiazines	Antacids, tea, coffee, milk, fruit juice, cholestyramine resin	Decreased phenothiazine effect	Impaired GI absorption
Thioridazine	Quinidine	Cardiac arrhythmias, myocardial depression	Additive myocardial and electrophysiologic effects
Chlorpromazine	Guanethidine, clonidine	Decreased antihypertensive effect	Chlorpromazine inhibits uptake mechanisms
Chlorpromazine	Cigarette smoking	Decreased antipsychotic effect	Increased chlorpromazine metabolism
Haloperidol	Methyldopa	Dementia	Dopamine blockade and decreased catecholamine synthesis
Chlorpromazine, thioridazine	Propranolol	Increased effect of both	Increased plasma levels
Haloperidol	Propranolol	No interaction	No interaction
Chlorpromazine	Captopril, enalapril	Hypotension	Vasodilation
Thioridazine	Phenylpropanolamine	Ventricular arrhythmias	Catecholamine release
Clozapine	Benzodiazepines	Circulatory collapse, respiratory arrest	Additive effect, mechanism unknown
Clozapine	Fluoxetine, fluvoxamine, paroxetine	Increased risk of seizures	Inhibition of clozapine metabolism by SSRIs

TRICYCLIC AND HETEROCYCLIC ANTIDEPRESSANTS

Although various mechanisms of action have been proposed for tricyclic and heterocyclic antidepressants, the most widely accepted is based on their ability to inhibit nerve reuptake of either norepinephrine or serotonin or both. Depressed patients respond differentially to drugs affecting one or the other of these transmitters. In addition to their different effects on reuptake mechanisms, they differ from one another in their propensity to produce various side effects. The tricyclic drugs, amitriptyline and doxepin; the tetracyclic antidepressant, maprotiline; and trazodone, are the most sedating and, are most likely to produce an additive interaction with other sedatives including barbiturates, benzodiazepines, and neuroleptics, potentially causing excessive drowsiness.

Tricyclic and heterocyclic antidepressant drugs all produce anticholinergic effects. Amitriptyline, imipramine, and trimipramine are relatively more anticholinergic than doxepin, amoxapine, maprotiline, trazodone, and desipramine as discussed in chapter 4. The anticholinergic actions of one type of medication are additive with the cholinergic receptor blocking effects of other drugs, be they neuroleptic, antiparkinsonian, or antisecretory. The central and peripheral manifestations of cholinergic blockade have been described in chapter 10. Physostigmine administration is a useful diagnostic test to assess anticholinergic toxicity due to antidepressant drugs. In prescribing medication for the elderly patient or the patient who must receive other anticholinergic agents, those drugs having the least anticholinergic potency are safest.

Since tricyclic antidepressants inhibit nerve reuptake of biogenic amines centrally as well as peripherally, they may increase myocardial norepinephrine; this in conjunction with their anticholinergic action, and their quinidinelike effect, may cause cardiac arrhythmias.[4,21] Arrhythmias can be characterized by the presence of atrial or ventricular premature beats and in some cases, the latter may be multifocal or give rise to short runs of ventricular tachycardia.[32] The arrhythmogenic effect of tricyclic antidepressants is more likely to occur in those individuals with underlying coronary or valvular heart disease, and particularly in patients who have had a recent myocardial infarction.[32,33] Patients who have had occasional extrasystoles may experience an increased frequency of these abnormal beats during the course of tricyclic antidepressant drug therapy. Patients receiving antidepressants in conjunction with sympathomimetic amines such as isoproterenol or ephedrine for asthma, or stimulants such as amphetamines, are more likely to experience cardiac arrhythmias.[4,21,33] Likewise, the elderly are more apt to experience the dysrhythmic effect of tricyclic antidepressants.

In contradistinction to these tricyclic effects, their ability to exert a quinidinelike membrane-stabilizing action may actually suppress atrial or ventricular premature beats.[32,33] Furthermore, the membrane-stabilizing effect of tricyclics may be additive with a similar mechanism produced by antiarrhythmic drugs including quinidine, procainamide, and disopyramide.

This additive interaction may not only suppress cardiac dysrhythmias, but may also cause depressed myocardial contractility and congestive heart failure.[21,32] Indeed, even when administered alone in conventional therapeutic dosage, tricyclic antidepressants may depress the myocardium with the resultant worsening of previously existing congestive heart failure or the appearance of heart failure de novo.[21] Tricyclic antidepressants and some neuroleptics, particularly thioridazine and chlorpromazine, may produce a variety of ECG changes including ST segment depression, and decreased voltage, inverted, or biphasic T waves.[34] Conduction disturbances may also occasionally occur in patients receiving tricyclic antidepressants or thioridazine.[32,34]

Although tricyclic antidepressants do not produce alpha-adrenergic blockade, they commonly cause postural hypotension, due to their ability to relax vascular smooth muscle, resulting in peripheral vasodilation.[32,34] This hypotensive effect of tricyclic antidepressants may be additive with a variety of vasodilator and antihypertensive medications, yielding uncomfortable or even dangerous hypotensive reactions.[4] Although hypertensive reactions have been attributed to the interaction of tricyclic with MAOI antidepressants, the risk of enhanced hypotension occurring with this combined regimen is greater than the risk of a hypertensive reaction.[4,6]

When tricyclic antidepressants are administered to patients receiving guanadrel, guanethidine, clonidine, bethanidine, or debrisoquin, the antihypertensive actions of these drugs are inhibited and blood pressure will increase.[3,4] This interaction is due to the ability of tricyclic drugs to inhibit nerve reuptake, not only of norepinephrine and serotonin, but also of these antihypertensive drugs.[4,15] It was reported previously that doxepin does not antagonize the antihypertensive action of these drugs. Pharmacologic evidence indicates that doxepin will antagonize those antihypertensive drugs that require active uptake into nerve endings.[15]

One useful drug-drug interaction involving tricyclic antidepressants and phenothiazines is the ability of phenothiazines to slow the metabolism of tricyclic antidepressants, thereby enhancing the therapeutic effects of the latter.[35] Some depressed patients who do not respond to tricyclic antidepressants when administered alone achieve a favorable response when these drugs are administered in combination with low doses of phenothiazines, as discussed in chapter 5.

Anticonvulsant drugs, including phenytoin and phenobarbital, may increase the rate of tricyclic antidepressant metabolism, thereby decreasing the antidepressant effect.[9] As in the case of chlorpromazine, clozapine, and other phenothiazines, the tricyclic antidepressants lower seizure threshold and may provoke seizures when used in ordinary therapeutic dosage in patients with convulsive disorders. Convulsions are a common manifestation of antidepressant drug overdose. Maprotiline, clomipramine, and bupropion have a greater ability to lower seizure threshold and provoke seizures than other antidepressants.[24,36] Stimulants, including amphetamines and methylphenidate, inhibit metabolism of tricyclic antidepressants, thereby increasing both tricyclic serum concentration and therapeutic response.[8]

Cimetidine and fluoxetine inhibit cytochrome P-450–mediated hepatic drug oxidation, thereby impairing the metabolism of many therapeutic agents, including benzodiazepines, neuroleptics, tricyclics, and phenytoin.[9] Cimetidine also reduces hepatic metabolism of high-clearance drugs such as propranolol, imipramine, and nortriptyline.[37] Hepatic metabolism of doxepin is also impaired by cimetidine.[38] Tricyclic antidepressant plasma levels are increased when these drugs are coadministered with cimetidine or fluoxetine which can cause adverse effects and potentially dangerous toxicity.[9] Disulfiram and isoniazid both inhibit metabolic degradation of tricyclic antidepressants and may thereby increase plasma levels and toxicity of tricyclic drugs.[8] Tobacco smoking, which is known to induce drug-metabolizing enzymes, may decrease plasma concentrations of tricyclic antidepressants along with levodopa and may produce agitation, tremor, and rigidity.[8] Table 12-3 reviews some of the interactions between tricyclic antidepressants and other drugs.

SEROTONIN-SELECTIVE REUPTAKE INHIBITORS

Fluoxetine, fluvoxamine, and paroxetine are potent inhibitors of cytochrome P-450 IID6 as is cimetidine, the latter drug however has a half-life of only 2 hours.[10,15] Fluoxetine and its metabolite, which is equiactive, have a combined half-life of approximately 7 days, while fluvoxamine and paroxetine have half-lives of 15 and 21 hours respectively with no active metabolites.[10] It can therefore be expected that these drugs will all have significant ability to inhibit the metabolism of any coadministered drug which is metabolized by oxidation utilizing the cytochrome P-450 enzyme system.[39,40] Since fluoxetine and its metabolite have such long half-lives, their impact on drug metabolism is certainly greater than cytochrome P-450 inhibitors with shorter half-lives.[10] Indeed, the half-life of fluoxetine indicates that some active drug may remain for 5 or more weeks after administration of the parent compound is discontinued, with longer-duration effects being present in patients who have received higher doses.[11] Coadministration of fluoxetine has been reported to increase serum concentrations of tricyclic antidepressants from to 2 to 11 times.[29,41,42] Likewise, serum concentrations of neuroleptics and benzodiazepines, with the exception of lorazepam and oxazepam which are metabolized by glucuronidation rather than oxidation, will be increased by fluoxetine.[11,28] The duration of significant serum concentrations of drugs which interact with fluoxetine will be prolonged.[42] Any adverse or toxic effect of any drug whose serum concentration is increased by fluoxetine, fluvoxamine, or paroxetine will be increased.[10,11,29] When used at ordinary therapeutic dosage, tricyclics and neuroleptics combined with fluoxetine will produce greater cardiovascular, autonomic, and convulsive effects.[29,41,42] Patients who take a modest overdose of a tricyclic antidepressant during or within a few weeks following

Table 12-3 Drug interactions: tricyclic antidepressants (TCAs)

Interacts with	Effect	Mechanism
Direct-acting sympathomimetics (epinephrine, norepinephrine)	Hypertension, arrhythmias	Inhibition of neuronal uptake mechanisms
Stimulants; amphetamines, methylphenidate	Increased antidepressant effect	Inhibition of TCA metabolism, increased brain levels of stimulants
Stimulants, including cocaine	Agitation, psychosis	Same mechanisms
Anticonvulsants	Decreased effect of TCA	Increased TCA metabolism
Anticonvulsants	Seizures	TCAs lower seizure threshold
CNS depressants: alcohol, anesthetics, barbiturates, benzodiazepines	Increased CNS depression, hypotension	Additive CNS depressant effects, adrenergic blockade and direct vasodilation
Alcohol, barbiturates, chloral hydrate	Decreased TCA effect	Lowered TCA serum concentration, enhanced TCA metabolism
Cimetidine, disulfiram, isoniazid	Increased TCA effect, toxicity	Inhibition of TCA metabolism
Levodopa	Agitation, tremor, rigidity	Dopaminergic effect
Tobacco smoking	Decreased TCA plasma level	Enzyme induction
Diazepam, antipsychotics, antiparkinsonian drugs, antisecretory drugs	Increased TCA effect, confusion, delirium, tachycardia, urinary retention, ileus	Decreased TCA metabolism, anticholinergic toxicity
Phenothiazines	Enhanced effects of both drugs	Decrease metabolism of each other
Antihypertensives: guanadrel, guanethidine, clonidine, bethanidine, debrisoquin	TCAs block antihypertensive effects; hypertension may occur	TCAs inhibit nerve uptake of these antihypertensive drugs
Antiarrhythmic drugs: quinidine, procainamide, disopyramide, lidocaine, propranolol, etc.	Myocardial depression, decreased contractility, dysrhythmias	Additive quinidinelike effects on myocardium and conduction system
Monoamine oxidase inhibitors (MAOIs)	Increased TCA effect; increase or decrease blood pressure	Monoamine oxidase inhibition with reuptake blockade
SSRIs: fluoxetine, fluvoxamine, paroxetine	Increased TCA effect and serum concentration; potentially serious TCA toxicity	Cytochrome P-450 inhibition by most SSRIs

fluoxetine therapy may have a fatal result, as has been reported in the literature and as I have observed in the course of clinical consultations.[29,41,42] Adverse interactions of fluvoxamine or paroxetine would not be expected to occur longer than 5 to 7 days following their discontinuation.[10] In severe obsessive-compulsive disorder, fluoxetine may be combined with clomipramine or in some cases with clozapine; it is important to recognize that both of these agents have considerable potential to induce seizures which will of course be increased if fluoxetine is included in the regimen.[23,24,25] Bupropion is a useful antidepressant which is associated with a significant convulsive risk in higher doses; therefore if a patient has been receiving fluoxetine and the regimen is changed to bupropion, the latter needs to be started at a lower than usual dosage with more gradual dosage titration.[11,24]

The most dangerous drug interaction in psychiatry is the combination of ANY serotonin-selective reuptake inhibitor, including fluoxetine, fluvoxamine, paroxetine, sertraline, venlafaxine, or the serotonergic TCA clomipramine, with ANY monoamine oxidase inhibitor, including phenelzine, tranylcypromine, selegiline, and moclobemide.[43] This drug interaction, which does not depend on cytochrome P-450 inhibition, consists of central nervous system, cardiovascular, and autonomic symptoms due to excessive serotonin activity, known as the serotonin syndrome as discussed in chapter 10.[43] In this syndrome, which is potentially fatal, there is confusion, agitation, myoclonus, hyperreflexia, diaphoresis, shivering, tremor, diarrhea, ataxia, headache, autonomic dysfunction with bradycardia or tachycardia, hypotension or hypertension, hyperpyrexia, and seizures which may progress to status epilepticus.[43,44] There may be associated myoglobinuria, renal failure, and disseminated intravascular coagulation.[45] A similar syndrome has long been known to occur when meperidine is combined with monoamine oxidase inhibitors.[46]

In addition to increasing serum concentrations and duration of pharmacologic effects of tricyclic antidepressants, bupropion, and benzodiazepines, fluoxetine also increases serum concentration and CNS depressant effects of barbiturates.[11] Fluoxetine also increases serum concentrations of valproate and carbamazepine, and may lead to toxic effects of either of these mood stabilizing drugs, which are often prescribed for patients who are also receiving antidepressant drugs such as fluoxetine.[47,48] Fluoxetine has been reported to potentiate calcium channel blockers[49] and to antagonize anxiolytic effects of buspirone.[50] Lithium is often combined with fluoxetine and may enhance its antidepressant effect;[51] however, lithium toxicity has also been reported when this ion is combined with fluoxetine.[52] Since lithium is excreted by the kidney and not metabolically changed in the body, the interaction of fluoxetine is not metabolic in nature but may result from additive neurotoxicity of these two drugs, particularly since signs of lithium toxicity in fluoxetine-treated patients often occur with ordinary therapeutic serum lithium concentrations and include CNS manifestations such as seizures. Sertraline has a minor ability to interact with tricyclics, which is terminated within days of discontinuing the drug,[53]

Table 12-4 Drug interactions: fluoxetine (may also occur with fluvoxamine and paroxetine)

Interacts with	Effect	Mechanism
Antidepressants: TCA, trazodone	Increased antidepressant effect and side effects; potentially serious toxicity with overdose	Inhibition of cytochrome P-450 (increased TCA serum concentration)
Clomipramine, maprotiline, bupropion, clozapine	Increased risk of seizures	Inhibition of cytochrome P-450, (increased serum drug concentration)
Barbiturates	Increased CNS depressant effects	Inhibition of cytochrome P-450
Benzodiazepines (except lorazepam and oxazepam)	Increased CNS depressant effects	Inhibition of cytochrome P-450
Haloperidol/neuroleptics	Increased EPS	Inhibition of cytochrome P-450, inhibition of DA release
Carbamazepine	Carbamazepine neurotoxicity Nausea, vomiting, vertigo, tinnitus	Inhibition of cytochrome P-450
Valproate	Increased effect	Inhibition of cytochrome P-450
Lithium	Lithium toxicity with or without increased Li serum level; enhanced therapeutic effect	Mechanism uncertain
Narcotics – especially pentazocine, meperidine, dextromethorphan	Increased narcotic effect, CNS depression	Mechanism uncertain, ? additive serotonergic effect
Phenytoin	Increased phenytoin effect	Cytochrome P-450 inhibition
Nifedipine, verapamil	Hypotension, additive effects	Mechanism uncertain
Monoamine oxidase inhibitors	Hyperpyrexia, hypertension or hypotension, rigidity, convulsions, coma, death (serotonin syndrome)	Excess CNS serotonin release, ? other unknown mechanisms

while fluvoxamine and paroxetine may interact to a greater extent than sertraline but to a lesser extent and of shorter duration than fluoxetine.[10]

MONOAMINE OXIDASE INHIBITOR ANTIDEPRESSANTS

Monoamine oxidase inhibitors produce their antidepressant action by blocking monoamine oxidase–catalyzed metabolic degradation of monoamine neurotransmitters.[15] Since blockade of reuptake mechanisms and inhibition of metabolic inactivation increase brain neurotransmitters, these two antidepressant mechanisms are complementary. It is theoretically possible that combined tricyclic-MAOI therapy could provoke a higher incidence of hypertensive reactions. Based on controlled studies and clinical observation, this drug combination does not appear to be associated with a high risk of hypertensive crises.[54,55] The most commonly encountered unwanted effect of MAOI antidepressants is the production of postural hypotension, which may be enhanced in some patients receiving tricyclics in combination with MAOIs. When combined therapy regimens are utilized, patients should be carefully monitored before and during treatment.

Tranylcypromine is a nonhydrazine, while phenelzine is a hydrazine compound. The hydrazine structure may be potentially hepatoxic, though the incidence of liver damage with phenelzine is exceedingly low. Tranylcypromine structurally resembles the amphetamines and may produce some direct stimulant action in addition to the pharmacologic effects resulting from enzyme inhibition. Although hypertensive reactions to tranylcypromine in the absence of food or drug interactions have been suggested, there is no convincing evidence that they do in fact occur. A patient who has been treated with phenelzine and subsequently abruptly started on tranylcypromine may experience a potentially fatal hypertensive reaction.[56] Therefore in changing treatment from phenelzine to tranylcypromine, a five- to ten-day drug-free interval is advised; when changing from tranylcypromine to phenelzine a drug-free interval is not required.

The most widely known drug interaction in psychiatry is the hypertensive reaction that may occur when tyramine-rich foods or beverages[57] are consumed by a patient being treated with an MAOI, as discussed in chapter 6 and appendix A. More dangerous than the interaction of tyramine-rich foods or pressor drugs with MAOIs, the serotonin syndrome, produced when meperidine or SSRIs are combined with MAOIs, is discussed above.

Patients being treated with MAOIs should generally limit their daily intake of caffeine-containing beverages, including coffee, tea, and cola drinks to three servings per day. If a patient consumes large quantities of these beverages, he or she should be advised to drink decaffeinated products. White wine or red wine consumption should be limited to 3 or 4 ounces per day, although Chianti, which is particularly high in tyramine, should be avoided.[57] Many beers contain significant amounts of tyramine, although generally patients can occasionally consume 4 to 6 ounces of canned or bottled beer, though they must avoid tap (draft) beers which are likely to contain much higher concentrations of tyramine.[58] Fermented liquors generally do not contain very much tyramine, although MAOIs may potentiate the pharmacologic effects of alcohol; therefore consumption of liquor should generally be limited to 1½ ounces and patients should be advised that the effect may be equivalent to what they previously experienced with twice the amount. Small quantities of sour cream, yogurt, cottage cheese, American cheese, or chocolate may be consumed during the course of MAOI therapy, generally without ill effect.

Patients receiving MAOI should be told to avoid nose drops, cold remedies, nasal decongestants, cough syrups, diet pills, and any prescription or over-the-counter remedy that may contain vasoconstrictor or stimulant-type drugs. The current epidemic of cocaine abuse indicates the necessity to specifically warn patients against the use of cocaine while taking an MAOI. I have seen two patients who have experienced this unfortunate drug interaction, which was manifested clinically by moderate hypertension and a pronounced but relatively transient acute psychosis. One of the patients experienced this reaction on several occasions despite strong warnings to avoid cocaine use. Asthmatic patients who may be medicated with ephedrine, epinephrine, or other bronchodilators have a risk of a drug-drug interaction during the course of MAOI antidepressant therapy. Therefore, generally, asthmatic patients should not receive this form of antidepressant treatment unless their asthma can be adequately controlled by the intermittent use of steroid inhalers such as beclomethasone. Meperidine may produce hypertension, hyperpyrexia, and death when administered to MAOI-treated patients.[15]

Patients who develop hypertensive reactions as a result of the combination of vasoactive substances with MAOI antidepressants frequently respond adequately to mild sedation administered in a quiet, darkened room. More severe hypertensive reactions generally are best treated by the IV administration of phentolamine (Regitine) in a dose of 5 mg. Propranolol, a β-adrenergic blocking agent administered slowly IV alone or in combination with the alpha-adrenergic blocking drug phentolamine, may also be useful in the presence of a severe hypertensive crisis. Sublingual nifedipine may also be useful in managing MAOI hypertensive crises.[59]

There are a number of potential drug interactions between MAOIs and antihypertensive medications. Guanethidine when initially administered causes the releases of norepinephrine from nerve endings.[15] An MAOI-treated patient who is started on guanethidine, guanadrel, or clonidine may experience a hypertensive reaction followed by severe hypotension. Hydralazine is likely to produce more pronounced tachycardia and possibly an elevation in blood pressure in an MAOI-treated patient.[9] Methyldopa can also provoke a hypertensive reaction in a patient receiving MAOI antidepressants.

The most common unwanted effect of MAOI antidepressants is a decrease in blood pressure, most prominent with postural change from a reclining or sitting position to a standing position.[15] Any vasodilator is likely to enhance the hypotensive reaction.[4,6] Phenothiazines, particularly low-potency agents such chlorpromazine, clozapine, and thioridazine, are particularly likely to provoke significant hypotensive reactions when given to patients receiving MAOIs. If a neuroleptic is necessary in conjunction with MAOI therapy, piperazine phenothiazines such as trifluoperazine or the butyrophenone haloperidol, are the safest drugs with the least likelihood of producing a hypotensive reaction. Levodopa, a common antiparkinsonian medication, may provoke pronounced CNS stimulation and hypertension in conjunction with MAOIs.[6,15] A similar reaction may occur with the respiratory center stimulant doxapram.[6]

Central nervous system depressants including alcohol, barbiturates, benzodiazepines, chloral hydrate, and opiates are generally potentiated by MAOIs, so that excessive sedation and CNS depression results.[4,6]

The narcotic analgesic meperidine, when administered to an MAOI-treated patient, may provoke a serious or fatal adverse reaction.[45] The MAOI-meperidine reaction is characterized by agitation, restlessness, headache, rigidity, and hyperpyrexia. It may be associated with profound hypotension or hypertension, convulsions may occur, the patient may become comatose and death may occur.[17,45] The administration of meperidine to MAOI-treated patients is absolutely contraindicated.

Although surgery under general anesthesia can be safely accomplished during MAOI therapy, many anesthesiologists prefer to delay elective surgical procedures for 1 to 2 weeks after discontinuing these drugs. In addition to the risk of a drug interaction involving the administration of pressor agents to an MAOI-treated patient during surgery, several drug interactions involving anesthetics have been reported. Halothane and enflurane have both been observed to produce muscle stiffness and hyperpyrexia in MAOI-treated patients.[17] Succinylcholine and related muscle relaxants may have their paralytic effect enhanced and prolonged as the result of MAO inhibition.[17] Barbiturates, including those used for general anesthesia may be potentiated and prolonged by MAOIs.[17] Table 12-5 delineates the spectrum of drug interactions involving MAOIs.

LITHIUM CARBONATE

Lithium carbonate, the simplest chemical substance used in psychiatric treatment, has been demonstrated to exert a therapeutic and prophylactic effect in manic illness, and depression as well as a variety of other psychiatric syndromes.[60] The physiologic actions of this ion are quite complex, and the mechanism of its therapeutic action is not yet well understood.[60]

Lithium is not metabolized by the body, but is filtered, reabsorbed, and excreted by the kidneys. The pharmacokinetics of lithium are intimately tied to the physiology of sodium, chloride, potassium, and fluid balance. Sodium depletion resulting from a salt-restricted diet or the administration of diuretics

Table 12-5 Drug interactions: monoamine oxidase inhibitor antidepressants (MAOIs)

Interacts with	Effect	Mechanism
Tricyclic antidepressants (TCAs)	Increased TCA effect; increased or decreased BP	MAO inhibition; blocks reuptake
Other MAOIs	Hypertension, hyperpyrexia	Sympathomimetic effect of tranyl-cypromine in presence of other MAOIs
Phenothiazines	Hypotension	Vasodilation and alpha-adrenergic blockade
Anesthetics: halothane enflurane	Muscle stiffness, hyperpyrexia	Impaired drug metabolism, increased catecholamines
Meperidine	Agitation, restlessness, hypotension, hypertension, headache, rigidity, hyperpyrexia, convulsions, coma, death	Elevation of brain serotonin levels by MAOI and impaired hepatic metabolism of narcotics due to enzyme inhibition of MAOI
Serotonin-selective reuptake inhibitors (SSRIs) and clomipramine	Serotonin syndrome: agitation, restlessness, hypotension, hypertension, hyperpyrexia, rigidity, coma, convulsions, death	Excess CNS serotonin release, inhibited drug metabolism, ? other unknown mechanisms
Benzodiazepines	Enhanced effect of benzodiazepines	Enzyme inhibition
Alcohol, barbiturates, chloral hydrate, opiates	CNS depression	Enzyme inhibition

Spinal anesthesia	Hypotension	Potentiated vasodilation
Doxapram	CNS stimulation, agitation, hypertension	Catecholamine release
Clonidine, guanethidine	Initial hypertension, subsequent hypotension	Catecholamine release, vasodilation
Levodopa	CNS stimulation, hypertension	Increased catecholamine synthesis
Sympathomimetics: amphetamines, cocaine, dopamine, ephedrine, epinephrine, metaraminol, norepinephrine, phenylpropanolamine, phenylephrine, tyramine, etc.	Hypertensive crisis, CNS stimulation, agitation, acute psychotic reaction	Impaired metabolism of endogenous catecholamines, and exogenous sympathomimetic compounds
Tyramine-rich foods: beer, wine, cheese, fermented meat and fish products, yeast derivatives, broad beans	Hypertensive crisis	Impaired GI degradation of tyramine and endogenous catecholamines
Succinylcholine, suxamethonium d-tubocurarine	Prolonged muscle relaxation, muscle paralysis	MAOI decreases plasma concentration of pseudocholinesterase

will increase lithium retention, increasing its serum concentration, and the risk of lithium toxicity. Hypokalemia, which may occur during the course of diuretic therapy, enhances the toxic potential of lithium.[60]

Thiazide diuretics and furosemide increase sodium and potassium excretion and lithium reabsorption, leading to increased serum lithium concentration.[61] The potassium-saving diuretics amiloride, spironolactone, and triamterene decrease renal clearance of lithium and may also increase lithium serum concentration.[61] The carbonic anhydrase inhibitor acetazolamide as well as sodium bicarbonate and sodium chloride increase renal lithium clearance, potentially decreasing serum concentration and therapeutic effect of lithium.[61]

Patients receiving stable diuretic regimens for hypertension or congestive heart failure whose serum potassium concentration remains normal can generally tolerate lithium therapy without ill effects or undue risk. Medically ill patients, particularly those receiving vigorous diuretic regimens for acute congestive heart failure or other serious conditions, may require temporary discontinuance of lithium. Hypokalemia during diuretic therapy may necessitate temporary discontinuance or dosage reduction. Hypokalemia not only increases the toxicity of lithium, but also increases the risk of digitalis intoxication.[61] Digitalis preparations such as digoxin may be used safely in conjunction with lithium provided that normal electrolyte balance is maintained and hypokalemia does not ensue. In the absence of excessive serum lithium concentration, lithium is not likely to produce cardiac arrhythmias or conduction disturbances. However, toxic serum concentrations of lithium may provoke atrial or ventricular premature beats and intraventricular conduction abnormalities.[64] Hypokalemia and digitalis toxicity likewise present the risk of cardiac dysrhythmias and may enhance the arrhythmogenic potential of lithium even when the latter is maintained at therapeutic serum concentration.[61,62]

Lithium interferes with iodine trapping by the thyroid gland and the formation of thyroid hormones.[60] In the course of lithium therapy, patients may develop goiter with normal thyroid hormone levels or may experience hypothyroidism in the absence of thyroid gland enlargement. In such cases, lithium carbonate therapy may be continued along with properly monitored thyroid hormone replacement.[61] It is useful to palpate the thyroid gland and obtain laboratory studies including triiodothyronine (T_3), thyroxine (T_4), and thyroid-stimulating hormone (TSH) prior to initiating lithium carbonate therapy.[61] These measurements should be repeated every year during treatment. Lithium has been reported to decrease glucose tolerance in some patients, although its ability to induce diabetes is doubtful.[61] There have been reports of the combined administration of phenothiazines with lithium potentially increasing the risk of hyperglycemia.[6] Not uncommonly, patients receiving lithium carbonate have elevated WBC counts, in the range of 14,000-16,000/mL or occasionally higher. There is no known significant adverse effect of lithium on the hematopoietic system and the occurrence of leukcocytosis does not suggest a need to modify the regimen.[60]

Two decades ago, a toxic syndrome was reported to occur when patients were treated simultaneously with lithium and haloperidol.[63] Subsequently, similar syndromes with abnormal EEG, confusion, impaired cognition and mentation, and a variety of autonomic symptoms were reported when lithium was used in conjunction with a variety of other neuroleptics including thioridazine and fluphenazine.[64] A review of 425 patients treated with the combination of haloperidol and lithium failed to confirm even one case of the previously described toxic syndrome.[65] In the experience of this author, such a syndrome does not exist. However, patients receiving neuroleptic drugs may develop neuroleptic malignant syndrome (NMS) that resembles the toxic syndromes attributed to combined therapy with neuroleptics and lithium. Many of these syndromes described findings consistent with lithium intoxication and, in the case of the initial reports involving haloperidol, the patients' serum lithium concentrations were all well above the generally accepted therapeutic range of 0.06-1.2 mEq/L.[63] Since lithium is most commonly used in conjunction with neuroleptic drugs in the treatment of acute manic psychosis, it would be inappropriate to delete this form of combination drug treatment from our therapeutic armamentarium.[60,61]

Numerous drugs when combined with lithium, are capable of increasing its serum concentration. Tetracycline increases serum lithium concentration and may provoke lithium intoxication either as a result of increased lithium absorption from the GI tract or impaired lithium renal excretion.[66] A variety of nonsteroidal antiinflammatory drugs, including diclofenac, ibuprofen, indomethacin, naproxen, sulindac, and piroxicam have been reported to increase serum lithium concentration and provoke lithium intoxication, apparently as a result of their ability to increase renal tubular reabsorption of the lithium ion.[67-70] Although some reports have indicated elevated lithium serum concentrations with phenylbutazone, this drug and aspirin appear to have minimal effects on lithium excretion or serum concentrations.[70]

Carbamazepine may enhance the therapeutic effect of lithium, and has also been reported to increase serum lithium concentration with the possibility of producing lithium toxicity.[71,72] There is a case report of a lithium-treated patient who experienced increased serum lithium concentrations during the course of marijuana smoking, the putative mechanism being that marijuana slowed GI motility, thereby increasing lithium absorption.[73] The combination of methyldopa with lithium has been reported to be associated with lithium toxicity, though the mechanism is uncertain, this interaction may depend more on neurotransmitter activity of the two drugs rather than on changes in drug absorption or excretion patterns.[74]

Prolonged muscle paralysis has been reported in lithium-treated patients who have received succinylcholine, pancuronium, or decamethonium as muscle relaxants during the course of surgical anesthesia.[17,61] The mechanism of interaction between lithium and these muscle relaxants appears to be a synergistic effect at the neuromuscular junction.[17] Hydroxyzine has been

Table 12-6 Drug interactions: lithium carbonate

Interacts with	Effect	Mechanism
Marijuana	Increased lithium concentration	Increased lithium absorption
Tetracyclines	Lithium intoxication	Enhanced lithium absorption, impaired lithium excretion
Muscle relaxants: succinylcholine, pancuronium, decamethonium	Prolonged muscle paralysis	Synergism at neuromuscular junction
Carbamazepine	Enhanced lithium effect Possible lithium toxicity	Synergistic effect Uncertain
Methyldopa	Lithium toxicity	Uncertain
Indomethacin, ibuprofen, piroxicam, diclofenac, sulindac, naproxen	Lithium toxicity	Increased tubular reabsorption of lithium
Hydroxyzine	Cardiac conduction disturbance	Increased effect of lithium on cardiac repolarization
Phenothiazines, neuroleptics	May enhance neurologic toxicity of each other, hyperglycemia	Additive effect—central dopamine blockade, effect on catecholamine turnover
Thiazide diuretics, furosemide	Increased lithium concentration	Increased Na and K excretion and lithium reabsorption
Amiloride, spironolactone, triamterene	Increased lithium effect	Decreased renal clearance of lithium
Acetazolamide, sodium bicarbonate, sodium chloride	Decreased lithium effect	Increased renal clearance of lithium
Cyclic antidepressants	Increased tremor	Neuromuscular irritability
Diltiazem, verapamil	Neurotoxicity, nausea, weakness, ataxia, tinnitus	Synergistic effect (resembles lithium toxicity, without elevated serum lithium level)
Lisinopril, enalapril, and other ACE inhibitors	Confusion, ataxia, dysarthria, tremor, ECG changes	Decreased renal clearance of lithium Sodium depletion
Fluoxetine (and ? other SSRIs)	Increased tremor, signs of Li toxicity with or without elevated serum Li levels	Mechanism uncertain, additive CNS serotonin effect?

reported to interact with lithium producing disturbances in cardiac conduction, presumably as a result of an increased effect of lithium on cardiac repolarization mechanisms.[13]

The calcium channel blockers, diltiazem and verapamil, when administered along with lithium, may provoke symptoms of lithium neurotoxicity without associated increased serum lithium concentration.[75,76] In the case of diltiazem, a patient developed a parkinsonian syndrome while receiving this drug along with lithium.[75] Another patient, who developed an adverse reaction to combined lithium and verapamil, experienced nausea, vomiting, muscular weakness, ataxia, and tinnitus.[76] It is unknown at this time whether other calcium channel blockers such as nifedipine may produce a similar syndrome. The potential interactions between calcium channel blockers and psychotropic drugs is of extreme importance currently because of the increased use of calcium channel blockers in the treatment of manic symptoms and other psychiatric syndromes.

Angiotensin converting enzyme (ACE) inhibitors, including enalapril, lisinopril, and captopril among many others, are used in the management of hypertension and cardiovascular disease. An interaction between enalapril and lithium has been reported, wherein the patient developed confusion, ataxia, dysarthria, and tremor, along with bradycardia, junctional rhythm, and T wave inversion.[77] These symptoms disappeared when lithium and enalapril were discontinued. Similar adverse reactions have been reported between lisinopril and lithium and are likely to occur with other ACE inhibitors as well.[78,79] This interaction appears to be due to ACE inhibitor reduction of renal function or depletion of sodium.[77] Lithium is frequently combined with fluoxetine and other SSRIs to increase antidepressant efficacy; however, lithium toxicity may occur in some patients who are simultaneously taking fluoxetine and perhaps other SSRIs as well.[80] Absence seizures have been reported with combinations of lithium and fluoxetine.[81] Table 12-6 reviews important drug interactions of lithium.

CARBAMAZEPINE

Carbamazepine, whose molecular structure is similar to that of the TCAs and phenytoin, was first marketed in the United States in the 1960s. This drug was originally used for the treatment of trigeminal neuralgia, and subsequently as an anticonvulsant. Since the late 1970s, the psychiatric use of carbamazepine has mushroomed. Initially used by psychiatrists for temporal lobe epilepsy and episodic dyscontrol disorders, carbamazepine is now being used with increasing frequency alone and in combination with lithium in the treatment of bipolar affective disorders. The most serious side effect of carbamazepine is its potential to produce leukopenia, thrombocytopenia, pancytopenia, and agranulocytosis. Fortunately, these side effects are rare; nevertheless, periodic CBCs must be done when carbamazepine is employed.[15] Because of the increasing psychiatric use of carbamazepine, its potential as a participant in drug-drug interactions is significant.[82,83]

Currently the most prevalent psychiatric use of carbamazepine is as an adjunct or replacement for lithium in the treatment and prophylaxis of mania. Carbamazepine may enhance the antimanic effect of lithium in treatment-refractory patients. Carbamazepine appears to enhance the synthesis and/or release of vasopressin, and it is perhaps through this mechanism that carbamazepine can inhibit lithium-induced polyuria.[15] Carbamazepine decreases renal clearance of lithium and may thereby increase serum lithium concentration and potentially cause lithium intoxication.[83] Some patients receiving lithium in conjunction with carbamazepine develop ataxia and dizziness, even in the absence of elevated serum concentrations of either drug.[84] Since carbamazepine is often used in the treatment of mania and behavioral dyscontrol syndromes, this drug is often combined with neuroleptics. There have been reports of the combined use of haloperidol and carbamazepine leading to decreased serum concentrations and effects of either drug.[85]

Carbamazepine has been reported to induce hyponatremia in some patients. The use of thiazide diuretics or furosemide in combination with carbamazepine may produce severe, symptomatic hyponatremia.[86] Patients receiving carbamazepine in conjunction with diuretics should have periodic serum electrolyte determinations. The combined use of carbamazepine, lithium, and diuretics should be managed with considerable caution because of the potential for electrolyte depletion, which may further enhance the risk of lithium intoxication.

Fluoxetine, cimetidine, isoniazid, and propoxyphene impair the metabolic degradation and clearance of carbamazepine, producing increased blood levels and potential toxicity of carbamazepine.[48,82] Erythromycin inhibits the metabolism of a variety of drugs, including tricyclic antidepressants, triazolam and carbamazepine.[87,88,89] Administration of conventional doses of erythromycin along with carbamazepine may provoke a toxic syndrome marked by somnolence, lethargy, dizziness, blurred vision, diplopia, ataxia, nausea, and nystagmus.[87] Because of the risk of carbamazepine intoxication, its use concomitantly with these other drugs should be approached cautiously and should be done only in conjunction with periodic carbamazepine serum level determinations.

Phenobarbital, phenytoin, and primidone induce enzymes and thus facilitate the metabolism of carbamazepine, leading to decreased serum concentrations and therapeutic actions of this drug.[8] Carbamazepine may decrease the serum concentration of clonazepam and tricyclic antidepressents and may thereby decrease their therapeutic effect, by inducing metabolizing enzymes.[8,90]

Neurotoxicity with dizziness, diplopia, headache, and nausea has been reported to occur with the combined use of verapamil and carbamazepine. It appears that the calcium channel blockers verapamil and diltiazem decrease hepatic metabolism of carbamazepine, thereby increasing its serum concentra-

Table 12-7 Drug interactions: carbamazepine

Interacts with	Effect	Mechanism
Lithium	Increased effect, lithium intoxication, ataxia, dizziness	Decreased lithium renal clearance, (intoxication may appear with normal levels of both)
Haloperidol	Inhibits lithium polyuria	Antidiuretic action of carbamazepine
Cimetidine, erythromycin, isoniazid, propoxyphene	Decreased effect of either	Decreased blood levels of either drug
	Somnolence, lethargy, dizziness, blurred vision, diplopia, ataxia, nausea, nystagmus	Increased carbamazepine serum levels, reduced metabolism and clearance of carbamazepine
Phenobarbital, phenytoin, primidone	Decreased carbamazepine effect	Enzyme induction, decreased carbamazepine serum levels
Clonazepam	Decreased clonazepam effect	Carbamazepine decreases clonazepam serum level
Verapamil, diltiazem (?other calcium channel blockers)	Neurotoxicity, dizziness, diplopia, headache, nausea	Decreased hepatic metabolism of carbamazepine, increased carbamazepine plasma level
Hydrochlorothiazide, furosemide	Hyponatremia	Carbamazepine may increase synthesis and/or release of vasopressin
Fluoxetine (? other SSRIs)	Somnolence, lethargy, dizziness, blurred vision, diplopia, ataxia, nausea, nystagmus	Cytochrome P-450 inhibition by fluoxetine with increased carbamazepine serum concentration and toxicity
Valproate (divalproex)	Carbamazepine reduces valproate serum concentration and effect; valproate increases accumulation of carbamazepine epoxide	Carbamazepine induces enzymes for VAL metabolism; VAL inhibits clearance of CBZ epoxide

tions.[91,92] The toxic interaction of carbamazepine with verapamil was observed in a series of six patients who received these drugs in combination for the treatment of their seizure disorder. In each case, the symptoms abated when the medications were discontinued. Two of these patients were rechallenged with this combination regimen and again developed neurotoxic symptoms.[91] It is conceivable that other calcium channel blockers, such as nifedipine, may produce a similar interaction with carbamazepine; however, these drug interactions have not yet been documented. The interactions of carbamazepine with other drugs are shown in Table 12-7.

VALPROATE

Increasing use of divalproex and related valproate analogues as mood stabilizing drugs has opened a new chapter of potential drug interactions in psychiatry. Initial concerns about potential hepatotoxicity of valproate primarily arose when this drug was used in conjunction with other anticonvulsants in young children. There is an important potential interaction between valproate and carbamazepine, wherein carbamazepine, through enzyme induction, reduces serum concentration and therapeutic effect of valproate.[93] In addition, coadministration of these drugs alters carbamazepine metabolism, with potential accumulation of the epoxide metabolite of carbamazepine, which is more hepatotoxic, particularly in children, than is the parent compound.[94] Accumulation of carbamazepine epoxide may well account for the hepatotoxicity previously observed with valproate combination anticonvulsant regimens in children. Valproate is known to displace phenytoin from protein binding sites, increasing the concentration of free drug and the possibility of adverse effects of phenytoin.[93] Thus far no clinically significant pharmacokinetic interactions between valproate and neuroleptics, tricyclic antidepressants, or lithium have been identified.[93] Fluoxetine, erythromycin, and cimetidine are all known to potentially increase valproate serum concentrations, probably due to inhibition of its metabolism.[9]

REFERENCES

1. Csernansky JG, Whiteford HA: Clinically significant psychoactive drug interactions, in Hales RE, Francis AJ (eds): *APA Annual Review.* Washington, DC, American Psychiatric Press, 1987, vol 6, pp 802-815.
2. Burrows GD, Norman TR: Psychotherapeutic drugs: Important adverse reaction and interactions. *Drugs* 1980;20:485-493.
3. Leipzig RM, Mendelowitz A: Adverse psychotropic drug-drug interactions. In Kane JM, Lieberman JA (eds): *Adverse effects of psychotropic drugs.* New York, Guilford Press, 1992, pp 13-76.
4. Bernstein JG: Drug interactions. In Cassem NH (ed): *Massachusetts General Hospital Handbook of general hospital psychiatry,* ed 3. St Louis, Mosby, 1991, pp 571-610.
5. Avant GR, Speeg KV, Freeman FR, et al: Physostigmine reversal of diazepam-induced hypnosis. *Ann Intern Med* 1979;91:53-55.
6. Blackwell B, Schmidt GL: Drug interactions in psychopharmacology. *Psychiatr Clin North Am* 1984;7:625-637.

7. Ruffalo RL, Thompson JF: Effect of cimetidine on the clearance of benzodiazepines. *N Engl J Med* 1980;303:753-754.

8. Glassman R, Salzman C: Interactions between psychotropic and other drugs: an update. *Hosp Community Psychiatry* 1987;38:236-242.

9. Rizack MA, Hillman CDM (eds): *The Medical Letter Handbook of drug interactions.* New Rochelle NY, Medical Letter, 1993.

10. van Harten J: Clinical pharmacokinetics of selective serotonin reuptake inhibitors. *Clin Pharmacokinet* 1993;24:203-220.

11. Ciraulo DA, Shader RI: Fluoxetine drug-drug interactions. II. *J Clin Psychopharmacol* 1990;10:213-217.

12. Malach M, Berman N: Furosemide and chloral hydrate. *JAMA* 1975;232:637-639.

13. Hollister LE: Hydroxyzine hydrochloride: possible adverse cardiac interactions. *Psychopharmacol Commun* 1975;1:61-65.

14. Sassim N, Grohmann R: Adverse drug reactions with clozapine and simultaneous application of benzodiazepines. *Pharmacopsychiatry* 1988;21:306-309.

15. Gilman AG, Rall TW, Nies AS, Taylor P (eds): *Goodman and Gilman's The pharmacological basis of therapeutics,* ed 8. New York, Pergamon Press, 1990.

16. Tesar GE, Murray GB, Cassem NH: Use of high-dose intravenous haloperidol in the treatment of agitated cardiac patients. *J Clin Psychopharmacol* 1985;5:344-347.

17. Janowsky EC, Risch C, Janowsky DS: Effects of anesthesia on patients taking psychotropic drugs. *J Clin Psychopharmacol* 1981;1:14-20.

18. Thornton WE: Dementia induced by methyldopa with haloperidol. *N Engl J Med* 1976;294: 1222-1223.

19. Demuth GW, Ackerman SH: Methyldopa and depression: a clinical study and review of the literature. *Am J Psychiatry* 1983;140:534-538.

20. Ovetsch RM, Achot RWP, Littin EM, et al: Depressive reactions in hypertensive patients. *Circulation* 1959;19:366-375.

21. Jefferson JW: A review of the cardiovascular effects and toxicity of tricyclic antidepressants. *Psychosom Med* 1975;37:160-179.

22. Donatini B, Le Blaye I, Krupp P: Transient cardiac pacing is insufficiently used to treat arrhythmia associated with thioridazine. *Clin Pharmacol* 1992;81:340-341.

23. Haller E, Binder RL: Clozapine and seizures. *Am J Psychiatry* 1990;147:1069-1071.

24. Schaul N, Degreef G, Ney GC: Psychotropic drugs and seizures. In Kane JM, Lieberman JA (eds): *Adverse effects of psychotropic drugs.* New York, Guilford Press, 1992, pp 321-337.

25. Centorrino F, Baldessarini RJ, Kando J, et al: Serum concentrations of clozapine and its major metabolites: Effects of cotreatment with fluoxetine or valproate. *Am J Psychiatry* 1994;151: 123-125.

26. Wood AJJ, Feely J: Pharmacokinetic drug interactions with propranolol. *Clin Pharmacokinet* 1983;8:253-263.

27. Silver JM, Yudofsky SC, Kogan M, et al: Elevation of thioridazine plasma levels by propranolol. *Am J Psychiatry* 1986;143:1290-1292.

28. Greendyke RM, Kanter DR: Plasma propranolol levels and their effect on plasma thioridazine and haloperidol concentrations. *J Clin Psychopharmacol* 1987;7:178-182.

29. Ciraulo DA, Shader RI: Fluoxetine drug-drug interactions. I. Antidepressants and antipsychotics. *J Clin Psychopharmacol* 1990;10:48-50.

30. Goff DC, Baldessarini RJ: Drug interactions with antipsychotic agents. *J Clin Psychopharmacol* 1993;13:57-67.

31. White W: Hypotension with postural syncope secondary to the combination of chlorpromazine and captopril. *Arch Intern Med* 1986;146:1833-1834.

32. Risch SC, Groom GP, Janowsky DS: Interfaces of psychopharmacology and cardiology. I. *J Clin Psychiatry* 1981;42:23-34.

33. Glassman AH, Preud'homme XA: Review of the cardiovascular effects of heterocyclic antidepressants. *J Clin Psychiatry* 1993;54(2 suppl):16-22.

34. Risch SC, Groom GP, Janowsky DS: Interfaces of psychopharmacology and cardiology, II. *J Clin Psychiatry* 1981;42:47-59.
35. Overo KF, Gram LF, Hansen V: Interaction of perphenazine with the kinetics of nortriptyline. *Acta Pharmacol Toxicol* 1977;40:97-105.
36. Dessain EL, Schatzberg AF, Woods BT, et al: Maprotiline in depression. *Arch Gen Psychiatry* 1986;43:86-90.
37. Henauer SA, Hollister LE: Cimetidine interaction with imipramine and nortriptyline. *Clin Pharmacol Ther* 1984;35:183-187.
38. Abernethy DR, Todd EL: Doxepin-cimetidine interaction: Decreased doxepine bioavailability during cimetidine treatment. *J Clin Psychopharmacol* 1986;6:8-12.
39. Shen WW, Lin KM: Cytochrome P-450 monooxygenases and interactions of psychotropic drugs. *Int J Psychiatr Med* 1991;21:47-56.
40. von Moltke LL, Greenblatt DJ, Harmatz JS, et al: Cytochromes in psychopharmacology. [Editorial.] *J Clin Psychopharmacol* 1994;14:1-3.
41. Cavanaugh SVA: Drug-drug interactions of fluoxetine with tricyclics. *Psychosomatics* 1990;31:273-276.
42. Rosenstein DL, Takeshita J, Nelson JC: Fluoxetine-induced elevation and prolongation of tricyclic levels in overdose. [Letter.] *Am J Psychiatry* 1991;148:807.
43. Sternbach H: The serotonin syndrome. *Am J Psychiatry* 1991;148:705-713.
44. Beasley CM, Masica DN, Heiligenstein JH, et al: Possible monoamine oxidase inhibitor-serotonin uptake inhibitor interaction: fluoxetine clinical data and preclinical findings. *J Clin Psychopharmacol* 1993;13:312-320.
45. Tackley RM, Tregaskis B: Fatal disseminated intravascular coagulation following a monoamine oxidase inhibitor/tricyclic interaction. *Anesthesia* 1987;42:760-763.
46. Browne B, Linter S: Monoamine oxidase inhibitors and narcotic analgesics: a critical review of the implications for treatment. *Br J Psychiatry* 1987;151:210-212.
47. Sovner R, Davis JM: A potential drug interaction between fluoxetine and valproic acid. [Letter.] *J Clin Psychopharmacol* 1991;11:389.
48. Pearson HJ: Interaction of fluoxetine with carbamazepine. [Letter.] *J Clin Psychiatry* 1990;51:126.
49. Sternbach H: Fluoxetine-associated potentiation of calcium-channel blockers. *J Clin Psychopharmacol* 1991;11:390. [Letter.]
50. Bodkin JA, Teicher MH: Fluoxetine may antagonize the anxiolytic actions of buspirone. *J Clin Psychopharmacol* 1989;9:150. [Letter.]
51. Pope HG, McElroy SL, Nixon RA: Possible synergism between fluoxetine and lithium in refractory depression. *Am J Psychiatry* 1988;145:1292-1294.
52. Salama AA, Shafey M: A case of severe lithium toxicity induced by combined fluoxetine and lithium carbonate. [Letter.] *Am J Psychiatry* 1989;146:278.
53. Preskorn SH, Alderman J, Chung M, et al: Pharmacokinetics of desipramine coadministered with sertraline or fluoxetine. *J Clin Psychopharmacol* 1994;14:90-98.
54. White K, Simpson G: Combined MAOI-tricyclic antidepressant treatment: a reevaluation. *J Clin Psychopharmacol* 1981;1:264-282.
55. Ranzani J, White KL, White J, et al: The safety and efficacy of combined amitriptyline and tranylcypromine antidepressant treatment: A controlled trial. *Arch Gen Psychiatry* 1983;46:657-661.
56. Bazire SR: Sudden death associated with switching monoamine oxidase inhibitors. *Drug Intell Clin Pharm* 1986;20:954-955.
57. Shulman KI, Walker SE, MacKenzie S, et al: Dietary restriction, tyramine, and the use of monoamine oxidase inhibitors. *J Clin Psychopharmacol* 1989;9:397-402.
58. Tailor SAN, Shulman KI, Walker SE, et al: Hypertensive episode associated with phenelzine and tap beer: a reanalysis of the role of pressor amines in beer. *J Clin Psychopharmacol* 1994;14:5-14.

59. Clary C, Schwetzer E: Treatment of MAOI hypertensive crisis with sublingual nifedipine. *J Clin Psychiatry* 1987;48:249-250.

60. Johnson FN (ed): *Depression and mania: modern lithium therapy*, Oxford, IRL Press, 1987.

61. Jefferson JW, Greist JH, Ackerman DS, et al: *Lithium encyclopedia for clinical practice*, ed 2. Washington DC, American Psychiatric Press, 1987.

62. Shom M: Electrocardiographic changes during treatment with lithium and with drugs of the imipramine type. *Acta Psychiatr Scand Suppl* 1963;169:258-259.

63. Cohen WJ, Cohen NH: Lithium carbonate, haloperidol, and irreversible brain damage. *JAMA* 1974;230:1283-1287.

64. Spring GH: Neurotoxicity with combined use of lithium and thioridazine. *J Clin Psychiatry* 1979;40:135-138.

65. Baastrup PC, Hollnagel P, Sorenson R, et al: Adverse reactions in treatment with lithium carbonate and haloperidol. *JAMA* 1976;236:2645-2646.

66. McGinnis AJ: Lithium-tetracycline: toxic interaction. *B Med J* 1978;1:1183.

67. Reimann IW, Diener U, Frolich JC: Indomethacin but not aspirin increases plasma lithium ion levels. *Arch Gen Psychiatry* 1983;40:283-286.

68. Kerry R, Owen G, Michaelson S: Possible toxic interactions between lithium and piroxicam. *Lancet* 1983;418-419.

69. Ragheb M, Powell AL: Lithium interaction with sulindac and naproxen. *J Clin Psychopharmacol* 1986;6:150-154.

70. Ragheb M: The clinical significance of lithium-nonsteroidal anti-inflammatory drug interactions. *J Clin Psychopharmacol* 1990;10:350-354.

71. Jefferson JW, Greist JH, Baudhuin M: Lithium: interaction with other drugs. *J Clin Psychopharmacol* 1981;1:124-134.

72. McGinness J, Kishimoto A, Hollister LE: Avoiding neurotoxicity with lithium-carbamazepine combinations. *Psychopharmacol Bull* 1990;26:181-184.

73. Ratey JJ, Ciraulo DA, Shader RI: Lithium and marijuana. *J Clin Psychopharmacol* 1981;1:32-33.

74. O'Regan JB: Adverse interactions of lithium carbonate and methyldopa. *Can Med Assoc J* 1976;115:385.

75. Valdiserri EV: A possible interaction between lithium and diltiazem: case report. *J Clin Psychiatry* 1985;46:540-541.

76. Price WA, Giannini AJ: Neurotoxicity caused by lithium-verapamil synergism. *J Clin Pharmacol* 1986;26:717-719.

77. Duoste-Blazy PH, Rostin, M, Livarek B, et al: Angiotensin converting enzyme inhibitors and lithium treatment. *Lancet* 1986;1:448.

78. Correa FJ, Eiser AR: Angiotensin-converting enzyme inhibitors and lithium toxicity. *Am J Med* 1992;93:108-110.

79. DasGupta K, Jefferson JW, Kobak KA, et al: The effect of enalapril on serum lithium levels in healthy men. *J Clin Psychiatry* 1992;53:398-400.

80. Noveske FG: Possible toxicity of combined fluoxetine and lithium. *Am J Psychiatry* 1989;146:1515. [Letter.]

81. Sacristan JA, Iglesias C, Arellano F, et al: Absence seizures induced by lithium: possible interaction with fluoxetine. [Letter.] *Am J Psychiatry* 1991;148:146-147.

82. Ketter TA, Post RM, Worthington K: Principles of clinically important drug interactions with carbamazepine. I. *J Clin Psychopharmacol* 1991;11:198-203.

83. Ketter TA, Post RM, Worthington K: Principles of clinically important drug interactions with carbamazepine. II. *J Clin Psychopharmacol* 1991;11:306-312.

84. Shukla S, Godwin CD, Long LEB, et al: Lithium carbamazepine neurotoxicity and risk factors. *Am J Psychiatry* 1984;141:1604-1606.

85. Kahn EM, Schulz SC, Perel JM, et al: Change in haloperidol level due to carbamazepine: a complicating factor in combined medication for schizophrenia. *J Clin Psychopharmacol* 1990;10:54-57.

86. Yassa R, Nastase C, Camille Y, et al: Carbamazepine, diuretics, and hyponatremia: A possible interaction. *J Clin Psychiatry* 1987;48:281-283.
87. Jaster P, Abbas D: Erythromycin-carbamazepine interaction. *Neurology* 1986;36:594-595.
88. Amsterdam JD, Maisline G: Effect of erythromycin on tricyclic antidepressant metabolism. *J Clin Psychopharmacol* 1991;11:203-206.
89. Miles MV, Tennison MB: Erythromycin effects on multiple-dose carbamazepine kinetics. *Ther Drug Monit* 1989;11:47-52.
90. Leinonen E, Lillsunde P, Laukkanen V, et al: Effects of carbamazepine on serum antidepressant concentrations in psychiatric patients. *J Clin Psychopharmacol* 1991;11:313-318.
91. MacPhee G: Verapamil potentiates carbamazepine neurotoxicity: A clinically important inhibitory interaction. *Lancet* 1986;1:700-703.
92. Eimer M, Carter BL: Elevated serum carbamazepine concentrations following diltiazem initiation. *Drug Intell Clin Pharm* 1987;21:340-342.
93. Bourgeois BFD: Pharmacologic interactions between valproate and other drugs. *Am J Med* 1988;84(suppl 1A):29-33.
94. Johnsen SD, Johns DW: Carbamazepine epoxide toxicity in children receiving carbamazepine and valproate. *Ann Neurol* 1991;230:491-493.

CHAPTER 13

Psychiatric Side Effects and Psychiatric Uses of Nonpsychotropic Drugs

OVERVIEW

Psychiatric Complications
of Nonpsychotropic Medications

Hormones

1. *Adrenal corticosteroids*
    Euphoria, mania, or depression with risk of suicide
2. *Thyroid hormones*
    Agitation, anxiety, psychosis resembling schizophrenia or mania
3. *Oral contraceptives*
    Estrogens — sense of well-being, may improve depressed mood
    Progesterone derivatives — depression
4. *Testosterone and anabolic steroids*
    Increased aggressive behavior, paranoia, depression, mania

Cardiovascular Drugs

1. *Digitalis*
    Weakness, apathy, depression, hallucinations, delirium
2. *Antiarrhythmic drugs*
    Quinidine — excitement, confusion, delirium, dementia
    Procainamide — weakness, giddiness, depression, delirium, psychotic reactions including hallucinations.
    Lidocaine — CNS stimulation, restlessness, tremors, seizures, disorientation, confusion, delirium, anxiety
    Propranolol — Depression, lassitude, insomnia, nightmares, toxic psychosis, confusion, disorientation, hallucinations.

Continued.

3. *Antihypertensive drugs*
   Reserpine — depression; may be severe with risk of suicide
   Methyldopa — clouding of consciousness, confusion, depression, dementia
   Prazosin — drowsiness, nervousness, depression
   Thiazide diuretics — weakness, hypokalemia, pseudo depression
   Guanethidine — Tricyclic antidepressants block the hypotensive effects of guanethidine, clonidine, and bretylium
   Clonidine — depression, hallucinations
   Angiotensin converting enzyme inhibitors (captopril, enalapril) — with chlorpromazine — severe hypotension; with lithium — lithium neurotoxicity
4. *Calcium channel blockers*
   All can produce depression
   Diltiazem — enhanced neurotoxicity of carbamazepine, lithium
   Nifedipine — psychosis, depression
   Verapamil — delirium, may decrease serum lithium concentration; enhanced neurotoxicity of carbamazepine and lithium

Respiratory Drugs
1. *Phenylpropanolamine, oxymetazoline* — anxiety
2. *Albuterol, terbutaline* — anxiety, psychosis
3. *Theophylline* — anxiety, restlessness, depression
4. *Dextromethorphan* — confusion, hallucinations

Anticonvulsant Drugs
1. *Phenytoin* — inappropriate affect, confusion, drowsiness, hallucinations

Antisecretory Drugs
1. *Cimetidine* — confusion, toxic delirium, hallucinations, depression, impaired elimination and prolonged effect of long-acting benzodiazepines such as chlordiazepoxide and diazepam
2. *Ranitidine* — infrequently produces similar effects

Gastrointestinal Motility Stimulant
1. *Metoclopramide* — drowsiness, anxiety, confusion, mania, parkinsonism, tardive dyskinesia

Continued.

Analgesics
1. *Propoxyphene* — clouding of consciousness, psychotic reactions, hallucinations, addiction
2. *Pentazocine* — psychotic reactions, addiction, withdrawal same as with narcotics, may hallucinate during withdrawal

Anti-inflammatory Drugs
1. *Indomethacin* — mental confusion, depression with suicidal attempts, acute psychosis with hallucinations
2. *Nonsteroidal anti-inflammatory agents* — all increase serum lithium concentration, lithium toxicity

Antibacterial Drugs
1. *Nalidixic acid* — mental clouding, confusion
2. *Nitrofurantoin* — mental clouding, confusion
3. *Isoniazid* — euphoria, impaired memory, impaired reality testing, loss of self-control, florid psychoses, may potentiate phenytoin by inhibiting its metabolism
4. *Tetracycline* — increased serum lithium concentration, risk of lithium toxicity
5. *Erythromycin* — carbamazepine neurotoxicity

Hypoglycemic Agents
1. *Oral and insulin* — anxiety, agitation (probably secondary to hypoglycemia)

Vitamins
1. *Niacin deficiency* — insomnia, depression, impaired memory, delusions, hallucinations, dementia, pellagra
2. *Folic acid deficiency* — irritability, sleeplessness, forgetfulness, depression dementia
3. *Pyridoxine deficiency* — hyperreflexia, myoclonus

Psychiatric Uses of Nonpsychotropic Drugs
Delineated in Table 13-2, page 386
1. Used to enhance efficacy of psychotropic drugs
2. Treatment of physiological symptoms of anxiety
3. Treatment and prophylaxis of mania
4. Treatment of movement disorders

Too often, physicians see psychiatric illness in isolation from medical illness. Indeed, many patients initially come to the attention of psychiatrists during the course of various medical problems. As is well known to physicians, numerous medical ailments have among their constellation of symptoms a variety of psychiatric complaints including anxiety, depression, insomnia, confusion, and hallucinations.[1] Some patients suffering from terminal illness, though they have no prior psychiatric history, may see a psychiatrist following a suicide attempt that occurred in reaction to a serious or incurable illness. It is beyond the scope of this volume to discuss the psychiatric aspects of medical diseases. However, since there is the potential for psychiatric symptoms to occur in response to an increasing number of potent and therapeutically useful nonpsychotropic drugs, the discussion of the psychiatric complications of these medications is of critical importance to the reader of this volume.

The number of isolated reports of adverse psychiatric effects of drugs is so extensive that it would be impossible to review each drug that at one time or another has been associated with psychiatric symptoms. On the other hand, there are a number of widely used pharmacologic agents whose risk of psychiatric sequelae is so great that the average psychiatrist will undoubtedly encounter one or more of these reactions in his practice. Since few patients receiving prescribed medication are taking a single drug or suffer from a single illness, the potential for interactions between medical drugs and psychiatric drugs is vast. Some of these drug interactions are of such critical importance that combined therapy with specific agents may prevent the therapeutic effect of one or the other, or may lead to severe toxic complications of one or both of the prescribed compounds. Furthermore, a significant majority of people medicate themselves with a variety of nonprescription over-the-counter drugs. Since so many over-the-counter drugs contain antihistamines, anticholinergics, and sympathomimetics, it is not surprising that there is a very high incidence of adverse behavioral complications associated with their use, particularly in the elderly and in those patients who may combine nonprescription products with potent prescribed medications for medical or psychiatric conditions.[2]

The development of effective therapeutic agents relies heavily on laboratory investigations and controlled clinical trials. Furthermore, many drugs that have proved to be clinically useful have had their therapeutic actions discovered quite by accident. Many compounds developed for one purpose, such as imipramine, originally developed as an antipsychotic agent, are later found to have other important and useful effects. The opportunity to observe unexpected therapeutic actions of previously marketed drug products has given rise to new and promising therapeutic agents for indications not initially considered when the drug was investigated or marketed. An example is the finding that the antiviral substance amantadine produced significant benefit in patients with parkinsonism. As the fertile mind of the physician courageously finds new applications for older drugs, our therapeutic armamentarium is strengthened, as is our potential understanding of the mechanisms of disease. The finding of new therapeutic uses for already marketed drugs is an exciting opportunity for the clinical investigator and the practicing physician. Many nonpsychotropic medications have been found to exert useful behavioral effects and in turn to possess potential for a new breed of psychotropic agents.

One example of such a compound is carbamazepine, originally marketed for the treatment of trigeminal neuralgia. It was subsequently found to exert important anticonvulsant effects in temporal lobe epilepsy and other seizure disorders, and has more recently been found to produce antidepressant and antimanic effects.[3] The treatment of anxiety is an important addition to the extensive list of clinical indications for the β-adrenergic blocking drug propranolol, although, as with so many nonpsychotropic medications with psychiatric benefits, this therapeutic indication has not yet been approved by the Food and Drug Administration.[4] The potential application of amino acids such as tryptophan and tyrosine in the treatment of depression and mood disorders,[5] and of other dietary substances such as choline and lecithin in the treatment of tardive dyskinesia and cognitive disorders, are promising areas of development in the future of psychopharmacology.[6] In this chapter I will review some of the psychiatric uses of nonpsychotropic medications. Since repeated well-controlled clinical investigations have demonstrated the ineffectiveness of several high-dosage vitamin regimens in the treatment of schizophrenia,[7] this topic is not discussed.

The clinician should be aware that the application of some drugs discussed in this chapter to the treatment of psychiatric illness has not received approval of the FDA. In discussing these potential applications of promising drugs we are dealing with unapproved indications for approved pharmaceutical products. The physician applying these newer approaches to the treatment of his patients should be aware of the lack of FDA approval; he should discuss this with the patient and document this information in the patient's medical record. The clinician may wish to refer appropriate patients to research centers doing controlled studies of these new indications of nonpsychotropic medications. In either case, consideration needs to be given to the use of new and promising approaches in patients who have failed to achieve a satisfactory benefit from a variety of previously tried therapeutic agents.

PSYCHIATRIC SIDE EFFECTS OF NONPSYCHOTROPIC DRUGS

To discuss even briefly all of the psychiatric side effects reported in association with nonpsychotropic medications would easily fill a volume several times the size of this one. Therefore, I have decided that it will be of more value to the practicing clinician to present those complications that have been well documented in the medical literature and those I have personally observed during the course of my own clinical practice. Of necessity, many psychiatric complications of non-psychotropic medications will not appear in this discussion. Their absence does not imply their nonexistence. Furthermore, in approaching a patient suffering from psychiatric symptoms that could possibly be connected with the medications they are receiving, it is critical for the physician to have a high index of suspicion. The most damaging thing a physician can do is to tell the patient that his reaction cannot possibly be due to the therapeutic agent in question. This is damaging because it blocks further inquiry into the problem, which may well resurface in the clinical experience of others. The most unfortunate aspect of this categorical denial, however, is the fear that it may engender in the patient. I recall seeing a patient a number of years ago in an emergency room. She was a middle-aged woman who had an acute psychotic illness several years previously. The day before I saw her, she had taken pentazocine prescribed by her internist. When she began to hallucinate she contacted her physician. He told her that this was not related to the medication he had prescribed, but was undoubtedly a recurrence of her psychotic illness, which had not resurfaced during the previous 15 years. When I was able to reassure this patient that her hallucinations were likely a result of the pentazocine,[8] she was immediately relieved and the symptoms disappeared within 48 hours of discontinuing the medication. The best clinical guideline therefore, is that even if you have not personally observed a particular reaction to the agent in question, discontinue the medication, and allow the patient to know that although you have not seen this reaction in the past, it is conceivably drug-related. Appropriate consultation or review of the literature should help to further clarify the question and provide an appropriate treatment approach.

Hormones

Adrenal corticosteroids widely used in the treatment of inflammatory disease, collagen vascular disease, and neoplastic disease, have long been recognized for their ability to produce mood changes. Prior to the clinical use of exogenously administered steroids, clinicians were aware that Cushing's disease, due to excessive endogenously produced corticosteroids, was often associated with depression, and in some patients, the appearance of euphoria, mania, or confusion.[1] When steroids are administered in the treatment of medical illnesses they may produce iatrogenic Cushing's syndrome, which is not infrequently associated with mood changes, including depression, euphoria, and mania.[9] Since the underlying illness of many patients receiving steroids may produce its own behavioral effects, such as systemic lupus erythematosus, it is important to differentiate the origin of the observed behavioral complications.[1] The affective symptoms associated with steroids tend to be proportional in both incidence and severity to the dose administered. Some patients receiving steroids become severely depressed, yet the treatment must continue. Therefore, the coadministration of antidepressant medications is not infrequently necessary in prolonged steroid therapy. Furthermore, the appearance of mania during treatment with either ACTH or adrenal corticosteroids may require the administration of haloperidol or other rapidly acting antimanic medication, with subsequent lithium maintenance during the remainder of the course of steroid treatment.[10] Although there is the clinical impression that those patients with underlying affective illnesses may be more vulnerable to mood effects of steroids, both severe depression with suicidal attempts, as well as in manic symptoms of psychotic proportion, are known to occur in patients with no previous personal or family history of psychiatric illness.[1,10]

Thyroid hormones, previously discussed from the standpoint of their ability to enhance the response to tricyclic antidepressants, may produce their own psychiatric complications. The most commonly seen psychiatric manifestation of the administration of thyroid preparations is the appearance of agitation and anxiety. Acute psychotic reactions similar clinically to either schizophrenia or mania are occasionally seen in patients receiving thyroid hormone replacement. While these reactions are somewhat more likely to occur when excessive dosages are employed, they may also occur when relatively moderate doses are administered.[1,9] Behavioral complications of thyroid hormones should lead the clinician to adjust the dosage of the administered medication or, if clinically appropriate, discontinue its use. It is often necessary to treat the patient with appropriate psychotropic medications along with continuing thyroid hormone replacement therapy.

Oral contraceptives have long been known to produce depression. One epidemiologic study reported a 7% incidence of depressive symptoms in patients taking oral contraceptives.[11] Progesterone is the component linked to depressive symptoms, and the risk of depression may be minimized by administering those preparations that contain minimal amounts of this hormone. A significant proportion of patients developing depression while taking oral contraceptives will need treatment with an antidepressant, though initially the birth control pill should be discontinued and the patient observed for a period of time. Estrogenic hormones, the other component of birth control pills, may improve the patient's sense of well-being and may exert a mild antidepressant effect. Some women whose response to conventional antidepressants is limited may achieve a further benefit when low doses of estrogenic hormones are administered under appropriate supervision by a gynecologist or internist. Estrogens have a monoamine oxidase inhibitory effect, which may partially be responsible for their salutary effect on mood.[9]

Testosterone, the male sex steroid, tends to increase aggressive behavior. This agent is occasionally administered to males suffering from impotence, and it may be associated with behavioral changes in these patients. Male heroin addicts and persons maintained on methadone have been reported to develop marked decreases in circulating serum testosterone.[9] Attempts to enhance the antidepressant response of imipramine by coadministration of methyltestosterone has been shown to provoke paranoia and increased aggression.[12]

Anabolic steroids are increasingly being used illicitly by athletes and bodybuilders to increase strength and muscle mass. Although testosterone and other anabolic steroids are now regulated by the DEA as Class III controlled substances, they appear to be quite available and their use is unfortunately quite popular even among teenagers. When used in relatively large doses as they are conventionally employed, anabolic steroids are very dangerous drugs with the potential of causing affective or psychotic symptoms, as well as violent behavior. One study of 41 bodybuilders and football players who had used steroids found that 22% of subjects met DSM-III-R criteria for an affective disorder, and 12% showed symptoms of psychosis in connection with their steroid use.[13] Among other reports, patients with severe depression with or without psychotic features, or with mania or other psychotic disorders, have appeared in the literature in the past decade and a half. I have seen several such patients and most often found it necessary to treat the steroid induced psychiatric syndrome while trying to support the patient's often reluctant gradual withdrawal from steroids. Quite often I have found lithium to be the optimal pharmacologic intervention, since in my experience, mood swings and hypomania have been the primary manifestation of psychiatric complications of anabolic steroid abuse.

Cardiovascular Drugs

Though many critics of psychotropic drug use have implied that these agents have a special place in respect to their overprescription, any experienced physician knows that digitalis has for centuries been widely prescribed, and not infrequently overprescribed, when not clinically necessary. Weakness and apathy are known to occur in association with digitalis intoxication, and it is less frequently appreciated that digitalis preparations may produce depression, hallucinations, and delirium, even at therapeutic plasma concentrations.[14] If it is suspected that this drug may be responsible for psychiatric symptoms in a patient receiving it without good therapeutic indications, its discontinuation may be considered as a first step in the treatment of the behavioral disturbance.

Quinidine, the oldest of the available antiarrhythmic drugs, has long been known to potentially produce excitement and confusion in some patients.[9] It may also produce delirium and a classical syndrome of dementia.[15,16] Although the psychiatric sequelae of antiarrhythmic drugs, including quinidine, may occur in individuals without prior psychiatric histories, a prior history of psychiatric illness often reduces the clinician's suspicion that the symptoms are drug-induced. Procainamide is known to produce weakness, giddiness, and depression in some patients. It may also produce delirium and psychotic reactions with associated hallucinations.[1,9] Lidocaine, when administered IV, may produce CNS stimulation, anxiety, restlessness, tremors, and the possibility of grand mal seizures.[9,17] Patients receiving lidocaine may also experience morbid ruminations, become disoriented and confused, and may develop a toxic delirium.[1,17] Phenytoin, a widely used anticonvulsant, may produce inappropriateness of affect, confusion, drowsiness, and occasionally, hallucinations.[18,19] This compound is also widely used in the management of cardiac arrhythmias, particularly those related to digitalis intoxication. Since the antiarrhythmic drugs are so commonly used in patients admitted to coronary care units and other intensive care unit settings, it must be borne in mind by the clinician that both the setting and the drug may contribute to the adverse behavioral effects observed.

Table 13-1 illustrates the electrophysiological and mechanistic characteristics of the increasingly wide spectrum of available antiarrhythmic drugs along with their potential psychiatric side effects.[9,20] It is interesting that one of the newer agents, moricizine, is a phenothiazine, which although apparently not associated with increased serum prolactin levels, may produce extrapyramidal side effects and depression.[9,20] Disopyramide, which is similar to quinidine in its therapeutic and adverse effects, also possesses anticholinergic activity.[9] Tocainide is an orally administered drug which has effects similar to lidocaine, which can only be administered parenterally.[20] Mexiletine, flecainide, and propaphenone are infrequent causes of depression and may also cause nervousness and tremor, the latter two agents being used primarily for serious ventricular arrhythmias.[20] Acebutolol, esmolol, and sotalol are beta adrenergic antagonists, whose psychiatric side effects are similar to those seen with propranolol.[9] Amiodarone has an indole nucleus, reminiscent of serotonin; it has a long half-life and the potential to inhibit the metabolism of and prolong the effects of many drugs; though not yet reported, its potential to interact with fluoxetine would be interesting, likely, and potentially dangerous.[9] The potential of amiodarone to produce confusion, ataxia, and movement disorders should alert the psychiatrist to potential interactions with neuroleptics. Bretylium, whose antiarrhythmic activity I studied many years ago, is a unique and fascinating compound which is actively taken up by noradrenergic nerve endings and inhibits release of norepinephrine; its antiarrhythmic activity will be inhibited by tricyclic antidepressants which prevent its nerve uptake.[21] Bretylium is unique among antiarrhythmic drugs since it has a positive inotropic effect.[21] Agitation, confusion, and depression are potential adverse

Table 13-1 Classification of antiarrhythmic drugs and their psychiatric side effects

Class	Action	Drug	Comment – side effects
I	Sodium Channel Blocker	Moricizine (atypical I B)	Phenothiazine, EPS, ?depression
IA	Moderate phase 0 depression	Quinidine	Anticholinergic, excitement, delirium
	Moderate conduction slowing	Procainamide	Depression, delirium
	Prolongs repolarization	Disopyramide	Anticholinergic, confusion, depression
IB	Minimal phase 0 depression	Lidocaine (IV)	Confusion, CNS excitation, seizures
	Shortens repolarization	Tocainide	Depression, psychosis, seizures
		Mexiletine	Tremor, nervousness, depression
		Phenytoin	Serum level increased by fluoxetine, confusion
IC	Marked phase 0 depression	Flecainide	Confusion, ?depression
	Marked conduction slowing	Propaphenone	Confusion, depression, ?psychosis
II	Beta-Blockers	Propranolol	Depression, confusion, toxic psychosis
		Acebutolol	Depression
		Esmolol	Confusion, agitation, depression
III	Prolong repolarization	Bretylium	Agitation, confusion, ?depression
		Amiodarone	Confusion, abnormal movements, ataxia
		Sotalol	Fatigue
IV	Calcium channel blockers	Verapamil	Depression, confusion
		Diltiazem	Depression, confusion

effects of bretylium.[21] The calcium channel blockers are both a blessing and a curse from the psychiatric standpoint, in that they may cause depression yet they may be useful adjuncts in the treatment or prophylaxis of mania.[9]

Propranolol, initially employed as an antiarrhythmic agent and subsequently used in the treatment of angina pectoris, hypertension, migraine headaches, and anxiety, may produce a variety of behavioral complications.[1,4] The two psychiatric syndromes associated with propranolol may be divided into dose-dependent reactions, wherein depression may occur in association with higher doses of the drug—generally above 80 mg/day.[22] Propranolol may also produce lassitude, insomnia, and nightmares, but these symptoms are more often associated with higher doses of drug.[1] A much rarer psychiatric complication of propranolol is the development of a toxic psychosis with associated confusion, disorientation, and hallucinations.[23] This tends to occur more commonly in the elderly and is not clearly dose-related, in that it may occur in patients receiving very small therapeutic doses. Patients developing a toxic psychosis or depression in response to propranolol should have the medication discontinued and replaced by a different β blocker. The more cardioselective β-blocking compounds, atenolol, metaprolol, and nadolol, are less likely to produce complications. Patients becoming depressed on propranolol may tolerate this medication in a lower dose or may require a different therapeutic agent such as a more cardioselective β-blocking drug. Since many newer β-blockers are less lipophyllic than propranolol, their ability to cross the blood-brain barrier and be potential sources of depression is diminished, although monitoring of patient mood remains important even when these drugs are employed.[24]

Antihypertensive Drugs

In hypertensive patients becoming depressed or confused while receiving propranolol, the clinician should consider the possibility that other antihypertensive agents may be contributing to the symptoms. Although thiazide diuretics are not ordinarily thought to be depressogenic, they often produce a reduction in both serum and intracellular potassium concentrations. Mild hypokalemia may be associated with decreased energy, weakness, and a clinical picture that resembles depression, though it may not in fact be associated with typical vegetative signs.[9,25] A series of eight thiazide-treated hypertensives who developed major depression meeting DSM-III criteria has been reported, although serum potassium data were unfortunately not provided.[26] Patients receiving thiazides who appear to become depressed should have serum potassium measurements done and may benefit by the oral administration of potassium chloride.

Probably the most widely known psychiatric complication of nonpsychotropic medication is the appearance of depression, which may be severe and associated with suicide attempts not infrequently violent in nature, in patients being treated with reserpine.[27] Rauwolfia compounds, including reserpine, were initially introduced for the treatment of hypertension and psychotic agitation in the early 1950s. At the present time, these compounds are rarely prescribed by psychiatrists, and most physicians believe that they have fallen into general disuse. Reserpine is a component of some combination tablets that are still prescribed for the treatment of hypertension. Although the doses of reserpine generally used now are lower than those previously employed, physicians should not have their anxiety about reserpine alleviated by the belief that severe depressive reactions occur only with larger doses. Clinically significant depression has been observed in patients receiving reserpine at doses as low as 0.25 mg daily,[27] and I see no evidence to deny that doses as low as 0.1 mg daily are capable of producing depression in susceptible individuals. Although some patients developing severe depression during reserpine treatment did have prior psychiatric histories, the literature documents the occurrence of severe affective illness in individuals with no prior personal or family history of psychiatric illness.

Despite the fact that methyldopa acts by modifying neurotransmitter function, the drug was widely used in hypertension for many years before clinicians recognized an association between it and the occurrence of depression. As an internist in the hypertension clinic at the Massachusetts General Hospital in the late 1960s I repeatedly observed prominent clinical signs of depression in patients receiving standard therapeutic doses of methyldopa. The literature now provides documentation of the ability of this drug to produce depression or to worsen previously existing depressive illness.[28] Methyldopa may produce excessive drowsiness and sedation in some patients receiving it alone or in combination with other medications.[1,5] Since this drug affects neurotransmitter function, it is not surprising that there is a potential for various interactions with psychotropic agents that similarly affect neurotransmitters or their receptor sites. Dementia has been reported as a complication of combined treatment with methyldopa and haloperidol.[29] Prazosin is another antihypertensive agent that may produce psychiatric effects including drowsiness, increased anxiety, and depression, the latter reported to occur in approximately 2.8% of treated patients.[9] The physician called on to treat depression in a hypertensive patient receiving either reserpine or methyldopa needs to work closely with that patient's internist to rearrange the antihypertensive regimen. Antidepressant drug therapy should not be initiated until treatment with reserpine or methyldopa is discontinued. The depressed hypertensive patient may be optimally treated with a thiazide diuretic in conjunction with oral potassium often in combination with another antihypertensive without depressogenic effects, such as an ACE inhibitor.

Guanethidine, guanadrel and clonidine are antihypertensive agents whose efficacy depends on their being taken up into nerve endings by the same transport mechanism responsible for norepinephrine and serotonin reuptake. Since reuptake mechanisms are blocked by tricyclic antidepressant drugs, these antihypertensives cannot be used simultaneously with tricyclic antidepressants.[25] One study suggested that doxepin does not interfere with these antihypertensive drugs. However, if doxepin is administered in a high-enough dose to inhibit reuptake mechanisms, there is no reason to believe that it can be used safely with these agents. I have clinically observed on a number of occasions an interaction between doxepin and clonidine, as well as guanethidine, similar to the interaction I have seen with other tricyclic antidepressants. The danger of this interaction is that if the patient is being treated for hypertension by an internist and for depression by a psychiatrist, and the physicians do not consult with each other, the patient remains in the middle, to be the repository of unfortunate drug interactions. I have repeatedly observed patients receiving guanethidine develop gradual and persistent blood pressure elevations with the administration of tricyclic antidepressants. If the physician prescribing the antihypertensive is unaware that the patient is receiving the contraindicated medication he will likely increase the dose of the antihypertensive agent in order to attain blood pressure control; subsequently, when the antidepressant is discontinued, the patient may develop a profound hypotensive reaction.[25] In addition to the interaction between clonidine, guanadrel and guanethidine with tricyclic antidepressants, clonidine itself may produce dementia,[30] or psychotic[31] symptoms, although it has been demonstrated to have a salutary effect in tardive dyskinesia and it may also possess antipsychotic action. Bretylium has both hypotensive and antiarrhythmic activity; tricyclic antidepressants inhibit the former but not the latter effect.[9]

Angiotensin, an endogenous polypeptide that is important in regulating vasomotor tone and circulatory homeostasis, contributes to the etiology of hypertension. Mechanisms for the synthesis and conversion of angiotensin exist in the kidney and in the brain. Angiotensin I is a decapeptide with weak hypertensive activity that is converted through the action of angiotensin coverting enzyme (ACE) to angiotensin II, which is an octapeptide with very potent pressor activity.[9] In addition to regulating vasomotor tone, there is evidence that angiotension II, released from nerve terminals in the brain, may have neurotransmitter or neuromodulary activity.[9]

Many newer antihypertensive drugs are ACE inhibitors which prevent conversion of the low-potency pressor peptide angiotensin I to the high-potency hypertensive peptide angiotensin II.[9] Inhibition of the formation of angiotensin II by these drugs lowers blood pressure in hypertensive patients.[32] Captopril and enalapril are the oldest and best studied ACE inhibitors, though many drugs including benazepril, fosinopril, lisinopril, quinapril, and ramipril, which belong to this group, have similar characteristics.[32] Adverse effects most often associated with ACE inhibitors include drowsiness, nervousness, depression, and decreased libido although these events appear less frequently and less prominently with ACE inhibitors than with older antihypertensive drugs.[33,34] Studies of the quality of life in treated hypertensive patients favor ACE inhibitors and calcium channel blockers.[34] There does appear to be a subtle advantage in terms of mood and positive feelings about life with captopril as compared to enalapril.[33] ACE inhibitors have at times been associated with significant psychotropic drug interactions.[35]

Severe hypotension has been reported in a patient receiving chlorpromazine and captopril simultaneously.[36] Another patient receiving enalapril and lithium simultaneously developed confusion, ataxia, dysarthria, and tremor, along with bradycardia and depression of the T-wave.[37] In the latter patient, signs of lithium toxicity were accompanied by an increase of the serum lithium concentration to 3.3 mEq/L.[37] In that patient, serum creatinine and BUN were elevated, and it appears that impaired renal function and sodium depletion, secondary to enalapril, were responsible for the observed lithium intoxication. I have, however, treated several patients with ACE inhibitors simultaneously with lithium and/or phenelzine without observing clinical or laboratory abnormalities. Since any drug that lowers blood pressure may produce an additive effect if used along with ACE inhibitors, enhanced hypotension may occur, necessitating careful patient monitoring. On a brighter note, three depressed patients have been reported to have experienced an antidepressant response during treatment with captopril.[38] Another patient without a prior affective history was reported to develop mania and subsequent depression when treated with captopril after sudden withdrawal of propranolol and the antihypertensive MAOI, pargyline.[39] In that latter patient, it is possible that the mania and subsequent depression were provoked by pargyline discontinuation rather than captropril, though both options need to be considered. Since the renin-angiotensin system is operative in the brain and there is some evidence for a transmitter role of angiotensin II, the possibility of ACE inhibitors as psychotropic drugs needs further exploration.

Calcium Channel Blockers

Extracellular and intracellular calcium plays an important regulatory role in a variety of metabolic and physiologic processes. Intracellular calcium concentration is tightly regulated.[40,41] Calcium enters cells from outside through macromolecular structures called calcium channels.[40,41] There are two or three types of receptors linked to the calcium channel and these receptors are selective for calcium channel blocking drugs, including verapamil, nifedipine, and diltiazem.[41] Lithium and thioridazine both appear to have some calcium channel blocking activity.[40] Since calcium channel blockers are so widely used in hypertension and cardiovascular disease, there has been an explosive development of drugs in this therapeutic class, including: amlodipine, bepridil, felodipine, isradipine, nicardipine, and nimodipine. The latter enters the CNS with greater ease than others and is used specifically to reduce ischemic deficits in patients with subarachnoid hemorrhage. Calcium channel blocking drugs are of interest in psychiatry because of their adverse behavioral effects, interactions with psychotropic drugs, and potential therapeutic use. Interactions with psychotropic drugs are only briefly mentioned here; the topic has been discussed in more detail in chapter 12. The therapeutic applications of calcium channel blockers is discussed later in this chapter.

Two cases of acute psychosis apparently triggered by nifedipine have been reported; one patient went on to develop agitation and depression.[42] I have observed two patients who developed depressive symptoms while taking nifedipine; in one patient symptoms abated after discontinuing the drug, but recurred 3 years later during treatment with verapamil. I have seen two patients who experienced severe depressive symptoms while taking diltiazem, one of whom required antidepressant pharmacotherapy.

Symptoms in the second patient began to abate three days after discontinuing the drug and were absent at the end of a week. Three of these four patients had no prior personal or family history of depression, while the patient who experienced a second depressive episode during treatment with verapamil had a previously treated depressive illness. Two patients with bipolar illness whom I treated with verapamil as a lithium alternative developed moderate depressive symptoms necessitating discontinuation of this drug and restabilization on lithium. Further experience with the calcium channel blockers is required in order to assess their risk as depressogenic drugs. Delirium has been reported in a patient receiving verapamil and I have observed this phenomenon in a patient under my care.[43] Reduced serum lithium concentration has been reported in a patient during verapamil therapy. Symptoms of lithium intoxication in the absence of elevated serum lithium concentrations has been reported during coadministration of either verapamil or diltiazem.[44] Simultaneous administration of verapamil and carbamazepine have been reported to produce dizziness, headache, diplopia and nausea.[45] Nifedipine, and presumably other calcium channel blockers can subtly impair learning and memory, particularly in elderly hypertensive patients.[46]

Respiratory Drugs

A variety of sympathomimetic drugs, including ephedrine, oxymetazoline, phenylephrine, and phenylpropanolamine are employed in prescription and nonprescription products for the treatment of asthma, allergic rhinitis, and colds. When used excessively, these compounds can produce anxiety and, infrequently, a toxic psychosis.[47] These drugs are discussed in greater detail later in this chapter. A large variety of sympathomimetic amines, including albuterol, isoetharine, isoproterenol, metaproterenol, and terbutaline are components of orally administered and inhalant products for the treatment of bronchial asthma. Each of these substances can produce tachycardia, tremor, anxiety, and, in rare instances, with large-dose administration, acute psychotic reactions.[47] Any of these compounds can provoke a hypertensive reaction when administered to a patient being treated with an MAOI. Theophylline, a commonly prescribed bronchodilator, can also provoke tachycardia, tremor, anxiety, and, infrequently, depression.[9,47] Although previous studies suggested that theophylline impaired school performance, more recent research indicates that neither asthma nor its treatment with theophylline impair cognitive function or school performance.[48] Dextromethorphan, a commonly used cough suppressant, can produce confusion and, rarely, hallucinations.[47]

Gastrointestinal Drugs

Prokinetic drugs

Metoclopramide, a cholinergic agonist and dopamine antagonist, increases motility and enhances gastric emptying.[49] Mania induced by metoclopramide has been reported.[50] This drug has also been reported to produce lethargy, sedation, restlessness, agitation, parkinsonism, and akathisia.[49,50] A number of cases of tardive dyskinesia have been reported in association with prolonged use of metoclopramide.[49,50]

Withdrawal dyskinesias are known to occur following abrupt discontinuation of metoclopramide therapy.[49] Simultaneous administration of neuroleptic drugs with metoclopramide would be likely to produce enhanced extrapyramidal and dyskinetic side effects.

Cisapride increases gastrointestinal motility and is primarily used in the treatment of gastroesophageal reflux. This agent lacks cholinergic and dopamine antagonist effects though it may facilitate acetylcholine release at the myenteric plexus without a concomitant cholinergic secretory effect.[51] Although generally used for GERD, this agent may eventually prove useful for management of constipation, including that induced by psychotropic drugs. Somnolence, fatigue, seizures, and abnormal movements are potential rare side effects of cisapride.[51]

Antiemetic drugs

Although neuroleptics are potent antagonists of the chemoreceptor trigger zone and often used as antiemetics, their side effects have been previously discussed and will not be reviewed here. Ondansetron is a serotonin 5-HT$_3$ receptor antagonist which has potent antiemetic activity and has been used to manage nausea and vomiting associated with antineoplastic chemotherapy.[51] Ondansetron, by virtue of its serotonin antagonist activity, has been reported to produce psychiatric side effects, including panic symptoms, fear, agitation and emotional lability.[52] Although the serotonin receptors which are best known in terms of activity of psychotropic drugs are 5-HT$_1$ and 5-HT$_2$, it is conceivable that patients being treated for psychiatric conditions with SSRIs who for unrelated reasons receive a 5-HT$_3$ antagonist such as ondansetron, may experience at least a partial reversal of therapeutic effects.

Antisecretory Drugs

Cimetidine, famotidine, nizatidine, and ranitidine are competitive antagonists of histamine H$_2$-receptors. These drugs block histamine-stimulated gastric acid secretion and may also indirectly block the action of gastrin and acetylcholine.[53] These compounds have found widespread clinical use in the treatment of duodenal ulcer, esophageal reflux, and the prevention of GI bleeding in seriously ill patients.

The duration of action of ranitidine is somewhat longer than other H_2 antagonists, however, all H_2 antagonists are capable of producing CNS side effects, including cognitive and mood changes, the incidence of which appears more related to the years of clinical use of the drug than to specific characteristics making one H_2 antagonist safer than another.[54] Delirium is the most common psychiatric side effect of H_2 antagonists and appears more frequently in patients who are elderly or more seriously ill, or in those with concurrent psychiatric conditions as well as in patients with hepatic or renal impairment.[53,54] Higher dose of H_2 antagonist or administration of other medications concomitantly may also be risk factors for psychiatric sequelae. Cimetidine is a potent inhibitor of cytochrome P-450, while ranitidine is only 1/5 to 1/10 as active against cytochrome P-450, and famotidine and nizatidine do not appear to inhibit this drug metabolizing enzyme.[53] Although I have not seen patients simultaneously receiving fluoxetine and cimetidine, one would certainly expect increased serum concentrations of both and potentially even greater than expected serum concentrations of any coaministered drugs whose metabolism utilizes cytochrome P-450.

Cimetidine-induced deliria appear within 24 to 48 hours of starting the drug and clear within 24 hours after its discontinuation.[55] Although toxic deliria, hallucinations, and confusion are more apt to occur in the acutely ill hospitalized patient, some outpatients receiving maintenance cimetidine have experienced depression with this drug.[56,57] Cimetidine-induced depression tends to begin 2 to 3 weeks after initiation of therapy. Ranitidine can also induce depression, but its onset often requires 4 to 8 weeks of treatment.[58] The half-life of long-acting benzodiazepines such as chlorazepate, chlordiazepoxide, and diazepam are significantly lengthened when these drugs are co-administered with cimetidine and, to a lesser extent, with ranitidine.[59] Short-acting benzodiazepines such as oxazepam and lorazepam, which do not undergo metabolic degradation, appear not to be affected by either cimetidine or ranitidine.

Analgesics

Propoxyphene may produce a clouding of consciousness, psychotic reactions, and hallucinations under conditions of ordinary therapeutic use.[9] These adverse effects are more likely to occur with excessive dosage or when the drug is administered IV by drug addicts seeking a hallucinogenic or narcoticlike effect. Propoxyphene is structurally similar to methadone; it is capable of inducing a true narcotic addiction that may require the patient to be detoxified under medical supervision.[9] Pentazocine is a moderately potent analgesic, initially marketed as a non-narcotic, nonaddicting substance. It exhibits both agonist and antagonist effects and may therefore provoke narcotic withdrawal symptoms when administered to patients addicted to narcotics.[8] Pentazocine itself is an addicting substance when administered by the oral or the IM route over a prolonged period of time.[8] This drug is also capable of producing hallucinations during the course of its administration. Furthermore, when patients addicted to pentazocine are suddenly withdrawn, they may develop a withdrawal syndrome identical to that seen with opiate drugs, except that pentazocine withdrawal often includes the appearance of hallucinations.[8] Patients addicted to this drug generally require detoxification under medical supervision, most commonly utilizing gradually decreasing doses of methadone.[8]

Anti-inflammatory Drugs

Indomethacin, which structurally has an indole nucleus, is a widely used agent in the treatment of arthritic and other inflammatory diseases. This compound occasionally produces mental confusion. It may produce depression, which at times is severe and associated with suicidal ideation or attempts.[25] Less frequently, patients receiving indomethacin may develop acute psychosis with visual or auditory hallucinations, requiring discontinuation of the medication and appropriate antipsychotic chemotherapy.[9,25] Drowsiness, fatigue, dizziness, and anxiety are infrequent side effects of nonsteroidal anti-inflammatory drugs, including ibuprofen, naproxen, piroxicam, sulindac, and tolmetin.[9] Depression is a rare side effect of naproxen and other non-steroidal antiinflammatory drugs (NSAIDs).[9]

Antibacterial Drugs

Nalidixic acid and nitrofurantoin are structurally unrelated antibacterial agents used in the treatment of urinary tract infection; they may both produce acute confusional states.[25] Isoniazid, an antituberculous drug chemically related to the first MAOI, iproniazid, may produce a variety of adverse behavioral effects. Patients receiving this drug may experience an impairment of memory, confusion, euphoria, and a florid psychotic reaction.[60,61] Psychotic reactions or other behavioral toxicity associated with isoniazid generally require discontinuation of the medication, and sometimes require administration of appropriate psychotropic medication. Isoniazid inhibits the metabolism of phenytoin, and may therefore lead to excessive blood levels and pharmacologic effects from this compound when they are simultaneously administered.[9] Tetracycline is an antibiotic that is widely used for a variety of infectious diseases and in the treatment of acne. Since patients receiving this drug for acne may take it over a prolonged period of time, its potential interaction with psychotropic drugs is of great importance. Tetracycline appears to effect the absorption and excretion of lithium and may increase serum lithium concentration in patients whose lithium blood levels were stable on a well-established dose of lithium carbonate.[62] The administration of tetracycline to patients receiving lithium should be avoided because of the increased risk of lithium intoxication. Patients receiving tetracycline for acne may be suitably managed by erythromycin instead, as it does not appear to interact with lithium, though it may provoke carbamazepine intoxication. Erythromycin and related drugs, including clarithromycin and azithromycin, may increase serum concentrations of carbamazepine, triazolam, and theophylline.[25]

Hypoglycemic Agents

Any drug capable of lowering serum glucose, whether it be an orally administered agent or parenterally administered insulin, may cause hypoglycemia, which may be associated with behavioral symptoms such as anxiety, agitation, and dysphoria.[1] Diabetic patients presenting with these complaints should generally have several random blood sugar determinations done to ascertain the appropriateness of their hypoglycemic treatment regimen prior to administering psychotropic medications.

Vitamins

Despite the claims of many proponents of megavitamin therapy in psychiatry, controlled clinical studies of the administration of large doses of niacin and other vitamins have failed to reveal the clinical value of this approach in the treatment of schizophrenia or other major mental disorders.[7] On the other hand, one of the longest-known medical conditions resulting from vitamin deficiency is pellagra, wherein patients may experience insomnia, depression, impairment of memory, delusions, hallucinations, and dementia, in conjunction with a variety of physical symptoms.[1] The administration of niacin to patients suffering from pellagra produces a dramatic therapeutic benefit, unlike its ill-defined efficacy in schizophrenia. Numerous studies of outpatients and hospitalized psychiatric patients have revealed a rather high incidence of folic acid deficiency. The administration of folic acid to patients with psychiatric complaints may produce an improvement in depression, irritability, and sleeplessness.[1,63] The high incidence of folic acid deficiency observed in previous studies of psychiatric patients suggests the possible value of serum folate determinations in psychiatric patients, particularly the elderly and those suffering from organic brain dysfunction. In the event that decreased serum folate levels are found the administration of folic acid in a dose of 0.5 to 1 mg daily is appropriate. Folic acid should not be administered until it has been determined that the patient's serum B_{12} level is normal, as the administration of folic acid to B_{12}-deficient patients may improve the megaloblastic anemia seen in both folic acid and B_{12} deficiency but will not correct the neurologic complications associated with B_{12} deficiency in patients with pernicious anemia.[1] Routine administration of megadoses of folic acid is not of clinical value and can be dangerous in the presence of B_{12} deficiency. Although there is no evidence that massive doses of vitamin C given to psychiatric patients has any clinical value, psychiatrists should be alerted to the fact that such are not uncommonly taken by patients and that this may be associated with severe epigastric pain or distress, and alter urinary excretion of psychotropic drugs. Pyridoxine deficiency may occur during treatment with phenelzine and isocarboxazid and produce hyperreflexia and myoclonus.[9,25]

Over-the-Counter Drugs

The variety of commercially available nonprescription pharmaceutical products is vast. Although discussions of renal damage produced by phenacetin and acetaminophen-containing analgesics and of the complications of salicylate intoxication are beyond the scope of this discussion, it should be pointed out that excessive use of salicylate-containing analgesics may cause organic brain dysfunction with hallucinations, delusions, delirium, disordered thinking, and agitation.[9] It is therefore important to include questions about nonprescription analgesics as well as other over-the-counter drugs in thoroughly evaluating a patient's current or prior drug exposure.

In addition to analgesics, nonprescription sedatives and patent remedies for the treatment of cough, colds, and allergic symptoms make up the bulk of nonprescription products taken by patients. All these remedies are likely to contain an antihistamine, alone or in conjunction with an anticholinergic compound such as scopolamine. Both antihistamines and anticholinergics are capable of producing atropine-like psychosis, more commonly known as anticholinergic delirium.[25] Patients may be confused, disoriented, have memory deficits, stuttering speech, agitation, and psychotic symptoms with auditory or visual hallucinations.[2] These patients may also have a variety of cardiovascular complications including tachycardia, and other autonomic symptoms including disturbances of sweating and bowel and bladder function.[25] The symptoms will disappear within one to several days after the offending agent is discontinued. In order to confirm the diagnosis of an anticholinergic delirium and produce mental clearing, physostigmine may be administered in a dose of 1 mg diluted to 10mL with normal saline, injected slowly IV over a period of three to five minutes. Use of short-acting nonanticholinergic sedatives such as lorazepam or oxazepam may be useful in the treatment of agitation associated with the anticholinergic syndrome. Patients who become frankly psychotic and agitated may require the cautious administration of low doses of haloperidol.

Cold and allergy remedies commonly contain phenylpropanolamine as a decongestant, and over-the-counter appetite suppressants generally include this compound as well. Since phenylpropanolamine is a sympathomimetic agent with weak amphetaminelike effects, one may observe excessive anxiety, agitation, and even a paranoid psychosis if large doses are taken.[2] Symptoms usually abate once the drug is discontinued, though the patient may need a temporary period of sedation with lorazepam or oxazepam, or may need a small dose of haloperidol. Low-potency antipsychotic agents such as thioridazine or chlorpromazine are to be avoided, since these compounds may produce significant hypotension in patients taking on phenylethylamine derivatives such as phenylpropanolamine.[25] The clinician must be aware that children may be unduly sensitive to anticholinergic agents or stimulants such as phenylpropanolamine, and that the elderly, particularly in the presence of organic brain dysfunction, are apt to be exceedingly sensitive and develop severe adverse reactions to these compounds commonly found in over-the-counter medications.[2,25]

Anticholinergic complications of psychotropic drugs have been discussed in chapter 10. The competent clinician needs to be cognizant that anticholinergic chemicals are ubiquitous in our environment. As described, a significant proportion of over-the-counter preparations, including the anticholinergics, and the majority of psychotropic drugs, have some anticholinergic effect. Furthermore, many prescription drugs used to treat GI conditions such as diarrhea, peptic ulcer disease, and irritable bowel syndrome, may contain anticholinergic compounds. In addition, there are a number of weeds and plants found throughout the United States and elsewhere that contain atropinelike substances. In this age of "health foods," when people are expressing concern about the safety of caffeine-containing beverages, numerous commercially available herbal teas are being promoted, which may, by virtue of atropinelike substances present in herbs, produce a more severe toxic reaction than the caffeine that many are trying to avoid.[66]

PSYCHIATRIC USES OF NONPSYCHOTROPIC DRUGS
(TABLE 13-2)
Cholinergic Agents

Many cyclic antidepressants, antipyschotic agents, non-psychotropic drugs and over-the-counter medications block brain acetylcholine receptors and can produce an acute toxic psychosis due to anticholinergic effects. The ability of physostigmine to rapidly reverse the central anticholinergic syndrome produced by psychotropic drugs has been discussed elsewhere. Although benzodiazepines such as diazepam are not strongly anticholinergic, they can produce confusion and persistent somnolence. The IV administration of physostigmine can reverse confusion and somnolence induced by diazepam, morphine and cimetidine.[67]

Physostigmine produces cholinergic stimulation by inhibiting the action of cholinesterase, the acetycholine-metabolizing enzyme. It has also been shown experimentally to improve long-term memory in normal humans,[68] and to enhance memory in a patient suffering from amnesia.[69] Unfortunately, the duration of action of physostigmine is about one hour; it is hoped the eventual availability of longer-lasting cholinesterase inhibitors may have considerable

Table 13-2 Psychiatric uses of nonpsychotropic drugs

Drug	Indications
Baclofen	Antianxiety, antipsychotic enhancer, dystonia, ?tardive dyskinesia
Bromocriptine	Antidepressant, NMS
Calcium channel blockers	Antimanic, ?antipanic, mood stabilizer, ?PMS
Carbamazepine	Antidepressant, antimanic, antipsychotic enhancer, mood stabilizer, ?PMS, dystonia
Clonazepam	Antianxiety, antipanic, antimanic, ?mood stabilizer, ?akathisia, ?Tourette's
Clonidine	Antimanic, antipanic, narcotic withdrawal, akathisia, ?tardive dyskinesia, Tourette's
Propranolol	Antianxiety, ?antipanic, ?antipsychotic, ?antipsychotic enhancer, akathisia, lithium tremors, ?tardive dyskinesia
Other β blockers	Antianxiety, antipanic, akathisia
Reserpine	Antipsychotic, antipsychotic enhancer, ?mood stabilizer
Valproate	Antimanic, antipsychotic, antipsychotic enhancer, ?PMS

? = studies or anecdotal reports indicate possible benefit; NMS = neuroleptic malignant syndrome; PMS = premenstrual syndrome.

therapeutic value. Galanthamine is an investigational compound that may answer this need.[70]

The peripheral manifestations of cholinergic blockade that are most troubling to patients receiving psychotropic medication include blurred vision, dry mouth, constipation, and difficulty urinating. The direct-acting cholinergic stimulant bethanechol is capable of reducing the severity of some of these peripheral anticholinergic side effects of cyclic antidepressants.[71] I have administered bethanechol tablets (5 or 10 mg) slowly dissolved in the mouth, and have seen efficacy in improving decreased salivation associated with psychotropic drugs. I have also utilized with some success a 1% solution of pilocarpine as a mouth rinse to improve salivary flow in patients receiving psychotropic drugs. Pilocarpine is a direct-acting cholinergic stimulant,[9] which is employed in the form of an ophthalmic solution in the treatment of glaucoma. It may also be used as a 1% eye drop solution for decreasing pupillary dilatation associated with psychotropic drugs, which is partially responsible for medication-associated blurred vision. Bethanechol in a dose of 10 mg orally or 5 mg IM or subcutaneously may be administered 3 or 4 times daily to improve urinary retention in patients receiving psychotropic agents, particularly the cyclic antidepressants.[71]

Reserpine

Although reserpine may produce depression and has only a limited value in medicine, it is still considered by some clinicians to be a useful antihypertensive agent. Several studies suggest that reserpine administered with antipsychotic medication may enhance the efficacy of neuroleptic compounds in the treatment of severely ill schizophrenic patients refractory to other treatment. Although this compound in conjunction with antipsychotics may increase the risk of postpsychotic depression, one group of investigators found reserpine potentially beneficial and worthy of trial in refractory psychotic patients.[72]

Beta-Adrenergic Antagonists

Since the mid-1960s, propranolol and other β-adrenergic antagonists have been studied and widely prescribed in England for the treatment of chronic anxiety.[4] Propranolol is not approved for this indication in the United States. Propranolol has also been shown to be effective when administered for short-term treatment of patients who become anxious prior to taking examinations.[4] I have had extensive experience with propranolol, metoprolol, and atenolol, used alone and in conjunction with low doses of benzodiazepines in the management of anxiety associated with prominent autonomic symptoms. These β-blocking drugs can be highly effective in eliminating tachycardia and other physiologic manifestations and may eliminate the necessity for benzodiazepine treatment in some patients, or reduce benzodiazepine dosage required by others. In the management of anxiety, propranolol is often effective at a dose of 10 to 20 mg 3 to 4 times daily and is unlikely to provoke depression at this dosage level. Metoprolol and atenolol have far less ability to cross the blood-brain barrier and are unlikely to provoke confusional states and depression, which occasionally occur with propranolol, particularly at higher doses. Some patients may experience sleep disturbance or increased or unpleasant dreams in association with propranolol or pindolol, though these effects are unlikely to occur with metoprolol and atenolol.

Several studies have been conducted over a number of years to assess the potential value of propranolol in the treatment of schizophrenia and other psychotic disorders. The doses employed for this purpose have been very high, ranging from 800 mg to 2000 mg or more daily. The available data suggests that, at best, propranolol in high dose has a modest antipsychotic action, and is unlikely to be useful for this indication in many patients.[73] As discussed in chapter 11, propranolol and, to a lesser extent, other β-adrenergic blocking drugs, are effective in the treatment of essential tremor and in tremors induced by lithium and tricyclic antidepressants. Propranolol and nadolol have both been found to be effective in controlling neuroleptic-induced akathisia, though these drugs are not promising in the management of tardive dyskinesia, as discussed in chapter 11. Propranolol, generally in higher doses of 160 to 600 mg daily, has been reported in various studies to be useful in the management of violent behavior, uncontrollable temper, and aggressive outbursts in children and adults, as discussed in chapter 15.[75]

Clonidine

Clonidine is an antihypertensive agent that stimulates presynaptic alpha-adrenergic autoreceptors in the brain, particularly in the locus ceruleus. This pharmacologic action results in a decrease in sympathetic outflow and a reduction in blood pressure.[9] Clonidine has been demonstrated by numerous studies to produce a variety of clinically useful effects in psychiatric disorders. Most notably, this drug supresses withdrawal symptoms associated with discontinuation of narcotic substances including heroin, methadone, narcotic analgesics, and propoxyphene.[76,77] The use of clonidine in the management of narcotic withdrawal and detoxification is discussed in chapter 17. In the management of opiate withdrawal, clonidine may be used in a dose of 5 μg/kg daily with gradual dosage reduction and eventual discontinuation. Since narcotic withdrawal is associated with noradrenergic hyperactivity, inhibition of this effect is the most likely mechanism to explain the efficacy of clonidine in alleviating narcotic withdrawal sysmptoms. Preliminary studies indicate that clonidine may suppress nicotine withdrawal symptoms and facilitate abstinence from tobacco.

Clonidine has been shown to have an antipsychotic effect as well as an antimanic effect in some patients. However, as discussed in chapter 8, controlled studies indicate clonidine is less effective than lithium in mania.[78] Early studies suggested that clonidine was of value in the management of tardive dyskinesia, though a more recent double-blind crossover study sheds doubt on the antidyskinetic activity of clonidine, which is further discussed in chapter 11.[79] Although sedation and hypotension are common side effects of clonidine, this drug is useful in the management of neuroleptic-induced akathisia in some patients.[80] Clonidine has been demonstrated to possess both antianxiety and antipanic activity in some patients.[77] A therapeutic trial of this drug in patients with panic disorder unresponsive to or intolerant of conventional therapeutic agents is indicated. However, the hypotensive activity of clonidine may limit its utility in these patients. Since clonidine, guanethidine, and bretylium require neural uptake mechanisms to be operative in order to exert their antihypertensive therapeutic effects, these drugs cannot be used simultaneously with cyclic antidepressants, which inhibit reuptake mechanisms. There have been occasional reports in the literature of clonidine worsening psychosis, provoking hallucinations, and inducing or worsening depression. Therefore it must be used with caution in psychiatric patients. Clonidine has also been shown to have a beneficial effect in Tourette's disorder, as discussed in chapter 15.

Yohimbine

Yohimbine is an antagonist of presynaptic alpha$_2$-adrenergic receptors producing effects which are opposite to those of clonidine, which is an agonist at alpha$_2$-adrenergic autoreceptors.[9] Mania has been reported in some patients treated with yohimbine.[81] Experience with yohimbine as a potential antidepressant has yielded mixed results, without a favorable response in some patients, while antidepressant activity or ability to enhance antidepressant efficacy has been observed in others.[82] Historically, yohimbine has been used for many years as an aphrodisiac, with uncertain beneficial results.[9] Several publications indicate that yohimbine is effective in improving psychopharmacologically induced reduction of libido and sexual function. Most notably, yohimbine, which is available in 5.4 mg tablets, has been used with considerable success in the treatment of reduced sex drive, erectile and orgasmic function in patients being treated with fluoxetine and other SSRIs which are the psychotropic agents most commonly associated with sexual dysfunction.[83,84] When used for sexual dysfunction, patients may take 1 to 2 tablets approximately 2 hours before intercourse or may be treated with a regular continuous regimen of 1 to 4 tablets daily.

Bromocriptine

Bromocriptine is a dopamine agonist that inhibits release of prolactin. As discussed in chapter 10, bromocriptine and the chemically unrelated antispasticity agent dantrolene are often useful in the management of neuroleptic malignant syndrome. Preliminary studies have also found bromocriptine to produce a clinically useful antidepressant effect in some patients.[85] Amantadine and Pemoline also have dopamine receptor agonist activity and may be useful in the treatment of some depressed patients as discussed in chapter 18. Some studies suggest that bromocriptine and amantadine may reduce symptoms of cocaine withdrawal and help cocaine abusers to remain abstinent from this drug, perhaps partially by reducing craving for cocaine.

Baclofen

Baclofen is a GABA derivative that crosses the blood-brain barrier and may affect central GABA receptors. This compound also appears to affect substance P receptors in the brain.[86] It is a potent antispastic drug that may produce dramatic reductions in spasticity in various neurologic conditions including cerebral palsy, multiple sclerosis, and torsion dystonia. Baclofen is of interest in psychiatry because of some observations that it may reduce abnormal movements associated with tardive dyskinesia.[86] Baclofen may also have an antipsychotic effect or may potentiate the antipsychotic action of conventional dopamine-blocking neuroleptics. One study, and occasional clinical observations, suggest that the addition of baclofen in a dose of 5 to 15 mg tid may enhance the response to antipsychotic drugs in patients who have had less than adequate therapeutic benefit from these agents.[87] Since baclofen appears to act on GABA and substance P, it may have some anxiety-relieving qualities. In a small number of patients in a non-blinded clinical trial, I observed some reduction of anxiety symptoms with baclofen in a dose of 20 to 40 mg daily.

Gabapentin

Originally synthesized as a structural analog of the inhibitory neurotransmitter gamma amino butyric acid (GABA), gabapentin does not interact with specific brain receptors for GABA but rather appears to act at system-L sites, which act as large neutral amino acid transporters.[88,89] Gabapentin has been recently marketed in the United States for treatment of partial seizures and as an add-on agent for convulsive disorders refractory to other pharmacotherapies.[88] Since this drug produces minimal side effects and shows little evidence of altering metabolism of other pharmacological agents, it may be a promising agent to try when attempting to modify symptom patterns which may involve GABA mediated mechanisms. Though clinical studies in psychiatry are yet to be done, this drug should be considered for investigation in the management of anxiety, tardive dyskinesia, and mania, conditions for which other anticonvulsants have been found useful.

Carbamazepine

Carbamazepine is chemically related to the antidepressant imipramine, and was initially introduced for the treatment of trigeminal neuralgia.[9] In the early experience with carbamazepine several cases of drug-associated agranulocytosis were reported, which led to concern about its safety.[9] Subsequently, the drug became increasingly used in the treatment of seizure disorders, particularly in patients with temporal lobe epilepsy.[90,91] As use of the drug expanded, two interesting observations emerged. First, although there were early reports of agranulocytosis, which made the drug appear frightening to many clinicians, with wider clinical use, the drug was not associated with a high incidence of serious hematologic complications, though some patients do develop mild, reversible, leukopenia. The other observation was that in 40 reports covering approximately 2500 patients with epilepsy, approximately 50% noted psychiatric improvement during carbamazepine treatment.[90]

A number of controlled studies have documented the psychiatric utility of this promising drug. Unlike the scientifically unsupported claims for the antidepressant efficacy of phenytoin, there are considerable data now available to support the antidepressant and antimanic action of carbamazepine.[91,92,93] This is based on multiple clinical observations and numerous well-designed

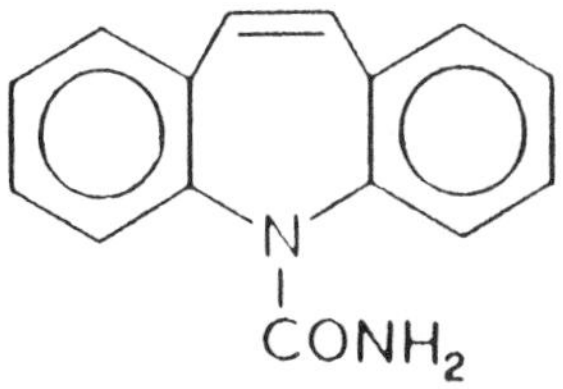

CARBAMAZEPINE

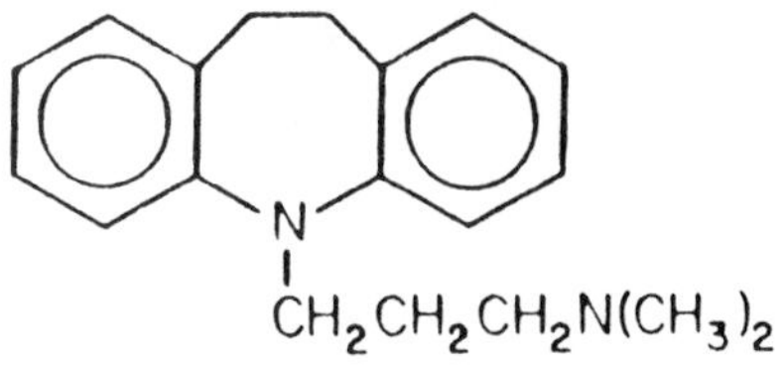

IMIPRAMINE

double-blind controlled studies as discussed in chapter 8. In patients unresponsive to lithium or unable to tolerate lithium, carbamazepine may have considerable prophylactic effect against recurrent mood symptoms.[92,93] Drowsiness is the most commonly reported side effect of this drug, and it can be minimized if a greater portion of the daily dose is administered at bedtime. Complete blood counts should be done prior to starting carbamazepine and every 1 to 2 weeks during the first month or two. Subsequently, blood counts done with decreasing frequency throughout the course of carbamazepine management are clinically useful to detect a reduction in WBC count. If this does occur, temporary dosage reduction or discontinuation is necessary, though the likelihood of this appears to be exceedingly small. Since many patients present to the psychiatrist with labile moods and impulsive behavior, with or without further signs suggesting temporal lobe epilepsy, a therapeutic trial of carbamazepine should be considered, particularly in those who have been unsuccessfully managed with lithium or other psychotropic agents.

Sodium Valproate

Sodium valproate and the related compounds valproic acid and divalproex have been used extensively for a number of years in the treatment of convulsive disorders. Individual case reports, studies of larger series of valproate-treated patients, and small controlled studies indicate that this compound has promising antipsychotic and antimanic effects.[94,95] In one uncontrolled series, 16 (44%) of 36 valproate-treated patients showed a moderate to marked therapeutic response to this drug. Patients with bipolar illness or schizoaffective disorder showed the most favorable response to valproate.[94] Many patients, who have not responded adequately to lithium, carbamazepine, or neuroleptics, have achieved a good response with valproate, which is discussed in more detail in chapter 8. One of the major factors that has discouraged more widespread clinical use of valproate has been the awareness of its potential hepatotoxicity and the small number of deaths that have occurred due to this complication.[96] In fact, the risk of hepatotoxicity is lower than many physicians realize. According to a retrospective review, the risk of fatalities primarily occurred in children 2 years old and younger, who were receiving multiple drugs simultaneously.[96] In that review, there were no fatalities in patients above the age of 10 years who were receiving valproate as their sole anticonvulsant.[96] Although the clinical efficacy of both carbamazepine and valproate are well established by extensive published studies and clinical experience, there is some controversy as to whether one of these drugs is superior to the other. Most evidence suggests that they are equally effective, although some patients respond preferentially to one or the other.

Calcium Channel Blockers

Of the multitude of currently available calcium channel blockers, verapamil, has been most extensively studied and used in psychiatry.[41] These drugs appear to share some common pharmacologic characteristics with the established antimanic agent lithium carbonate.[40] Verapamil has been used in doses of 80-320 mg/day in a large number of acutely manic patients. Side effects with this drug are relatively infrequent and generally mild.[41] Some hypotension and drowsiness are occasionally observed. Clinical studies have found verapamil frequently to be comparable to lithium in efficacy, and of occasional benefit in manic patients who neither tolerate nor respond to lithium. One double-blind crossover study in 20 patients noted a more favorable antimanic response to verapamil than to clonidine.[97] Preliminary experience suggests that verapamil may be useful not only in the treatment of acute mania, but as a maintenance drug in patients with bipolar affective illness. The applications of calcium channel blockers in the treatment of mania are further discussed in chapter 8. Verapamil has also been demonstrated to be useful in conjunction with imipramine in a patient with recurrent unipolar depression who failed to respond previously to imipramine alone or in combination with lithium carbonate.[98] Although some investigators have reported a favorable response to verapamil in schizophrenia, a study of seven schizophrenic patients was unable to confirm a beneficial effect.[99]

Experience with a smaller number of patients indicates potential usefulness of calcium channel blocking drugs, primarily verapamil, in a variety of psychiatric conditions, including Tourette's syndrome, PCP intoxication, premenstrual dysphoria, and migraine headaches. Further clinical experience and more extensive controlled studies are necessary to further define the role of this interesting group of drugs in psychiatric disorders. One of the many unanswered questions is whether there may be differential responsiveness to different calcium channel blockers. The possibility that this may be true is suggested by evidence that there are two or three distinct receptors sensitive to calcium channel blocking drugs.[41] Another novel use of a calcium channel blocker, nifedipine, is in the treatment of hypertensive crises in MAOI-treated patients. The relative safety of the calcium channel blockers should encourage their continuing use and exploration in the management of psychiatric patients.

Although these indications are not approved by the FDA, properly selected patients, given adequate information and offering their consent to treatment, may achieve beneficial therapeutic results with these medications.

REFERENCES

1. Jefferson JW, Marshall JR: *Neuropsychiatric Features of Medical Disorders*, New York, Plenum Medical Book, 1981.
2. Gardner ER, Hall RCW: Psychiatric symptoms produced by over-the-counter drugs. *Psychosomatics* 1982;23:186-190.
3. Ballenger JC, Post RM: Carbamazepine in manic-depressive illness: A new treatment. *Am J Psychiatry* 1980;137:782-790.
4. Johnson JM: Psychiatric uses of antiadrenergic and adrenergic blocking drugs. *J Nerv Ment Dis* 1984;172:123-132.
5. Wurtman RJ, Wurtman JJ (eds): *Nutrients and the Brain*, New York, Raven Press, 1986, vol. 7.
6. Wurtman RJ: Nutrients affecting brain composition and behavior. *Integrative Psychiatry* 1987;5:226-257.
7. Wittenborn JR, Weber ESP, Brown M: Niacin in the long-term treatment of schizophrenia. *Arch Gen Psychiatry* 1973;28:308-315.
8. Brogden RN, Speight TM, Avery GS: Pentazocine: A review of the pharmacological properties, therapeutic efficacy and dependence liability. *Drugs* 1973;5:6-91.
9. Gilman AG, Rall TW, Nies AS, Taylor P (eds): *Goodman and Gilman's The pharmacological basis of therapeutics*, ed 8, New York, Pergamon Press, 1990.
10. Lewis DA, Smith RE: Steroid-induced psychiatric syndromes: A report of 14 cases and a review of the literature. *J Affective Disord* 1983;5:319-332.
11. Malek-Ahmadi P, Behrmann PJ: Depressive syndrome induced by oral contraceptives. *Dis Nerv Syst* 1976;37:406-408.
12. Wilson IC, Prange AJ, Lard PP: Methyltestosterone in men: Conversion of depression to paranoid reaction. *Am J Psychiatry* 1974;131:21-24.
13. Pope HG, Katz DL: Affective and psychotic symptoms associated with anabolic steroid use. *Am J Psychiatry* 1988;145:487-490.
14. Eisendrath SJ, Sweeney MA: Toxic neuropsychiatric effects of digoxin at therapeutic serum concentrations. *Am J Psychiatry* 1987;144:506-507.
15. Gilbert GJ: Quinidine dementia. *JAMA* 1977;237:2093-2094.
16. Eisenman DP, McKegney FP: Delirium at therapeutic serum concentrations of digoxin and quinidine. *Psychosomatics* 1994;35:91-93.
17. Saravay SM, Marke J, Steinberg MD, et al: "Doom anxiety" and delirium in lidocaine toxicity. *Am J Psychiatry* 1987;144:159-163.
18. Franks RD, Richter AJ: Schizophrenia-like psychosis associated with anti-convulsant toxicity. *Am J Psychiatry* 1979;136:973-974.
19. Tollefson G: Psychiatric implications of anticonvulsant drugs. *J Clin Psychiatry* 1980;41: 295-302.
20. Naccarelli GV, Dougherty AH, Nappi J, *et al:* Pharmacological therapy of arrhythmias. In Naccarelli GV (ed): *Cardiac arrhythmias: a Practical Approach*, Mount Kisco, NY, Futura Publishing Co, 1991.
21. Bernstein JG, Koch-Weser J: Clinical evaluation of bretylium tosylate in refractory ventricular arrhythmias. *Circulation* 1972;45:1024-1034.
22. Petrie WM, Maffucci RJ, Woosley RL: Propranolol and depression. *Am J Psychiatry* 1982;139:92-93.
23. Gershon ES, Goldstein RE, Moss AJ, et al: Psychosis with ordinary doses of propranolol. *Ann Intern Med* 1979;90:938-939.
24. Bright RA, Everitt DE: Beta-blockers and depression. Evidence against an association. *JAMA* 1992;267:1783-1787.

25. Bernstein JG: Drug Interactions. In Cassem NH (ed): *Massachusetts general hospital handbook of general hospital psychiatry,* ed 3, St Louis, Mosby, 1991.
26. Okada F: Depression after treatment with thiazide diuretics for hypertension. *J Clin Psychiatry* 1985;142:1101-1102.
27. Quetsch RM, Achor RWP, Litin EM: Depressive reactions in hypertensive patients. *Circulation* 1959;19:366-375.
28. Whitlock FA, Evans LEJ: Drugs and depression. *Drugs* 1978;15:53-71.
29. Thornton WE: Dementia induced by methyldopa with haloperidol *N Engl J Med* 1976;294:1222.
30. Lavin P, Alexander CP: Dementia associated with clonidine therapy. *Br Med J* 1975;1:628.
31. Brown M, Salmon D, Rendell M: Clonidine hallucinations. *Ann Intern Med* 1980;93:456-457.
32. Gengo FM, Gabos C: Central nervous system considerations in the use of Beta-blockers, angiotensin-converting enzyme inhibitors, and thiazide diuretics in managing essential hypertension. *Am Heart J* 1988;116:305-310.
33. Testa MA, Anderson RB, Nackley JA, *et al:* Quality of life and antihypertensive therapy in men: A comparison of captopril and enalapril. *N Engl J Med* 1993;328:907-913.
34. Materson BJ, Reda DJ, Cushman WC, *et al:* Single-drug therapy for hypertension in men: A comparison of six antihypertensive agents with placebo. *N Engl J Med* 1993;328:914-921.
35. Williams GH: Converting-enzyme inhibitors in the treatment of hypertension. *N Engl J Med* 1988;319:1517-1525.
36. White W. Hypotension with postural syncope secondary to the combination of chlorpromazine and captopril. *Arch Intern Med* 1986;146:1833-1834.
37. Duoste-Blazy PH, Rostin M, Livarek B, et al: Angiotensin converting enzyme inhibitors and lithium treatment. *Lancet* 1986;1:448.
38. Zubenko GS, Nixon RA: Mood-elevating effects of captopril in depressed patients. *Am J Psychiatry* 1984;141:110-111.
39. McMahon T: Bipolar affective symptoms associated with use of captopril and abrupt withdrawal of pargyline and propranolol. *Am J Psychiatry* 1985;142:759-760.
40. Dubovsky SL, Frank RD: Intracellular calcium ions in affective disorders: A review and an hypothesis. *Biol Psychiatry* 1983;18:781-797.
41. Pollack MH, Rosenbaum JF, Hyman SE: Calcium channel blockers in psychiatry. *Psychosomatics* 1987;28:356-369.
42. Ahmad S: Nifedipine-induced psychosis. *J Am Geriatr Soc* 1984;32:408.
43. Jacobsen FM: Delirium induced by verapamil. *Am J Psychiatry* 1987;144:248.
44. Price WA, Giannini AJ: Neurotoxicity caused by lithium-verapamil synergism. *J Clin Pharmacol* 1986;26:717-719.
45. MacPhee G: Verapamil potentiates carbamazepine neurotoxicity: A clinically important inhibitory interaction. *Lancet* 1986;1:700-703.
46. Skinner MH, Futterman A, Morrissette D, *et al:* Atenolol compared with nifedipine: effect on cognitive function and mood in elderly hypertensive patients. *Ann Int Med* 1992;116:615-623.
47. Hall RCW, Beresford TP, Stickney SK, et al: Psychiatric reactions produced by respiratory drugs. *Psychosomatics* 1985;26:605-616.
48. Lindgren S, Lokshin B, Stromquist A, *et al:* Does asthma or treatment with theophylline limit children's academic performance? *N Engl J Med* 1992;327:926-930.
49. Lieberman DA, Keefe EB: Treatment of severe reflex esophagitis with cimetidine and metachlopramide. *Ann Intern Med* 1986;104:21-26.
50. Ritchie KS, Preskhorn SH: Mania induced by metoclopramide: Case report. *J Clin Psychiatry* 1984;45:180-181.
51. Patel AR, Snape WJ: Prokinetic agents and antiemetics. In: Wolfe MM (ed): *Gastrointestinal pharmacology,* Philadelphia, 1993, Saunders.
52. Mitchell KE, Popkin MK, Trick W, *et al:* Psychiatric complications associated with ondansetron. *Psychosomatics* 1994;35:161-163.

53. Lichtenstein DR, Wolfe MM: Histamine H_2-receptor antagonists. In Wolfe MM (ed): *Gastrointestinal Pharmacotherapy*, Philadelphia, 1993, Saunders.

54. Cantu TG, Korek JS: Central nervous system reactions to histamine-2 receptor blockers. *Ann Intern Med* 1991;114:1027-1034.

55. Strauss A: Cimetidine and delirium: Assessment and management. *Psychosomatics* 1982;23:49-53.

56. Adler LE, Sadja L, Wilets G: Cimetidine toxicity manifested as paranoia and hallucinations. *Am J Psychiatry* 1980;137:1112-1113.

57. Jefferson JW: Central nervous system toxicity of cimetidine: A case of depression. *Am J Psychiatry* 1979;136:346.

58. Billings R, Stein M: Depression associated with ranitidine. *Am J Psychiatry* 1986;143:915-916.

59. Desmond PV, Patwardhan RV, Schenker S: Cimetidine impairs elimination of chlordiazepoxide in man. *Ann Intern Med* 1980;93:266-268.

60. Reilly DK: Isoniazid-related CNS toxicity. *Drug Ther* 1979;9:187-188.

61. Duncan H, Kerr D: Toxic psychosis due to isoniazid. *Br J Dis Chest* 1962;56:131-138.

62. McGinnis AJ: Lithium-tetracycline interaction. *Br Med J* 1978;1:1183.

63. Reynolds EH, Preece JM, Bailey J, et al: Folate deficiency in depressive illness. *Br J Psychiatry* 1970;117:287-292.

64. Howard JS: Folate deficiency in psychiatry practice. *Psychosomatics* 1975;16:112-119.

65. Thornton WE, Thornton BP: Folic acid, mental function and dietary habits. *J Clin Psychiatry* 1978;39:314-322.

66. Siegel RK: Herbal intoxication. *JAMA* 1976;236:473-477.

67. Bourke DL: Physostigmine effectiveness as an antagonist of respiratory depression and psychomotor effects caused by morphine or diazepam. *Anesthesiology* 1984;61:523-528.

68. Sitaram N, Weingartner H, Gillin JC: Physostigmine: Improvement in long-term memory processes in normal humans. *Science* 1978;201:272-276.

69. Peters BH, Levin HS: Memory enhancement after physostigmine treatment in the amnestic syndrome. *Arch Neurol* 1977;34:215-219.

70. Baraka A, Harik S: Reversal of central anticholinergic syndrome by galanthamine. *JAMA* 1977;238:2293-2294.

71. Pollack MH, Rosenbaum JF: Management of antidepressant-induced side effects. *J Clin Psychiatry* 1986;48:3-8.

72. Berlant JL: Neuroleptics and reserpine in refractory psychoses. *J Clin Psychopharmacol* 1986;6:180-184.

73. Manchanda R, Hirsch SR: Does propranolol have an antipsychotic effect? A placebo-controlled study in acute schizophrenia. *Br J Psychiatry* 1986;148:701-707.

74. Lipinski JF, Zubenko GS, Cohen BM, et al: Propranolol in the treatment of neuroleptic-induced akathisia. *Am J Psychiatry* 1984;141:412-415.

75. Kuperman S, Stewart MA: Use of propranolol to decrease aggressive outbursts in younger patients. *Psychosomatics* 1987;28:315-319.

76. Gold MS, Pottash AC, Sweeney DR, et al: Opiate withdrawal using clonidine. *JAMA* 1980;243:343-346.

77. Bond WJ: Psychiatric indications for clonidine: The neuropharmacologic and clinical basis. *J Clin Psychopharmacol* 1986;6:81-87.

78. Freedman R, Bell J, Kirsch D: Clonidine for coexisting psychosis and tardive dyskinesia. *Am J Psychiatry* 1980;137:629-630.

79. Browne J, Silver H, Marin R, et al: The use of clonidine in the treatment of neuroleptic-induced tardive dyskinesia. *J Clin Psychopharmacol* 1986;6:88-82.

80. Adler LA, Angrist B, Peselow E, et al: Clonidine in neuroleptic-induced akathisia. *Am J Psychiatry* 1987;144:235-236.

81. Price LH, Charney DJ, Heninger GR: Three cases of manic symptoms following yohimbine administration. *Am J Psychiatry* 1984;141:1267-1268.

82. Pollack MH, Hammerness P: Adjunctive yohimbine for treatment in refractory depression. *Biol Psychiatry* 1993;33:220-221.

83. Hollander E, McCarley A: Yohimbine treatment of sexual side effects induced by serotonin reuptake blockers. *J Clin Psychiatry* 1992;53:207-209.

84. Jacobsen FM: Fluoxetine-induced sexual dysfunction and an open trial of yohimbine. *J Clin Psychiatry* 1992;53:119-122.

85. Waehren J, Gerlach J: Bromocriptine and imipramine in endogenous depression: A double-blind controlled trial in outpatients. *J Affective Disord* 1981;3:193-202.

86. Simpson GM, Lee JH, Shrivastava RK, et al: Baclofen in the treatment of tardive dyskinesia and schizophrenia. *Psychopharmacol Bull* 1978;14:16-18.

87. Frederiksen PK: Baclofen in the treatment of schizophrenia. *Lancet* 1975;1:702-703.

88. Chadwick D (ed): *New trends in epilepsy management: The role of gabapentin.* London, Royal Society of Medicine Services, 1993.

89. Suman-Chauhan N, Webdale L, Hill DR, *et al:* Characterization of ³(H)gabapentin binding to a novel site in rat brain: homogenate binding studies. *Eur J Pharmacol-Molecular Pharmacology Section* 1993;244:293-301.

90. Penry JK, Daly DD (eds): Complex partial seizures and their treatment, New York, Raven Press, 1975.

91. McElroy SL, Pope HG (eds): *Use of anticonvulsants in psychiatry: recent advances.* Clifton, New Jersey, Oxford Health Care, 1988.

92. Post RM, Leverich GS, Rosoff AS *et al:* Carbamazepine prophylaxis in refractory affective disorders: A focus on long-term follow-up. *J Clin Psychopharmacol* 1990;10:318-327.

93. Stuppaeck CH, Barnas C, Schwitzer J, *et al:* Carbamazepine in the prophylaxis of major depression: A 5-year follow-up. *J Clin Psychiatry* 1994;55:146-150.

94. McElroy SL, Keck PE, Pope HG Jr: Sodium valproate: Its use in primary psychiatric disorders. *J Clin Psychopharmacol* 1987;7:16-24.

95. McElroy SL, Keck PE, Pope HG, *et al:* Valproate in the treatment of bipolar disorder: literature review and clinical guidelines. *J Clin Psychopharmacol* 1992;12:42S-52S.

96. Dreifuss FE, Santilli N, Langer DH, et al: Valproic acid hepatic fatalities: A retrospective review. *Neurology* 1987;37:379-385.

97. Giannini AJ, Loiselle RH, Price WA, et al: Comparison of antimanic efficacy of clonidine and verapamil. *J Clin Pharmacol* 1985;25:307-308.

98. Pollack MH, Rosenbaum JF: Verapamil in the treatment of recurrent unipolar depression. *Biol Psychiatry* 1987;22:779-782.

99. Pickar D, Wolkowitz OM, Doran AR, et al: Clinical and biochemical effects of verapamil administration to schizophrenic patients. *Arch Gen Psychiatry* 1987;44:113-118.

CHAPTER 14

Psychotropic Drugs in Pregnancy and Lactation

OVERVIEW

1. Because of potential teratogenicity, drugs should be avoided during the first trimester if possible.
2. Women of childbearing age receiving psychotropic drugs should be urged to use effective birth control.
3. Lithium taken in the first trimester increases the risk of cardiac anomalies, but to a lesser extent than initial data indicated.
4. Carbamazepine and valproate increase the risk of neural tube anomalies (eg: spina bifida); carbamazepine may be employed, if ultrasound and elective termination are options before 20 weeks of gestation.
5. Current evidence indicates that tricyclic antidepressants and fluoxetine do not present a significant risk of anomalous development. Fetal risk of maternal MAOI therapy is uncertain.
6. Fluphenazine, haloperidol, perphenazine, and trifluoperazine present minimal risk of teratogenicity.
7. Benzodiazepines may increase the risk of cleft lip and cleft palate, probably to a very limited extent; clonazepam appears to be safest.
8. Optimally lithium and probably benzodiazepines should be discontinued 1 to 2 months before attempting to conceive and should not be restarted until after the first trimester.
9. If pregnancy is suspected during lithium treatment, lithium should be discontinued if clinically feasible. Benzodiazepines should be tapered and discontinued or changed to clonazepam as soon as pregnancy is suspected.
10. Breast-feeding should generally be avoided if psychotropic medications must be continued.

O ver the years, clinical wisdom has dictated the avoidance of medications during pregnancy because of their potential risk to the developing fetus. Unfortunately, chemicals are ubiquitous in our environment, whether they be in the air we breathe or as additives in the food we eat. Women may unknowingly consume substances which may adversely affect the fetus. Certainly, the effect of alcohol on fetal development is well known in the form of the fetal alcohol syndrome.[1] Many people do not consider over-the-counter remedies to be medications, yet OTC agents may contain pharmacologic substances that can adversely affect the developing fetus. Pregnant women and women who contemplate pregnancy should be alerted to the potential risks, not only of prescribed medications, but of the many substances that are taken for granted as a part of modern life. Indeed, it is difficult to ascertain the precise risks of psychotropic drugs in view of the fact that so many other substances may be consumed simultaneously.[2]

The psychiatrist is likely to become involved in providing information and making recommendations to the patient who has been maintained on a psychotropic medication regimen and decides to become pregnant. Likewise, some patients who are being maintained on medication will consult the psychiatrist when they learn that they have become pregnant. Although the incidence of psychiatric illness does not appear to be dramatically different during pregnancy, some pregnant women will experience their first episode of psychosis or depression during pregnancy. The treating psychiatrist will then need to make a decision regarding the safest course of therapy to be followed, both from the standpoint of the needs of the mother and that of the developing child. The psychiatrist's advice is also likely to be sought in respect to the effect of medications on the infant at the time of delivery and during the course of breast-feeding in the case of a mother who is being maintained on psychotropic medication. In many instances, the risk of a psychiatrically ill mother may outweigh the relatively low risk of commonly prescribed psychotropic medications on fetal development, labor, and the newborn infant.[3]

The psychiatrist may also be consulted when a woman with a known psychiatric illness contemplates pregnancy. Investigators have shown that there is a 27% risk of the offspring developing either bipolar or unipolar affective disorder in adulthood when one parent has either type of illness. The risk increases to more than 50% if both parents have an affective illness. There is an estimated 10% risk that offspring will develop schizophrenia in adulthood if one parent has schizophrenia; the risk is approximately 46% if both parents are affected.[4] Although these factors should be kept in mind when contemplating pregnancy, they should not be seen as an absolute contraindication to bearing a child. It is important for the psychiatrist to discuss this issue openly with a woman who consults him about potential pregnancy. It is also important that the psychiatrist provide thorough information and opportunity for discussion regarding the potential effects of psychotropic medications on fetal development.

Although no specific effects of psychotropic drugs on fertility have been identified, chromosomal gaps or breaks, and haploid cells in the embryo have been reported with perphenazine, thioridazine, and lithium. An increased risk of spontaneous abortion has not been found with the use of psychotropic drugs, which one might expect if severe chromosomal defects, grossly affecting the fetus, were present.[5] The greatest risk of medication-induced dysgenesis occurs in the first 2 months of pregnancy.[2,5] Nervous system development is most affected from the tenth to the 25th day of gestation, cardiac development from the 20th to the 40th day, and limb development between the 24th and 26th day.[5] Metabolic changes in the pregnant woman may affect drug disposition and metabolism.[5,6] Furthermore, immature enzyme systems in the developing fetus and newborn may enhance drug effects by impairing metabolic degradation and excretion of medications.[5,6] This chapter reviews the effects of some commonly prescribed psychotropic drugs on fetal development and on the newborn, who may receive medication through the placenta prior to delivery and through breast milk following parturition.

SEDATIVE AND ANTIANXIETY DRUGS

A relatively early study of the teratogenic potential of psychotropic drugs in the first trimester of pregnancy reported a 12.1% incidence of severe congenital anomalies in meprobamate-treated mothers.[7] The same study found an 11.4% incidence of congenital anomalies associated with chlordiazepoxide. The control group utilized in that study had a 2.6% incidence of anomalies. A retrospective study of 30 mothers of children with cleft palates found that 6.3% had used diazepam in the first trimester of pregnancy compared to 1.1% of the controls.[8] The risk of in utero exposure to diazepam was evaluated in a case control study involving 445 infants with cleft lip with or without cleft palate and

160 infants with cleft palate alone, who were compared to 2498 control infants having other birth defects. The study concluded that first-trimester exposure to diazepam does not materially affect the risk of cleft lip with or without cleft palate or of cleft palate alone.[9]

Recent reports raise further questions about the safety of maternal exposure to benzodiazepines from the standpoint of fetal development and physiology.[10] Seven of 36 infants whose mothers were exposed to high-dose benzodiazepines during pregnancy showed signs of abnormal development or physiology. In those cases in which the dosage was documented, two mothers had been receiving oxazepam 75 mg/day, three had been receiving diazepam 30-50 mg/day, and two, whose doses were not known, had exceedingly high serum diazepam concentrations.[10]

A recent publication reviewed 441 reports of in utero exposure to alprazolam or triazolam.[11] These represented prospective reports to the pharmaceutical manufacturer regarding first-trimester use of these benzodiazepines. Most of the 441 patients discontinued alprazolam as soon as pregnancy was diagnosed. Data are unavailable on 235 of these pregnancies, either because the patients were still pregnant at the time of publication or because patients dropped out of the study or elected to have abortions. Over one half of the cases that went to term resulted in the delivery of a normal child without complications.[11] Twenty children had normal birth weight and experienced perinatal events not thought to be drug-related. There were 16 reports of spontaneous abortion or miscarriage. One infant with multiple congenital anomalies had only a single-dose alprazolam exposure in the mother during pregnancy, and another with multiple anomalies involved a single-dose exposure to triazolam in the mother. One mother who had taken 0.5 mg of alprazolam daily for the first 2 months of pregnancy gave birth to an infant with anomalous development. Five infants whose mothers had been exposed to alprazolam had minor abnormalities, including pyloric stenosis, tongue-tie, umbilical hernia, ankle inversion, and clubfoot. There were two cases of withdrawal symptoms in infants of mothers who had taken alprazolam throughout pregnancy; in one case the daily dose was 3 mg and in the other, 7 to 8 mg.[11]

Clonazepam has been used extensively for many years as an anticonvulsant, and considerable experience has accumulated regarding its use throughout pregnancy. Based on the clinical track record of this drug, it appears to have minimal potential to cause anomalous fetal development.[12] Patients who require a benzodiazepine during pregnancy would probably best be treated with clonazepam, employing the lowest effective dosage. Patients who have been receiving high doses of alprazolam are likely to respond well to clonazepam with potentially greater safety for mother and baby. Clearly, if benzodiazepines are not clinically necessary, it is preferable to discontinue them prior to pregnancy or as early as possible when pregnancy is confirmed.

Benzodiazepines given at the end of gestation may depress fetal and neonatal respiration in a dose-dependent fashion. Doses of diazepam greater than 30 mg given during labor have been reported to produce neonatal hypotonia, hypothermia, low Apgar scores, and reluctance to feed.[5] Low doses of benzodiazepines given during labor are unlikely to adversely affect an otherwise healthy infant. Because of the relatively long half-life of long-acting benzodiazepines such as diazepam, effects may be present for several weeks in the neonate whose mother received significant doses of these drugs during the latter phase of pregnancy. Indeed, immature drug-metabolizing enzymes in the infant may cause the effects of even short-acting benzodiazepines, such as lorazepam, to be prolonged.[6] The addictive potential of benzodiazepines is significant in the newborn; mothers receiving these drugs in substantial doses over prolonged periods of their pregnancy may expose their infant to the risk of a drug withdrawal syndrome following parturition. Neonatal withdrawal symptoms, including irritability, jitteriness, tremors, diarrhea, vomiting, and high-pitched crying, have been reported following maternal ingestion of diazepam 15-20 mg/day for at least 12 weeks during the second and third trimesters.[13] These symptoms are similar to those seen in association with neonatal narcotic withdrawal.

Benzodiazepines are excreted in breast milk and present a significant risk of lethargy and impaired temperature regulation in infants that are being breast-fed. These drugs are not metabolized in the fetal liver or intestine, and in the first four days of life the infant is unable to conjugate them with glucuronic acid, which may result in an increased risk of jaundice.[5] Phenobarbital use by nursing mothers has been reported to have little or no effect on the infant with the exception of enhanced hepatic drug-metabolizing enzymes.[5]

Although the risk of low doses of benzodiazepines in terms of fetal development does not appear to be great, it is probably advisable to avoid their use during the first trimester of pregnancy. In the event that a woman has been maintained on benzodiazepines and becomes pregnant, it would be appropriate in most instances to taper and discontinue benzodiazepine administration, though the inadvertent use of these drugs early in pregnancy should not be cause for alarm with respect to the probability of anomalous fetal development. Since alprazolam tends to be utilized in relatively large doses in the treatment of panic disorder, the dose of this drug should be gradually tapered to the minimal tolerated level and discontinued if pregnancy is contemplated. The occurrence of pregnancy in a woman being maintained at a high dosage of alprazolam should guide the physician toward gradual dosage reduction. The risk of abrupt discontinuation of benzodiazepine therapy to both mother and fetus must be kept in mind when a decision is made to alter the therapeutic regimen. Imipramine[5] and fluoxetine[14] appear to have less teratogenic potential than does high dose benzodiazepine therapy, therefore these agents may be preferable for the management of panic disorder in the pregnant patient. It is inadvisable for women taking substantial doses of benzodiazepines to nurse their infant. Those who wish to nurse should be helped to taper their drug dosage in order to do so.

ANTIPSYCHOTIC DRUGS

Phenothiazines and other neuroleptic drugs have been used extensively in pregnancy for many years, both for the treatment of nausea and vomiting as well as various psychotic disorders. Data presented in various studies of their teratogenic potential are conflicting; some studies have reported significant risk,[13] whereas others maintain that the effects on fetal development are minimal.[12,15]

In a retrospective French study of 12,764 births, there was a 1.6% incidence of congenital malformations unrelated to chromosomal abnormalities in the control subjects. Of the 315 women who took phenothiazines during the first trimester of pregnancy, 3.5% gave birth to malformed infants.[16] The French study suggested a higher incidence of malformations in association with aliphatic phenothiazines, such as chlorpromazine. The California Child Health and Development Project, a study of 19,000 births between 1959 and 1966, reported no increase in congenital anomalies associated with phenothiazine use during pregnancy.[17] Re-analysis of the data revealed a 5.4% incidence of congenital anomalies in infants born of phenothiazine-treated mothers as compared with a 3.2% incidence in a population with no drug exposure.[18] A multicenter study of 5282 pregnancies found no increased incidence of congenital malformations in 1309 infants born of phenothiazine-treated mothers.[19]

Although occasional case reports of congenital anomalies in association with haloperidol, loxapine, molindone, and thiothixene have appeared in the literature, current evidence does not support their teratogenicity. Large studies have not revealed a significant increase in fetal abnormalities in infants whose mothers received thioridazine, perphenazine, trifluoperazine, fluphenazine, or haloperidol.[5,20] Although the safety of molindone and loxapine in pregnancy has not been adequately documented, there is thus far no striking evidence that they are teratogenic.[5]

Clozapine and risperidone have not been systematically studied in pregnancy, and their use is thus far too limited to determine whether they have any unique advantages or disadvantages in terms of fetal development. The autonomic and leukopenic potential of clozapine would favor its avoidance in pregnant women.

Extrapyramidal reactions have been reported in neonates exposed to neuroleptic drugs in utero.[5,15] These effects may last for several weeks after birth. Fluphenazine decanoate administered to a pregnant woman has been associated with a late-occurring extrapyramidal syndrome.[6] Low-potency strongly hypotensive antipsychotic agents such as chlorpromazine, thioridazine, and mesoridazine should be avoided at the end of pregnancy since they may complicate delivery by producing excessive sedation and hypotension in the mother. Neuroleptic drugs administered during the last trimester of pregnancy have been associated with hypertonicity, hyperreflexia, vasomotor instability, and excessive crying in newborns.[5,6] Potential adverse effects on the newborn may be minimized by cautious use of the lowest possible dose of antipsychotic medication during the latter phase of pregnancy.

All neuroleptic drugs are excreted in breast milk, and therefore may exert pharmacologic actions on the breast-fed infant. All antipsychotic drugs have some potential to produce extrapyramidal side effects, which may be marked in the infant by rigidity, restlessness, and tremor. The anticholinergic action of neuroleptic drugs may reduce bowel tone and motility and cause constipation in the breast-feeding infant. The alpha-adrenergic blocking activity of phenothiazines such as chlorpromazine, thioridazine, and mesoridazine may predispose the infant to vasomotor instability. These latter neuroleptic agents are also more likely to produce excessive sedation and lethargy in breast-fed infants than high-potency agents such as trifluoperazine and haloperidol. All neuroleptic drugs affect hypothalamic temperature-regulating mechanisms and thus may impair temperature-regulation in suckling newborns.[5,15]

Current evidence suggests that in the presence of established psychotic illness, the benefits of neuroleptic drugs outweigh the risk of producing fetal malformation. These drugs, however, are not indicated in the treatment of non-psychotic mental disorders in pregnant women. It is advisable to utilize the lowest possible dosage of high-potency neuroleptics such as haloperidol, perphenazine, and trifluoperazine in the treatment of psychosis during pregnancy. More strongly sedating and more strongly anticholinergic agents such as chlorpromazine, thioridazine, and mesoridazine are probably less desirable than the previously mentioned drugs. The risk of extrapyramidal side effects can be minimized by utilizing the lowest possible dosage of neuroleptics. Benztropine and diphenhydramine have been used effectively in managing extrapyramidal side effects should they occur in the newborn.[6] It is advisable to avoid breast-feeding by mothers who are receiving high dosages of any neuroleptic medication. Breast-feeding can be undertaken cautiously by mothers being maintained on low-dose regimens of antipsychotic medication, provided they are alert and carefully observe their infant for signs of lethargy, bowel dysfunction, and extrapyramidal symptoms.[5]

ANTIDEPRESSANT DRUGS

Although occasional reports in the literature have suggested possible teratogenic effects of tricyclic antidepressants, the evidence from large-scale studies is to the contrary. A Finnish study of 2784 cases of birth defects found no link between fetal deformities or limb dysgenesis in infants born of mothers who had taken tricyclic antidepressants during pregnancy.[21] An English study of 10,000 pregnancies and a Scottish study of 15,000 pregnancies found no association between tricyclic antidepressant administration during pregnancy and the occurrence of fetal abnormalities.[22,23] Although no data exist regarding the teratogenic potential of MAOI-type antidepressants, these drugs have been demonstrated to be teratogenic in animals.[24]

Fluoxetine, by virtue of the absence of common tricyclic side effects, has revolutionized the pharmacotherapy of depression, making this form of treatment acceptable to patients who previously rejected antidepressants because of intolerance to side effects. Consequently, in its relatively short period of use, this drug has been employed in approximately 10,000,000 people worldwide. Extensive use of this drug has included large numbers of pregnant women who have taken fluoxetine at various times during pregnancy. Postmarketing experience reported by the manufacturer identified 12 infants with major malformations among 485 pregnancies with outcome data available taken from a total of 1031 pregnancies which occurred during fluoxetine treatment.[25] This series included 59 spontaneous abortions, which is similar to what would be expected in a non-drug treated population. In a series of 72 pregnancies which occurred in patients participating in clinical trials of fluoxetine, there were 7 spontaneous abortions and only one infant with major malformations, data which is similar to what could be expected in the absence of drug therapy.[25] As of March 15, 1993, 28 retrospective reports of fetal abnormalities were received by the manufacturer, with no pattern of preponderance of any particular anomaly. Again the numbers are very low in light of the previously noted number of patients who have been treated with fluoxetine.[25] A published study followed 128 women treated with fluoxetine, a similar number of matched controls who received non-teratogenic drugs, and 74 women who were treated with tricyclic antidepressants.[14] In that study the three groups did not differ significantly in terms of occurrence of major fetal anomalies following first-trimester treatment with any of the agents studied.[14] The risk of miscarriage was 13.5% for fluoxetine, 12.2% for tricyclics and 6.8% for drugs considered nonteratogens.[14] Evidence based on perhaps the most extensive prenatal exposure of any drug suggests that the risk of anomalous development due to fluoxetine is insignificantly different from what would be expected in non-drug treated pregnancies. This data cannot be extrapolated to other SSRIs, however, since they are chemically diverse though mechanistically similar. There is thus far no data to support or deny the occurrence of anomalous development with other SSRIs. One caveat is that the potent cytochrome P-450 inhibition produced by fluoxetine would be likely to increase fetal and maternal serum concentrations of a variety of coadministered drugs, and may alter developing enzyme systems. The absence of sedative, hypotensive, and autonomic side effects with fluoxetine may make this drug more desirable than tricyclics in depressed pregnant women. A case report of restlessness, jitteriness, increased muscle tone, and temperature instability in a neonate whose mother had received fluoxetine throughout pregnancy suggests that it may be good clinical practice to use lower doses of fluoxetine in pregnant women or to reduce medication dosage for 2 to 4 weeks before delivery is anticipated.[26] In that neonate significant serum concentrations of fluoxetine and norfluoxetine were found.[26] Since many patients respond well to fluoxetine at daily doses of 5 mg, this dosage may be preferable to the usual daily dose of 20 mg which the mother of that child was receiving. The long half-life of fluoxetine and its active metabolite, norfluoxetine, indicate that dosage reduction 2 to 4 weeks before delivery may increase the safety of this drug for babies born of fluoxetine treated mothers. Clinical symptoms attributed to fluoxetine in the neonate described in the above mentioned report disappeared as the drug was cleared from the baby.[26]

Like all other psychotropic drugs, tricyclic and SSRI antidepressants freely pass the placental barrier and may therefore affect fetal physiology. There have been occasional case reports of urinary retention and other manifestations of the anticholinergic effect of tricyclic drugs in neonates whose mothers were receiving tricyclic antidepressants in the third trimester of pregnancy.[13] A more generalized neonatal distress syndrome has been reported in an infant who experienced respiratory distress, peripheral cyanosis, and hypertonia with tremor, clonus, and spasm, which may be related to a combination of anticholinergic action and adrenergic supersensitivity induced by the tricyclic drug.[6]

Although tricyclic antidepressants are excreted in breast milk, the concentration is variable and may not produce significant plasma levels or toxicity in the infant.[27] Since the effects of tricyclic drugs on the developing neurotransmitter systems in the newborn are poorly understood, the risk of drug exposure must be weighed carefully against the potential benefits of breast-feeding.[5] Since patients with a prior history of significant depressive illness may be at increased risk of a recurrence of depression during the postpartum period, clinical judgment would generally favor continuation of antidepressant drug therapy and avoidance of breast-feeding, as opposed to discontinuation of necessary antidepressant medication. Furthermore, in patients who experience an initial episode of depression during the postpartum period, the benefit to both mother and child that is available through tricyclic antidepressant drug therapy is likely to override the beneficial effect of breast-feeding. A depressed mother is likely to have a significantly impaired ability to care for her newborn.[5]

Tricyclic antidepressant drugs appear to be safe from the standpoint of potential risks of anomalous fetal development. When antidepressants must be administered during the first trimester of pregnancy, it is preferable to use agents that have longer established safety records, specifically imipramine, amitriptyline, desipramine and fluoxetine. Since drugs with greater sedative and anticholinergic potency may have a more adverse effect on the newborn, imipramine, desipramine and fluoxetine may be preferable to amitriptyline when antidepressant drug therapy must be initiated late in pregnancy. In a woman who has been maintained throughout her pregnancy on amitriptyline, it is probably reasonable to use the lowest effective dose of this medication during the latter phase of pregnancy and then increase the dosage following parturition if clinically necessary.

It is likely that MAOIs may adversely affect developing enzyme systems in the fetus. The hypotensive potential of MAOIs may present an additional risk at the time of delivery.[13] Women who must remain on antidepressant drug therapy during the postpartum period should generally be encouraged not to nurse their infants.[27] In those situations where nursing is of great importance to the mother, antidepressant drug therapy may be continued and the infant observed carefully.

LITHIUM

Among psychotropic drugs, lithium has been more strongly associated with congenital anomalies than have other agents. In spite of this well-known association, many normal, healthy babies have been born of mothers who have received lithium throughout their pregnancy. Considerable controversy thus exists as to the proper approach to pregnancy in a woman who requires lithium therapy. Schou reported on six normal babies whose mothers were continuously on lithium treatment from conception through pregnancy and birth.[28] Another report by the same investigator found no higher incidence of physical or mental abnormalities in children whose mothers had received lithium during pregnancy.[29] In contradistinction to these favorable reports, numerous publications indicate an increased incidence of cardiovascular abnormalities, particularly an increase in Ebstein's anomaly in infants born of lithium-treated mothers.[5,15] Central nervous system anomalies and external ear malformations have also been reported in association with lithium.

The *International Register of Lithium Babies* was last reviewed in 1979 and provided data on 225 babies whose mothers received lithium during pregnancy. This review found 25 children with malformations, 18 of which involved the heart and great vessels. Six of these children had Ebstein's anomaly, a malformation of the tricuspid valve that is usually associated with an atrial septal defect.[30,31] Eleven per cent of the 225 lithium babies, reviewed in 1979 when the lithium register was terminated, had visible malformations at birth which is considerably in excess of the 2% found in the general population.[32] The risk of lithium-associated congenital abnormalities suggests that lithium be discontinued prior to conception and be avoided during the first trimester of pregnancy. In a patient with a severe unstable affective disorder, discontinuation of lithium may be associated with a recurrence of psychotic illness. Therefore, the decision as to the safety of discontinuing lithium versus maintaining lithium treatment and proceeding with a planned pregnancy must be carefully weighed by patient and physician together.

It was initially hoped that alternative antimanic agents would be more benign in terms of anomalous fetal development and that these agents could replace lithium in pregnant bipolar patients. The dominant view at the time of publication of the second edition of this book was that carbamazepine was safer than lithium. A review of 94 infants exposed to carbamazepine in utero revealed no evidence of teratogenicity.[32] Several case reports preceding and following that publication pointed out carbamazepine induced malformations. Most recent publications indicate a significant potential of carbamazepine-associated congenital defects, primarily neural tube defects, with 0.9% of carbamazepine-exposed fetuses having spina bifida.[33] Cardiac anomalies, cleft lip, and cleft palate are also seen with carbamazepine, although these are rare.[34] One of the major concerns with anticonvulsant use in pregnancy has been neurodevelopmental and I.Q. impairment by these drugs, most notably phenytoin. Recent studies indicate that these abnormalities are unlikely to occur with carbamazepine.[35] Valproate can also cause neural tube anomalies, with 1% to 2% of infants exposed in utero to this drug having spina bifida.[36] Other valproate-associated fetal abnormalities include cardiac, skeletal, and facial defects, although the incidence appears quite low.[37] Increasing assessment of the risks of alternative antimanic agents, based largely on experience with these drugs in the treatment of maternal seizure disorders, and continuing review of more recent experience with lithium, suggest that lithium may be no more dangerous than its alternatives and may be safer in terms of fetal development than earlier reports indicated.[38] If an alternative to lithium is required, carbamazepine may be slightly safer than valproate. Clonazepam and neuroleptics are safest of the alternatives. If carbamazepine is used, administration of smaller divided doses, avoidance of high serum concentration, and potential use of folic acid supplements may all contribute to its safety. Some studies have correlated anticonvulsant fetal effects with folic acid deficiency.[34]

Since the relative risks of lithium and carbamazepine to fetal development are not clearly proven, the decision to use alternative antimanic therapy must be fully discussed with the prospective mother, including the possibility that carbamazepine will be less effective than lithium in maintaining the stability of the affective disorder. In those situations where the prospective mother is relatively stable, it would be far preferable to discontinue lithium and avoid pharmacotherapy entirely for 1 to 2 months prior to conception and throughout the first trimester of pregnancy.

Since dramatic metabolic, fluid, and electrolyte changes occur throughout pregnancy, it is important to carefully monitor a patient who is being maintained on lithium throughout the course of pregnancy. Excessively high lithium dosage, salt restriction, and diuretic therapy all contribute to increased serum lithium concentration in the mother and the potential consequences of lithium intoxication in the fetus. Lithium intoxication has been reported in newborns of mothers who took lithium during the third trimester of pregnancy.[39] Lithium-toxic neonates may show hypotonia, lethargy, cyanosis, poor sucking reflex, shallow respirations, and cardiac arrhythmias. Elevated lithium concentrations may persist for over a week in newborns who have been exposed in utero to lithium during the latter phase of pregnancy. Transient hypothyroidism and nephrogenic diabetes insipidus have been reported in neonates whose mothers were taking lithium at the end of pregnancy.[13,39]

Lithium passes freely into breast milk, the concentration being approximately one half of the maternal plasma concentration.[5] Although it has been reported that nursing mothers can safely take lithium, toxic reactions including hypotonia, lethargy, and cyanosis have occurred in infants whose mothers were being maintained on lithium.[5,39] It is therefore advisable that lithium-treated mothers not nurse their infants. Since carbamazepine is also excreted in breast milk, its use would also preclude nursing, particularly since this drug could conceivably produce hematologic abnormalities, including leukopenia, in the newborn.

It is prudent to recommend that lithium-treated women of childbearing age cautiously use birth control and plan their pregnancies. Women should be advised to discontinue lithium 1 to 2 months prior to attempting conception and to remain off this medication during the first trimester. During the second and third trimesters, lithium therapy may be reinstituted if affective symptoms occur. During the last two trimesters of pregnancy, maintaining the patient at the lowest effective serum level of lithium, while being certain that fluid and electrolyte balance is maintained, is likely to avoid the consequences of lithium toxicity in both the pregnant woman and her fetus. Lithium-treated mothers of newborns should be advised not to nurse their infants. If the affective illness is sufficiently stable, it may be clinically desirable to discontinue lithium treatment and allow the mother to nurse her infant. In those instances where pregnancy is a strongly desired goal, individual circumstances may suggest carbamazepine rather than lithium maintenance during pregnancy. In a non-medication-maintained patient who develops acute manic symptoms during pregnancy, it may be preferable to initiate treatment with the lowest possible dose of a high-potency neuroleptic and continue that treatment throughout the first trimester of pregnancy, instituting lithium once the woman is clearly into her second trimester.

Lithium has been associated with an 11% to 12% incidence of fetal abnormality. It is thus the psychotropic medication of greatest concern during the first trimester of pregnancy.[40] Although the exact risk associated with benzodiazepines is unknown, these agents should be avoided whenever possible during pregnancy. Neuroleptic drugs are clearly indicated for the treatment of acute psychosis and for the prevention of psychotic relapse; their potential role as teratogens seems minor, and thus they may be used cautiously when indicated in a pregnant patient. Current evidence suggests that fluoxetine and tricyclic antidepressants, specifically imipramine and amitriptyline, are quite safe from the standpoint of teratogenicity, and are therefore not contraindicated during pregnancy. Women who suffer from acute psychiatric disturbances, be they affective disorders or psychoses, are likely to be less able to carry through a pregnancy, remain well compensated, and take on the responsibility of caring for a newborn; therefore the risk of illness versus the risk of drug therapy must be constantly weighted in making treatment decisions.[3] There is evidence that psychotic women have a significantly higher risk of fetal loss than do normal women.[3] Decisions to provide or withhold treatment are difficult and must involve frank discussions with the woman and her husband. The occurrence of

Table 14-1 Psychotropic drugs in pregnancy and lactation

Drug	Teratogenicity (first trimester)	Effect on newborn (last trimester)	Lactation
Sedative/antianxiety			
Barbiturates	Oral clefts, growth retardation	Potential drug withdrawal symptoms	Present in milk
Benzodiazepines	Cleft lip, cleft palate	Neurologic depression; low Apgar; potential drug withdrawal symptoms	Breast-feeding contraindicated; lethargy, jaundice, impaired temperature regulation
Meprobamate	Severe anomalies in 12% of newborns	Potential drug withdrawal symptoms	Present in milk
Antipsychotic			
Phenothiazines, especially chlorpromazine	Some risk of anomalies if used during weeks 6-10	Extrapyramidal symptoms (EPS), excessive crying, hyperreflexia	Present in milk; nursing should be discouraged; EPS may occur in infants
Fluphenazine Haloperidol Perphenazine Trifluoperazine	Little or no risk; probably safest neuroleptics in pregnancy	EPS, excessive crying, hyperreflexia	Present in milk; nursing should be discouraged; EPS may occur in infant
Antidepressants			
Tricyclics	No evidence of teratogenicity	Tachycardia, autonomic lability; respiratory distress may occur if large doses used just prior to delivery	Present in milk; nursing should be discouraged but can be done if infant is carefully observed
Fluoxetine	No evidence of teratogenicity	Restlessness, jitteriness, increased muscle tone, temperature instability	Present in milk, nursing should be discouraged. Restlessness, lethargy, increased muscle tone may occur, impaired temperature regulation
Monoamine oxidase inhibitors	Teratogenic in animals	May affect developing enzyme systems	Not recommended

Continued.

Table 14-1 Psychotropic drugs in pregnancy and lactation—cont'd.

Drug	Teratogenicity (first trimester)	Effect on newborn (last trimester)	Lactation
Mood-stabilizing drugs			
Lithium carbonate	Chromosomal gaps and breaks; 11-12% risk of anomalies; higher incidence of congenital heart anomalies, especially Ebstein's anomaly	Carefully monitored lithium level in mother can allow safe use; higher blood levels may cause hypotonia, lethargy; use throughout pregnancy may reduce thyroid function in fetus and lead to goiter	Breast-feeding contraindicated
Carbamazepine	0.9% risk of spina bifida	May produce CNS depression, ? leukopenia	Present in milk; nursing should be discouraged, lethargy, leukopenia
Valproate	1-2% risk of spina bifida	May produce CNS depression, ? hepatotoxicity	Present in milk; nursing should be discouraged, lethargy, hepatotoxicity

an inadvertent pregnancy while a woman is being maintained on psychotropic drugs will not necessarily be associated with abnormal fetal development, yet it should at least open the channels of communication between doctor and patient and allow for discussion of the availability of genetic counseling. Effects of psychotropic drugs on the fetus and neonate are shown in Table 14-1.

REFERENCES

1. Council Report: Fetal effects of maternal alcohol use. *JAMA* 1983;249:2517-2521.
2. Beeley L: Adverse effects of drugs in the first trimester of pregnancy. *Clin Obstet Gynecol* 1986;13:177-196.
3. Oates MR: The treatment of psychiatric disorders in pregnancy and the puerperium. *Clin Obstet Gynecol* 1986;13:385-395.
4. Weissman MM, Gershon ES, Kidd KK, et al: Psychiatric disorders in the relatives of probands with effective disorders. *Arch Gen Psychiatry* 1984;41:13-21.
5. Robinson GE, Stewart DE, Flak E: The rational use of psychotropic drugs in pregnancy and postpartum. *Can J Psychiatry* 1986;31:183-190.
6. Beeley L: Adverse effects of drugs in later pregnancy. *Clin Obstet Gynecol* 1986;13:197-214.
7. Milkovich L, Van den Berg BT: Effects of prenatal meprobamate and chlordiazepoxide hydrochloride on human embryonic and fetal development. *N Engl J Med* 1974;291:1268-1271.
8. Aaskog D: Association between maternal intake of diazepam and oral clefts. *Lancet* 1975;2:921.
9. Rosenberg L, Mitchell AA, Parsells JL, et al: Lack of relation of oral clefts to diazepam use during pregnancy. *N Engl J Med* 1983;309:1282-1285.
10. Laegreid L, Olegard R, Wahlstrom J, et al: Abnormalities in children exposed to benzodiazepines in utero. *Lancet* 1987;1:108-109.
11. Barry WS, St Clair SM: Exposure to benzodiazepines in utero. *Lancet* 1987;1:1436-1437.
12. Cohen LS, Heller VL, Rosenbaum JF: Treatment guidelines for psychotropic drug use in pregnancy. *Psychosomatics* 1989;30:25-33.
13. Hauser LA: Pregnancy and psychiatric drugs. *Hosp Community Psychiatry* 1985;36:817-818.
14. Pastuszak A, Schick-Boschetto B, Zuber C, et al: Pregnancy outcome following first-trimester exposure to fluoxetine (Prozac). *JAMA* 1993;269:2246-2248.
15. Nurnberg HG, Prudic J: Guidelines for treatment of psychosis during pregnancy. *Hosp Community Psychiatry* 1984;35:67-71.
16. Rumeau-Rouquette C, Goujard J, Huel C: Possible teratogenic effects of phenothiazines in human beings. *Teratology* 1977;15:57-64.
17. Milkovich L, Van den Berg BJ: An evaluation of the teratogenicity of certain antinauseant drugs. *Am J Obstet Gynecol* 1976;125:244-248.
18. Edlund MJ, Craig TJ: Antipsychotic drug use and birth defects: an epidemiologic reassessment. *Compr Psychiatry* 1984;25:32-37.
19. Slone D, Suskind V, Heinonen OP, et al: Antenatal exposure to the phenothiazines in relation to congenital malformations, perinatal mortality, birth weight and intelligence quotient score. *Am J Obstet Gynecol* 1977;128:486-488.
20. Ananth J: Congenital malformations with psychopharmacologic agents. *Compr Psychiatry* 1975;16:437-445.
21. Idanpaan-Heikkila J, Saxen L: Possible teratogenicity of imipraminechloropyramine. *Lancet* 1973;2:282-284.
22. Crombie DL, Pinsent RJ, Fleming DM, et al: Fetal effects of tranquilizers in pregnancy. *N Engl J Med* 1975;293:198-199.
23. Kuenssberg EV, Knox JD: Imipramine in pregnancy. *Br Med J* 1972;2:292.
24. Poulson E, Robson JM: Effect of phenelzine and some related compounds on pregnancy. *J Endocrinol* 1964;30:205-215.
25. Goldstein DJ: Personal communication, July 13, 1994.

26. Spencer MJ: Fluoxetine hydrochloride (Prozac) toxicity in a neonate. *Pediatrics* 1993;92: 721-722.
27. Stancer HC, Reed KL: Desipramine and 2-hydroxydesipramine in human breast milk and the nursing infant's serum. *Am J Psychiatry* 1986;143:1597-1600.
28. Schou M: Special review: lithium in psychiatric therapy and prophylaxis. *J Psychiatr Res* 1968;6:67-95.
29. Schou M: What happened to the lithium babies: a follow-up of children without malformations. *Acta Psychiatr Scand* 1976;54:193-197.
30. Weinstein MR, Goldfield MD: Cardiovascular malformations with lithium use during pregnancy. *Am J Psychiatry* 1975;132:529-531.
31. Schou M: Lithium treatment during pregnancy, delivery and lactation: An Update. *J Clin Psychiatry* 1990;51:410-413.
32. Niebyl JR, Blake DA, Freeman JM, et al: Carbamazepine levels in pregnancy and lactation. *Obstet Gynecol* 1979;53:139-140.
33. Rosa FW: Spina Bifida in infants of women treated with carbamazepine during pregnancy. *N Eng J Med* 1991;324:674-677.
34. Delgado-Escueta AV, Janz D: Consensus guidelines: Preconception counseling, management, and care of the pregnant woman with epilepsy. *Neurology* 1992;42(suppl 5):149-160.
35. Scolnik D, Nulman I, Rovet J, *et al:* Neurodevelopment of children exposed in utero to phenytoin and carbamazepine monotherapy. *JAMA* 1994;271:767-770.
36. Martinez-Frias ML: Clinical manifestations of prenatal exposure to valproic acid using case reports and epidemiologic information. *Am J Med Genet* 1990;37:277-282.
37. Nau H, Hauck RS, Ehlers K: Valproic acid-induced neural tube defects in mouse and human: Aspects of chirality, alternative drug development, pharmacokinetics and possible mechanisms. *Pharmacol Toxicol* 1991;69:310-321.
38. Cohen LS, Friedman JM, Jefferson JW *et al:* A reevaluation of risk of in utero exposure to lithium. *JAMA* 1994;271:146-150.
39. Spielvogel A, Wile J: Treatment of the psychotic pregnant patient. *Psychosomatics* 1986;27: 487-492.
40. Whittle MJ, Hanretty KP: Prescribing in pregnancy: identifying abnormalities. *Br Med J* 1986;293:1485-1488.

Psychopharmacology in Children and Adolescents

OVERVIEW

1. Pharmacologic nihilism will preclude a favorable treatment response.
2. Use medications with documented safety and efficacy in this age group.
3. Medication dosage must be individualized; higher than expected doses may be required because of more efficient drug metabolism and excretion in younger patients.
4. Depression, which may present as acting out behavior or substance abuse in children and adolescents, is relatively common and often requires pharmacotherapy.
5. Eating disorders, panic disorder, school phobia, and enuresis often respond to antidepressants.
6. Obsessive compulsive related disorders are not uncommon in children and adolescents and often respond well to clomipramine and SSRIs.
7. Lithium-responsive mania occurs in children and adolescents; often, relatively high lithium doses are required.
8. Attention-deficit hyperactivity disorder (ADHD) begins in young children, continues through adolescence into adult life, and often responds dramatically to stimulants and tricyclic antidepressants.
9. Tourette's syndrome is a frequently missed diagnosis which responds favorably to haloperidol, pimozide, or clonidine; SSRIs may be beneficial.
10. Acute psychosis in adolescents should be treated with low doses of high-potency neuroleptics.
11. Pervasive developmental disorder patients may have symptomatic improvement with pharmacotherapy (e.g. SSRIs may reduce stereotypes).
12. Aggressivity and impulsivity may benefit from neuroleptics, lithium, carbamazepine, and propranolol.

Drug therapy of children and adolescents has been one of the most controversial areas in psychopharmacology.[1] There are many reasons for this controversy. In part, diagnostic categorization in this age group is often more difficult than it is in adults. Furthermore, there are gray areas between one diagnostic category and another in young persons undergoing the process of maturation and change. Many behavioral symptoms seen in children and adolescents may be either variations in the maturation process or symptoms of an underlying or developing psychiatric disorder.[2] Variations of behavior in children and adolescents over time often make clear diagnostic categorization difficult. Indeed, psychiatric illnesses well known in the adult population, such as affective disorders and OCD, have been underappreciated in child psychiatry. Symptom patterns consistent with major depressive disorder are now more frequently being described in young preadolescent children. Likewise, mania is being more frequently described in the literature, even in very young children, and certainly in adolescents. Unfortunately, the newspapers and the psychiatric literature remind us all too frequently that adolescent suicide is not as uncommon as it was once thought to be. The burgeoning rate of suicide in the adolescent population is a painful reminder that major depressive disorders do, indeed, afflict this population.[3]

In addition to diagnostic vagaries, there are many other reasons for the controversial nature of psychopharmacologic treatment of children and adolescents. The rate of growth and physiologic change occurring from early childhood through adolescence is more rapid and more extensive than at any other period in life. In the face of rapidly changing psychological, behavioral, and physiologic events, there is concern about the potential of drugs to alter the normal developmental process. As enzyme systems and neurotransmitters are evolving in early childhood, there is the concern that the administration of potent pharmacologic agents to the young child will adversely affect these systems, perhaps irreversibly. There is concern that psychotropic effects during development may influence behavioral, affective, and cognitive processes later in life. The possibility of endocrine, immunologic, and other somatic consequences of drug administration to children has also concerned clinicians and researchers.[1]

Despite the potential risks of drug therapy on physiological and psychological development, pharmacotherapy can reduce suffering of the afflicted child, allowing him or her a greater chance of a more successful voyage through the vicissitudes of the developmental process. A child with attention-deficit hyperactivity disorder (ADHD) may not be able to achieve satisfactory school performance and developmental goals in the nonmedicated state, but with proper pharmacologic intervention he or she may successfully pursue school work and development toward a stable adult life.[4] Children with separation anxiety disorder may be so crippled by school phobia that they cannot even attend school, let alone perform in that environment. This situation can often be reversed by pharmacologic intervention with drugs such as imipramine. An adolescent suffering through a painful depressive disorder, and contemplating suicide, if diagnosed and treated early with antidepressant medication, may proceed through the developmental process into adulthood rather than become another statistic in the adolescent suicide epidemic.[3]

Another concern that has often been voiced with respect to pharmacologic intervention in children and adolescents is the possibility that medical management may predispose the child to drug abuse or dependence. This problem must be considered with some seriousness in making choices and recommendations regarding pharmacotherapy. Stimulant drugs such as dextroamphetamine and methylphenidate may be addicting, although drug abuse and addiction have not been reported in medically monitored children and adolescents receiving these therapeutic agents for hyperactivity disorders.[1] Stimulants may retard physical growth of children and adolescents, yet they often allow a child suffering from ADHD to function normally at home and in the classroom. Thus the risks of these medications are most often outweighed by their benefits.[4]

Benzodiazepine dependence is a potential problem when these drugs are used in the treatment of anxiety disorders in both adults and children. Nevertheless, if there are clear indications for their use, and dosage as well as duration of treatment are carefully limited and monitored, the risk of dependency is not likely to be overwhelming. If nonaddicting anxiety-relieving drugs are effective, they may be preferable to the use of benzodiazepines in children. In some instances, tricyclic antidepressants or sedating antihistamines such as diphenhydramine or hydroxyzine may alleviate anxiety or insomnia in a child or adolescent without the need for a benzodiazepine.[1] Neuroleptic drugs such as phenothiazines and butyrophenones may, with long-term or high-dose use, cause tardive dyskinesia. When used cautiously, they have unique therapeutic benefits, and allow for better integration and function of children and adolescents who might otherwise be aggressive, assaultive, or self-mutilating.[1] Therapeutic decisions must be made on an individual basis, however in spite of concerns about potential long-term effects, pharmacologic interventions may offer therapeutic advantages that far outweigh their risks.

The principles of good psychopharmacologic practice in the treatment of children and adolescents are similar to those employed in adult practice. Careful diagnostic evaluation of the patient must be undertaken. When a proper clinical diagnosis is established, pharmacologic treatment, if indicated, should proceed utilizing those agents most likely to benefit the patient, while producing minimal side effects. In some cases, it is necessary to use medications for treatment of specific behavioral or cognitive symptoms, before a definite diagnosis can be established. It is important to titrate the dosage of medication gradually while observing the child for evidence of therapeutic effects and unwanted side effects. In most instances, it is appropriate to start pharmacotherapy with a single agent and titrate the dosage appropriately prior to the addition of secondary or tertiary medications. It is important not to make abrupt changes from one medication to another without careful consideration of potential drug interactions or symptoms that may be associated with withdrawal of the first agent.

Although careless polypharmacy is to be avoided, there are indeed clinical situations in which the combination of two or more medications simultaneously is necessary in order to achieve the desired therapeutic result. For example, some severely depressed adolescents may require the simultaneous administration of an antidepressant, a low dose of a neuroleptic, and lithium. In some impulse disorders with associated violence, it may be necessary to employ propranolol, haloperidol, and lithium or carbamazepine.[5] Once a patient receiving multiple pharmacologic agents is stabilized, it may be appropriate to gradually reduce the dosage in an attempt to discontinue individual agents in order to achieve the simplest effective pharmacologic regimen. As in adult psychopharmacology, the occurrence of inexplicable symptoms during the course of pharmacotherapy should raise the clinician's suspicion regarding a potential drug interaction or an unexpected adverse drug effect, the initial treatment of which may require drug discontinuation and reassessment of the patient in the drug-free state.

This chapter reviews some of the more common psychiatric disturbances of children and adolescents, for which there is evidence for a therapeutic benefit of pharmacologic intervention. Since the pharmacologic characteristics of the various psychotropic drugs have been discussed elsewhere in this book, this chapter presents only brief discussions of the pharmacology and dosages of these compounds relevant to their therapeutic use in children and adolescents. Indications for psychotropic drugs in the treatment of children and adolescents are shown in Table 15-1.

AFFECTIVE DISORDERS
Depression

Depression is one of the most common illnesses for which adults seek psychiatric attention. Depressive disorders which meet DSM-IV criteria for

Table 15-1 Psychotropic drugs in children and adolescents (with preferred drugs)*

Clinical indications	Tricyclic antidepressants (Imipramine, Desipramine, Amitriptyline)	Monoamine oxidase inhibitors (Phenelzine, Tranylcypromine)	Stimulants (Methylphenidate, Dextroamphetamine, Pemoline)	Neuroleptics (Haloperidol, Trifluoperazine, Perphenazine, Chlorpromazine)	Mood stabilizers (Lithium, Carbamazepine)	Others (see below)
ADHD	TCA	?MAOI	Stimulant			? SSRI (Fluox)
Aggression				H,C	Li,C	Propranolol
Anorexia	TCA					Cyproheptadine
Anxiety	TCA					Alprazolam, diphenhydramine
Bulimia	TCA	MAOI			Li,C	?Fluox
Conduct disorder	?TCA		?Stimulant	H,T,P,C	Li	?Fluox, ?Valp
Cyclothymia					?Li	
Depression, acute	TCA	MAOI			?Li	SSRI (Fluox)
Depression, recurrent	TCA	MAOI			Li	SSRI (Fluox)
Enuresis	TCA					
Impulsivity			?Stimulant	H,T,P	Li,C	
Insomnia						Oxazepam, diphenhydramine
Mania					Li,C	Valproate
Night terror						Oxazepam, diphenhydramine
OCD						Clom, Fluox, Fluvox
Panic	TCA	MAOI				Alprazolam, ?SSRI
Pervasive developmental disorder				H,T,P,C	?Li;?C	Clom, Fluvox, ?Fluox, ?clonidine, ?Fenfluramine

Continued.

Table 15-1 Psychotropic drugs in children and adolescents (with preferred drugs)*—cont'd.

Clinical indications	Tricyclic antidepressants (Imipramine, Desipramine, Amitriptyline)	Monoamine oxidase inhibitors (Phenelzine, Tranylcypromine)	Stimulants (Methylphenidate, Dextroamphetamine, Pemoline)	Neuroleptics (Haloperidol, Trifluoperazine, Perphenazine, Chlorpromazine)	Mood stabilizers (Lithium, Carbamazepine)	Others (see below)
Psychosis				H,T,P	?Li,?C	
Rage				H	Li,C	Propranolol, ?oxazepam
Seizures, TLE					C	
Sleep walking						Oxazepam, diphenhydramine
School phobia	TCA	?MAOI				
Social phobia						SSRI, alprozolam
Tourette's disorder				H		Clonidine, SSRI, Fluox, Clom

*TCA = tricyclic antidepressant; MAOI = monoamine oxidase inhibitor; H = haloperidol; C = chlorpromazine; T = trifluoperazine; P = perphenazine; C = carbamazepine; Clom = clomipramine; Fluox = fluoxetine; Fluvox = fluvoxamine; Valp = Valproate; ADHD = attention-deficit hyperactivity disorder; TLE = temporal lobe epilepsy; OCD = obsessive compulsive disorder; ? = studies or anecdotal reports indicate possible benefits.

major depression and dysthymic disorder are now being more commonly recognized in children and adolescents than previously.[6,7] A recent multicenter study reported a 6-month prevalence rate ranging from 4.6% to 6.5% for all affective disorders in adults.[8] A community sample study recently reported a prevalence of 1.8% for major depression in a group of 9-year-old children.[8] In another study, it was found that more than 40% of the adolescents interviewed expressed feelings of depression and misery.[10] A more recent study of 150 14- to 16-year-old boys and girls attending public school reported that nearly 50% of them expressed some dysphoric mood state. In that investigation, 4.7% of the children met diagnostic criteria for major depression and 3.3% met criteria for dysthymic disorder.[7]

The prevalence of depressive disorders is significantly higher among adolescents exhibiting acting out behavior and substance abuse and those who are children of affectively ill parents. Many investigators have reported that among younger children with depressive disorders, there is often coexistence of separation anxiety disorder or conduct disorder. The DSM-IV criteria for major depression and dysthymic disorder are similar for adults and children. In clinical practice, depressed children are more likely to cry and look sad or to present with school failures, aggressive acting out behaviors, defiance toward parents, and substance abuse. Depressed children may or may not experience changes in appetite or body weight, and not uncommonly, depressed adolescents will gain weight. The clinician's best ally in diagnosing depression in a child or adolescent is a high index of suspicion, even in the face of a relatively negative or unconvincing history. Neuroendocrine testing of depressed children is not likely to be of major diagnostic help, although nonsuppression has been reported in dexamethasone suppression tests in depressed children.[4]

Tricyclic antidepressants are the mainstay of pharmacologic intervention in depressive disorders of children and adolescents. Imipramine is the antidepressant that has been most extensively studied, both in children and in adolescents. Amitriptyline, desipramine, and to a lesser extent, nortriptyline, have also been studied and found to be effective in depressed children and adolescents.[11-14] Of these agents, amitriptyline produces the greatest sedative and anticholinergic effect and is thus more likely to produce drowsiness, dry mouth, constipation, and tachycardia. Desipramine is the least sedating and anticholinergic, and therefore may be associated with a lower incidence of side effects. Imipramine is intermediate between these two compounds in terms of sedative and anticholinergic side effects, and is the agent that has been employed most extensively in young children and in adolescents.[11] In those instances in which sleep disturbances are prominent, amitriptyline may be preferable, while in those depressed children who sleep excessively or complain of low daytime energy levels, desipramine may be better tolerated. Since bupropion, doxepin, protriptyline, trimipramine, maprotiline, trazodone, and amoxapine have not been studied extensively in the younger age group, there is no evidence to encourage their use in these patients. Seizures are more often provoked by antidepressants in children and adolescents than in adults, therefore agents with greater epileptogenic potential such as bupropion and maprotiline should generally not be used in children.

Hepatic metabolism of tricyclic antidepressants is more rapid in children. Relatively higher TCA doses therefore need to be administered to children than to adults in order to achieve therapeutic effects.[1] Unfortunately, serum concentrations of tricyclic antidepressants in children and adolescents do not always correlate as well with dosage and therapeutic response as indicated by studies in adults.[1,12] More rapid metabolism of tricyclic antidepressants, particularly by younger children, results in these drugs having a shorter half-life, thus requiring not only a higher relative dosage, but also often a longer duration of administration in order to achieve a clinically discernible antidepressant effect.[1] In adults, most tricyclic antidepressants produce their maximal therapeutic response after 2 to 4 weeks of administration, whereas in children, 4 to 6 weeks of treatment may be required.[1] In adults, an antidepressant response can generally be achieved with a dosage of 2-3 mg/kg body weight. In children under the age of 14 years doses of 5 mg/kg are often required to achieve a satisfactory response.[1,11] In older adolescents, the kinetics, metabolism, and therapeutic dosage of tricyclic antidepressants are more similar to those observed in adults. In children, hydroxylated metabolites of imipramine constitute almost 50% of the total active metabolic product of orally administered imipramine.[1] Since commercial measurements of serum tricyclic concentration generally do not report hydroxylated metabolites, the usefulness of these measurements in following antidepressant drug therapy in children is limited.[1]

As in adults, tricyclic drugs can effect cardiac rate, rhythm, and conduction. The PR interval may be increased and the QRS complex may be widened. Since blood levels are often unreliable in following antidepressant drug therapy, particularly in young children, it is useful to get a baseline ECG prior to initiating antidepressant drug therapy, and then to repeat the ECG every 1 to 2 weeks, particularly when higher doses of antidepressants are being administered, or approximately 48 hours after each dosage increment as the dose is increased above 3.5 mg/kg/day.[1,4] If the PR interval on the ECG exceeds 0.21 second or the QRS widening exceeds 30% of the pretreatment duration, the antidepressant dosage should be decreased. Desipramine, which has been seen as having milder autonomic side effects than other tricyclics, has been rather frequently used in childhood depression and ADDH, however, several reports of sudden collapse and sudden death in children remind us that this drug, particularly when used in higher doses, is far from benign, and may be a source of dangerous arrhythmias.[16] Postural hypotension is a relatively common side effect of tricyclic antidepressant drug therapy, which can often be managed by advising the patient to avoid standing up abruptly. However, the persistence of postural hypotension with dizziness may require dosage reduction.

Children with seizure disorders or abnormal EEGs should be observed closely during antidepressant drug therapy, particularly as the dosage is titrated upward. Although all tricyclic antidepressants may lower seizure threshold and increase the risk of convulsions, this phenomenon is most likely to occur in children with a prior seizure history or abnormal EEG.[1,4] The occurrence of seizures during antidepressant drug therapy may require temporary dosage reduction and initiation of phenytoin, carbamazepine, or other suitable anticonvulsant medication followed by gradual and cautious titration of the antidepressant dosage as clinically indicated.[1]

In children, tricyclic antidepressants may provoke anger outbursts, which may be related to the manic symptoms that are occasionally provoked in tricyclic-treated adults.[1]

When initiating tricyclic antidepressant drug therapy in children and adolescents, it is generally appropriate to start with a test dose of 10 mg in a child or 25 mg in an adolescent. Assuming no significant adverse effects occur, the dosage then may be gradually titrated upward by 25 mg every second to fourth day, observing the patient for evidence of a therapeutic response, as well as adverse drug effects.[1,4] Once a clinically significant mood improvement has been achieved, the therapeutic dose of antidepressant should be maintained for approximately 3 months, after which the dosage may be gradually decreased while observing the patient for evidence of recurrent depressive symptoms that may necessitate upward dosage titration, a further period of treatment, and a subsequent attempt at downward dosage titration and discontinuation.[1,4]

Serotonin selective reuptake inhibitors (SSRIs) have become increasingly popular and indeed dominant in the treatment of depression, panic disorder, social phobia, and obsessive compulsive disorder in adult patients, yet none of these agents has been approved by the U.S. FDA in the treatment of children and adolescents. The relative absence of autonomic, sedative, cardiovascular, and convulsive side effects of these drugs makes them logical choices for the treatment of a variety of disorders of childhood and adolescence. Indeed fluoxetine and clomipramine have been rather widely used clinically and have been studied in a number of controlled investigations in children and adolescents, where they have been employed primarily as antidepressants and anti-obsessional agents.[16,17,18] Fluoxetine has also been studied in children with ADHD.[19] Clinical experience and studies of fluoxetine and clomipramine in children, have generally found them to be well tolerated and effective in the broad range of disorders for which they have been used in adult patients. Clomipramine has the disadvantage of being a tricyclic and thus presenting the usual tricyclic risks of autonomic, cardiovascular, and sedative effects of other tricyclics, with a greater risk of provoking seizures than other drugs in this group. Experience with fluoxetine has been more extensive than with other SSRIs such as fluvoxamine, paroxetine, sertraline, and venlafaxine in children and adolescents. The long half-life of fluoxetine has the advantage of reducing consequences of missed doses, and the disadvantage of requiring a longer time interval to dissipate if adverse effects occur. Since children are much less likely than adults to be receiving other medications simultaneously, the significant potential of drug interactions with fluoxetine and its general lack of significant adverse effects, along with its ease of administration using a single daily dose regimen, makes it appear to be the optimal SSRI in children and adolescents. Most studies and clinical use have employed 20 mg daily, although, particularly in anxiety disorders, and in younger children, it would be most prudent to initiate fluoxetine at a daily dose of 2.5 to 5 mg, with gradual dosage titration if necessary. Efficacy of fluoxetine in childhood depression and OCD has been documented in published studies.[16,17] It is appropriate to discuss the lack of FDA approval of this and related SSRIs with parents before prescribing these agents for children and to closely follow patients during treatment and document favorable and unfavorable effects in the medical record.

Affective-Spectrum Disorders and Anxiety-Spectrum Disorders

Many psychiatric conditions in adults simultaneously have features of both affective and anxiety disorders, and appear to bridge the spectrum between seemingly distinct groups of illnesses. Similar disorders are beginning to be recognized in the pediatric age group. These disorders in both adults and children share a common responsivity to imipramine and other tricyclic antidepressants. Many of these disorders in adults are highly responsive to treatment with MAOIs such as phenelzine and tranylcypromine. Since these drugs inhibit monoamine oxidase and perhaps other enzymes as well, and since they have not been extensively studied in younger children, they should be used with caution in this age group. On the other hand, in adolescents with ADHD, depressive illness, eating disorders, panic, and phobic disorders, there may be an appropriate place for the judicious use of MAOIs.[20-22] Thus far, limited studies have appeared indicating the potential usefulness and safety of these drugs in adolescents. The necessity for strict compliance with dietary restrictions may, however, further complicate the use of MAOIs in adolescents.

Phobic symptoms, which usually relate to specific objects, places, and events in younger children, generally do not require drug therapy since they may be part of the developmental process and resolve spontaneously or with psycho-therapeutic intervention. The presence of more severe or disabling phobic symptoms in adolescents may require pharmacologic intervention and be quite responsive to imipramine therapy. School phobia, which is one source of school absences in children, is generally seen as a manifestation of separation anxiety disorder. Children with separation anxiety disorder may indeed be phobic and may also suffer from panic disorder. The presence of other depressive symptoms should be sought in a child with prominent symptoms of separation anxiety disorder. Forcing such children to attend school may be associated with increased anxiety and potentially aggressive behavior. Children who are school-phobic often present with a variety of somatic complaints, which may be a manifestation of the underlying disorder or may be feigned to facilitate the avoidance of school attendance.[1]

Several well-controlled studies have reported a significant, and often dramatic, response in school-phobic children to treatment with imipramine.[23] Imipramine treatment of separation anxiety disorder may yield a rapid response within 1 week or may require 4 to 6 weeks of treatment.[4,24] Generally, in younger children the dosage of imipramine needs to be gradually titrated upward to 5 mg/kg/day, although many children will respond to a lower dosage. Often, children will be totally symptom-free after a 3- to 4-month course of drug treatment, and may then have their medication gradually decreased and eventually discontinued.[4] Some school-phobic children will also experience anticipatory anxiety as the time to go to school nears. Although low doses of benzodiazepines have been suggested for short-term treatment of this anticipatory anxiety, it is probably preferable to avoid the use of benzodiazepines in children because of their potential for inducing dependence, as well as the risk of dulling the child's ability to participate and learn in the school setting.[25,26] Very often, as the phobic and panic symptoms ameliorate with imipramine treatment, the anticipatory anxiety symptoms will also diminish or disappear.

Panic disorder, which may include hyperventilation, restlessness, nausea, dizziness, and trembling, often along with a mixture of fear, anger, anxiety, and confusion, are beginning to be recognized in children and adolescents.[1] Panic disorder is more likely to occur in children who also have coexisting phobic or depressive disorders. Likewise, a family history of panic disorder, phobias, and affective illness is more likely to be seen in children and adolescents with panic disorder.[1] Fortunately, clinical experience and studies both support a favorable therapeutic response to imipramine in children and adolescents with panic disorder, similar to the therapeutic response observed in adults.[1,4]

Social phobia is becoming increasingly recognized as a source of impaired work and social functioning in adults, and although somewhat responsive to treatment with benzodiazepines and beta blockers, is more often responsive to treatment with MAOIs and SSRIs. In social phobia, adult patients fear social or performance situations in which they will be exposed to scrutiny and potential embarrassment or humiliation. Indeed children and adolescents may experience similar fears of embarrassment or humiliation with peers or in the school environment, which may actually be the provocateur of school phobia or panic disorder. This condition may become most symptomatic when the child is expected to read or recite in the classroom and thus lead to school failure, chronic tardiness, or attempts to avoid school attendance or participation in social situations with peers. Cautious short-term use of benzodiazepines has been recommended, however, use of low doses of SSRIs, such as fluoxetine, is likely to be more beneficial and associated with fewer adverse effects.[25]

Obsessive compulsive disorder, once thought to be a rare phenomenon in adults and children, is likely to occur in at least 1 or 2 percent of people, regardless of age. Although certain ritualistic behaviors may be part of the developmental process in children, persistence of repetitive behaviour or obsessional thinking in a child or adolescent should make the clinician suspect this disorder and thoroughly evaluate the patient using the Yale-Brown Obsessive Compulsive Scale (Y-BOCS), child versions of the Y-BOCS or similar instruments. OCD is more common in children with family histories of affective disorders and OCD, and affected children and adolescents often suffer simultaneously from depressive disorders.[25] Symptoms of OCD often coexist with tic disorders and probably occur in a majority of patients with Tourette's Syndrome.[25] Conventional doses of imipramine and other tricyclics are often beneficial in OCD, however, clomipramine and SSRIs such as fluoxetine are likely to be significantly more effective than standard TCAs in children and adolescents with OCD whether or not there are associated tics or signs of Tourette's Syndrome.[17,18] Depending on the age and size of the child or adolescent patient, the fluoxetine dose is likely to be between 5 and 20 mg per day, although occasionally higher doses are necessary. Just as some adults respond better to one antiobsessional agent than another, some younger patients will respond more favorably to clomipramine (25 to 150 mg per day) than to fluoxetine.

Eating disorders, including anorexia nervosa and bulimia, often begin during the adolescent years, with females being more frequently affected than males. These eating disorders also occasionally occur in younger children. Anorexia and bulimia often respond favorably to SSRIs, including fluoxetine and sertraline, and to tricyclics such as desipramine, imipramine, and amitriptyline.[25,28,29] Phenelzine is often beneficial in the treatment of bulimia in young adults, although experience and studies in adolescents are more limited with this drug.[30] Biological mechanisms associated with affective disorders, and pharmacologic interventions in eating disorders are more fully discussed in chapter 9.

Nocturnal enuresis, although apparently not related to the affective disorders, often responds favorably to antidepressant drug therapy. If enuresis is a persistent problem in a child in whom organic causes of bladder dyscontrol are not found, medication may be a useful adjunct to the treatment regimen, which should also include behavioral approaches to bladder training. Imipramine is generally the standard pharmacologic intervention for enuresis, and therapeutic responses may occur within a few days of initiating treatment at a low dosage, of 10 to 75 mg nightly.[1] Therapeutic responses in enuresis are often achieved at doses far lower than conventional antidepressant doses. Amitriptyline and MAOIs also have an antienuretic effect. Though the mechanism of action is unclear, it has been hypothesized that these drugs act by correcting a developmental lag of neural control mechanisms governing bladder sphincter function.[1] DDAVP, a synthetic analogue of 8-arginine vasopressin, administered by nasal spray, is a potent antidiuretic agent which is often very effective in the management of nocturnal enuresis.[25]

Mania

Manic disorders are rare in prepubertal children but have been reported as early as the age of 4 years. Mania is being recognized more commonly during adolescence. Indications are, however, that mania is often missed in adolescent patients, who, if they present with psychotic symptoms, agitation, belligerence, and expansiveness, may be seen by many clinicians as suffering from a schizophrenic disorder. Indeed, retrospective review of many adolescents diagnosed as schizophrenic reveals evidence of a manic disorder. Periodicity of symptoms and a marked affective component should alert the clinician to the possibility of adolescent mania.[1] A family history of bipolar affective disorder should further raise the clinician's suspicion of mania in an adolescent. Indeed, studies indicate that the presence of affective illness in the child's family predict a favorable response to lithium.[31]

Commonly, lithium-responsive manic illness in childhood does not present with hallucinations, delusions, or overt psychotic features. Impulsivity, aggressivity, obliviousness, and temper tantrums in a cyclical pattern are suggestive of the presence of mania. Low self-esteem, episodes of depression, and angry interpersonal interactions are also suggestive of a manic disorder. Some features of attention-deficit disorder, including overactivity, distractibility, and impaired school performance, may also be seen in juvenile mania.[1,24] A family history of affective illness, alcoholism, substance abuse, violence, and disintegration within the family is not uncommonly found in adolescents with manic disorders.[1]

Since lithium renal clearance is higher in children than in adults, younger patients may require higher dosages in order to achieve therapeutic blood levels. Many children and adolescents will be responsive to lithium dosages which maintain serum concentrations of 0.5 mEq/L, whereas others will fail to respond until they achieve serum concentrations of up to 2.0 mEq/L. Relatively higher oral doses of lithium carbonate may be required in order to achieve therapeutic serum concentrations of lithium in children and adolescents.[1,31]

Prior to initiating lithium treatment in children, a baseline ECG, CBC, serum creatinine, T_3, T_4, and TSH should be done. Once lithium therapy is initiated, lithium serum concentration should be measured on a weekly basis during the first month. During the second month, lithium measurements every 2 weeks are generally adequate and, subsequently, lithium levels may be measured approximately once monthly.[1,4]

In children who are reluctant to have frequent blood level determinations done, simultaneous serum lithium concentration and salivary lithium concentrations may be done initially and periodically during the course of treatment. Regular and more frequent follow-up may be done utilizing the salivary lithium concentration as discussed in chapter 8. If the course of lithium is prolonged in a child or adolescent, it is advisable to measure serum creatinine, T_3, T_4, and TSH approximately every 6 months during the course of lithium treatment. It may also be appropriate to periodically determine creatinine clearance since lithium has been reported to produce renal changes in some adults.[32] Thus far, as discussed in chapter 8, there is no reason for major concern about lithium-induced renal changes.[32] Nevertheless, caution is appropriate in dealing with the pediatric age group. Failure to achieve a satisfactory therapeutic response to lithium during an initial 2 to 3 month trial with adequate dosage and serum concentrations suggests that an alternate treatment, including the possible use of carbamazepine, valproate, or neuroleptics, would be more appropriate.[25,27] In a child or adolescent who has had a favorable response to lithium, it may be appropriate after 6 months to 1 year of treatment to contemplate a drug-free interval in order to determine the necessity of continuing lithium maintenance.[1]

ATTENTION-DEFICIT HYPERACTIVITY DISORDER (ADHD)

Attention-deficit hyperactivity disorder (ADHD) generally begins in young children, may persist throughout childhood into adolescence, and may continue with a modified symptom complex into adult life. Some aspects of ADHD suggest a relationship to affective disorders. Indeed, some children with this disorder are lithium-responsive.[1,33] Furthermore, adults who present with symptoms of hypomania and a previous history of ADHD in childhood may experience a favorable therapeutic response to lithium therapy.[1]

The severity of ADHD is quite variable and is likely to worsen in situations which demand sustained effort or which provide limited structure. Secondary symptoms, such as poor frustration tolerance, poor peer relations, aggressivity, and poor academic performance, also occur in this syndrome. Abnormal findings in EEG, neurologic examinations, or psychometric tests are not helpful in diagnosing ADHD.[34] Box 15-1 presents DSM-IV criteria for the diagnosis of attention deficit/hyperactivity disorder (ADHD).[34]

Pharmacologic Treatment of ADHD

The first major psychopharmacologic intervention described in children was the finding of dramatic therapeutic benefits of amphetamine in hyperactivity in 1937. Since that time, numerous controlled studies have repeatedly documented the therapeutic efficacy of a variety of stimulant medications, including dextroamphetamine, methylphenidate, and, pemoline in ADHD.[2,22] Studies of children with ADHD have indicated a response rate as high as 90%. When treatment is fully effective, the hyperactive child becomes indistinguishable from a normal child.[4] A study of a group of normal boys showed a decrease in motor activity, increased vigilance, and improvement on learning tasks when they were treated with dextroamphetamine; thus this treatment cannot be seen as a specific diagnostic indicator of ADHD.[35] Improvement in attention following stimulant treatment does not necessarily imply improvement in

Box 15-1 DSM-IV criteria for ADHD

Diagnostic criteria for attention-deficit/hyperactivity disorder

A. Either (1) or (2):

  (1) six (or more) of the following symptoms of **inattention** have persisted for at least 6 months to a degree that is maladaptive and inconsistent with developmental level:

  Inattention

   (a) often fails to give close attention to details or makes careless mistakes in schoolwork, work, or other activities
   (b) often has difficulty sustaining attention in tasks or play activities
   (c) often does not seem to listen when spoken to directly
   (d) often does not follow through on instructions and fails to finish schoolwork, chores, or duties in the workplace (not due to oppositional behavior or failure to understand instructions)
   (e) often has difficulty organizing tasks and activities
   (f) often avoids, dislikes, or is reluctant to engage in tasks that require sustained mental effort (such as schoolwork or homework)
   (g) often loses things necessary for tasks or activities (e.g., toys, school assignments, pencils, books, or tools)
   (h) is often easily distracted by extraneous stimuli
   (i) is often forgetful in daily activities

  (2) six (or more) of the following symptoms of **hyperactivity-impulsivity** have persisted for at least 6 months to a degree that is maladaptive and inconsistent with developmental level:

  Hyperactivity

   (a) often fidgets with hands or feet or squirms in seat
   (b) often leaves seat in classroom or in other situations in which remaining seated is expected
   (c) often runs about or climbs excessively in situations in which it is inappropriate (in adolescents or adults, may be limited to subjective feelings of restlessness)
   (d) often has difficulty playing or engaging in leisure activities quietly
   (e) is often "on the go" or often acts as if "driven by a motor"
   (f) often talks excessively

  Impulsivity

   (g) often blurts out answers before questions have been completed
   (h) often has difficulty awaiting turn
   (i) often interrupts or intrudes on others (e.g., butts into conversations or games)

B. Some hyperactive-impulsive or inattentive symptoms that caused impairment were present before age 7 years.

C. Some impairment from the symptoms is present in two or more settings (e.g., at school [or work] and at home).

Continued.

DSM-IV CRITERIA

Box 15-1 DSM-IV criteria for ADHD — cont'd.

D. There must be clear evidence of clinically significant impairment in social, academic, or occupational functioning.

E. The symptoms do not occur exclusively during the course of a Pervasive Developmental Disorder, Schizophrenia, or other Psychotic Disorder and are not better accounted for by another mental disorder (e.g., Mood Disorder, Anxiety Disorder, Dissociative Disorder, or a Personality Disorder).

Code based on type:

314.01 Attention-Deficit/Hyperactivity Disorder, Combined Type: if both Criteria A1 and A2 are met for the past 6 months

314.00 Attention-Deficit/Hyperactivity Disorder, Predominantly Inattentive Type: if Criterion A1 is met but Criterion A2 is not met for the past 6 months

314.01 Attention-Deficit/Hyperactivity Disorder, Predominantly Hyperactive-Impulsive Type: if Criterion A2 is met but Criterion A1 is not met for the past 6 months

---

Coding note: For individuals (especially adolescents and adults) who currently have symptoms that no longer meet full criteria, "In Partial Remission" should be specified.

From American Psychiatric Association: *Diagnostic and statistical manual of mental disorders*, ed 4 [DSM-IV]. Washington DC, American Psychiatric Press, 1994.

---

acquisition of specific skills such as reading, arithmetic, or memory.[4] Some studies, however, have indicated improvement in learning and intellectual accomplishment among ADHD children treated with stimulants.[36,37] Several studies have found tricyclic antidepressants, including imipramine, amitriptyline, and desipramine, to produce favorable therapeutic responses in children with ADHD.[4,38] In some instances, children who have had less than an optimal therapeutic response to stimulants have been found to be responsive to desipramine.[38] Preliminary studies also indicate efficacy of fluoxetine in ADHD.[19]

In some studies in which there was a comparable initial therapeutic response to imipramine and methylphenidate, symptoms recurred after about 6 weeks of imipramine treatment.[4,39] From 10% to 30% of ADHD children may be refractory to stimulant drug therapy.[4] Favorable responses to neuroleptic drugs, most often chlorpromazine or thioridazine, have been found in some clinical studies of ADHD.[4] These drugs, however, tend to decrease overactivity but not to improve distractibility.[40] Some ADHD children have been found to be partially responsive to haloperidol.[41] Although cognitive impairment by neuroleptics has been reported anecdotally, this observation is not based on objective data.[4] The major disadvantage of neuroleptics in this condition is the potential development of tardive dyskinesia as well as the occurrence of a response generally less robust than that seen with stimulants.

The short half-life and duration of action of dextroamphetamine and methylphenidate are major disadvantages to their therapeutic use in ADHD.

Onset of therapeutic action of these drugs generally occurs 30 to 60 minutes after a dose is administered, lasts for four to eight hours, and may be associated with symptom aggravation at ten to 20 hours after a dose.[1] Thus when dextroamphetamine and methylphenidate are utilized they most often must be administered in two or three daily doses or be prescribed in the somewhat more expensive sustained-release preparations, which are available for both of these drugs.

Although previously thought to require 2 to 8 weeks to achieve a therapeutic response in ADHD, pemoline in more recent studies appears to have an onset of action which is not dissimilar to that seen with methylphenidate and dextroamphetamine.[42] This latter investigation found an onset of action within 2 hours for standard methylphenidate, sustained-release methylphenidate, sustained-release dextroamphetamine and pemoline.[42] Each of these medications produced comparable therapeutic benefits in children with ADHD, with the finding that medications with longer durations of action including sustained-release preparations of stimulants and pemoline may be easier for patients to utilize.[42] Pemoline, which has a duration of action of 24 hours, may be administered once daily in the morning. All long acting stimulants may produce sleep disturbances in some patients, and do not differ from shorter acting medications in terms of potential appetite suppression. Therapeutic responses to stimulants do not correlate well with serum concentrations.[1]

Pemoline has a lesser psychostimulant effect than do dextroamphetamine or methylphenidate, thus lessening its abuse potential.[4,43] Reduced appetite and delayed sleep onset occur in 30% of children receiving moderately high doses of stimulants.[1,4] Infrequently, adverse mood changes, including sadness and increased interpersonal sensitivity, may occur in stimulant-treated children. These latter effects diminish over time, and may also be responsive to dosage adjustment. Both dextroamphetamine and methylphenidate can suppress body growth, yielding less rapid weight gain and height increase in children. Dextroamphetamine is more likely to produce this effect than is methylphenidate, and pemoline is least likely to affect growth.[1,4] Following discontinuation of stimulants, rebound growth acceleration occurs and height and weight gains approach normal. The mechanism of this growth inhibition is not understood, though it has been suggested to involve inhibition of somatomedins.[4] A major disadvantage of pemoline is its potential to form hepatotoxic metabolites in 1% to 3% of treated children.[1] This may result in hepatocellular injury and is associated with elevated hepatic transaminases (SGPT, SGOT). These enzyme elevations gradually appear over the initial 6 months of treatment and return to normal following discontinuation of medication.[1] The presence of decreased appetite, fatigue, or stomach fullness after several months of pemoline therapy may indicate a hepatotoxic effect and suggest the necessity for performing liver function tests.[1] During treatment with stimulants, patients should be carefully monitored for evidence of adverse drug effects, adequacy of dosage, and indications of noncompliance or abuse of the prescribed medication.

Dextroamphetamine is generally prescribed in a daily dosage range of 10 to 40 mg (0.1-0.8 mg/kg in divided doses). Methylphenidate is generally administered in a daily dose of 20 to 60 mg (0.5-2.0 mg/kg in divided doses). Magnesium pemoline is generally administered in a daily dosage of 37.5 to 112.5 mg (1.0-2.5 mg/kg). Therapy with these agents should be started at 5 mg daily for dextroamphetamine, 10 mg daily for methylphenidate, and 37.5 mg daily for pemoline. Dosage may then be gradually increased every two to four days with dextroamphetamine and methylphenidate given in a twice-daily regimen and pemoline given in a single dose each morning.[1,4]

When tricyclic antidepressants are utilized in the treatment of ADHD, they may be given in a single bedtime dose.[38,39] Imipramine, desipramine, or amitriptyline may be initiated at 10 mg nightly at bedtime with gradual increments as required up to 75 mg at bedtime. Response to tricyclics in ADHD may occur within a few days or may require several weeks of treatment.[1,4] If the initial response diminishes, the dosage must be titrated upward to achieve continuing therapeutic benefit. The long duration of action of tricyclic drugs, allowing for their administration once daily as well as their lack of abuse potential, makes them desirable therapeutic agents in those ADHD patients who are responsive.[4] Children who have a positive family history of affective illness may respond more favorably to tricyclic drugs and should, perhaps, have an initial therapeutic trial with these agents prior to contemplating stimulant drug therapy.[4] Although clinical experience and research data are thus far limited, preliminary work suggests that fluoxetine is beneficial in some children with ADHD, when employed at daily doses of 20 to 40 mg.[19] If further data confirms the initial findings, the advantages of this drug in producing minimal side effects and having no potential for abuse and dependency would be a bright star on the difficult ADHD horizon.

There are no well-defined criteria for the duration of pharmacologic treatment of ADHD. Experienced clinicians and investigators in the field support the notion that the drugs be continued for as long as there is a need for them and they demonstrate clinical benefit. Drug holidays may be of some value in assessing the continuing need for these medications. During school vacations, medications may be withdrawn and the child's behavior assessed in the drug-free state. In some instances, it is useful to provide children a drug-free period on the weekend, both to assess the continuing need for medication and to reduce the likelihood of tolerance developing.[1,4] Preliminary clinical studies indicate that clonidine, an alpha$_2$-noradrenergic agent which reduces the frequency of firing in the locus ceruleus, thus decreasing norepinephrine release, is effective, particularly in reducing hyperactivity, in some children and adolescents with ADHD.[44]

TOURETTE'S DISORDER (SYNDROME)

Tourette's disorder, or syndrome (TS) typically begins in childhood and presents with multiple motor tics and one or more vocal tics, which may appear simultaneously or at different periods of the illness. The tics occur many times daily nearly every day. Typically, tics involve the head and, frequently, other parts of the body, including the torso and limbs. In approximately one half of cases, initial symptoms consist of bouts of a single tic, most frequently eye blinking. Initial symptoms may also include tongue protrusion, squatting, sniffing, hopping, skipping, throat clearing, stuttering, uttering of various sounds and words, and coprolalia. Vocal tics commonly include various sounds, such as clicks, grunts, yelps, barks, sniffs, and coughs. Coprolalia, the involuntary utterance of obscenities, is a well-known symptom of Tourette's disorder, but may occur in only a third of cases, and is not necessary for the diagnosis. Patients with Tourette's disorder may repeatedly touch objects, engage in compulsive acts, and experience obsessional thoughts. Increasing clinical experience with TS indicates that symptoms of OCD are likely to be more prevalent and disturbing than is coprolalia, which is now recognized to be present in a minority of patients rather than in the majority which was the previous teaching. This disorder may appear as early as the first year of age, but the median age of onset is 7 years, and the majority of cases occur before the age of 14.[34] Tic disorders are more common among first-degree biological relatives of patients with Tourette's disorder. There is some evidence that obsessive-compulsive disorder is more common in first-degree biological relatives of persons with Tourette's disorder.[45] Occasionally, Tourette's disorder and ADHD coexist, which presents a significant therapeutic problem, since psychostimulants are known to provoke or worsen the tics of Tourette's disorder.[46] This disorder is believed to be related to an abnormality in central neurotransmission, most likely involving dopamine or norepinephrine or both. The severity of symptoms varies considerably from day to day and from month to month and may fluctuate in response to external circumstances.[46]

Neuroleptic drugs that block dopamine receptors have become established as the most effective treatment for Tourette's disorder. Specifically, haloperidol, has become established as the standard pharmacologic treatment for Tourette's disorder.[46] Generally, children and adolescents will respond favorably and promptly to low doses of haloperidol, most often ranging between 0.5 and 5.0 mg per day. Significant extrapyramidal side effects seldom occur when dosage is initiated at the low end of the spectrum and very slowly titrated upward to achieve symptom control. The more sedating and less dopamine-specific low-potency agents such as chlorpromazine and thioridazine are generally not desirable in the treatment of Tourette's disorder. Pimozide is a dopamine blocking neuroleptic drug approved in the United States only for the treatment of Tourette's disorder.[47] Controlled studies using this drug indicate a high degree of clinical success in the management of Tourette's symptoms and, in some cases, efficacy in haloperidol-refractory patients.[47] The major disadvantage of pimozide is its potential cardiovascular toxicity.

Ten percent of pimozide-treated patients have developed ECG abnormalities. Therefore, periodic ECGs are necessary in monitoring patients treated with this medication. The ECG abnormalities reported with pimozide include T wave and U wave abnormalities, as well as prolongation of the QTc interval.[48] The latter abnormality may increase the risk of a potentially fatal arrhythmia such as torsade de pointes.[1] Cardiac arrhythmia was suspected as the cause of sudden death of two schizophrenic patients during acute titration of pimozide up to 70-80 mg/day.[48] One study of 40 patients with Tourette's disorder found prolongation of the QTc interval on the ECGs of pimozide-treated patients, but no other evidence of adverse cardiac effects or changes in rate, rhythm, or ECG wave form.[48] In that study, no ECG changes were found in haloperidol-treated patients.

In prescribing pimozide for Tourette's disorder, the initial dose should be 1 mg/day with gradual dosage titration as necessary to control symptoms. Most patients with Tourette's disorder are maintained on doses of less than 0.2 mg/kg/day or a daily dose of 10 mg, whichever is less. In no case should a dosage in excess of 0.3 mg/kg/day or 20 mg/day be administered.[46] The commonly recognized neuroleptic side effects are likely to be similar for haloperidol and pimozide. Clinical judgment therefore suggests that prior to initiating treatment with pimozide an attempt should first be made to control Tourette's symptoms with conventional low-dosage haloperidol regimens.

Clonidine, which decreases release of norepinephrine in the locus ceruleus and other brain structures, has been found to be therapeutically useful in the management of patients with Tourette's disorder who do not respond to or tolerate haloperidol. Controlled studies have reported comparable therapeutic efficacy of clonidine and haloperidol.[49,50] Clonidine, which is marketed as an antihypertensive agent, is not approved by the FDA for the treatment of Tourette's disorder. In addition to lowering blood pressure, clonidine may also slow the heart rate and produce dizziness, dry mouth, and drowsiness. More rarely, clonidine may exacerbate depression or provoke hallucinations.[49] In the treatment of Tourette's disorder, clonidine may be initiated in a dose of 0.05 mg twice daily with gradual dosage increments as necessary and as tolerated by the patient, up to 0.1 or 0.2 mg twice daily. In some instances, where blood pressure remains stable, adverse effects have not occurred, and a desirable therapeutic result has not been obtained, dosage increments may be cautiously made up to 0.3 mg twice daily to achieve the desired therapeutic result.

In some patients with Tourette's disorder, who do not tolerate neuroleptics or clonidine, the anticonvulsant carbamazepine may be tried. Carbamazepine is, at times, effective, particularly if there is a preexisting EEG abnormality. The benzodiazepine, clonazepam may also be therapeutically beneficial with or without EEG abnormality in a patient with Tourette's disorder who does not tolerate neuroleptics or clonidine. Clonazepam may be started at 0.25 to 0.5 mg daily and gradually increased as tolerated. Drowsiness is the most common side effect of clonazepam, which lacks hypotensive and extrapyramidal side effects. Preliminary trials indicate that the calcium channel blockers verapamil and nifedipine may benefit some patients who have Tourette's disorder.[51] This finding is particularly interesting since the neuroleptic pimozide possesses calcium channel blocking activity in addition to its dopamine receptor antagonism.[48]

Since obsessive compulsive symptoms are so often a major disturbing feature of Tourette's disorder, preliminary findings of the anti-obsessional activity of fluoxetine in patients with TS are very encouraging.[52] This drug which lacks autonomic and extrapyramidal side effects should be considered for initial treatment of many TS patients, thus potentially providing symptomatic improvement without the risk of tardive dyskinesia.[52] Studies suggest an initial fluoxetine dose of 20 mg daily which may be increased if necessary, although I have seen benefits at doses of 10 to 20 mg daily.

PSYCHOTIC DISORDERS

The adult form of schizophrenia may first appear during the mid- to late teenage years. As in the case of adult patients, dopamine blocking neuroleptic agents are the drugs of choice. These compounds may reduce or eliminate paranoia, delusions, hallucinations, and other psychotic manifestations. These medications may also facilitate better adjustment of the patient by reducing aggressive and inappropriate behavior patterns. The pharmacology and techniques in the clinical use of antipsychotic drugs are discussed in chapter 4 and are applicable in treating an adolescent with adult-type schizophrenia. High-potency antipsychotic drugs, such as haloperidol, trifluoperazine, fluphenazine, perphenazine, and thiothixene, are generally preferred because of their more specific antipsychotic dopamine blocking activity. These high-potency drugs produce less drowsiness and hypotensive action and may thus be better tolerated by patients. On the other hand, high-potency antipsychotic drugs may be associated with a greater potential for acute dystonic and other extrapyramidal side effects.[53]

As in the case of adult psychopharmacology, it is desirable to use the lowest effective dose of antipsychotic medication and the shortest duration of drug exposure in order to minimize the potential risk of developing tardive dyskinesia. Young male patients have a somewhat higher incidence of acute dystonic reaction when receiving high-potency neuroleptic drugs. Several controlled studies have suggested the therapeutic benefits of the coadministration of antiparkinsonian medications along with high-potency neuroleptics to reduce the occurrence of extrapyramidal side effects.[54] Low-potency agents such as chlorpromazine and thioridazine may be more likely to produce sedation, hypotension, dry mouth, and constipation, and may also be more likely to provoke sexual dysfunction, which may be particularly alarming to a psychotic adolescent male. Thioridazine is a particular offender in this area, since it may impair potency and ejaculatory function and produce retrograde ejaculation, an alarming symptom in a young male trying to come to terms with his own sexuality. In many instances, acute psychosis in the adolescent may represent a single episode and be responsive to neuroleptic medication. Acute psychosis in the adolescent may also be drug-induced, and may not require neuroleptic treatment with the exception of PCP psychosis, which may benefit from low-dose haloperidol administration. Some cases of adolescent psychosis represent the beginning phase of a schizophrenic process and may require more prolonged administration of neuroleptic medication. Acute psychosis in the adolescent should raise the clinician's suspicion of a possible manic disorder, which may be lithium-responsive, and thus preclude long-term neuroleptic treatment.[53]

PERVASIVE DEVELOPMENTAL DISORDERS

Pervasive developmental disorder and autistic disorder in children and adolescents benefit only minimally from neuroleptic treatment.[2] These disorders are likely to become apparent very early in childhood and represent a failure to achieve normal developmental processes, rather than an interruption of normal development by an acute psychotic disturbance.[1] Autistic children lack normal responsiveness to other persons and exhibit gross deficits in language development. If present, speech is abnormal, consisting of patterns such as immediate and delayed echolalia, metaphorical language, and pronominal reversals.[34] Finally, the child may show an interest in or fascination with unusual objects and refuse to allow any changes or disruption from his or her attachment to them. Social and emotional functioning are extremely limited and behavior may be bizarre and marked by extreme mood changes, self-mutilation, peculiar mannerisms, hyperactivity, and lethargy.[34]

Pharmacologic treatment of these children involves the use of neuroleptics to control marked agitation, hyperactivity, and destructive behavior. Successful pharmacologic response may allow the child to be maintained at home, rather than in an institution. More sedating low-potency neuroleptics, such as chlorpromazine and thioridazine, may be useful in severely agitated children.[4] More specific dopamine blocking agents such as haloperidol may, in some cases, be therapeutically superior and produce less drowsiness and sedation than the low-potency agents.[55,56] In children with known convulsive disorders, chlorpromazine has an ability to lower seizure threshold in excess of that seen with other neuroleptic drugs. Thioridazine and haloperidol appear to be the safest neuroleptics in a patient with a convulsive disorder because of their lesser likelihood of provoking seizures. Children with pervasive developmental disorders present with stereotypes, mannerisms, or tics, which may disappear when neuroleptics are administered. These movements may recur during withdrawal of neuroleptic medication and should not be confused with withdrawal-emergent dyskinesia or tardive dyskinesia.[1,4]

In pervasive developmental disorder (PDD), repetitive stereotypic behaviors are suggestive of obsessive compulsive disorder, as is the so commonly observed fascination with unusual objects and intolerance to change, when imposed from outside. These symptoms may be reduced significantly by a variety of serotonergic drugs, including clomipramine, fluvoxamine, fluoxetine, and sertraline.[57] The potential utility of serotonergic agents in autism and PDD was first seen with fenfluramine, prior to the availability of the now more commonly used SSRIs.[58] Fenfluramine was found in many but not all studies to improve social relatedness, reduce stereotypic behavior, lessen overactivity, and improve attention span.[58] Concerns about potential neurologic damage from prolonged administration of fenfluramine, as observed in animal but not human studies, has discouraged more extensive use of this agent, however, it appears that the potential for adverse effects of fenfluramine were emphasized beyond the reliability of available data.[58] Extensive use of fluoxetine in more than 10 million patients with a variety of disorders supports the safety of this compound and favors more extensive use of this drug in child and adolescent psychiatry, and particularly in the management of stereotypic behavior and OCD-like symptoms seen in PDD and autism. The extent of clinical experience with fluoxetine suggests that this SSRI should be seriously studied and used to control those PDD symptoms, which have been demonstrated to be responsive to serotonergic drugs.[57] In addition to fluoxetine, fluvoxamine and sertraline have been shown to reduce stereotypic behavior and improve interactive abilities of children and adults with PDD.[57] Although clomipramine has also been found effective in reducing stereotypic behavior in PDD, its autonomic, cardiovascular, and potential epileptogenic side effects would generally make it a less desirable agent in patients with this complex and poorly understood disorder or family of disorders, than are the SSRIs. Fluoxetine, which may be used in daily doses of 5 to 60 mg, has the disadvantage of a long half-life, requiring weeks to clear if adverse effects occur as well as the potential for a variety of drug interactions. Fluvoxamine, which has a short half-life, also has the potential to interact with a variety of drugs, while sertraline, which has been least extensively studied in PDD, has a half-life of only 1 day and the least potential for drug interactions. It would therefore appear that if further studies document efficacy for sertraline in PDD stereotypic behaviors, this agent may be a better choice than fluoxetine.

TARGET SYMPTOM PHARMACOTHERAPY IN CHILDREN AND ADOLESCENTS

As stated at the outset, it is preferable to employ specific pharmacologic intervention in the management of specific disease entities and syndromes. In some instances, however, symptoms responsive to pharmacotherapy may cut across diagnostic lines. In the remaining section of this chapter, I discuss briefly the use of therapeutic agents for symptomatic treatment.

Aggressive and nonaggressive conduct disorders appear in children and adolescents. Several investigators have found an association between conduct disorder and affective illnesses and have described favorable therapeutic responses to antidepressant medication.[4] Aggressive symptoms may coexist with a depressive illness and be responsive to the judicious administration of neuroleptics, lithium, carbamazepine, and propranolol.[1,5,59,60] Agitated, aggressive, belligerent behavior may occur in the context of a psychotic illness and be responsive to neuroleptics alone or in combination with lithium or carbamazepine. Similar behavior can appear in conjunction with pervasive developmental disorders in children who have not developed functionally beyond a primitive level of understanding of reality. In such patients, neuroleptics cannot be expected to achieve the same therapeutic efficacy as that observed in adolescents and adults experiencing an acute episode of psychosis. In these instances, the goal of pharmacotherapy may be to control the unacceptable and dangerous behavior, rather than to repair an irreparable underlying pervasive disorder. Likewise, there is no evidence that any pharmacologic intervention will improve the intellectual function of a mentally retarded child or adolescent. Yet, behavior patterns in retarded individuals may be favorably affected by pharmacologic intervention.[61] Mentally retarded patients may indeed experience depressive disorders, and thus achieve a favorable therapeutic response when treated with tricyclic drugs.[61] Hallucinations, paranoia, and agitation, as well as belligerent behavior, may be favorably influenced by the use of neuroleptic drugs and on occasion, by administration of lithium, even in the absence of a clear-cut manic disorder. Mania does occur in mentally retarded patients and lithium responsiveness has been demonstrated in these individuals.[48] When lithium is employed in the mentally retarded, organic brain changes may increase sensitivity to the drug and enhance side effects, thus suggesting the employment of lower-than-conventional therapeutic doses and blood levels.[61]

Aggressive and assaultive behaviors in retarded or nonretarded patients unresponsive to neuroleptics or lithium may respond to a therapeutic trial of carbamazepine.[61] Patients who are aggressive or assaultive but have normal EEGs are generally less responsive to anticonvulsant drugs than those whose EEGs are abnormal. The beta-adrenergic blocking agent propranolol may be the drug of choice in the management of aggressive and assaultive behaviors unrelated to affective illness, schizophrenia, and ADHD.[5,22,60] Propranolol may be effective in managing belligerent behavior associated with acute or chronic brain trauma, organic brain dysfunction, mental retardation, autism, and conduct disorder.[22] Since propranolol may lower blood pressure and decrease heart rate, it is important to monitor these parameters prior to and at intervals during treatment, particularly when the dosage is increased.

In the absence of initial bradycardia or hypotension, propranolol may be initiated at a dose of 10 to 20 mg twice daily with gradual dosage increase, depending on the patient's body size, degree of aggressivity, and behavioral and physiologic response to the medication. Favorable therapeutic responses may be seen in younger children at doses as low as 20 mg daily or in older and larger adolescents at doses as high as 200 mg daily.[5,60] Self-destructive and self-injurious behaviors in children and adolescents, with or without mental retardation, may be responsive to neuroleptics, lithium, carbamazepine, valproate or propranolol.[4,22,61] Impulse control disorders in children and adolescents are worthy of a therapeutic trial of lithium, carbamazepine, or valproate which may facilitate better impulse control and allow the child to adapt more successfully to external limits and social conventions.[1,4]

Overanxious disorder of childhood, which is similar to generalized anxiety in adults, may, from time to time, require short courses and relatively low doses of benzodiazepines, preferably shorter-acting drugs such as oxazepam or alprazolam.[1,26] Since these drugs have a potential for producing tolerance and dependence, their use in children should be limited to very brief courses of therapy, necessitated by escalating anxiety in the face of acute external traumatic events. If more prolonged treatment of generalized anxiety is necessary in childhood, consideration should be given to the use of nonaddicting, more strongly sedating antihistamines such as diphenhydramine or hydroxyzine.[1] These drugs, given intermittently or regularly in relatively low dosage, may reduce the severity of generalized anxiety symptoms. They may, however, cause excessive drowsiness, which may interfere with school work and social interactions, and may give rise to feelings of fogginess, dullness, or "spaciness" as manifestations of their sedative and anticholinergic action.[1] These sedating antihistamines may also be of value in childhood insomnia, sleep disturbances, and night terrors. If larger doses must be employed to induce sleep, however, the anticholinergic side effects of these drugs may, on occasion, worsen symptoms of night terror. If these drugs are found ineffective in childhood sleep disturbances, low doses of short-acting benzodiazepines administered intermittently or for brief periods of time may be of therapeutic value.[1,4,22]

REFERENCES

1. Campbell M, Spencer EK: Psychopharmacology in child and adolescent psychiatry: A review of the past five years. *J Am Acad Child Adolesc Psychiatry* 1988, 27:269-279.
2. Popper CW: Child and adolescent psychopharmacology, in Michels R, Cavenar JO, Brodie HKH (eds): *Psychiatry*. Philadelphia, Lippincott 1985, vol 2, ch 59, pp 1-23.
3. Slaby AE, McGuire PL: Prevention of child and adolescent suicide. *Psychiatry Lett* 1986;4:65-74.
4. Gittelman R, Kanner A: Overview of clinical psychopharmacology in childhood disorders, in Bernstein JG (ed): *Clinical Psychopharmacology*, ed 2. Boston, John Wright-PSG, 1984, pp 189-210.
5. Kuperman S, Stewart MA: Use of propranolol to decrease aggressive outbursts in younger patients. *Psychosomatics* 1987;28:315-319.
6. Kashani JH, Carlson GA: Seriously depressed pre-schoolers. *Am J Psychiatry* 1987;144:348-350.
7. Kashani JH, Carlson GA, Beck NC, et al: Depression, depressive symptoms and depressed mood among a community sample of adolescents. *Am J Psychiatry* 1987;144:931-934.
8. Myers JK, Weissman MM, Tischler GL, et al: Six month prevalence of psychiatric disorders in three communities. *Arch Gen Psychiatry* 1984;41:959-967.
9. Kashani JH, McGee RO, Clarkson SE, et al: Depression in a sample of 9 year old children. *Arch Gen Psychiatry* 1983;40:1217-1223.
10. Rutter M, Graham P, Chadwick OF, et al: Adolescent turmoil: fact or fiction. *J Child Psychol Psychiatry* 1976;17:35-56.
11. Puig-Antich J, Perel JM, Lupatkin W, et al: Imipramine in prepubertal major depressive disorders. *Arch Gen Psychiatry* 1987;44:81-89.
12. Geller B, Cooper TB, Chestnut EO, et al: Preliminary data on the relationship between

nortriptyline plasma level and response in depressed children. *Am J Psychiatry* 1986;143:1283-1286.

13. Kashani J, Shekion WO, Reid JC: Amitriptyline in children with major depressive disorder. *J Am Acad Child Psychiatry* 1984;23:348-351.

14. Kramer E, Feiguine R: Clinical effects of amitriptyline in adolescent depression. *J Am Acad Child Psychiatry* 1984;23:636-644.

15. Riddle MA, Nelson JC, Kleinman CS, et al: Sudden death in children receiving Norpramin®: a review of three reported cases and commentary. *J Am Acad Child Adolesc Psychiatry* 1991;30:104-108.

16. Simeon JD, Dinicola VF, Ferguson HB, et al: Adolescent depression: a placebo-controlled fluoxetine treatment study and follow-up. *Prog Neuropsychopharmacol Biol Psychiatry* 1990;14:791-795.

17. Riddle MA, Scahill L, King RA, et al: Double-blind, crossover trial of fluoxetine and placebo in children and adolescents with obsessive-compulsive disorder. *J Am Acad Child Adolesc Psychiatry* 1992;31:1062-1069.

18. DeVeaugh-Geiss J, Moroz G, Biederman J, et al: Clomipramine hydrochloride in childhood and adolescent obsessive-compulsive disorder- A multicenter trial. *J Am Acad Child Adolesc Psychiatry* 1992;31:45-49.

19. Barrickman L, Noyes R, Kuperman S, et al: Treatment of ADHD with fluoxetine: A preliminary trial. *J Am Acad Child Adolesc Psychiatry* 1991;30:762-767.

20. Zametkin A, Rapoport JL, Murphy DL, et al: Treatment of hyperactive children with monoamine oxidase inhibitors. *Arch Gen Psychiatry* 1985;42:962-966.

21. Ryan ND, Puig-Antich J, Rabinovich H, et al: MAOIs in adolescent major depression unresponsive to tricyclic antidepressants. *J Am Acad Child Adolesc Psychiatry* 1988;27:755-758.

22. Biederman J: Psychopharmacology in children and adolescents. In Wiener J (ed): *Comprehensive textbook of child and adolescent psychiatry.* Washington, DC, 1991, American Psychiatric Press. pp 545-570.

23. Gittelman-Klein R, Klein DF: Controlled imipramine treatment of school phobia. *Arch Gen Psychjatry* 1981;25:204-207.

24. Biederman J, Jellinek MS: Psychopharmacology in children. *N Engl J Med* 1984;310:968-972.

25. Rosenberg DR, Holttum J, Gershon S (eds): *Textbook of pharmacotherapy for child and adolescent psychiatric disorders.* New York, Brunner/Mazel, 1994.

26. Simeon JG, Ferguson HB, Knott V, et al: Clinical, cognitive, and neuropysiological effects of alprazolam in children and adolescents with overanxious and avoidant disorders. *J Am Acad Child Adolesc Psychiatry* 1992;31:29-33.

27. Papatheodorou G, Kutcher SP: Divalproex sodium treatment in late adolescent and young adult acute mania. *Psychopharmacol Bull* 1993;29:213-219.

28. Hughes PL, Wells LA, Cunningham CJ, et al: Treating bulimia with desipramine. *Arch Gen Psychiatry* 1986;43:182-186.

29. Halmi KA, Eckert E, La DO, et al: Anorexia nervosa: treatment efficacy of cyproheptadine and amitriptyline. *Arch Gen Psychiatry* 1986;43:177-181.

30. Walsh BT, Stewart JW, Roose SP: Treatment of bulimia with phenelzine. *Arch Gen Psychiatry* 1984;41:1105-1109.

31. McKnew DH, Cytryn L, Buchsbaum MS, et al: Lithium in children of lithium-responding parents. *Psychiatr Res* 1981;4:171-180.

32. DePaulo JR, Correa EI, Sapir DG. Renal function and lithium: a longitudinal study. *Am J Psychiatry* 1986;143:892-895.

33. Biederman J, Munir K, Knee D, et al: High rate of affective disorders in probands with attention deficit disorder and in their relatives. *Am J Psychiatry* 1987;44:330-333.

34. American Psychiatric Association: *Diagnostic and Statistical Manual of Mental Disorders,* ed 4, [DSM IV]. Washington, DC, American Psychiatric Press, 1994.

35. Rapoport JL, Buchsbaum MS, Weingartner H, et al: Dextroamphetamine: its cognitive and

behavioral effects in normal and hyperactive boys and normal men. *Arch Gen Psychiatry* 1980;37:933-943.

36. Pelham WE, Bender ME, Caddell J: Methylphenidate and children with attention deficit disorder: dose effects on classroom academic and social behavior. *Arch Gen Psychiatry* 1985;42:948-952.

37. Famularo R, Fenton T: The effect of methylphenidate on school grades in children with attention deficit disorder without hyperactivity. *J Clin Psychiatry* 1987;48:112-114.

38. Biederman J, Gastfriend DR, Jellinek MS: Desipramine in the treatment of children with attention deficit disorder. *J Clin Psychopharmacol* 1986;6:359-363.

39. Quinn PO, Rapoport JL: One year follow-up of hyperactive boys treated with imipramine or methylphenidate. *Am J Psychiatry* 1975;132:244-245.

40. Werry JS, Weiss G: Studies on the hyperactive child III: The effect of chlorpromazine upon behavior and learning ability. *J Am Acad Child Psychiatry* 1966;5:292-312.

41. Werry J, Aman MG: Haloperidol and methylphenidate in hyperactive children. *Acta Paedopsychiatr (Basle)* 1976;42:26-40.

42. Pelham WE, Greenslade KE, Vodde-Hamilton M, et al: Relative efficacy of long-acting stimulants on children with attention deficit/hyperactivity disorder: A comparison of standard methylphenidate, sustained-release methylphenidate, sustained-release dextroamphetamine, and pemoline. *Pediatrics* 1990;86:226-237.

43. Zametkin AJ, Linnoila M, Karoum F, et al: Pemoline and urinary excretion of catecholamines and indoleamines in children with attention deficit disorder. *Am J Psychiatry* 1986;143:359-362.

44. Hunt RD: Treatment effects of oral and transdermal clonidine in relation to methylphenidate: an open pilot study in ADD-H. *Psychopharmacol Bull* 1987;23:111-114.

45. Pauls DL, Towbin KE, Leckman JF, et al: Gilles de la Tourette's syndrome and obsessive-compulsive disorder: evidence supporting a genetic relationship. *Arch Gen Psychiatry* 1986;43:1180-1182.

46. Leckman JF, Cohen DJ: Tourette's disorder and other stereotyped movement disorders, in Michels R, Cavenar JO, Brodie HKH (eds): *Psychiatry*. Philadelphia, Lippincott, 1985, vol 2, ch 38, pp 1-8.

47. Shapiro AK, Shapiro E: Controlled study of pimozide vs placebo in Tourette's syndrome. *J Am Acad Child Psychiatry* 1984;23:161-173.

48. Fulop G, Phillips RA, Shapiro AK: ECG changes during haloperidol and pimozide treatment of Tourette's disorder. *Am J Psychiatry* 1987;144:673-675

49. Cohen DJ, Detlor J, Young JG: Clonidine ameliorates Gilles de la Tourette syndrome. *Arch Gen Psychiatry* 1980;37:1350-1357.

50. Leckman JF, Ort S, Caruso KA, et al: Rebound phenomena in Tourette's syndrome after abrupt withdrawal of clonidine. *Arch Gen Psychiatry* 1986;43:1168-1176.

51. Walsh TL, Larenstein B, Licamele WL: Calcium antagonists in the treatment of Tourette's disorder. *Am J Psychiatry* 1986;143:1467-1468.

52. Riddle MA, Hardin MT, King R, et al: Fluoxetine treatment of children with Tourette's and obsessive compulsive disorders: preliminary clinical experience. *J Am Acad Child Adolesc Psychiatry* 1990;29:45-48.

53. Teicher MH, Glod CA: Neuroleptic Drugs: Indications and guidelines for their rational use in children and adolescents. *J Child Adolesc Psychopharmacology* 1990;1:33-56.

54. Winslow RS, Stillner V, Coons DJ, et al: Prevention of acute dystonic reactions in patients beginning high-potency neuroleptics. *Am J Psychiatry* 1986;143:706-710.

55. Campbell M, Anderson LT, Meier M, et al: A comparison of haloperidol and behavior therapy and their interaction in autistic children. *J Am Acad Child Psychiatry* 1978;17:640-655.

56. Anderson LT, Campbell M, Grega DM: Haloperidol in the treatment of infantile autism: effects on learning and behavioral symptoms. *Am J Psychiatry* 1984;141:1195-1202.

57. McDougle CJ, Price LH, Volkmar FR: Recent advances in the pharmacotherapy of autism and related conditions. *Child Adolescent Psychiatric Clinics of North America* 1994;3:71-89.

58. Aman MG, Kern RA: Review of fenfluramine in the treatment of the developmental disabilities. *J Am Acad Child Adolesc Psychiatry* 1989;28:549-565.
59. Campbell M, Small AM, Green WH, et al: Behavioral efficacy of haloperidol and lithium carbonate: a comparison in hospitalized aggressive children with conduct disorder. *Arch Gen Psychiatry* 1984;41:650-656.
60. Ratey JJ, Mikkelson E, Sorgi P, et al: Autism: the treatment of aggressive behaviors. *J Clin Psychopharmacol* 1987;7:35-41.
61. Rogoff ML: Psychotropic medications and mentally retarded patients, in Bernstein JG (ed): *Clinical Psychopharmacology,* ed 2. Boston, John Wright-PSG, 1984, pp 211-231.

CHAPTER 16

Geriatric Psychopharmacology and the Dementias: Alzheimer's and HIV

OVERVIEW

1. Changes in drug metabolism, distribution, and brain receptors accompany the normal aging process and must be considered for optimal pharmacotherapy.
2. Dementia, whether due to Alzheimer's, HIV, or other causes, results in altered brain response and potential adverse effects of psychotropic and other drugs.
3. Elderly and physiologically compromised patients should be started on the lowest possible dose of medication.
4. Titrate dosage upward slowly, monitor pulse, BP, and ECG as indicated.
5. The total effective safe daily dosage is nearly always lower in elderly than in younger patients.
6. Be aware of interactions of psychotropic medications.
7. The elderly are more likely to be receiving multiple nonpsychotropic medications and thus present a greater risk of drug interactions with psychotropic medications.
8. Temporary discontinuation of medications is one of the most effective techniques to evaluate an unfavorable clinical course or potential adverse drug reaction.
9. Avoid longer-acting benzodiazepines such as diazepam and flurazepam; if necessary, small doses of lorazepam, or oxazepam may be used. Cumulative effects and dependency may occur.
10. Neuroleptics with greater hypotensive and anticholinergic effects such as chlorpromazine, mesoridazine, and thioridazine should be avoided. Low doses of high-potency agents such as haloperidol, risperidone, perphenazine, and trifluoperazine, are preferred.

Continued.

11. Among cyclic antidepressants, desipramine and trazodone are safer than more strongly anticholinergic drugs such as amitriptyline. MAOIs which lack anticholinergic effect are useful but produce postural hypotension. Low doses of SSRIs are often effective with minimal side effects, but fluoxetine has a prolonged effect and the risk of drug interactions is high; sertraline is likely to be safest.

12. Lithium carbonate may be used safely in the elderly, generally at lower dosage, maintaining blood levels of 0.4-0.6 mEq/L. Diuretics must be administered with caution since they may increase serum lithium concentration or produce hypokalemia, which may increase the risk of lithium intoxication.

People 65 years of age and over currently make up 12% of the population in the United States, yet they account for 25% to 30% of the health care costs. Age-related physiologic changes and the increased likelihood of multiple medical conditions add to the complexity of providing medical care and pharmacologic management of the elderly.[1] All people, young and old, tend to self-medicate, and often do not scrupulously follow recommendations of the treating physician, yet the compliance problem tends to be of far greater impact when it occurs in concert with the physiologic changes of aging.

Although people aged 65 and over make up 12% of the population, they receive approximately 25% of the prescriptions for psychotropic medications and 30% of all prescriptions.[2,3,4] One survey revealed that the average older person receives 13 prescriptions per year.[4] In a study of 700 hospitalized patients, drug-induced illness was found in 25% of patients over age 80, compared with 12% in the 41- to 50-year age group.[4]

A study of medication orders written in a general hospital in a single day revealed that of a total census of 348 patients, 195 were over the age of 60. In this group 32% were receiving psychotropic drugs. Flurazepam was ordered for 63% of the patients over age 60, while 29% had orders for diazepam; neuroleptics were prescribed for nonpsychotic indications in 52% of the patients over age 60.[4]

Most data reported on medication misadventures of the elderly have been based on nursing home populations.[5] Attempts to decrease inappropriate use of psychotropic drugs in these patients through physician and staff education have, when employed experimentally, been gratifyingly successful resulting in no impairment of behavior.[5] More recent studies of elderly patients living independently have shown that they too are often medicated inappropriately.[2] The latter study found elderly patients to be frequently receiving long acting benzodiazepines such as chlordiazepoxide, diazepam, and flurazepam; the strongly anticholinergic antidepressant amitriptyline; and depressogenic anti-hypertensive agents including propranolol, methyldopa, and reserpine.[2] It was also found that many elderly patients living in the community are receiving medications with doubtful efficacy and considerable potential for adverse effects including ergoloid mesylates for Alzheimer's disease, diphenhydramine for insomnia, and dipyridamole and vasodilators for dementia.[2,3]

GENERAL CONSIDERATIONS

Pharmacologic management of psychiatric illness in elderly patients is more complicated and subject to more unwanted effects than is the treatment of young healthy persons. Because of extreme biological variability, it is impossible to define elderly by any concrete numerical age. Typically, persons 65 and over are considered elderly, though many individuals 5 or 10 years their junior may show more evidence of biological aging. On the other hand, many people in their seventies are neither physiologically nor functionally elderly. As the population (and medical authors) age, there is increasing discomfort with 65 as a definition of elderly, thus such terms as "old old" and "very old" have begun to be employed for people over 75, and "frail elderly" for people whose physiology reveals their age. There are a number of physiologic characteristics of elderly persons that may contribute to increased risks of adverse drug effects.[6] As people age, their likelihood of experiencing adverse drug effects increases and the incidence of side effects is also greater.[7]

As individuals age, their metabolic organs (liver, kidneys, and lungs) become less efficient, so that the usual adult medication dosages may produce toxic effects.[6] In addition, aging is associated with an increased ratio of fat-to-lean body mass.[6] This favors increased retention of lipid-soluble drugs, including psychotropic agents such as sedatives, antidepressants, and antipsychotic agents.[8]

Many drugs are bound to plasma proteins, which are synthesized along with a variety of drug-metabolizing enzymes in the liver.[8] Age-associated diminution in liver parenchyma may thus reduce the availability of both plasma protein drug-binding sites and drug-metabolizing enzymes, leading to increased and prolonged serum drug concentrations.[8] Cardiac output may diminish with aging, delaying circulation time and consequently affecting the tissue distribution of drugs.[6] In the elderly, marked diminution in renal blood flow, glomerular filtration rate, and renal tubular secretion are seen, favoring the persistence of pharmacologic agents in the body.[6] In addition to these metabolic factors, changes in brain tissue may be in part responsible for the variation of drug effects seen in geriatric patients. The aging process is associated with the replacement of neurons by glial cells in the brain, and this anatomical change may be partly responsible for variations in drug responsiveness and sensitivity in elderly patients.[4,9]

Along with the normal physiologic changes of aging, individuals become more susceptible to a variety of diseases. The incidence of disease affecting virtually all organ systems increases with advancing age. Some diseases may make a patient particularly vulnerable to unwanted drug effects. For example, coronary arteriosclerosis can increase the risk of arrhythmogenic effects of tricyclic antidepressants. Elderly persons are more likely to be receiving a variety of medications for illnesses coexistent with their psychiatric condition. In this population, therefore, we are more likely to encounter problems related to drug interactions, as in a hypertensive patient receiving guanethidine for hypertension who becomes depressed and requires pharmacologic management.[10]

In the elderly, an adverse drug effect may have a greater overall effect on the patient's welfare than in a young healthy individual. For example, postural hypotension, which may occur with antipsychotic and antidepressant drugs, may have little consequence other than momentary discomfort in a young person, while the same effect in the geriatric patient may predispose to the person falling and fracturing his hip.[10] The clinical symptomatology of psychiatric disturbances in old age may differ from the patterns seen in younger individuals affected with similar illnesses.[11] Furthermore, the tendency to attribute mental symptoms to senility in the elderly is, unfortunately, all too great. If the clinician is too quick to attribute psychiatric symptoms in the elderly to senility, the patient may not be treated properly and may be prevented from the potential of pharmacologic recovery or cure.[9] I have treated many patients previously labeled as having organic brain syndromes of aging, with antidepressant drugs, and have seen a dramatic recovery with return to productive life.

Perhaps more than any other population in psychiatry, the elderly need to be managed by clinicians with sophisticated knowledge of both medicine and psychiatry. Careful history, physical examination, and laboratory studies must precede any pharmacologic intervention in the elderly. A detailed drug history, taking into account the entire drug experience and response (therapeutic and adverse), as well as information about current drug therapy (nature of medication, dosage, and duration of treatment), must precede the prescription of psychopharmacologic agents. Patients must be asked specifically about use of over-the-counter medications, since these often contain anticholinergic substances and are frequently excluded from even careful drug histories. The best approach to psychopharmacologic intervention in the elderly can be described as cautiously aggressive; the physician must be willing to try this therapeutic approach even in doubtful circumstances, since a favorable outcome may be achieved, while nontreatment may relegate the patient to the hopeless category of "senile organic brain disease." The treating physician must use the safest drugs possible, starting with one medication at a time, beginning with very low (often subtherapeutic) dosages, and increasing the dose slowly while remaining vigilant for the development of any unwanted adverse effects.[4,7,10]

Having considered some of the factors that alter drug response in the elderly, we now proceed to a review of specific psychotropic drugs in the management of cognitive and behavioral disturbances in geropsychiatry.

SEDATIVE AND ANTIANXIETY DRUGS

Currently the most widely prescribed antianxiety drugs belong to the chemical group known as benzodiazepines. The various compounds in this group vary considerably in their duration of action, half-life, and dosage. The anxiolytic action of benzodiazepines is linked to their interaction with specific neuronal benzodiazepine receptors rather than to a nonspecific CNS depressant effect. Anxiolytic potency of various benzodiazepines correlates with receptor binding affinity. γ-Aminobutyric acid (GABA) is a naturally occurring inhibitory neurotransmitter which can increase the affinity of benzodiazepines for the receptor site. Benzodiazepines increase the frequency with which anion channels open in response to GABA. Opening of anion channels produces hyperpolarization of the postsynaptic neuron, potentially decreasing the frequency of neuronal firing. Since most of the effects of GABA are mediated through changes in anion channels, anionic effects on benzodiazepine binding may be mediated at sites close to the channel. The ability of benzodiazepines to modulate the neurotransmitter activity of GABA in the brain is an important part of their action. The inhibitory neurotransmitter action of GABA as well as the interaction of benzodiazepines with the GABA system suggest a correlation of this system with the mechanisms of anxiety.[12]

Most comparative studies of antianxiety drugs have found benzodiazepines to be superior to placebo, barbiturates, meprobamate, sedative-type antihistamines, and neuroleptics in controlling symptoms of anxiety.[12,13] Animal studies and some human studies have found neuroleptics to alleviate anxiety. However, the potential risk of tardive dyskinesia would suggest that this use of neuroleptics be minimized or avoided.[12,13] Buspirone, a nonbenzodiazepine antianxiety drug, with mixed agonist-antagonist effects at 5-HT$_{1A}$ serotonin receptors has been found to be equivalent to diazepam in some studies of anxious patients.[20] Other studies have found that patients with severe chronic anxiety, who have previously been treated with benzodiazepines, do not achieve satisfactory control of anxiety with buspirone.[21]

With the exception of buspirone, antihistamines, antidepressants, and antipsychotic drugs, other antianxiety agents are capable of inducing tolerance, physical dependence, and addiction.[10] When barbiturates, benzodiazepines, and meprobamate are administered for a prolonged period of time at moderate to high dosage, and suddenly discontinued, patients may develop a withdrawal syndrome marked by confusion, delirium, and seizures.[10] For this reason, their dosage and duration of administration must be limited. In the elderly, metabolism of these compounds is slowed, and they are likely to persist at higher concentrations than they would under comparable conditions in a younger person.[8] Since sedation is an important clinical action of antianxiety drugs, and since drug metabolism is impaired in the geriatric population, there is likely to be excessive CNS depression when these drugs are administered to elderly patients.[50] Clinical evidence of CNS depression from antianxiety agents may take many forms including ataxia, dysarthria, diplopia, blurred vision, confusion, dizziness, vertigo, nystagmus, muscle weakness, incoordination, somnolence, and respiratory depression.[7,13] Antipsychotic drugs and sedative-type antihistamines can produce anticholinergic effects, which may be manifested by blurred vision, dry mouth, urinary retention, constipation, and tachycardia.[7,10,13] Drugs with anticholinergic effects administered to elderly individuals, particularly those with underlying organic brain dysfunction, may produce an acute toxic delirium.[9] Signs of excessive CNS depression or anticholinergic effect are particularly likely to occur in elderly persons, because of their sensitivity to these actions and impaired ability to metabolize the drugs. Also, they may be receiving a variety of other medications that produce similar effects, and the clinician is likely to see many additive-type drug interactions in this population.[10] For example, the antihypertensive agent methyldopa can produce sedation which may add to the sedative action of a coadministered antianxiety agent. Antiarrhythmic agents such as quinidine have anticholinergic effects that may add to the sedative action of a coadministered antianxiety agent. Antiarrhythmic agents such as quinidine have anticholinergic effects that may add to the anticholinergic action of a coadministered psychotropic agent.[10]

Chronic obstructive pulmonary disease is rather common in elderly individuals. Barbiturates, benzodiazepines, and meprobamate are capable of depressing the respiratory center, particularly when present in excessive serum concentrations.[13] These agents may produce clinically significant impairments in respiratory function in elderly individuals. Sedative-type antihistamines and antipsychotic agents are not likely to impair respiratory function when used cautiously. Some geriatric patients present with anxiety as a result of hypoxia secondary to chronic pulmonary disease. Excessive daytime or nighttime use of sedative-type drugs is likely to worsen the hypoxia and thereby increase anxiety and insomnia.[7,13] If this cycle is allowed to continue, by increasing the dosage of sedative in order to control the anxiety or insomnia, a dangerous level of CNS depression may result.

Antianxiety drugs generally have long half-lives. The half-life of chlordiazepoxide is approximately one to two days, while that for diazepam and flurazepam approximates three days at steady state.[13,22] Alprazolam, lorazepam, and oxazepam have half-lives of approximately 12 hours.[13] The half-life of meprobamate is about ten hours, while that of the sedative-type antihistamines is about four to six hours.[13] The half-life of any given drug can be expected to increase as the age of the patient increases, due to decreased efficiency of drug metabolism and excretion.[1,8] Therefore, drugs known to have longer duration of action should be used with extreme caution in geriatric patients.[7]

If medications are administered to geriatric patients in standard adult dosage, therapeutic misadventures can be expected to occur. Since barbiturates may produce dangerous levels of CNS depression and can cause paradoxical agitation in elderly patients, particularly those with organic brain dysfunction, they should generally be avoided.[7] Because of the long half-life of chlordiazepoxide, flurazepam, and diazepam, and the potential of benzodiazepines to occasionally produce paradoxical agitation or violent behavior, these drugs should be avoided.[7,10] Oxazepam and lorazepam have shorter half-lives and may be less likely to induce paradoxical agitation, making them potentially safer in older patients.[7] Triazolobenzodiazepines should generally be avoided in the elderly since they inhibit platelet aggregation factor (PAF), a property not shared by other benzodiazepines.[14] Inhibition of PAF could adversely alter cerebral and coronary blood flow, particularly in a patient whose cardiovascular system is compromised.[14] The FDA has received reports suggesting an increased risk of adverse cerebrovascular events associated with triazolam.[14] Although a cause and effect relationship has not been established, there are ample reasons not to use triazolam or alprazolam in the elderly, including evidence that the triazolobenzodiazepines present significant addictive potential and greater difficulty in detoxification than other benzodiazepines.[15,16] Triazolam, which has the enticing quality of the shortest half-life among marketed benzodiazepines, would seem to be ideal in elderly patients where the goal is to employ short half-life drugs. In reality, its very short half-life may contribute to its excellent ability to encourage physiological dependence. Triazolam has also been shown to induce a variety of behavioral abnormalities including black-outs, next-day confusion and disinhibition in both young and old patients, even with infrequent and low dose administration.[17] It is beyond my understanding that the FDA continues to allow triazolam to be marketed in the United States when it has been eliminated from use in most other countries of the world. Indeed, it seems irrational to allow distribution of a proven dangerous drug while at the same time the same regulatory agency is waging war against vitamins and dietary supplements, whose risk in overdose is likely to be a fraction of that encountered with minimal doses of certain approved pharmaceuticals. To simplify the issue, triazolam should never be prescribed for the elderly. If alprazolam is used, caution should be employed, and dosage, frequency, and duration of treatment should be strictly limited.

Eztazolam is another triazolobenzodiazepine marketed for treatment of insomnia, which like triazolam, has no place in the management of elderly patients. Zolpidem, which is chemically not a benzodiazepine, binds to the omega-1 benzodiazepine receptor through which it induces sleep without muscle relaxant or anticonvulsant activity. Although zolpidem has the advantage of a short half-life approximating that of triazolam, it too can impair short and long term memory and psychomotor performance. The ability of zolpidem, thus far with limited clinical use, to provoke confusion, behavioral disinhibition, and psychotic reactions distinguishes this compound as one to avoid in elderly patients.[18] Zopiclone, marketed throughout the world except in the United States, is a non-benzodiazepine which has sedative, anticonvulsant, muscle relaxant, and anxiolytic effects, through its action at the benzodiazepine receptor.[19] Zopiclone, which is unrelated to zolpidem, has a half-life of approximately 6 hours and thus far appears to be a promising agent in the management of insomnia in both young and elderly patients with a tolerable level of side effects.[19]

There is no evidence that meprobamate is particularly effective, and its use in the elderly is to be discouraged. Sedating antihistamines, particularly diphenhydramine, have been widely used to induce sleep in elderly patients for many years. Though somewhat effective, and lacking central nervous system and respiratory depressant effects, diphenhydramine and related compounds have potent anticholinergic activity and may produce toxin deliria, even at conservative doses.[13] Diphenhydramine should be used very cautiously, if at all, in the elderly, and avoided in patients with organic brain dysfunction.

When medications are used to treat anxiety in the elderly, the dosage should be as small as possible. It should be increased as required, but at a slower rate in these patients than in younger persons because of the possibility of drug buildup in the presence of impaired drug metabolism.[8] The dosages listed in Table 16-1 are suggested as general guidelines for the use of antianxiety agents in the elderly. Obviously, dosage must be individualized to the needs of each patient.

The nonbenzodiazepine buspirone is sometimes effective in controlling persistent anxiety in the elderly. This drug must, however, be continually

Table 16-1 Dosage range of antianxiety drugs

	Adult dose (mg/day)	Geriatric dose (mg/day)
Benzodiazepines		
Alprazolam (Xanax)	0.25-4.0	0.125-0.5
Chlordiazepoxide (Librium)	10-100	5-30*
Diazepam (Valium)	5-30	1-10*
Lorazepam (Ativan)	1-4	0.5-1.5
Oxazepam (Serax)	10-60	10-30
Hypnotic		
Triazolam (Halcion)	0.125-0.25	0.00
Propanediol carbamate		
Meprobamate (Equanil)	400-1200	200-400
Antihistamine		
Diphenhydramine (Benadryl)	50-100	0-10
Hydroxyzine (Altarax)	25-100	0-10

*The exceedingly long half-lives of these drugs in the elderly suggest that for optimal safety their use should be avoided in geriatric patients. If a benzodiazepine must be used, the shorter half-lives of drugs such as alprazolam, lorazepam, or oxazepam would favor their selection in preference to drugs with longer half-lives.

administered and cannot be used on an as-needed basis. Buspirone requires at least one week of treatment to begin working. An appropriate dose in the elderly would be 2.5 to 5.0 mg 3 times daily, although higher doses may be required. Dizziness, nausea and nervousness are the most common side effects of this drug, which generally does not produce drowsiness and therefore is not useful in insomnia.[14,20]

Before prescribing sedatives for the relief of insomnia, it is important to realize that the need for sleep may diminish with age.[23] Medical causes of insomnia such as cerebral atherosclerosis, hypoglycemia, hypoxia, polyuria, and paroxysmal cardiac arrhythmias must also be ruled out.[23] Psychiatric conditions, most notably depression, can cause insomnia in the elderly and should be treated specifically, rather than by the administration of sedatives. If nighttime sedation is necessary for insomnia, 500 mg chloral hydrate upon retiring may be safely employed. However, this drug affects the binding and metabolism of anticoagulant agents and should not be employed in a patient who is receiving these agents. Lorazepam (0.5 mg), oxazepam (10 mg), or temazepam (15 mg), may be used cautiously to induce sleep; they do not interact with anticoagulants, though excessive drug buildup may occur if administered frequently over a prolonged period of time. Although caution must be exercised because of the anticholinergic potential of antihistamines, occasionally diphenhydramine used intermittently at a dose of 10 mg is useful for insomnia.

As we gain greater understanding of human physiology, we become better equipped to design safe and effective pharmacologic interventions. Melatonin is a hormone secreted by the pineal gland which is thought to be the naturally occurring modulator of sleep and wakefulness.[24] It is well established that with aging there is reduced secretion of melatonin, therefore the most physiological intervention in the management of idiopathic insomnia, not due to medical or psychiatric causes in the elderly, would be the administration of exogenous melatonin. It has been demonstrated in numerous studies that melatonin administration can reduce sleep latency and improve the quality of sleep without producing significant side effects, hangover, or drug dependency.[24] Although not approved as a drug, melatonin is available in many health food stores, labeled as a dietary supplement. In clinical practice, administration of a single 1 mg commercially available melatonin capsule approximately 3 hours before retiring can induce a non-drug-feeling sleep with reduced likelihood of night-time or early morning awakening and without daytime hangover. Experimental studies have demonstrated sleep inducing effect of even lower doses, and although much higher doses have been studied, there is no need to employ them clinically.[24]

ANTIPSYCHOTIC DRUGS

Antipsychotic drugs alleviate many of the clinical signs and symptoms of psychosis, such as hallucinations, delusions, disordered thinking, and inappropriate behavior.[25] All drugs with antipsychotic efficacy share the ability to block brain dopamine receptors.[25] Evidence suggests that psychotic processes are based on disordered dopamine neurotransmission.[25] Despite the fact that the various antipsychotic drugs differ from one another chemically, and can be divided into seven distinct groups based on differences in molecular structure, these drugs all share the ability to block dopamine receptors. Clinical and laboratory evidence demonstrates that the potency of antipsychotic drugs parallels their ability to antagonize dopamine receptors.[25] In addition, antipsychotic drugs exert other pharmacologic effects, and most of them produce some sedation, although their antipsychotic efficacy is independent of sedative potency. In treating elderly psychotic patients, it is preferable to minimize sedation and maximize control of psychotic symptoms. Among the antipsychotic drugs, clozapine, chlorpromazine and thioridazine produce the most sedation and drowsiness. Trifluoperazine, thiothixene, haloperidol, and risperidone produce considerably less sedation with greater antipsychotic efficacy.[26,27]

Antipsychotic drugs also produce alpha-adrenergic blockade, which leads to peripheral vasodilatation and possible hypotension.[27] Clozapine, chlorpromazine, and thioridazine are most likely to produce hypotensive reactions. Trifluoperazine, perphenazine, thiothixene, and risperidone produce less alpha-adrenergic blockade and are less likely to produce hypotension. Haloperidol has the least ability to produce vasodilatation and hypotension.[27,28] Since cardiovascular homeostasis is considerably more fragile in elderly persons, it is preferable to avoid strongly hypotensive antipsychotic agents.[10] Furthermore, because an elderly individual is more apt to fall and sustain serious physical injury (such as hip fractures) if he has a hypotensive response to

Table 16-2   Dosage range of antipsychotic drugs

	Adult dose (mg/day)	Geriatric dose (mg/day)
Phenothiazine		
Aliphatic		
Chlorpromazine (Thorazine)	100-1600	25-200
Piperidine		
Thioridazine (Mellaril)	100-600	25-200
Piperazine		
Trifluoperazine (Stelazine)	5-60	2-15
Thioxanthene		
Piperazine		
Thiothixene (Navane)	5-60	2-15
Butyrophenone		
Haloperidol (Haldol)	2-100	0.25-15
Benzisoxazole		
Risperidone (Risperdal)	2-6	0.5-2

medication, it is safer to use drugs such as trifluoperazine, thiothixene, perphenazine, risperidone and haloperidol in the elderly.[10,29]

Unfortunately, the more potent antipsychotic agents, which have the advantage of less sedation and less hypotension, are more likely to produce extrapyramidal (parkinsonian) symptoms than are drugs such as chlorpromazine and thioridazine.[26] Nevertheless, if the potent antipsychotic agents are used cautiously in elderly patients, the possibility of extrapyramidal effects can be minimized by dosage adjustment or judicious use of antiparkinsonian medication. Extrapyramidal reactions, if they do occur, are less likely to produce serious clinical problems than excessive drowsiness or hypotension in a geriatric patient. Because of the potential for producing unwanted physiologic and behavioral complications of cholinergic blockade, conventional antiparkinsonian medication such as benztropine and trihexyphenidyl should generally be avoided in the elderly. Even 1 or 2 mg of these antiparkinsonian drugs may produce a toxic delirium, particularly if there is underlying organicity.[7,10] Small doses of lorazepam (0.25 to 0.5 mg once or twice daily), diphenhydramine (10 mg 2 or 3 times daily), or amantadine (50-100 mg once or twice daily), along with careful dosage adjustment of antipsychotic medication, will generally adequately control extrapyramidal reactions.[27] Because of the sensitivity of elderly persons to anticholinergic effects of antiparkinsonian drugs, these agents should never be used prophylactically in geriatric patients. Antipsychotic drugs exert their own anticholinergic effects. Thioridazine is the most potent anticholinergic agent among antipsychotic medications, and may itself produce, even at low dosage (25-100 mg daily), an anticholinergic delirium in elderly patients, particularly those with organicity. Chlorpromazine and clozapine are also strongly anticholinergic, while trifluoperazine, perphenazine, and thiothixene have less anticholinergic action, and haloperidol has the least anticholinergic action of all available antipsychotic drugs.[7,10] The phenothiazines, particularly thioridazine and chlorpromazine, may produce ECG changes in normal persons as well as those with preexisting cardiac disease. The ECG changes produced by phenothiazines resemble those seen with ischemic coronary heart disease, such as T wave flattening, ST segment depression, and changes in intraventricular conduction.[30,31] Haloperidol has not been demonstrated to produce ECG changes.[10,28,32]

Although risperidone has not been extensively studied in the elderly, pharmacologically, this agent appears to be a potentially ideal antipsychotic in patients of advanced age. Risperidone has minimal sedative action, insignificant affinity for cholinergic receptors, limited hypotensive activity, and at low doses minimal extrapyramidal side effects. An appropriate initial dose in the elderly is 0.5 mg per day with increases as needed up to 0.5 to 1.0 mg twice daily.

In administering antipsychotic drugs to elderly patients, it is best to avoid those which are strongly hypotensive. If chlorpromazine or thioridazine are given, the blood pressure should be monitored before drug administration and at intervals thereafter, the dosage should be kept to a minimum, and IM administration of chlorpromazine should be avoided. Because of the absence of cardiovascular toxicity, haloperidol appears to be a safe antipsychotic for elderly patients.[27,28,32] Nevertheless, when antipsychotic drugs are given, baseline ECGs and blood pressure measurements should be done if possible.[27] During the course of treatment it is good clinical practice to monitor blood pressure periodically and to administer the lowest effective dosage. Table 16-2 presents comparative dosages of antipsychotic drugs for adults and geriatric patients. These dosages are intended only as suggested guidelines. Indeed, some patients will require and tolerate dosages many times greater than the maximum tabulated dose.

ANTIDEPRESSANT DRUGS

Depression is among the most common illnesses for which patients consult physicians. The elderly frequently suffer from depression. Unfortunately, an elderly person presenting with symptoms otherwise suggestive of depression is all too often seen as suffering simply from old age or Alzheimer's disease.[11] Since many older patients with sleep and appetite disturbance, anxiety, confusion, and lassitude are labeled as senile, they may miss the potential dramatic benefit of pharmacologic intervention. If drugs are carefully administered and patients are adequately monitored, there is little risk associated with antidepressant medication. If an elderly patient does not receive such treatment, he or she may be consigned to a nursing home and may approach the end of life in despair. This is not to say that antidepressant drugs are without risk. All effective antidepressants produce a variety of desired, as well as undesired, pharmacologic effects. Cyclic antidepressants have been the most widely used. They exert their beneficial effect by inhibiting nerve reuptake of serotonin and norepinephrine.[13,27] MAOIs produce their antidepressant action by increasing the availability of neurotransmitters in the brain through inhibition of their metabolism.[13,27]

Serotonin selective reuptake inhibitors (SSRIs) are rapidly becoming the most widely used antidepressants, and these drugs, which lack anticholinergic, cardiovascular, and sedative side effects, are generally better tolerated by the elderly. The major risk of SSRIs in elderly patients, who are likely to be taking multiple medications, is that they inhibit metabolism of a wide variety of drugs, potentially increasing their pharmacologic and toxic effects. Among SSRIs, drug interactions are likely to be less of a problem with sertraline and venlafaxine.[33]

Tricyclic antidepressants possess sedative potential that may be beneficial in alleviating nighttime sleep disturbances but they also can cause excessive daytime drowsiness. Among the cyclic drugs, amitriptyline and trazodone produce the most sedative effect, doxepin is somewhat less sedating, and imipramine still less sedating. Other tricyclic agents such as amoxapine, desipramine, nortriptyline, and protriptyline are less sedating than the previously mentioned compounds. Maprotiline is a tetracyclic antidepressant with high sedating and low anticholinergic properties. The cyclic antidepressants all produce anticholinergic actions. Amitriptyline is most potent; amoxapine, desipramine, bupropion and trazodone are least anticholinergic, and imipramine is intermediate in cholinergic blocking potency.[7,27,34] Because of their anticholinergic effect, tricyclic antidepressants must be used very cautiously in the elderly. These drugs can produce a variety of side effects associated with cholinergic blockade, the most serious being their ability to produce tachycardia, which may lead to decreased cardiac output.[35] Furthermore, tricyclic antidepressants are capable of directly depressing myocardial contractility and thereby lowering cardiac output.[36] Some patients receiving tricyclic antidepressants develop peripheral edema. The mechanism of this is uncertain, but perhaps it is due to increased capillary permeability or mild congestive heart failure.[27] Tricyclic antidepressants, though they do not produce alpha-adrenergic blockade, may cause hypotension, possibly secondary to diminished cardiac output or to a direct peripheral vasodilator effect.[13,36] Tricyclic antidepressants may also exert a quinidinelike effect and thus have some antiarrhythmic potential.[37] By virtue of their ability to inhibit nerve reuptake of norepinephrine and to block the action of acetylcholine, these drugs may be arrhythmogenic, particularly in individuals with underlying coronary heart disease.[35,36] They may produce atrial or ventricular premature beats or worsen a preexisting arrhythmia.[38] Because of their effect on cardiac rhythm and conduction, tricyclic antidepressants must be used cautiously in patients with recent myocardial infarction or unstable coronary heart disease and in those receiving digitalis or antiarrhythmic drugs. In patients with stable coronary heart disease, these agents can be used quite safely.[35,39]

Patients with unstable heart disease, including those who have had a recent uncomplicated myocardial infarction, and those with unstable angina or moderately compensated congestive heart failure should generally be treated with SSRIs. If a cyclic antidepressant is necessary, agents with lesser anticholinergic activity, low-dose regimens, and very gradual dosage titration must be employed.[27] In these patients pulse and blood pressure should be monitored frequently and the physician should look for evidence of peripheral edema and other signs of congestive heart failure as well as any change in the pattern, including frequency and severity, of chest pain. These patients may also require serial ECGs as well as laboratory determinations of serum electrolytes, and serum concentration of antidepressant and any other relevant drug, including antiarrhythmic agents and digoxin.

It was originally hoped, based on initial clinical investigations, that trazodone, one of the second generation cyclic antidepressants, would be free of cardiovascular side effects. Unfortunately, as further experience has been gained with trazodone, there is evidence that this drug may also provoke ventricular arrhythmias, and a case of heart block has been reported.[40,41] Bupropion, a structurally unique antidepressant, increases dopaminergic and probably noradrenergic neurotransmission, and is relatively free of sedative and anticholinergic side effects. Extensive studies of the cardiovascular pharmacology of bupropion reveals it to be quite benign with respect to effects on cardiac contractility, conduction, and rhythm and to not significantly increase or decrease blood pressure.[42] The serotonin selective antidepressants (SSRIs) have generally been found to be free of effects on cardiac contractility, conduction, and rhythm, and with one possible exception to be devoid of effects on blood pressure.[43,44,45] Venlafaxine, when used in higher doses, may occasionally increase systolic or diastolic blood pressure by 5 mm to 10 mm. I have not observed significant alterations in blood pressure however, even in elderly or hypertensive patients, yet it is good medical practice to monitor blood pressure in the sitting and standing positions in any patient receiving antidepressants, particularly in the elderly. Two patients were reported to develop bradycardia, each with a heart rate of 50 beats/minute, one of whom experienced syncope, during fluoxetine treatment. In both cases the heart rate returned to normal with no further symptoms following drug discontinuation or dosage reduction.[46] The rapid resolution of bradycardia in these patients suggests that the observed abnormality may not have been directly due to fluoxetine, since the drug has such a long half-life that drug induced side effects would be expected to take a week or more to clear. It must be again emphasized that inhibition of drug metabolism by SSRIs, particularly fluoxetine, fluvoxamine, and paroxetine, may increase the serum concentration, therapeutic and adverse effects of many coadministered drugs, including antiarrhythmic agents, antihypertensives, tricyclics, and benzodiazepines. Thus, when SSRIs are combined with other potent therapeutic agents, it may be necessary to monitor serum concentrations of potentially interacting drugs, and to follow the patient closely clinically.

The major behavioral consequence of the anticholinergic action of tricyclic antidepressants is that these agents may produce a toxic delirium when administered in normal therapeutic doses to individuals who have underlying organic brain disease. Furthermore, patients receiving other anticholinergic agents may experience an additive effect when tricyclic drugs are given, and thus may have a greater likelihood of developing toxic delirium. Elderly persons may be receiving anticholinergic agents for the treatment of GI symptoms, antipsychotic agents, antiparkinsonian drugs, antiarrhythmic drugs, antihistamines, sedatives, and antihypertensive agents, all of which may produce additive interactions with the anticholinergic effects of tricyclic antidepressants.[10]

Guanethidine, guanadrel and clonidine are antihypertensive drugs that are taken up into nerve endings by a mechanism similar to norepinephrine reuptake. The antihypertensive action of these drugs is reduced or completely obliterated by concurrent administration of any of the tricyclic antidepressant drugs.[10] Although there is no evidence that other antihypertensive drugs are antagonized by antidepressants or other psychoactive agents, methyldopa and reserpine may produce clinically significant depression.[10] It is also conceivable that these drugs may make the treatment of depression in individuals receiving them more difficult. Methyldopa and reserpine lower blood pressure through changes in biogenic amines. It has been reported that dopamine blocking drugs such as haloperidol may interact with methyldopa and produce a toxic dementia.[47]

In treating depression in the elderly, it is often preferable to administer medication in divided doses throughout the day, while single daily dosage at bedtime is generally preferable in young healthy persons. Divided-dose administration is advantageous because it reduces the risk of anticholinergic effects in those who may be particularly susceptible.[7,10] An elderly person, or one with underlying cardiac disease, is less likely to have pronounced hypotension, tachycardia or cardiac rhythm disturbance when receiving 25 mg of a tricyclic 4 times daily than if he is given 100 mg as a single bedtime dose. Elderly patients generally achieve higher serum concentrations of tricyclic drugs than younger persons receiving comparable doses.[48] Although most healthy adults will require tricyclic drugs in daily doses of 150 to 200 mg, elderly patients receiving this dosage level often experience severe side effects and excessive serum concentrations. Some elderly patients do require higher doses of these drugs. Anticholinergic potency and suggested dosage ranges for tricyclic antidepressants in elderly patients are given in Table 16-3. In the elderly, or in patients with medical conditions which make them particularly sensitive to anticholinergic drug effects, SSRIs, bupropion, nortriptyline, desipramine, and trazodone are

Table 16-3 Anticholinergic potency and dosage range of antidepressant drugs

	Adult dose (mg/day)	Geriatric dose (mg/day)	Anticholinergic potency*
Tricyclic (tertiary amine)			
Amitriptyline (Elavil)	75-200	30-100	+ + + + +
Imipramine (Tofranil)	75-200	30-100	+ + + +
Doxepin (Sinequan)	75-300	30-150	+ + +
Tricyclic (secondary amine)			
Desipramine (Norpramin)	75-250	50-150	+
Tricyclic (dibenzoxapine)			
Amoxapine (Asendin)	75-250	25-100	+ +
Tetracyclic			
Maprotiline (Ludiomil)	75-200	50-100	+ +
Triazolopyridine			
Trazodone (Desyrel)	100-300	50-150	+ +
Monoamine oxidase inhibitor			
Phenelzine (Nardil)	30-60	15-45	0
Tranylcypromine (Parnate)	20-40	10-20	0

*Relative anticholinergic potencies are derived from a composite of several laboratory and clinical investigations.

probably the safest agents to use,[7,34] starting cyclic antidepressants at 10 to 25 mg 2 or 3 times daily, and gradually increasing as tolerated and as required to achieve a therapeutic response. Some patients will complain of excessive sedation with trazodone, while SSRIs, bupropion, nortriptyline, and desipramine are much less sedating. If the patient does not respond, a trial of imipramine or amitriptyline is appropriate, although the greater anticholinergic and sedative potential must be kept in mind. Just as a young person may preferentially respond to a particular antidepressant, the same is true in geriatric patients.

Increasing clinical experience and studies in elderly patients suggest that SSRIs should often be the first choice antidepressant in elderly patients, although bupropion has shown promise also in the management of geriatric depression. The latter drug has the advantage of not interacting significantly with other drugs and of not producing sexual dysfunction which is common with SSRIs, particularly in older patients. All of these drugs have the advantage of freedom from anticholinergic side effects, and minimal risk of sedation or adverse cardiovascular effects. Potential of drug interactions with fluoxetine and most SSRIs is an important consideration if the patient is receiving or is likely to receive other medications. As in the case of all other drugs given to geriatric patients, dosage must start low, and be increased only gradually if clinically indicated. In most instances, sertraline at an initial dose of 25 mg each morning would be the optimal starting medication; if side effects occur the dose may be decreased to 12.5 mg daily; while the absence of response after 2 to 3 weeks of treatment would suggest that dosage be increased to 50 mg once daily. Alternatively venlafaxine at an initial dose of 12.5 mg twice daily may be administered with gradual dosage titration, if clinically indicated up to 25 to 37.5 mg 2 to 3 times daily. If fluoxetine is used, dosage should be started at 5 mg daily and not increased until at least 2 to 3 weeks of therapy has been completed. Paroxetine, which is somewhat more likely to induce tremors than other SSRIs, should be started at no more than 10 mg daily, and not increased unless no response has been observed following 2 to 3 weeks of continuous administration.

MONOAMINE OXIDASE INHIBITORS

Monoamine oxidase inhibitor-type antidepressants are important therapeutic agents for some depressed patients who do not tolerate or respond to cyclic antidepressants.[10] MAOIs carry an increased risk, however, in that they may trigger a hypertensive crisis or cerebrovascular accident in patients taking them in conjunction with tyramine-containing foods or medications containing phenylethylamine derivatives. Whenever MAOIs are prescribed, the patient should be thoroughly informed about the potential for adverse effects, and he should be instructed carefully about dietary restrictions. Patients taking these drugs must not eat pickled herring, sardines, anchovies, chicken livers, canned or processed meats, pods of broad beans, canned figs, yeast extract, or fermented cheeses. Alcoholic beverages, particularly chianti wine and tap beer, must be avoided during MAOI therapy. Likewise, coffee consumption should be limited to three cups daily. Nasal decongestants, patent cold remedies, bronchodilators, and all phenylethylamine-containing medications must be avoided in conjunction with MAOI therapy. The most dangerous drugs, which can produce a fatal interaction with MAOIs, are meperidine and ALL SSRIs. The latter drugs, if coadministered with MAOIs or given before or following MAOIs can produce hyperpyrexia, hypertension, seizures, and the serotonin syndrome. At least 2 weeks should elapse after discontinuing all SSRIs, and at least 5 weeks after fluoxetine before initiating MAOI therapy.

Monoamine oxidase inhibitors have been used extensively for many years in elderly patients. MAOI antidepressants appear to be as effective in the geriatric age group as in younger patients, with a similar incidence of adverse effects,[49] although the elderly, in whom circulatory homeostasis may be impaired, appear to be somewhat more subject to postural hypotension during MAOI therapy.[7] The absence of anticholinergic activity often makes MAOI antidepressants better tolerated than cyclic antidepressants with less risk of memory impairment, confusion, tachycardia, and urinary retention.[10] The lack of anticholinergic effect may allow some demented depressed patients to achieve a satisfactory antidepressant response without drug induced confusion.[50] MAOIs are often effective in elderly patients who fail to respond to other antidepressants or who experience intolerable side effects with alternative therapeutic agents. Dosage ranges for MAOI antidepressants are shown in Table 16-3.

Selegiline (deprenyl) has been used experimentally for many years in the treatment of both young and elderly depressed patients, generally with variable results. This drug is a selective inhibitor of MAO-B, and when used in lower doses of 10 mg daily, maintains this selectivity, eliminating the need for tyramine dietary precautions. It must be emphasized that regardless of the dose, selegiline cannot be used simultaneously with SSRIs or clomipramine, as is the case with all other MAOIs, including the reversible inhibitors of MAO-A. Although often effective at doses of 5 mg twice daily, in young patients and geriatric patients, and frequently useful in managing depression in patients with Parkinson's disease and Alzheimer's disease, many patients fail to respond to these doses. A recently reported study of selegiline at 60 mg daily in 16 treatment-resistant depressed patients between 55 and 78 years of age found significant clinical improvement in 50% of patients, all of whom had failed to receive significant benefit from previous intensive pharmacotherapy or electroconvulsive therapy.[51] It should be emphasized that tyramine dietary precautions must be followed when daily doses of selegiline exceed 15 to 20 mg.

If depressive illness is severe, and unresponsive to pharmacotherapy, electroconvulsive therapy may need to be considered. In elderly patients who have difficulty with conventional antidepressants, methylphenidate (Ritalin) in doses of 5 to 10 mg 2 to 3 times daily may produce a useful antidepressant effect.

Dextroamphetamine in doses of 5 mg 2 to 3 times daily may also be an effective short-term antidepressant in elderly patients.[52] Alprazolam appears to have an antidepressant effect in younger persons.[53] Low doses of this compound (0.25-0.50 mg 2 to 3 times daily) may improve mood in elderly patients without producing a significant anticholinergic effect, although drowsiness may be excessive. Alprazolam is a unique benzodiazepine in that it may induce mania.[54] Although some have found alprazolam to have antidepressant activity, I have generally not found it to be a useful alternative to conventional antidepressant drugs in young or elderly patients.

LITHIUM CARBONATE

Lithium carbonate is an effective mood-stabilizing drug which is beneficial in the treatment of acute mania and in the prophylaxis of recurrent mania. The ability of this drug to facilitate recovery from depression and protect against recurrence is also clinically important, though less firmly established than its antimanic action.[27,55] Lithium may be safely used in elderly patients if the clinician is cautious. The half-life of lithium in elderly persons is 36 to 48 hours, compared with 24 hours in younger adults.[55] The longer half-life of the drug in the elderly is related to renal aging, since lithium is excreted by the kidney, and glomerular filtration rate decreases by about 30% in the elderly. Geriatric patients are also more likely to show signs of lithium toxicity at serum levels conventionally employed therapeutically in younger patients.[7,55]

One of the primary areas wherein lithium has been used successfully is in the enhancement of efficacy of heterocyclic, MAOI, and SSRI antidepressants in patients of varying age groups. Indeed many patients who achieved partial or minimal responses to antidepressants have gone on to full recovery from depression as a result of coadministration of lithium. Lithium has also proven effective in improving responsiveness to antidepressants in elderly patients; one study found complete recovery in 7 of 14 patients following the addition of lithium to the previous antidepressant regimen.[56] In that study, 3 patients showed a partial response following the addition of lithium. Although a total of 5 patients had tremor or other neurological side effects, these were relieved with dosage reduction in 2 and required lithium discontinuation in 3 patients.[56] It should be noted that the 3 patients requiring lithium discontinuation were receiving high doses of trazodone (2 patients), or relatively high doses of doxepin (1 patient). Patients in that study were maintained at serum lithium levels of 0.7 to 1.1 in most cases, and it is likely that less tremors and other side effects would have been encountered with more conservative lithium dosage. Two elderly patients were reported to have lithium induced neurotoxicity during its use to augment antidepressants; my review of those case reports suggests that one patient had a psychotic depression and needed neuroleptics rather than lithium. The other, a 73-year-old lady, was receiving 1 to 3 mg of clonazepam along with 20 to 40 mg of fluoxetine, which in combination were more likely to have caused the reported ataxia and tremor than was lithium at a serum concentration of 0.4 mEq/L.[57]

Because lithium may alter the ECG, it is important to record a baseline ECG before starting therapy. Lithium may also reduce thyroid function, and baseline thyroid function tests (T_3, T_4, and TSH) should be obtained. Of greatest importance is the measurement of serum creatinine levels before initiating lithium therapy, as this measurement offers an estimate of renal function and may help to guide lithium dosage adjustment.[7,55] Lithium serum levels must be done frequently at the onset of treatment, particularly in the elderly. The generally accepted therapeutic serum concentration for lithium is 0.6-1.2 mEq/L. In the elderly, it may be preferable to aim for serum lithium levels of 0.4-0.6 mEq/L.[7,55] If this range is not effective, gradual dosage increases should be undertaken while monitoring lithium levels. In an elderly person with a normal serum creatinine, it is appropriate to begin therapy with 150 to 300 mg lithium carbonate twice daily, measure serum lithium levels every three to seven days, and gradually increase the dosage to achieve the desired lithium concentration.[27] After the initial week or two of treatment, it is adequate to measure lithium levels weekly for the next month, gradually increasing the interval between blood level determinations during the course of subsequent therapy. Cachectic individuals must be treated more cautiously with lithium, and adequate fluid intake and urinary output must be established and maintained throughout its use. I have safely treated people in their eighties with lithium over a period of many years.

Since diuretic drugs tend to increase serum lithium concentration and cause potassium loss, concurrent administration of diuretics with lithium may present an increased risk.[55] Nevertheless, if adequate fluid intake is maintained, serum electrolytes are measured periodically, and conservative lithium dosage is administered, diuretics are not an absolute contraindication to lithium. The clinician must be alert to the development of hypokalemia, as lowered serum potassium (and consequently intracellular potassium depletion) may increase the risk of lithium intoxication.[55] Generally, the side effects of lithium are not different in the elderly when therapy is carefully managed. Patients may complain of increased thirst, polydipsia, polyuria, hand tremor, nausea, and diarrhea. These symptoms generally diminish or disappear when patients become accustomed to lithium and the blood level is adequately regulated. Occasionally, these symptoms may persist and require dosage reduction and maintenance at a lower serum lithium concentration. Infrequently, persistence of lithium side effects necessitates discontinuation of the drug. In some individuals, reinstituting lithium after a week or two off the medication may allow treatment to continue without the recurrence of unwanted effects. The adverse effects of lithium are shown in Table 8-1.

Carbamazepine and valproate have been widely used in place of lithium or as adjuncts to lithium in the treatment and prophylaxis of mania in younger patients. These drugs are also useful in the management of elderly patients with bipolar disorder, if used cautiously, at conservative doses, with appropriate clinical and laboratory monitoring. It must be emphasized that potential drug interactions are more important in elderly patients, who are likely to be receiving multiple medications, as discussed in chapter 12. Carbamazepine, which has been used in the treatment of agitation and dyscontrol in adolescents and adults, is often useful in managing behavior problems in the elderly, particularly those with Alzheimer's disease.[58] Whenever agitation or dyscontrol occurs in elderly patients, the physician must first look for medical causes such as hypoxia, hypoglycemia, and brain tumor as well as potential adverse effects of medications that the patient is receiving at the onset of agitation. Carbamazepine may in some cases be more effective for agitation and assaultive behavior than neuroleptics and does not carry the risk of extrapyramidal side effects or tardive dyskinesia.[58] It is important to not overuse neuroleptics in the elderly for non-specific indications since these drugs can cause extrapyramidal effects and neuroleptic malignant syndrome. Another anticonvulsant widely used in adolescent and adult psychiatry in the management of anxiety and panic disorder, clonazepam may be useful in some geriatric patients. Clonazepam, however, has a long-half life and is more likely to accumulate and cause excessive central nervous system depression or ataxia in the elderly than in younger individuals, therefore dosage must be low, generally not exceeding 0.5 to 0.75 mg per day, and extreme caution must be exercised if an SSRI such as fluoxetine is coadministered since these agents will impair degradation of clonazepam and increase the risk of oversedation and ataxia.

MISCELLANEOUS DRUGS

In addition to the conventional psychotropic drugs which have demonstrated clinical efficacy in the treatment of discrete problems of aging such as anxiety, psychosis, and depression, a variety of other medications have been clinically useful. Although antipsychotic drugs are often beneficial for disturbed behavior including agitation, confusion, and paranoid ideation, many elderly people have organic brain syndromes which are less responsive to pharmacologic intervention. Often, acute confusional states marked by anxiety, agitation, belligerence, and paranoid ideation occur in the elderly without obvious psychological or environmental precipitants. Not infrequently, these behavioral changes are manifestations of coexisting medical illnesses. Therefore, behavioral changes of acute onset must be initially approached by a thorough medical evaluation to rule out the possibility of medical problems, such as stroke, hypertension, electrolyte imbalance, hypoglycemia, hyperglycemia, hypoxia, azotemia, hepatic encephalopathy, or other medical and metabolic disturbances. It is of great importance in investigating acute behavioral changes to be certain the patient is not suffering from an adverse reaction to medication that is being given for psychiatric or nonpsychiatric indications. Although pharmacologic factors in the etiology of acute behavioral change are more often associated with recent changes in medication regimens, not infrequently an individual has been receiving the same medication or group of medications over a prolonged period of time and has developed an adverse reaction, perhaps through impaired ability to metabolize or excrete the previously well-tolerated medication.

Vasodilators such as cyclandelate, isoxsuprine, and papaverine have been used in an attempt to produce vasodilatation in the cerebral circulation, thereby improving mental functioning in patients with cerebral arteriosclerotic disease. None of these vasodilators has been proven beneficial by controlled studies. Although some patients may benefit from these agents, it is not possible to recommend their use, because of the lack of proven efficacy and the potential risk of producing peripheral vasodilatation, with consequent decreased perfusion of the myocardium and cerebral circulation.[7,13] Since impaired brain function in the elderly is often due to sclerotic blood vessels and reduction in cerebral neurons, it seems unlikely that these agents could produce significant improvement in cerebral metabolism or function.[7,13]

Ergoloid mesylates (Hydergine), a combination of three dihydro derivatives of ergot alkaloids, is unlikely to be beneficial in improving symptoms of mental dysfunction in elderly patients with Alzheimer's or other degenerative syndromes. In animals, this drug improves cerebral blood flow and oxygen utilization, but it is doubtful that this mechanism applies clinically. This drug may reduce vascular tone, slow the heart rate, and produce peripheral alpha-adrenergic blockade with associated hypotension and dizziness.[59] There is no convincing data to recommend the clinical use of ergoloid mesylates for cognitive dysfunction in the elderly.

ALZHEIMER'S DISEASE

Alzheimer's disease was first described in the early 1900s, and for many years was considered a relatively uncommon dementing illness of relatively early onset, affecting people in their forties and fifties. In more recent years, the definition of Alzheimer's disease has changed and the eponym is now applied to dementing illness of uncertain etiology having its onset at any age from the thirties to late adult life. Alzheimer's disease is to be differentiated from a variety of other dementing illnesses, including those induced by chemicals, such as alcohol, and from multi-infarct dementia (MID), resulting from hypertension.[60] Patients with multi-infarct dementia have a history of abrupt onset with stepwise deterioration, and have often had cerebrovascular accidents, small strokes, or transient ischemic attacks. Patients with MID, in addition to being demented, are often depressed and have emotional lability, focal neurologic signs, and often, episodic psychotic symptoms.[60]

Alzheimer's disease, also known as senile dementia, Alzheimer's type (SDAT), has an insidious onset with gradual progressive deterioration of mental function.[7,61] Alzheimer's disease may occur relatively early in life, beginning in the thirties or forties; more commonly, it has its onset in the sixties, seventies, and eighties.[7] Although the etiology of Alzheimer's disease is not known, there is evidence of a genetic predisposition and this condition develops in virtually everyone with Down's syndrome.[62] There are differences in genetic heritability, rate of progression, and clinical course, depending on whether the onset of dementia is earlier or later in life.[63]

Earlier in our knowledge of Alzheimer's disease, this condition was seen as a degenerative brain disease, whose hallmark was the development of neurofibrillary tangles within the cerebral cortex.[7] As our knowledge of the histopathology of this disorder developed, the neuritic plaques that form in the brains of patients with Alzheimer's disease were identified as amyloid.[63]

Although more questions remain unanswered, with increasing research, newer evidence points to additional etiologic mechanisms, including the finding that inflammatory and immune mechanisms are involved in neuronal destruction in Alzheimer's.[64] Serum elevations of acute phase proteins and their deposition around senile plaques are newer mechanistic findings.[64] Additionally, complement components including the membrane attack complex have been found around dysphoric neurites and neurofibrillary tangles.[64] This recent research suggests that clinical investigation of anti-inflammatory and immunosuppressive drugs would be useful in determining whether alterations in these mechanisms could slow the progression of this devastating disorder.[64]

Alzheimer's research has revealed impaired synthesis, release and receptor site activity of a wide variety of neurotransmitters.[65,66] In Alzheimer's disease, there is deficient synthesis of acetylcholine, which is associated with increased sensitivity to anticholinergic drugs.[67] The disturbance of cholinergic neurotransmission in patients with Alzheimer's disease accounts for the high incidence of adverse anticholinergic effects of a variety of psychotropic drugs given to these patients.[7,27] The disturbance of cholinergic neurotransmission has also been a clue for possible therapeutic interventions. Numerous investigators have attempted to enhance central cholinergic activity by the use of choline or lecithin, which act as precursors for synthesis of acetylcholine. Some of those studies have found memory or cognitive improvement and others have been negative.[68,69] Favorable responses to acetylcholine precursors have been more often reported when these substances were administered along with physostigmine or other cholinesterase inhibitors.[68]

The only cholinesterase inhibitor currently marketed in the United States specifically indicated for the treatment of Alzheimer's Disease (AD) is tacrine (tetrahydroaminoacridine, or THA). In a disease which is becoming more prevalent as the population ages, the need for an effective treatment is obvious. Furthermore, evidence of impaired cholinergic function in AD supports the theoretical potential of tacrine. Indeed, the first published double-blind study of this compound, THA, revealed a more favorable response in all 14 study patients to the drug than to placebo.[70] Subsequently 215 of 632 Alzheimer's patients in a multicenter study showed some improvement, and the patients who improved were randomly assigned to receive either placebo or their best dose of tacrine (10 or 20 mg four times daily).[71] After 6 weeks, the tacrine treated patients showed a smaller decline in the cognitive subscale of the AD Assessment Scale than did placebo treated patients.[71] In that study the tacrine group had a significantly smaller decline in activities of daily living, and the major side effects were headache and elevation of liver enzymes (aminotransferase).[71] It should be emphasized that the patients had relatively early, more mild manifestations of AD, and that the study duration was only 6 weeks. Another multicenter study of 663 AD patients yielded 263 patients with evaluable data at the end of a 30 week study of high dose tacrine.[72] Tacrine at a daily dose of 160 mg was statistically superior to placebo on objective-performance based tests, clinician and caregiver rated global evaluations, and measures of quality of life.[72] The major deterrent to widespread use of tacrine is its relatively limited beneficial effects, generally seen only in early or mild Alzheimer's Disease and the significant risk of its causing abnormalities of liver function. Additionally tacrine is costly to administer and has a number of other potentially annoying side effects including nausea, vomiting, diarrhea, dizziness, and headache.[71,72] Assessment of liver function abnormalities in 2446 patients receiving tacrine in several multicenter clinical trials found elevated levels of serum alanine aminotransferase (ALT, formerly known as SGPT) on at least one occasion in 49% of patients.[73] ALT levels greater than 3 times normal occurred in 25% of patients and greater than 20 times normal in 2% of patients. Therefore it is very important to titrate dosage gradually, monitoring liver function tests weekly, and avoiding coadministration of other potentially hepatotoxic drugs or drugs which could impair metabolic degradation of tacrine, thereby increasing its serum concentration.

Carbamazepine, or valproate, which may be indicated for behavioral dyscontrol in AD, may add to the risk of hepatotoxicity. SSRIs, particularly fluoxetine, fluvoxamine, and paroxetine could potentially increase the serum concentration and possibly increase adverse effects of tacrine. Although serum concentrations of tacrine are likely to be higher if taken between meals, it may be better tolerated when taken with food. Ordinarily, tacrine is started at 10 mg four times daily, and may be gradually increased after the initial 6 weeks of therapy. The next dosage plateau would be 20 mg four times daily, and subsequently the dose is increased at 6 week intervals to 30 mg four times daily and eventually to 40 mg four times daily with careful observation of the patient and weekly monitoring of liver function, including ALT. It is more likely to be effective at higher doses and in the interest of safety needs to be slowly titrated to achieve the more commonly effective dose of 80 to 160 mg daily.

It is unlikely that alteration of cholinergic neurotransmission will be the total answer in the treatment of Alzheimer's disease since many other neurotransmitter systems are involved. In addition to deterioration of the cholinergic basal forebrain system, there is also variable alteration in noradrenergic and serotonergic neurotransmission.[65,66,74] Perhaps further work with noradrenergic and serotonergic precursors, MAOIs, reuptake inhibitors, and novel receptor agonists may positively alter these neurotransmitter dysfunctions and have a beneficial effect on the course of Alzheimer's disease. A variety of neuropeptides, including somatostatin, corticotropin releasing factor, neuropeptide Y, and substance P, have also been found to be altered in this condition.[66] Thus far, our knowledge of neuropeptide neurotransmission is in its infancy and we have relatively few experimental compounds which may alter activity of these substances in the brain.

In evaluating and treating a patient with Alzheimer's disease, it is important for the clinician to realize that the rate of progression is variable, but that there are specific behavioral and cognitive symptoms which may facilitate the

Table 16-4 Stages of Alzheimer's Disease

Stage 1: No cognitive decline
Stage 2: Very mild cognitive decline
        Complaints of forgetfulness
        Forgets names
        Loses items
        No objective deficits in employment or social situations
        Patient displays appropriate concern
Stage 3: Mild cognitive decline
        May remember little of passage read from a book
        Decreased performance in demanding employment and social situations
        Coworkers become aware of patient's relatively poor performance
        Difficulty finding words and names
        May get lost when traveling to unfamiliar locations
        Anxiety is common
        Denial is likely
Stage 4: Moderate cognitive decline
        Clear-cut deficits
        Concentration deficits, e.g., poor serial sevens
        Decreased knowledge of recent events in their lives and of current events
        Difficulties traveling alone and in handling personal finances
        Remains oriented to time and person
        Recognizes familiar persons and faces
        Can still travel to familiar locations, eg, corner drugstore
        Withdrawal from challenging situations
        Denial becomes dominant defense
Stage 5: Moderately severe cognitive decline
        Patient can no longer survive without some assistance
        May forget address or telephone number and names of close family members,
          eg, grandchildren
        Frequently disoriented to time or place
        Remembers own names and names of spouse and children
        May clothe themselves improperly, eg, shoe on wrong foot
        Need no assistance with eating or toileting
Stage 6: Severe cognitive decline
        Occasionally forgets spouse's name
        Largely unaware of all recent events and experiences in their lives
        Unaware of surroundings, season, or year
        Sleep patterns frequently disturbed
        Personality and emotional changes frequent (often occur at earlier stages)
          Delusions, eg, spouse is an imposter, imaginary visitors, talks to own reflec-
            tion in mirror
          Repetitive behaviors — continual cleaning, raking leaves, or lawn mowing
          Anxiety, agitation, occasional violent behavior
          Loss of initiative, abulia, apathy
Stage 7: Very severe cognitive decline
        Late dementia
        Inability to communicate, grunting
        Incontinent of urine
        Needs assistance with toileting and eating
        May be unable to walk
        Focal neurological signs and symptoms common

From Jenike MA: *Geriatric psychiatry and psychopharmacology: a clinical approach.* Chicago, Yearbook, 1989.

Box 16-1 Diagnostic criteria for dementia of the Alzheimer's type

A. The development of multiple cognitive deficits manifested by both
   (1) memory impairment (impaired ability to learn new information or to recall previously learned information)
   (2) one (or more) of the following cognitive disturbances:
       (a) aphasia (language disturbance)
       (b) apraxia (impaired ability to carry out motor activities despite intact motor function)
       (c) agnosia (failure to recognize or identify objects despite intact sensory function)
       (d) disturbance in executive functioning (i.e., planning, organizing, sequencing, abstracting)
B. The cognitive deficits in Criteria A1 and A2 each cause significant impairment in social or occupational functioning and represent a significant decline from a previous level of functioning.
C. The course is characterized by gradual onset and continuing cognitive decline.
D. The cognitive deficits in Criteria A1 and A2 are not due to any of the following:
   (1) other central nervous system conditions that cause progressive deficits in memory and cognition (e.g., cerebrovascular disease, Parkinson's disease, Huntington's disease, subdural hematoma, normal-pressure hydrocephalus, brain tumor)
   (2) systemic conditions that are known to cause dementia (e.g., hypothyroidism, vitamin B_{12} or folic acid deficiency, niacin deficiency, hypercalcemia, neurosyphilis, HIV infection)
   (3) substance-induced conditions
E. The deficits do not occur exclusively during the course of a delirium.
F. The disturbance is not better accounted for by another Axis I disorder (e.g., Major Depressive Disorder, Schizophrenia).

Code based on type of onset and predominant features:
   With Early Onset: if onset is at age 65 years or below
   290.11 With Delirium: if delirium is superimposed on the dementia
   290.12 With Delusions: if delusions are the predominant feature
   290.13 With Depressed Mood: if depressed mood (including presentations that meet full symptom criteria for a Major Depressive Episode) is the predominant feature. A separate diagnosis of Mood Disorder Due to a General Medical Condition is not given.
   290.10 Uncomplicated: if none of the above predominates in the current clinical presentation
   With Late Onset: if onset is after age 65 years
   290.3 With Delirium: if delirium is superimposed on the dementia
   290.20 With Delusions: if delusions are the predominant feature
   290.21 With Depressed Mood: if depressed mood (including presentations that meet full symptom criteria for a Major Depressive Episode) is the predominant feature. A separate diagnosis of Mood Disorder Due to a General Medical Condition is not given.
   290.0 Uncomplicated: if none of the above predominates in the current clinical presentation
Specify if:
   With Behavioral Disturbance

Coding note: Also code 331.0 Alzheimer's disease on Axis III.

From American Psychiatric Association: *Diagnostic and statistical manual of mental disorders*, ed 4 [DSM-IV]. Washington DC, American Psychiatric Press, 1994.

diagnosis of this condition. Generally, there is impairment of abstraction and judgment, personality change, and in up to 50% of patients, significant depression. Patients with Alzheimer's may also experience aphasia, apraxia, and agnosia. In Alzheimer's disease, there are not uncommonly delusional thoughts, paranoia, and considerable emotional lability. Specific mental status changes and symptoms appear at various stages throughout the course of the development of Alzheimer's disease. The characteristics of the various phases of this condition have been clearly elucidated by Reisberg's group.[61] These criteria for the stages of Alzheimer's disease are presented in Table 16-4. The DSM-IV criteria for the diagnosis of Alzheimer's Disease are shown in Box 16-1.

Unfortunately, the routine pharmacologic management of Alzheimer's disease is neither highly effective nor routine. I have reviewed some of the experimental studies of substances which may delay cognitive deterioration or improve memory and cognition in this condition. Unfortunately, none of them has proved uniformly effective nor are any of them available on the market. At this point, the pharmacotherapy of Alzheimer's disease focuses primarily on symptomatic improvement of the patient. Patients who are paranoid, delusional, or hallucinatory may benefit from judicious use of low doses of neuroleptic medications, as described earlier in this chapter. Though there are conflicting opinions regarding the incidence of depression in Alzheimer's disease — some investigators consider it to be rare, while others consider it to be almost always present. Depression does indeed occur in this condition, and may be responsive to antidepressant drugs. Many patients with Alzheimer's disease will benefit from judicious use of SSRIs, cyclic antidepressants or MAOIs.[7] In the case of both neuroleptics and antidepressants, those agents with minimal anticholinergic activity should be employed, that is, haloperidol, risperidone, sertraline, desipramine, and trazodone. This is important because Alzheimer's patients are exquisitely sensitive to anticholinergic drugs. Lithium may occasionally benefit emotional lability in Alzheimer's disease; however, the risk of neurotoxicity and enhanced confusion, even at low doses and low blood levels of lithium, must be kept in mind. Agitation, which is not responsive to tolerable doses of neuroleptics, may benefit from low doses of carbamazepine.[58,75] Although some have claimed favorable results with ergoloid mesylates, the evidence is not convincing and the risk of postural hypotension, fainting, and falls may exceed the likelihood of benefit.[59]

SLEEP APNEA

Sleep apnea is a relatively common but underrecognized problem, which may produce daytime hypersomnia and disturbed nocturnal sleep. The most common form of this disorder is obstructive sleep apnea, caused by an obstruction of air flow related to narrowing of the airways in the pharynx and hypopharynx. Obstructive sleep apnea most typically occurs in middle-aged overweight men who have excessive daytime somnolence.[76] Moderate to heavy alcohol intake and hypertension are relatively more common in patients with obstructive sleep apnea. It has been suggested that the apnea itself may contribute to the elevation of blood pressure. There is increasing evidence to suggest that various forms of sleep apnea become more common with advancing age. In addition to obstructive sleep apnea (OSA) some patients experience central sleep apnea (CSA) which results from a failure of the CNS to activate the muscles that produce respiratory movement. Mixed sleep apnea (MSA) is the occurrence of both obstructive and central forms of apnea in the same patient.

Generally, the diagnosis of this condition is made in a sleep laboratory, where respiratory activity and EEG are simultaneously monitored throughout the night. An interesting study, utilizing home sleep recordings on 358 randomly selected elderly volunteers, found that 24% of the subjects, whose mean age was 72 years, suffered from some form of sleep apnea. Seventeen percent had predominantly OSA, 6% had predominantly CSA, and 1% had MSA.[77] Despite early reports that OSA patients tend to complain of hypersomnia while those with CSA more often complain of insomnia, the two forms of sleep apnea cannot clearly be clinically differentiated. Laboratory or home recordings of sleep in which apneic events can be identified represent the only means of establishing the diagnosis. As in the case of middle-aged persons with sleep apnea, affected geriatric patients are likely to be overweight. Snoring is a common finding in sleep apnea, though not a reliable indicator of the presence of OSA.

Patients with OSA and to some extent those with CSA also, commonly complain of excessive daytime sleepiness, reduced energy, and insomnia. They often find their way to psychiatric treatment because of the presumed presence of a depressive disorder. Though there was no difference in depression scores between groups of patients with different forms of sleep apnea, there was a strong correlation between number of apneic events and ratings on a depression scale in elderly volunteers with OSA.[77] Some patients treated for depression with tricyclic antidepressants report decreased daytime sleepiness, improved nocturnal sleeping, and decreased snoring and, when studied in the sleep laboratory, may actually have fewer apneic events. The tricyclic antidepressant, protriptyline, in conventional dosage, has been found to be useful in many patients with OSA.[78] Decreased oxygenation in OSA is a likely cause of impaired alertness and daytime sleepiness; evidence that nortriptyline reduces diurnal and nocturnal hypoxemia in patients with chronic obstructive pulmonary disease adds credence to its use in OSA.[79] Progesterone generally in high doses of approximately 60 mg/day, has also been shown to produce beneficial effects in sleep apnea, presumably as a result of its ability to stimulate the respiratory center of the brain.[80] Nocturnal administration of oxygen may also decrease apneic events in some patients.[76] When the diagnosis of sleep apnea is made, the physician must urge the patient to discontinue alcohol use and begin a stringent diet, since weight loss is the most reliably effective treatment for OSA. A study of 15 hypersomnolent patients with moderately severe OSA found a decline from a mean of 55 to 29 apneic episodes per hour following a mean weight loss of 10 kg.[76] In patients with severe sleep apnea unresponsive to pharmacotherapy and weight loss, surgical procedures, including tracheostomy and uvulo-palatopharyngoplasty, may be necessary.[81]

NARCOLEPSY

Narcolepsy is a relatively uncommon condition which may occur at any age, but may be particularly problematic in the elderly. Narcolepsy is characterized by attacks of irresistible sleepiness which disrupt the patient's daily life. Cataplexy, a bilateral sudden motor paresis without loss of consciousness, is virtually pathognomonic of this condition.[82] The physician can help the narcoleptic patient by developing a predictable routine of bedtimes, arising times, and planned daytime naps. Stimulating tricyclic antidepressants such as protriptyline may be helpful in narcolepsy, as it is in sleep apnea, a condition that may be confused with narcolepsy. Methylphenidate 5 to 10 mg 2 to 3 times daily is also often beneficial and may be used alone or in combination with a cyclic antidepressant. Other stimulants, including dextroamphetamine and magnesium pemoline, may be helpful to narcolepsy patients who do not tolerate or respond favorably to methylphenidate.[82] Since dextroamphetamine has a relatively short duration of action, it generally must be administered in three to four divided daily doses, while pemoline, which is a long-acting psychostimulant, may be administered in a single daily dose.

ACQUIRED IMMUNODEFICIENCY SYNDROME (AIDS)

Recognizing the AIDS epidemic, any current text in psychopharmacology must consider the broad spectrum of disorders that may result from human immunodeficiency virus (HIV) infection and potentially beneficial pharmacologic interventions. A thorough discussion of these disorders, their pathology and medical management, is beyond the scope of this volume, but very well reviewed elsewhere.[83] Inclusion of HIV disease in this chapter results from the recognition that affected patients are physiologically compromised and require gentle and cautious pharmacological management, analogous to that required in the elderly who must also be conservatively treated. Infection with the HIV virus results in selective destruction of blood cells and neurons which possess the CD4 receptor.[84] In the course of illness, AIDS patients are likely to have impaired renal, hepatic, circulatory and brain function, all of which result in increased sensitivity to medications, including psychotropic drugs, and greater potential for clinically significant adverse drug reactions.[84] These patients will often be receiving multiple medications and are therefore likely to have a significant risk of drug interactions. HIV infected patients commonly experience anxiety and depression as a reaction to knowledge that they are infected and may be ill or may become seriously and terminally ill, even if they are at the moment feeling well. When ill, these patients may experience anxiety and depression as an emotional reaction to their illness or as a result of a previously existing major depression or one triggered possibly biologically by their HIV disease.[84] Likewise psychotic illness or substance abuse problems which pre-dated HIV infection may be exacerbated during the course of AIDS and require cautious pharmacologic intervention. As the neurodestructive process of AIDS progresses, cognitive dysfunction, encephalopathy, and dementia become increasingly common and devastating components of the illness, further impairing the quality of life and calling for whatever benefit that pharmaco-therapy can provide.[85] The AIDS patient is likely to be receiving a variety of potentially toxic antiretroviral drugs and antibiotics which may add to the cognitive and behavioral symptoms of HIV disease.[86] The psychiatrist who endeavors to treat HIV infected patients must broaden his or her medical knowledge of this condition, its complications and medical treatment, and must guard against being nihilistic in terms of both psychotherapeutic and pharmacologic interventions. The psychiatrist who cannot be sensitive to the medical and psychosocial plight of these patients should probably elect not to treat them.

Anxiety is prevalent in HIV patients who are not ill as well as in patients in various stages of AIDS. There is likely to be increased sensitivity to cumulative sedative effects of long-acting benzodiazepines, which should generally be avoided, in favor of using limited doses of shorter acting drugs such as lorazepam or oxazepam.[84] These latter agents can also be useful in the short-term management of insomnia, which is not uncommon and may also occur as a side effect of antiretroviral drugs including AZT, ddI, ddC, and d4T.[86] Although buspirone has been somewhat helpful in the management of anxiety in patients with HIV disease, its lack of rapid onset and nighttime sedation limits its usefulness.[84] Since many HIV patients have been drug dependent, additional cautions may need to be considered when prescribing benzodiazepines. Trazodone, which has significant sedative activity with relatively minimal anticholinergic effect, has proven useful at doses of 25 to 200 mg per day in the long-term treatment of stress-distress symptomatology and chronic anxiety in HIV disease.[84] Mild to moderate depression may also respond favorably to trazodone.[84]

As in the elderly, patients with AIDS are likely to be more sensitive to cognitive disturbances and deliria when given more strongly anticholinergic drugs, including tricyclic antidepressants such as amitriptyline and imipramine, and antipsychotics such as chlorpromazine, clozapine and thioridazine. Likewise these patients, similar to geriatric patients, may have a greater risk of symptomatic hypotension, congestive heart failure, or cardiac arrhythmias when treated with antidepressants and antipsychotic drugs such as the above mentioned drugs. Because of potential interactions with concurrent pharma-cotherapy, particularly AZT (which can inhibit catecholamine-o-methyl-transferase) and "alternative" dietary treatments, MAOI antidepressants should probably be avoided, except in those patients who have had a uniquely beneficial response to these drugs prior to developing AIDS.[84]

Depression in HIV infected patients is probably most safely treated with low-anticholinergic cyclic drugs such as desipramine or trazodone, or with serotonin selective antidepressants. When SSRIs are chosen, their potential to increase and prolong serum concentrations of other coadministered drugs must be considered. At the present there have not yet been adequate controlled trials of the newer antidepressants including SSRIs and bupropion in AIDS, however clinical experience supports their efficacy and safety.[84] Fluoxetine would be appropriate in an HIV positive individual who is well and not receiving a complicated pharmacologic regimen, however, with the onset and progression of illness and the need for other pharmacotherapies, sertraline, with less potential for drug interactions would be likely to be a safer alternative, with equal efficacy. Sertraline would be best initiated at a daily dose of 25 mg and either increased or decreased depending on clinical response. The SSRIs and bupropion have the advantage of lacking anticholinergic activity, sedative side effects, and cardiovascular and hemodynamic effects. Stimulant drugs including methylphenidate and dextroamphetamine have been successfully used in the short-term and long-term treatment of depression in AIDS patients, even those with advanced disease and encephalopathy.[84] Generally adverse effects of stimulants are relatively mild and responsive to dosage reduction. Treatment with methylphenidate by mouth, feeding tube, or rectally can be initiated at 5 to 10 mg daily with dosage titration as clinically indicated.[84] Lithium carbonate can be safely used in patients with HIV disease if serum levels are closely monitored, electrolyte imbalance is avoided, and adequate renal function is maintained. In patients with renal impairment, electrolyte disturbances or severe encephalopathy, lithium dosage may need to be reduced or interrupted and more frequently monitored by serum lithium level determinations. Carbamazepine and valproate have also been effective in the management of mood disorders and impulsive behavior, although serum concentration, hepatic function, and white blood cell counts need to be closely followed.

Psychotic symptoms in AIDS are best managed with low doses of high potency neuroleptics such as haloperidol, carefully monitoring patients for extrapyramidal side effects which may be more safely treated by dosage reduction or concurrent use of lorazepam than by coadministration of antiparkinsonian drugs or propranolol. AIDS patients may become psychotic as a result of pervasive brain disease due to HIV infection or as a result of coadministered therapies including antiretroviral drugs, cycloserine adminis-tered for tuberculosis or steroid therapy.[84,85,86] Patients with these disorders may respond to low doses of haloperidol, or in the case of steroid-induced mood disorders, may benefit from lithium carbonate. Delirium not uncommonly occurs with the progression of AIDS, and may be responsive to cautious intravenous administration of haloperidol. As in any other patient with delirium, the physician should look for iatrogenic causes, and where possible try to eliminate any drugs which are not absolutely essential and may be playing an etiologic role in the delirium.[84]

Epidemiological studies suggest that among homosexual men, whether HIV infected or not there appears to be a higher incidence of major depression, and that major depression may occur in association with HIV infection in the absence of HIV central nervous system disease.[87] On the other hand, studies of HIV-associated psychosis indicate that patients so affected were more likely to have histories of previous stimulant or sedative/hypnotic abuse and that new-onset psychosis in these patients may be at least in part a manifestation of HIV-associated encephalopathy.[88]

Previous research indicates that subcortical dementia is the main manifes-tation of the cognitive deficit in patients with AIDS.[85] Neurologic complications occur in 40% of patients with AIDS, and in 10% of patients represent the first sign of disease.[85] Neurologic involvement in AIDS results largely from immunosuppression with the appearance of CNS lymphoma and opportunistic infections as well as direct CNS infection by the HIV virus.[85] HIV infection of the brain is manifested as a subacute encephalitis or diffuse HIV encephalopathy, characterized clinically by a progressive subcortical dementia without focal neurologic signs.[85] HIV dementia may occur without, before, or independently of AIDS.[85] Antiretroviral medications have been effective in halting and reverting the dementing process, which is therefore better conceptualized as an HIV organic mental disorder rather than AIDS dementia complex, a term previously employed.[85] HIV dementia may be manifested by subtle mood changes, inattentiveness, difficulty concentrating, distractibility, forgetfulness, and apathy, features that are similar to those seen in depression.[85] The interplay of symptoms of depression and HIV dementia, both of which may present with similar symptoms, often make treatment decisions difficult. Since functional improvement may occur, with cautious use of non-anticholinergic antidepressants such as SSRIs or bupropion and with stimulants such as methylphenidate, a therapeutic trial of one of these interventions is generally in order since there is no specific pharmacotherapy for the dementia and improvement of the depressive component may improve the quality of life of the patient. Additionally, use of antiretroviral agents to attempt to arrest the dementing process as well as use of appropriate medications to control opportunistic infections may contribute to slowing the debilitating process.

REFERENCES

1. Montamat SC, Cusack BJ, Vestal RE: Management of drug therapy in the elderly. *N Engl J Med* 1989;321:303-309.
2. Wilcox SM, Himmelstein DU, Woolhandler S: Inappropriate drug prescribing for the community-dwelling elderly. *JAMA* 1994;272:292-296.
3. Gurwitz JH: Suboptimal medication use in the elderly: The tip of the iceberg. (Editorial) *JAMA* 1994;272:316-317.
4. Salzman C (ed): *Clinical geriatric psychopharmacology*. ed 2 Baltimore, 1992.
5. Avorn J, Soumerai SB, Everitt DE, et al: A randomized trial of a program to reduce the use of psychoactive drugs in nursing homes. *N Engl J Med* 1992;327:168-173.
6. Isselbacher KJ, Braunwald E, Wilson JD, et al (eds): *Harrison's Principles of Internal Medicine*, ed 13, New York, McGraw-Hill, 1994.
7. Jenike MA: *Geriatric psychiatry and psychopharmacology: a clinical approach*. Chicago, Yearbook, 1989.
8. Greenblatt DJ, Sellers EM, Shader RI: Drug disposition in old age. *N Engl J Med* 1982;306:1081-1088.
9. Crook T: Pharmacotherapy of cognitive deficits in Alzheimer's disease and age-associated memory impairment. *Psychopharmacol Bull* 1988;24:31-38.
10. Bernstein JG: Drug interactions, in Cassem NH (ed): *Massachusetts General Hospital Handbook of General Hospital Psychiatry*, ed 3, St. Louis, Mosby Yearbook, 1991, PP571-610.
11. Feinberg T, Goodman B: Affective illness, dementia and pseudodementia. *J Clin Psychiatry* 1984;45:99-103.
12. Bernstein JG: Anxiety, drug therapy, in Adelman G (ed): *Encyclopedia of Neuroscience*. Boston, Birkhauser, 1987, pp 59-60.
13. Baldessarine RJ: Drugs and the treatment of psychiatric disorders. in Gilman AG, Rall TW, Nies AS, *et al* (eds): *Goodman and Gilman's The Pharmacological Basis of Therapeutics*, ed 8, New York, Pergamon, pp 383-435.

14. Ayd FJ: Prescribing anxiolytics and hypnotics for the elderly. *Psychiatric Annals* 1994;24:91-97.
15. Schneider LS, Syapin PJ, Pawluczyk S: Seizures following triazolam withdrawal despite benzodiazepine treatment. *J Clin Psychiatry* 1987;48:418-419.
16. Fyer AJ, Liebowitz MR, Gorman JM et al: Discontinuation of alprazolam treatment in panic patients. *Am J Psychiatry* 1987;144:303-308.
17. Wysowski DK, Barash D: Adverse behavioral reactions attributed to triazolam in the Food and Drug Administration's spontaneous reporting system. *Arch Intern Med* 1991;151:2003-2008.
18. Gelenberg AJ: Zolpidem-withdrawal reactions and CNS effects. *Biol Therp in Psychiatry Newsletter* 1993;16:46-47.
19. Musch B, Maillard F: Zopiclone, the third generation hypnotic: A clinical overview. *Int Clin Psychopharmacol* 1990;5(suppl 12):147-158.
20. Rickels K, Weisman K, Norstad N, et al: Buspirone and diazepam in anxiety: A controlled study. *J Clin Psychiatry* 1982;43:81-86.
21. Olajide D, Lader M: A comparison of buspirone and diazepam in anxiety: A controlled study. *J Clin Psychiatry* 1982;43:81-86.
22. Hollister LE, Muller-Oerlinghausen B, Rickels K, et al: Clinical uses of benzodiazepines. *J Clin Psychopharmacology* 1993;13:1S-169S.
23. Regestein QR. Treatment of insomnia in the elderly, in Salzman C (ed): *Clinical Geriatric Psychopharmacology.* ed. 2, Baltimore, Williams and Wilkins, 1992, pp 235-253.
24. Dollins AB, Zhdanova IV, Wurtman RJ, et al: Effect of inducing nocturnal serum melatonin concentrations in daytime on sleep, mood, body temperature, and performance. *Proc Natl Acad Sci* 1994;91:1824-1828.
25. Creese I. Dopamine and antipsychotic medications, in Hales RE, Frances AJ (eds): *APA Annual Review.* Washington, DC, American Psychiatric Press, 1985, vol 4, pp 17-36.
26. Levinson DF, Simpson GM. Antipsychotic drug side effects, in Hales RE, Frances AJ (eds): *APA Annual Review.* Washington, DC, American Psychiatric Press, 1987, vol 6, pp 704-723.
27. Bernstein, JG: Psychotropic drug prescribing in Cassem NH (ed): *Massachusetts General Hospital Handbook of General Hospital Psychiatry* ed 3. St Louis, Mosby Yearbook, 1991, 527-569.
28. Tesar GE, Murray GB, Cassem NH: Use of high-dose intravenous haloperidol in the treatment of agitated cardiac patients. *J Clin Psychopharmacol* 1985;5:344-347.
29. Ray WA, Griffin MR, Schaffner W, et al: Psychotropic drug use and the risk of hip fracture. *N Engl J Med* 1987;316:363-369.
30. Axelsson R, Aspenstrom G: Electrocardiographic changes and serum concentrations in thioridazine-treated patients. *J Clin Psychiatry* 1982;43:332-335.
31. Risch SC, Groom GP, Janowsky DS: The effects of psychotropic drugs on the cardiovascular system. *J Clin Psychiatry* 1982;43:16-31.
32. Fulop G, Phillips RA, Shapiro AK: ECG changes during haloperidol and pimozide treatment of Tourette's disorder. *Am J Psychiatry* 1987;144:673-675.
33. Preskorn SH, Alderman J, Chung M, et al: Phararmacokinetics of desipramine coadministered with sertraline or fluoxetine. *J Clin Psychopharmacol* 1994;14:90-98.
34. Bernstein JG: Pharmacotherapy of geriatric depression. *J Clin Psychiatry* 1984;45(10, sec 2):30-34.
35. Salzman C: Pharmacologic treatment of depression in the elderly. *J Clin Psychiatry* 1993;54(2, suppl):23-28.
36. Glassman AH, Preud'homme XA: Review of the cardiovascular effects of heterocyclic antidepressants. *J Clin Psychiatry* 1993;54(2,suppl):16-22.
37. Bigger JT, Giardina EGV, Perel JM, et al: Cardiac antiarrhythmic effect of imipramine hydrochloride. *N Engl J Med* 1977;296:206-208.
38. Fowler NO, McCall D, Chou TC: Electrocardiographic changes and cardiac arrhythmias in patients receiving psychotropic drugs. *Am J Cardiol* 1976;37:223-230.
39. Veith RC, Raskind M, Caldwell JH, et al: Cardiovascular effects of tricyclic antidepressants in depressed patients with chronic heart disease. *N Engl J Med* 1982;306:954-959.

40. Janowsky D, Curtis G, Zisook S, et al: Trazodone aggravated ventricular arrhythmias. *J Clin Psychopharmacol* 1983;3:372-376.
41. Rausch JL, Paulinac DM, Newman PE: Complete heart block following a single dose of trazodone. *Am J Psychiatry* 1984;141:1472-1473.
42. Roose SP, Dalack GW, Glassman AH, *et al:* Cardiovascular effects of bupropion in depressed patients with heart disease. *Am J Psychiatry* 1991;148:512-516.
43. Stokes PE: Fluoxetine: A five-year review. *Clin Therapeutics* 1993;15:216-243.
44. Cohn CK, Shrivastava R, Mendels J, et al: Double-blind, multicenter comparison of sertraline and amitriptyline in elderly depressed patients. *J Clin Psychiatry* 1990;51(12, suppl B):28-33.
45. Dunner DL, Cohn JB, Walshe T, et al: Two combined, multicenter double-blind studies of paroxetine and doxepin in geriatric patients with major depression. *J Clin Psychiatry* 1992;53(2,suppl): 57-60.
46. Ellison JM, Milofsky JE, Ely E: Fluoxetine-induced bradycardia and syncope in two patients. *J Clin Psychiatry* 1990;51:385-386.
47. Thornton WE: Dementia induced by methyldopa and haloperidol. *N Engl J Med* 1976;294:1222.
48. Nies A, Robinson DS, Friedman MJ, et al: Relationship between age and tricyclic antidepressant plasma levels. *Am J Psychiatry* 1977;134:790-793.
49. Ashford W, Ford CV: Use of MAO inhibitors in elderly patients. *Am J Psychiatry* 1979;136:1466-1476.
50. Jenike MA: Monoamine oxidase inhibitors as treatment for depressed patients with primary degenerative dementia (Alzheimer's disease). *Am J Psychiatry* 1985;142:763-764.
51. Sunderland T, Cohen RM, Molchan S, et al: High-dose selegiline in treatment-resistant older depressive patients. *Arch Gen Psychiatry* 1994;51:607-615.
52. Chiarello RJ, Cole JO: The use of psychostimulants in general psychiatry. *Arch Gen Psychiatry* 1987;44:286-295.
53. Feighner JP, Aden GC, Fabre, et al: Comparison of alprazolam, imipramine, and placebo in the treatment of depression. *JAMA* 1983;249:3057-3064.
54. Goodman WK, Charney DS: A case of alprazolam, but not lorazepam, inducing manic symptoms. *J Clin Psychiatry* 1987;48:117-118.
55. Jefferson JW, Greist JH, Ackerman DL, et al: *Lithium Encyclopedia for Clinical Practice,* ed 2. Washington, DC, American Psychiatric Press, 1987.
56. Lafferman J, Solomon K, Ruskin P: Lithium augmentation for treatment-resistant depression in the elderly. *J Geriatr Psychiatry and Neurol* 1988;1:49-52.
57. Austin LS, Arana GW, Melvin JA: Toxicity resulting from lithium augmentation of antidepressant treatment in elderly patients. *J Clin Psychiatry* 1990;51:344-345.
58. Gleason RP, Schneider LS: Carbamazepine treatment of agitation in Alzheimer's outpatients refractory to neuroleptics. *J Clin Psychiatry* 1990;51:115-118.
59. Hollister LE, Yesavage J: Ergloid mesylates for senile dementias: Unanswered questions. *Ann Intern Med* 1984;100:894-898.
60. Cummings JL: Multi-infarct dementia: Diagnosis and management. *Psychosomatics* 1987;28: 117-126.
61. Reisberg B, Ferris SH, deLeon MJ et al: The stage specific temporal course of Alzheimer's disease: Functional and behavioral concomitants based upon cross-sectional and longitudinal observation. *Prog Clin Res: Alzheimer's Disease and Related Disorders* 1989;317:23-41.
62. Mohs RC, Breitner JCS, Silverman JM, et al: Alzheimer's disease: Morbid risk among first-degree relatives. *Arch Gen Psychiatry* 1987;44:405-408.
63. Bondareff W, Mountjoy CQ, Roth M, et al: Age and histopathologic heterogeneity in Alzheimer's disease: evidence for subtypes. *Arch Gen Psychiatry* 1987;44:412-418.
64. Aisen PS, Davis KL: Inflammatory mechanisms in Alzheimer's disease: Implications for therapy. *Am J Psychiatry* 1994;151:1105-1113.
65. Price DL, Whitehouse PJ, Struble RG: Cellular pathology in Alzheimer's and Parkinson's disease trends. *Neuroscience* 1986;9:29-33.

66. Whitehouse PJ, Kellar KJ: Nicotine and muscarinic cholinergic receptors in Alzheimer's disease and related disorders, in Wurtman RJ, Corkin SH, Growdon JH (eds): *Alzheimer's Disease: Advances in Basic Research and Therapies.* Cambridge, Mass, Center for Brain Sciences and Metabolism Charitable Trust, 1987, pp 169-179.

67. Sunderland T, Tariot PN, Cohen RM, et al: Anticholinergic sensitivity in patients with dementia of the Alzheimer's type and age matched controls. *Arch Gen Psychiatry* 1987;44: 418-426.

68. Thal LJ, Fuld PA, Masur DM, et al: Oral physostigmine and lecithin improve memory in Alzheimer's disease. *Psychopharmacol Bull* 1983;19:454-456.

69. Heyman A, Schmechel D, Wilkinson W, et al: Failure of long term high-dose lecithin to retard progression of early-onset Alzheimer's disease, in Wurtman RJ, Carkin SH, Growdon JH (eds): *Alzheimer's Disease: Advances in Basic Research and Therapies.* Cambridge, Mass, Center for Brain Science and Metabolism Charitable Trust, 1987, pp 293-304.

70. Summers WK, Majovski LV, Marsh GM, et al: Oral tetrahydroaminoacridine in long term treatment of senile dementia, Alzheimer's type. *N Engl J Med* 1986;315:1241-1245.

71. Davis KL, Thal LJ, Gamzu ER, et al: A double-blind, placebo-controlled multicenter study of tacrine for Alzheimer's Disease. *New Engl J Med* 1992;327:1253-1259.

72. Knapp MJ, Knopman DS, Solomon PR, et al: A 30-week randomized controlled trial of high-dose tacrine in patients with Alzheimer's Disease. *JAMA* 1994;271:985-991.

73. Watkins PB, Zimmerman HJ, Knapp MJ, et al: Hepatotoxic effects of tacrine administration in patients with Alzheimer's Disease. *JAMA* 1994;271:992-998.

74. Whitford GM: Alzheimer's disease and serotonin: A review. *Neuropsychobiology* 1986;15: 133-142.

75. Essa M: Carbamazepine in dementia. *J Clin Psychopharmacol* 1986;6:234-236.

76. Smith PL, Gold AR, Meyers DA, et al: Weight loss in mildly to moderately obese patients with obstructive sleep apnea. *Ann Intern Med* 1985;103:850-855.

77. Ancoli-Israel S, Kripke DF, Mason W: Characteristics of obstructive and central sleep apnea in the elderly: An interim report. *Biol Psychiatry* 1987;22:741-750.

78. Brownell LG, West P, Sweatmen P, et al: Protriptyline in obstructive sleep apnea: A double-blind trial. *N Engl J Med* 1982;307:1037-1042.

79. Series F, Cormier Y: Effects of protriptyline on diurnal and nocturnal oxygenation in patients with chronic obstructive pulmonary disease. *Ann Int Med* 1990;113:507-511.

80. Strohl KP, Hensley MJ, Saunders NA, et al: Progesterone administration and progressive sleep apneas. *JAMA* 1981;245:1230-1232.

81. Fujita S, Conway W, Zorick F, et al: Surgical correction of anatomic abnormalities in obstructive sleep apnea syndrome: uvulopalatopharyngoplasty. *Otolaryngol Head Neck Surg* 1981;89: 923-934.

82. Regestein QR, Reich P, Mufson MJ: Narcolepsy: an initial clinical approach. *J Clin Psychiatry* 1983;44:166-172.

83. Fauci AS, Lane HC: Human immunodeficiency virus (HIV) disease: AIDS and related disorders. in: Isselbacher KJ, Braunwald E, Wilson JD, et al: *Harrison's Principles of Internal Medicine.* ed 13, New York, McGraw-Hill, 1994, pp 1566-1618.

84. Fernandez F, Levy JK: Psychopharmacology in HIV spectrum disorders. *Psychiatr Clin North Am* 1994;17:135-148.

85. Pajeau AK, Roman GC: HIV encephalopathy and dementia. *Psychiatr Clin North Am* 1992;15:455-466.

86. Katz MH: Effect of HIV treatment of cognition, behavior, and emotion. *Psychiatr Clin North Am* 1994;17:227-230.

87. Perkins DO, Stern RA, Golden RN, et al: Mood disorders in HIV infection: Prevalence and risk factors in a nonepicenter of the AIDS epidemic. *Am J Psychiatry* 1994;151:233-236.

88. Sewell DD, Jeste DV, Atkinson JH, et al: HIV-associated psychosis: A study of 20 cases. *Am J Psychiatry* 1994;151:237-242.

CHAPTER 17

The Self-Medicated Patient: Recreational Drug Use and Addiction

OVERVIEW

1. *Alcohol:* Liver damage may impair ability to metabolize any administered drug. During withdrawal, short-acting benzodiazepines may reduce risk of seizures. Chlorpromazine which can cause seizures and hypotension should be avoided. Haloperidol is the safest agent to control agitation and psychotic symptoms.

2. *Marijuana:* Detoxification is not required; chronic users may be depressed and require antidepressants.

3. *Hallucinogens:* LSD is rapidly increasing in frequency of use, "bad trips" may require lorazepam and infrequently haloperidol. PCP is widely used; adverse reactions are best treated with haloperidol. Chlorpromazine and thioridazine, which can worsen autonomic effects, should be avoided. Prolonged effects of PCP may require several months of haloperidol maintenance. Chlorpromazine can increase risk of seizures, and diazepam may provoke dangerous impulsive behavior. Street purchases of THC, LSD, and mescaline often contain PCP.

4. *Amphetamines:* Users may be paranoid and require haloperidol. Detoxification is not required; depression, which can be severe and require pharmacotherapy, commonly occurs during withdrawal from amphetamines and similar drugs.

5. *Cocaine* has similar effects to amphetamines and related compounds; depression is common during withdrawal; detoxification is not required.

6. *Anticholinergics:* Physostigmine, by slow IV injection, is useful to confirm diagnosis. Avoid medicating patients with anticholinergic drugs; sedation with small doses of lorazepam may be required.

Continued.

7. *Narcotics (opiates and synthetics):* Detoxification using methadone or clonidine reduces discomfort of drug discontinuation. Abrupt discontinuation produces an unpleasant flulike syndrome but is not dangerous. Estimate methadone dosage schedule by evaluation of response to methadone 5 to 10 mg administered orally, observing change in pupil size, postural blood pressure change, autonomic signs, and other withdrawal symptoms.

8. *Sedatives (barbiturates, benzodiazepines, miscellaneous CNS depressants):* Abrupt withdrawal can be fatal due to status epilepticus, hyperthermia, and disseminated intravascular coagulation, if large doses have been used over a prolonged period of time. Do not rely on history for determination of detoxification dosage. Patients must have a pentobarbital tolerance test to determine severity of addiction and dose schedule for detoxification from barbiturates, benzodiazepines, or other CNS depressants. Detoxification employs gradually diminishing dosage of phenobarbital based on pentobarbital tolerance test (30 mg phenobarbital is equivalent to 100 mg pentobarbital). Major withdrawal symptoms tend to occur five to seven days after barbiturate discontinuation, and may occur ten to 21 days after stopping long-acting benzodiazepines. Tissue and blood content of drug at time of tolerance test may yield spurious test result. Long-term use of low doses of sedatives may produce discomfort when drug use is stopped; patients require careful observation; they may not require detoxification.

The problem of drug abuse is as old as human history. As recounted in an ancient Jewish legend, the tree in the Garden of Eden was actually a vine.[1] According to this legend the fruit given to Eve by the serpent was not an apple, as is commonly believed, but rather a grape. The assumption that can be made based on this legend is that somehow Eve became intoxicated by the fruit of the tree (or vine) of knowledge, and thus all of human history was affected by the banishment of Adam and Eve from the Garden of Eden. Throughout the Bible we find numerous instances of intoxication leading to a variety of human tragedies.[1] Throughout ancient and modern history we find recurrent tales of important political and military figures being intoxicated and eventually meeting their downfall. In modern times we read repeatedly about prominent persons becoming intoxicated, by alcohol, cocaine or other drugs, leading to their embarrassment, loss of prominence, or loss of life itself.

Drug abuse in the broadest sense includes inappropriate prescribing of medications by physicians and improper use of prescribed medications by patients. Drug abuse includes the use of not only prescription drugs and over-the-counter drugs, but also other freely available substances including alcohol, marijuana, heroin, cocaine, and phencyclidine. This chapter focuses on some aspects of the evaluation and treatment of patients suffering from common forms of drug abuse. The signs and symptoms of drug use are presented in Table 17-1.

Drug abuse, which implies the improper use of drugs, can be extended further to a consideration of drug addiction, wherein an individual becomes physically dependent on a specific chemical compound. The physical characteristics of addiction entail the development of tolerance; that is, the individual requires progressively increasing doses of the drug to achieve the same pharmacologic effect.[2] By definition addiction also includes the development of physical dependence, wherein a withdrawal syndrome develops following abrupt discontinuation of the chemical to which he or she has become physically addicted. Although an in-depth review of the neuro-chemistry of the addictive process is beyond the scope of this book, we know that those substances capable of inducing addiction produce changes in brain chemistry that accommodate to the continuous administration of the substance. When the addicting substance is withdrawn, the neurochemical changes that take place during the process of addiction persist, causing a new set of symptoms defined as a withdrawal syndrome. During alcohol intoxication and withdrawal an increase in urinary excretion of catecholamines has been well documented. Furthermore, studies in rodents and primates have suggested that noradrenergic hyperactivity mediates the syndrome of opiate withdrawal.[2] Hallucinogens, including LSD, PCP, and MDMA, alter serotonin synthesis, release, and receptor site sensitivity.[3] Drugs, such as CNS depressants including barbiturates and benzodiazepines, as well as narcotics, are capable of inducing addiction, marked by tolerance and a withdrawal syndrome.[3] Other drugs, such as the neuroleptics, though they may be administered in large doses over a prolonged period of time, do not produce the classic withdrawal syndrome seen with CNS depressants. Withdrawal of neuroleptics, however, may be associated with a disturbance in autonomic nervous system function and the appearance of dyskinetic movements in some patients. Neuroleptics, antidepressants, and lithium do not produce tolerance and do not cause the kind of withdrawal symptoms that are associated with addiction.

ALCOHOL

Ethyl alcohol, the pharmacologically active component of a variety of beverages, is a CNS depressant whose actions are dose-dependent. Persistent use

Table 17-1 Signs and symptoms of drug use

Drug	Pulse	Blood pressure	Tendon reflexes	Temperature	Skin	Eyes	Behavioral/other
Marijuana (hashish)	Increased	Postural hypotension	Unchanged	May be decreased	No change	Conjunctival injection	Increased appetite; distortion of time and space; paranoia; hallucinations may occur
Hallucinogens (PCP, LSD)	Increased	Elevated	Hyperactive	May increase (PCP)	Flushed face (PCP)	Pupils may dilate	Euphoria, panic, agitation, paranoia, perceptual distortions; depersonalization, hallucinations; PCP may cause convulsions
Stimulants (amphetamines, cocaine)	Increased	Elevated	Hyperactive	May increase	Sweating	Pupils dilated	Dry mouth, tremors, confused or hyperacute sensorium, paranoid, hyperactive, impulsive, may hallucinate

Drug							Clinical findings
Anticholinergics (atropine, OTC drugs, plant products, psychotropics)	Increased	Labile	Increased or decreased	Increased	Dry, flushed	Pupils dilated	Drowsiness, coma, or agitation, amnesia, sensorium clouded, body image distorted, visual hallucinations
Narcotics (heroin, methadone, propoxyphene, pentazocine, etc.)	No consistent change	Decreased, shock may occur	Slowed or absent	May decrease	Cyanosis with overdose	Pupils constricted	Depressed respiration, drowsiness, coma, obtundation; propoxyphene—convulsion; pentazocine—hallucinations
Sedatives (barbiturates, benzodiazepines, and miscellaneous others including alcohol)	No consistent change	Decreased, shock may occur	Decreased or absent	May decrease	Cyanosis with overdose	No change or small pupils	Lateral gaze nystagmus, depressed respiration, confusion, ataxia, slurred speech; drowsiness to coma; seizures and delirium after discontinuation in addicted patients

PCP = phencyclidine.

of alcohol in any form may be associated with a variety of medical complications, including hepatic disease and organic brain dysfunction. The repeated use of alcoholic beverages produces gradually increasing tolerance and the individual will require larger doses to achieve the same effect over a period of time. Once alcohol use is discontinued in a steady drinker, a variety of new symptoms arise, characterized as a withdrawal syndrome with autonomic hyperactivity, tremulousness, irritability, and in more extreme forms, withdrawal delirium, which may be associated with seizures.[5] Disulfiram has been recommended by some as a deterrent to persistent alcohol intake. The use of alcohol by a patient taking disulfiram may provoke an adverse reaction characterized by flushing, throbbing in the head and neck, headache, respiratory distress, sweating, tachycardia, vomiting, and extreme discomfort. The basis for the recommendation of disulfiram in the treatment of chronic alcohol abusers is that the individual may experience this adverse reaction and thereby lose his desire to continue drinking.[2] In reality this is not a very practical approach in the treatment of alcoholism, since the reaction itself may be dangerous or life-threatening. Furthermore, the alcoholic individual who wishes to continue his alcohol intake has simply to discontinue disulfiram several days prior to drinking, thus avoiding the serious reaction and allowing himself to continue the process of alcohol abuse.

Since the introduction of benzodiazepines into psychiatry, these compounds have been widely recommended for their ability to alleviate anxiety and presumably reduce the need for continuous alcohol use. There is no evidence to suggest that the use of these drugs in alcoholics provides any particular deterrent to drinking. Furthermore, these drugs have their own addiction-producing liabilities, and may produce an additive, and at times serious, CNS depressant effect when combined with alcohol.[5]

Though psychotherapy has some value in helping alcoholic patients to reduce their alcohol consumption, the approaches used by Alcoholics Anonymous are likely to be more effective than conventional psychotherapy.[5] Many persons who become alcohol-dependent actually have a significant underlying psychiatric illness, particularly an affective illness, with the tendency to have recurrent depression and mood swings, including mania. If there is any group of therapeutic agents that may be of value in discouraging continuous alcohol abuse it is to be found among the antidepressant drugs and lithium, which can improve the underlying affective illness and lead to decreased need for continual alcohol consumption.[6]

Acutely intoxicated individuals may become extremely agitated and combative. Administration of barbiturates or benzodiazepines to these patients may enhance their intoxication and potentially increase the risk of their dangerousness. The use of low-potency antipsychotic agents in alcohol-intoxicated persons may provoke profound autonomic side effects including considerable hypotension. In an agitated combative alcohol-intoxicated patient the safest pharmacologic agent to employ is haloperidol, using it initially in a dose of 2 to 5 mg, with gradual dosage titration as necessary to provide behavioral control.[7]

Patients admitted to hospitals for alcoholism or for unrelated medical problems who have been drinking consistently will often require detoxification from alcohol. Chlordiazepoxide and diazepam have been widely used in the treatment of acute alcoholism and in detoxification of alcoholic patients. Both of these drugs have long durations of action that will be further lengthened by impaired hepatic function, which is likely to exist in alcoholic patients.[2,7] They suppress seizure activity, and therefore are effective in reducing the morbidity of alcohol withdrawal. Although it has been standard practice to prescribe a fixed-dose benzodiazepine regimen for alcohol detoxification, a more recent controlled study has found that when chlordiazepoxide is administered in response to symptoms during detoxification, patients may require shorter courses of treatment and only about 1/4 of the usual total benzodiazepine dose. In that study, there were no significant differences in withdrawal symptoms, including seizures and delirium tremens.

Benzodiazepines, with the exception of lorazepam, should not be administered IM, since their IM absorption is erratic and may lead to either excessive or inadequate plasma concentrations.[9] If a benzodiazepine is to be administered to a patient to suppress alcohol withdrawal and for subsequent detoxification, the agents of choice are oxazepam and lorazepam, short-acting benzodiazepines that do not produce pharmacologically active metabolites. These drugs are less likely to enhance aggressive behavior than diazepam and can be administered by the oral route, in a dose of 10 to 30 mg, or 1 to 2 mg respectively, 4 times daily initially, with gradual reduction during the course of detoxification.

Chlorpromazine should never be given alone or in combination with benzodiazepines during alcohol withdrawal.[10] It will lower seizure threshold — increasing the risk of convulsions — and produce a dramatic hypotensive response in a patient whose circulatory homeostasis and autonomic nervous system function are already impaired as a result of alcohol withdrawal.

Haloperidol, which has little effect on seizure threshold, blood pressure, and autonomic function, is the antipsychotic agent of choice in patients withdrawing from alcohol who become agitated and develop psychotic symptoms.[6,10] It may be administered orally or IM, generally in doses of 2 to 5 mg 2 to 4 times daily, with gradual titration as dictated by the clinical situation. Propranolol and atenolol have been shown to be beneficial in reducing the tachycardia and other manifestations of sympathetic nervous system hyperactivity associated with alcohol withdrawal.[11] Carbamazepine is potentially useful in the management of alcohol withdrawal, particularly in patients, who have had seizures previously when withdrawing from alcohol and in individuals with a convulsive disorder unrelated to alcohol.[12] Patients being withdrawn from alcohol should have their temperature and other physiologic signs monitored several times daily, and they should generally receive thiamine in a dose of 100 mg/day orally in addition to other vitamin and nutritional supplements.[2]

MARIJUANA

Marijuana *(Cannabis sativa)* has been used for centuries as a recreational drug to modify mood and behavior.[4] It was also used during the eighteenth and nineteenth centuries as a medication to produce a variety of effects, including sedation.[4] The primary active component of marijuana is delta-9-tetrahydrocannabinol (THC). Marijuana is generally used by smoking the leaves and flowering portion of the plant in a pipe or cigarette. Marijuana is also taken orally in baked products, and at times a highly potent volatile oil extracted from the cannabis plant is used as an intoxicant. Within minutes after smoking, perceptual, emotional, and behavioral changes, commonly known as a "high," appear. THC is metabolized to both active and inactive forms and excreted, although THC derivatives are lipid-soluble and may persist in the body for several days after heavy intake. THC is ostensibly sold in pure form on the street. However, the considerable instability of this compound makes it very unlikely that illicitly obtained THC is genuine. Substances sold as THC are usually phencyclidine or other mind-altering drugs.[13]

A variety of psychiatric complications associated with marijuana use have been reported from controlled clinical studies as well as from uncontrolled clinical observations. There is increasing clinical evidence to suggest that marijuana use presents considerable risk, from both the psychiatric and the physiologic actions of the drug.

Under some circumstances cannabis will produce an acute toxic delirium, characterized by clouding of mental processes, disorientation, confusion, and memory impairment.[14] It occurs most commonly with high doses, and is not unlike toxic deliria produced by other psychoactive agents. Patients who develop deliria in response to marijuana complain of feeling apprehensive, fearful, and paranoid. They may have poorly organized delusions, as well as illusions and hallucinations. During the delirium patients experience a variety of physiologic signs and symptoms including restlessness, tremor, slurred speech, nystagmus, gait disturbances, repeated swallowing, and drowsiness. Toxic deliria are relatively rare with commonly available marijuana preparations, but are more likely to occur with hashish and products containing higher concentrations of THC.[14]

Acute panic reactions similar to non-drug-induced panic anxiety are the most common psychiatric complications of marijuana use.[14] Panic reactions occur most frequently in inexperienced users and in persons utilizing more potent preparations. During a panic reaction the individual may feel that he is becoming psychotic; he may have pronounced paranoid ideation with impaired reality testing. Preexisting personality disorder or psychiatric illness, particularly previous psychotic states, appear to increase the risk of marijuana-associated panic reactions.

Heavy persistent use of marijuana has been reported to trigger an acute psychosis that can last for 6 weeks or longer.[14] Psychotic reactions to the drug are particularly likely to occur in persons with prior psychotic disturbances.

Studies of schizophrenic patients using marijuana indicate that these individuals are more likely to experience psychotic reactions to the drug.[13]

When marijuana use began to be more common on college campuses, a marijuana-related amotivational syndrome was described. Individuals experiencing this syndrome tend to become complacent and withdrawn, and have a decrease both in their interest in activities as well as in their ability to work consistently at a task. One study suggested that the amotivational syndrome was associated with a decrease in work productivity, apparently related to a reduction in time spent at work-related tasks.[15] In the comprehensive Harvard study of the biological and behavioral effects of marijuana, we observed a decrease in work output by subjects utilizing operant task performance to earn marijuana cigarettes.[16] Clinical experience with depressed teenagers and young adults reveals a high incidence of marijuana use. My own clinical experience, in addition to data in the literature, strongly suggests a possible depressogenic effect of persistent marijuana use. It appears that the previously described amotivational syndrome associated with marijuana may in fact be a manifestation of the depression sometimes observed in chronic marijuana users.[14,15] Those who experience depression and subsequently decrease or discontinue their marijuana use during treatment of the depression often describe a worsening of their depressed state as they resume use of marijuana. Some depressed persons report a transient mood elevation following marijuana smoking.

The clinical psychiatrist treating patients who are habitual users of marijuana would be well advised to recommend the discontinuation of its use. Evidence suggests that marijuana is a greater risk to patients who have suffered psychotic illness and to those who have had major affective illnesses.[14] Clinical experience suggests that depressed individuals who are heavy marijuana users may be less responsive to conventional pharmacologic treatment of their depression.

There is no evidence to prove that marijuana is addicting. However, studies by our group suggest that the duration of marijuana intoxication decreases somewhat with frequent usage.[13] Some of our data also suggest the rapid development of tolerance to the tachycardiac effect of marijuana when larger quantities are used.[17] Likewise, with heavy use of marijuana, many subjects report a diminution of the subjective level of intoxication as drug use is continued. A specific marijuana-associated withdrawal syndrome has not been confirmed, although dysphoric states and irritability that occur in association with discontinuation of marijuana,[18] or the subsequent use of other psychoactive drugs, may in fact be evidence of some form of withdrawal. It is conceivable that many persons continue the use of marijuana in order to attempt to suppress this dysphoria and irritability.

There are some physiologic effects produced by marijuana, including tachycardia, to which the regular user becomes somewhat tolerant. Propranolol is capable of inhibiting marijuana-induced tachycardia, suggesting a sympathetically mediated effect. Some studies have shown that propranolol may also inhibit the learning impairment associated with marijuana use and minimize the subjective high produced by the drug.[13] Minor ECG changes and premature atrial or ventricular beats occasionally occur with heavy marijuana use.[19] Probably the most significant medical complication of chronic marijuana use is its ability to produce irritation of the bronchopulmonary epithelium, and in many persons to produce clinically significant bronchitis. The Harvard study group was the first to report significant reduction in vital capacity and FEV_1 in chronic marijuana users. These changes were noted in 14 of the first 20 subjects we studied and were confirmed in a number of subsequent subjects participating in the study.[13,19] Although acute administration of marijuana has been associated with bronchodilatation, the more important effect, associated with chronic use, is impairment in pulmonary function reported by our group and other investigators.[13,19,20] Although some studies suggest that marijuana might produce a beneficial bronchodilator effect in asthmatic patients, risk of long-term adverse pulmonary effects of the drug would be likely to cause eventual worsening of the asthmatic patient's pulmonary status.[13]

Although the findings from endocrine studies of marijuana users have been inconsistent, gynecomastia has occasionally been associated with the drug. Marijuana may enhance sexual interest when administered in small doses, but chronic use of larger doses appears to decrease sexual interest and potency in male subjects.[13] Marijuana has been shown to produce an increase in appetite and weight gain in several clinical studies.[21] A craving for sweets is often prominent among regular users of marijuana. Both marijuana smoking and the oral administration of THC are capable of lowering body temperature.[13]

A number of neurologic signs and symptoms have been reported in association with marijuana, including dizziness, weakness, paresthesias, hot and cold sensations, nausea, dry mouth, hunger, and thirst.[22] In addition to producing a lability of mood — at times associated with intense laughter and at other times associated with dysphoria — marijuana may disturb an individual's sense of time, so that events appear to be occurring very slowly. Visual and auditory perceptions are sometimes sharpened, while with larger doses there may be perceptual distortions including hallucinations, even in the absence of a frank psychotic state. Difficulty with concentration, thinking, and expression, as well as feelings of depersonalization, have also been reported with marijuana.[22] Attention span and short-term memory functions are impaired by marijuana. Most clinical studies of marijuana were done in the 1970s and used experimental material with a THC content of 1 to 1.5%. Currently, much of the commonly used marijuana has a THC content of 7 to 11%. The higher potency material is known as sinsemilla, and has been shown to have a more striking ability to impair recent (short-term) memory.[23] It is likely that a teenager with a learning disability will have more significant impairment of learning if consuming marijuana.[23]

Subjects consuming moderate to large amounts of marijuana may experience incoordination, ataxia, tremors, involuntary movements, dilatation of the pupils, nystagmus, conjugate deviation of the eyes, blurred vision, photophobia, headaches, and paresthesias.[22] Convulsions rarely occur in response to marijuana, but persons with a prior seizure history may convulse when using large amounts of this drug. Marijuana or its active component THC is capable of increasing stage 4 sleep and decreasing REM sleep, similar to the effect of lithium on sleep. THC has been shown to produce dysphoric symptoms in patients with unipolar depression but not in those with bipolar affective illness.[13] A number of years ago pneumoencephalographic abnormalities were reported in a series of marijuana users. In retrospect, these abnormalities were more likely related to concurrent neurologic conditions, since careful evaluations utilizing computed transaxial tomography have not shown structural abnormalities of the brain in marijuana users.[13]

Marijuana-Drug Interactions

A variety of pharmacologic agents have been reported to interact with marijuana in both humans and animals. Marijuana is frequently smoked in conjunction with alcohol use, and may be associated with nausea, vomiting, dysphoria, and increased autonomic nervous system lability.[13] Secobarbital may produce increased impairment of psychomotor performance in persons smoking marijuana.[13] Since marijuana generally increases heart rate and may produce variable effects on blood pressure, it is not surprising that the coadministration of amphetamines can enhance this effect.[13] Physostigmine decreases both tachycardic response and conjunctival injection produced by marijuana. There is some evidence to suggest that THC may potentiate the actions of narcotic drugs.

HALLUCINOGENS

A wide variety of drugs capable of producing psychedelic effects are known. These agents yield a heightened awareness of sensory input, but simultaneous diminution in control over what is experienced.[2] The environment may be perceived as distorted in a pleasurable way under psychedelic drugs.[2] The user's attention is turned inward and there is an apparent increase in clarity of one's thinking processes, though they may in reality be quite distorted.[22] The individual may experience illusions, hallucinations, delusions, and paranoid ideation, as well as alteration of mood and thought processes that may resemble the experiences of an individual during a psychotic state.[2] A wide variety of hallucinogenic or psychedelic compounds are known and have been studied both clinically and in the laboratory. Many different hallucinogens are readily available in the streets and school playgrounds throughout the United States, yet lacking an underground FDA, many illicit drugs actually consist partially or entirely of phencyclidine (PCP) since it is inexpensive and easy to make.[24]

$$CH_3O$$
$$CH_3O-\langle\!\!\!\rangle-(CH_2)_2-NH_2 \quad . H_2SO_4$$
$$CH_3O$$

MESCALINE

Therefore whenever a hallucinogen ingestion is encountered, the clinician must look for signs of PCP intoxication, regardless of what the patient thinks he has taken.

Many hallucinogens are structurally similar to neurotransmitters.[2] LSD is related to serotonin while mescaline is structurally related to the catecholamines. Mescaline, derived from the peyote cactus, is used in ancient Indian rituals in Mexico and the southwestern United States.

LSD

The hallucinogenic properties of lysergic acid diethylamide (LSD) were discovered by accident in the 1940s. Throughout the 1950s LSD was widely used in animal and clinical studies in attempts to unravel the mysterious connection between behavior and neurochemistry.[2] During this time many psychiatrists and neuroscientists experimented with LSD by observing their own behavior under the influence of this drug. In the 1960s LSD spread to college campuses and was widely used by persons attempting to enhance their perception or their intellectual or artistic creativity. Throughout the 1970s and early 1980s there was a decline in the availability and use of LSD.[25] Indeed, during that period, street samples of LSD procured by law enforcement agencies most often contained phencyclidine, amphetamine, or other compounds unrelated to LSD.[2] Since the mid-1980s there has been a steady increase in availability and use of LSD and apparently less misbranding of PCP as LSD.[25] Unfortunately the age of LSD users is declining, and the doses being employed are often larger than those used in the 1960s, both factors increasing potential dangers of this psychedelic substance.[25,26]

By the middle of this century, structural similarity of LSD to serotonin and of mescaline to the catecholamines suggested interactions at these respective receptors as the mechanism of hallucinogenic activity. Indeed, shortly after its discovery, LSD was found to antagonize peripheral serotonin receptors. More recent work and the recognition of multiple serotonin receptors in the central nervous system, helps to clarify mechanisms of action of these hallucinogens. LSD is a potent agonist at 5-HT_{1A} autoreceptors, as is buspirone, which lacks psychedelic properties, yet mescaline is inactive at these receptors.[27] Both LSD

$$CON(C_2H_5)_2$$

LYSERGIC ACID DIETHYLAMIDE

and mescaline are $5\text{-}HT_2$ agonists, and through this mechanism activate the locus coeruleus (LC).[27] This latter mechanism offers a potential unitary explanation of psychedelic and hallucinogenic activity of a wide range of indolamine and phenylethylamine derived compounds. MDMA (methylene-dioxymethamphetamine), also known as ecstasy, an extremely dangerous and toxic amphetamine-derived psychedelic compound, is an indirect serotonergic agonist which releases serotonin, and subsequently inhibits both reuptake and synthesis of serotonin, effectively producing a massive serotonin discharge, followed by depletion of serotonergic activity.[28]

Both mescaline and LSD have relatively short durations of action, and though they usually produce perceptual distortions and a mild psychotic state, some individuals will experience a "bad trip" in response to LSD, particularly when larger doses are taken.

Reactions to psychedelic drugs usually do not require specific treatment. They are most often self-limited and the patient may be aided in his recovery by a sympathetic professional calmly "talking him down."[2] In the event of an LSD bad trip, which may be associated with prominent signs of sympathetic nervous system hyperactivity, mild sedation with lorazepam may be useful.[22] In the case of a bad trip with LSD or mescaline, a neuroleptic may be necessary, and haloperidol, a potent antipsychotic with minimal autonomic side effects, is the agent most often employed. Evidence that hallucinogenic properties of LSD and mescaline are mediated through the $5\text{-}HT_2$ receptor, suggests that risperidone, which is a more potent antagonist of $5\text{-}HT_2$ than D_2 receptors, may be a more effective antidote to bad trips.[27]

There is no way of predicting who will experience a bad trip; many persons who have previously had pleasant uncomplicated LSD experiences will from time to time experience a bad trip, with enhanced psychotic symptoms and an intense feeling of panic.[2] Some persons will experience "flashbacks," or the recurrence of the drug-induced experience without readministration of the drug. Frequent and severe flashbacks generally respond favorably to relatively low doses of potent antipsychotic agents. Individuals who have repeatedly used LSD may develop prolonged psychotic episodes that are often indistinguishable from a schizophrenic illness.[22] There is no clear evidence to prove that LSD produces schizophrenia or a schizophrenialike state, despite these observations of persistent psychotic episodes following repeated administration of LSD. It is conceivable that those who utilize LSD repeatedly, perhaps "tripping" daily or several times a week over a period of several years, may have an underlying propensity to develop schizophrenia.[22] It is possible that rather than LSD causing the schizophrenia, these individuals have chosen to use LSD in an attempt to alter their perception and perhaps to block out symptoms that professionals might recognize as premonitory evidence of a developing schizophrenic process.

Several persons whom I have seen with massive and persistent exposure to LSD have had histories and clinical presentations very suggestive of a long-standing underlying psychotic illness. Regardless of the source of the LSD-associated schizophreniform psychosis, these individuals tend to require ongoing treatment with neuroleptic drugs and a lengthy period of maintenance to prevent recurrence of symptoms not dissimilar to those seen in ordinary schizophrenic illnesses. Although in the early years of work with LSD it was often recommended as an aid to psychotherapy and as an adjunct to the treatment of various psychiatric illnesses including alcohol and opiate dependency, its therapeutic value is far from proven, and there seems to be no basis for employing it in the treatment of any psychiatric or behavioral disorder at the present time.[2]

PHENCYCLIDINE (PCP)

Phencyclidine, an arylcyclohexylamine, is structurally and mechanistically unique among hallucinogenic drugs. PCP antagonizes the NMDA (N-methyl D-aspartate) receptor and thereby blocks chloride and sodium channels of the neuronal membrane.[3] These channels are normally activated by the neurotransmitter, glutamate, for which NMDA sites are one type of receptor.[3] In fact a number of non-hallucinogenic NMDA antagonists are now being developed as potential therapeutic agents to inhibit neuronal damage from stroke and other forms of brain injury. Glutamate is highly neurotoxic when present in excess or when neuronal function is impaired, and NMDA antagonists have been shown to reduce cell damage by blocking glutamate activity.[3] The role of NMDA antagonism is not necessarily a factor in the psychedelic mechanisms of PCP, which also antagonizes acetylcholine and serotonin and enhances central dopaminergic activity.[3,24,29]

PCP, which is easily and inexpensively manufactured, is therefore readily available on the illicit drug market. Initially developed and used as a human and veterinary anesthetic, PCP produced a high incidence of postanesthesia

PHENCYCLIDINE

delirium, and this coupled with its abuse potential has ended its career as a legitimate pharmaceutical. Phencyclidine is known by a variety of names, including PCP, angel dust, dust, peace pill, hog, and animal tranquilizer.[2] PCP is most commonly taken either by being smoked with tobacco or marijuana that has been "dusted," or by the oral use of very small crudely made tablets known as "microdots." The drug is commonly used by teenagers and young adults, though use in younger children and older adults is not unknown.[24] Not uncommonly users who believe they have purchased LSD, mescaline, or THC have obtained intentionally mislabeled phencyclidine.

Some individuals who use PCP in relatively low dosage several times a week, or even several times a day over prolonged periods of time, achieve a relatively mild hallucinogenic state with associated euphoria, emotional lability, and a feeling of numbness.[29] There seems to be some tolerance to the effect of PCP,[24] and habitual users do not generally experience the severe, persistent, and dangerous psychotic reaction that more commonly occurs in novice users or those who unknowingly take a large dose of this substance, the purity and potency of which varies considerably.[2] Persons who use small doses of PCP habitually do not usually come to psychiatric attention. However, there is evidence suggesting that these individuals may gradually develop a limited or pervasive thought disorder and symptoms of depression.[29] Chronic PCP users who develop these unwanted psychiatric complications may require pharmacologic intervention for their thought disorder or depressive illness, but they are likely to respond very slowly because of the presence of PCP in body tissues, which can persist for several months after heavy use.

The more serious toxic psychoses that result from PCP often occur in persons using the drug for the first time, or in those who have used it only a few times. These reactions are usually associated with larger doses of 10 mg or more. Patients may experience bodily distortions and disturbances of proprioception. Pain and touch sensations are blunted and verbal communication is impaired.[29] These patients appear to be flooded by external stimuli and the inner turmoil may make them mute. They are disoriented to time, place, and other persons, and may appear either restless or withdrawn.[30] At times they seem to move about purposelessly, making no contact with their environment. One common, apparent purposeful behavior associated with PCP toxic psychosis is the patient's tendency to isolate himself from external stimuli.[29] These patients will be more comfortable in a quiet, darkened room, with as few people around as possible. They will often crawl into the darkest, most isolated area of the room, such as the corner of a closet.[29]

Behavior during a PCP psychosis tends to be exceedingly primitive. I have observed numerous patients crawl around the floor of the room, not uncommonly into the bathroom, and attempt to drink out of the toilet bowl. In my observation of numerous cases of PCP intoxication I would consider this type of behavior to be a classic manifestation of an acute severe PCP psychosis. These patients are generally unresponsive to verbal messages from others apprising them of the inappropriateness of their behavior. Psychotherapy or various attempts to "talk down" such individuals is useless. Not uncommonly, during the course of acute PCP psychosis, the patient will develop what has been termed a stuporous catatonia, with mutism, grimacing, repetitive movements of the extremities or body, posturing, or the waxy flexibility seen in classic catatonia.[29] At other times, excited catatonia emerges, marked by psychomotor agitation, incoherent profuse speech, and unpredictable, often destructive behavior. During PCP-induced excited catatonia the patient may suddenly, and without reason, attempt to assault a bystander or clinician. These patients will often run aimlessly, unresponsive to any external verbal messages. During this state, PCP-toxic individuals may suddenly attempt to leap out of windows, apparently believing that they can fly. Not infrequently patients with this reaction have met an untimely death because of their inability to recognize their human limitations or the dangerousness of a task that they attempt.

In relationship to this distorted sense of reality, patients having a severe reaction to PCP may make dangerous, and at times successful, suicide attempts. Visual hallucination and a state resembling an organic psychosis are typical. However, subjects who have taken large amounts of PCP may at times show a psychotic state difficult to differentiate from paranoid schizophrenia, wherein they experience auditory hallucinations, ideas of reference, and feelings of unreality.[29] The pressure of speech and grandiosity, which is not infrequently seen during a PCP reaction, may make the clinician believe that his patient is having an acute manic psychosis and miss the fact that he is reacting to a toxic hallucinogenic substance. With massive doses of PCP, generally in the neighborhood of 50 to 1000 mg, prolonged comatose states and fatalities have been reported. With relatively large doses of PCP the patient may be unresponsive to painful stimuli and show decerebrate rigidity or opisthotonos.[29]

Of all drugs currently being abused, the autonomic nervous system manifestations associated with PCP are the most dramatic and potentially the most confusing to clinicians, as physiologic manifestations may suggest stimulation or antagonism of a variety of receptor sites on both sides of the autonomic system.[29] Sympathomimetic effects including tachycardia, hypertension, and increased deep tendon reflexes are often quite dramatic. Not infrequently, hypotension may occur during an acute PCP reaction. Simultaneously with the pronounced adrenergic stimulation, there is almost always profound cholinergic activity marked by sweating, flushing, drooling, and pupillary constriction. Cerebellar signs including dizziness, ataxia, dysarthria, and nystagmus are also commonly seen.

During a PCP psychosis the individual appears unable to sort and process sensory information, and there is a profound loss of ego boundaries and reality-testing, as well as disorganization of both intellectual and emotional function.[31] In addition to coma, which not uncommonly occurs with massive doses of PCP, grand mal seizures that may progress to status epilepticus may occur.[29] Toxic reactions to large doses of PCP may cause cardiac or respiratory distress, and there may be a hypertensive crisis with death occurring as a result of intracranial bleeding.[29] Table 17-2 presents some of the common behavioral and physiologic effects of PCP.

Not only is PCP one of the most commonly abused and dangerous hallucinogens, the treatment of PCP reactions is one of the most controversial issues in psychopharmacology. Numerous experts have recommended diazepam or other benzodiazepines as the treatment of choice for acute PCP reactions.[30] Although this treatment may be beneficial in alleviating the discomfort of a mild hallucinogenic reaction to a small dose of PCP, this approach could result in a serious or fatal outcome if given for more serious reactions. Diazepam has a long duration of action, and once given, an adverse effect is not rapidly reversed. By virtue of its high lipid solubility, PCP is also long-acting.[32] Since the behavioral manifestations of PCP reactions include a disturbance in the processing of sensory information and cause a dissolution of ego boundaries and judgment, it is likely that benzodiazepines, which disinhibit higher centers of control, would increase the risk of PCP-intoxicated patients performing violent or dangerous acts. In PCP psychosis, the sensorium is severely disturbed.[29,31] Administration of a long-acting sedative could increase that disturbance.

Benzodiazepines have no antihallucinatory effect, so that the major manifestations of this toxic psychosis would not be eliminated. Based on extensive clinical experience with severe PCP reactions, I would strongly urge against the use of benzodiazepines in this form of toxic psychosis. Even more dangerous than these drugs in a patient having an adverse reaction to PCP would be the administration of chlorpromazine, which will further lower the seizure threshold in a patient who is already prone to the development of convulsions.[11] Chlorpromazine's pronounced anticholinergic effect and alpha-adrenergic blocking actions would worsen PCP-induced autonomic dysfunction.[11] It appears to me that, based on the known reactions to PCP and the pharmacology of chlorpromazine, the administration of this drug to PCP-intoxicated patients is indefensible.[10,29,30] The high-potency antipsychotic agents have less autonomic side effects, and therefore would be safer.

Based on my clinical experience and the observations of others, haloperidol, with its minimal anticholinergic and hypotensive action and its limited

Table 17-2 Phencyclidine intoxication

Intoxication (severity/dose)	Clinical findings	Treatment
Mild (<5 mg)	Euphoria lasting a few hours	Place patient in darkened, quiet, nonthreatening environment with nonintrusive observer; pharmacotherapy generally not necessary.
Moderate (5-10 mg)	Noncommunicative, may progress to stupor or coma; may be agitated; horizontal and vertical nystagmus; muscle rigidity; diaphoresis; increased bronchial and oral secretions; hyperreflexia; tachycardia; hypertension; may be unresponsive to pain	If patient alert and intoxication recent, induce emesis with syrup of ipecac. Continuous nasogastric suction may be used. Provide adequate oral or IV fluid intake. Acidification of urine will facilitate PCP excretion. Maintain patient in dark, quiet, nonthreatening environment with a trained but nonthreatening observer. AVOID LOW-POTENCY NEUROLEPTICS that will worsen autonomic dysfunction and lower blood pressure, and may provoke seizures. Generally avoid diazepam and related drugs which may enhance PCP-induced dyscontrol. Haloperidol in low dose (2-5 mg 1 to 4 times daily) is safest agent to control agitation and psychotic symptoms with least autonomic side effects. Risperidone 1 mg orally, may be an effective alternative.
Severe (≥20 mg)	More severe form of above manifestations; opisthotonic posturing; deepening coma; generalized convulsions; respiratory arrhythmia or arrest; cardiac arrhythmias, hypertensive crisis; consciousness and severity of physiologic symptoms may fluctuate considerably over a period of several days	Treatments as described above are indicated. Acidify urine with ascorbic acid (2-4 g/day) or similar dose of ammonium chloride to facilitate excretion of PCP. Haloperidol for hallucinations, agitation, and psychotic symptoms. Avoid low-potency neuroleptics and diazepam for above reasons. Support ventilation as necessary. If severely hypertensive, lower BP with slow IV drip of trimethaphan or rapid IV injection of diazoxide (2-5 mg/kg)

potential to lower seizure threshold, appears to be the drug of choice in PCP toxic psychoses.[10,29] Haloperidol should generally be started in a relatively low dose, most commonly 2 mg 4 times daily, and slowly titrated upward to achieve control of the psychotic symptoms, while continuing to monitor peripheral signs of autonomic function. Most PCP psychoses will respond to this drug in doses ranging from 5 to 20 mg daily. Although not yet extensively studied in drug-induced psychoses, risperidone, which has minimal anticholinergic, hypotensive, and extrapyramidal side effects, in low doses, may be useful in PCP psychoses. The relatively greater $5\text{-}HT_2$ versus D_2 antagonism of risperidone may allow this drug to be useful in hallucinogen induced psychoses, starting at 1 mg orally once or twice daily.

Because of the considerable disarray of the autonomic and central nervous systems during a PCP reaction, antiparkinsonian medication should not be given prophylactically to these patients. If acute extrapyramidal reactions occur, diphenhydramine in a dose of 25 to 50 mg may be cautiously administered IM or IV. PCP psychoses may take several days or weeks for symptoms to clear, even with haloperidol treatment, although there is usually some significant clinical improvement in the first few days of pharmacotherapy. I have seen numerous severe PCP psychoses following a course of diazepam or, unfortunately, at times chlorpromazine, which steadily improved once the inappropriate medications were discontinued and treatment with haloperidol was instituted.

After a sizable dose of PCP has been taken there is relatively rapid clearing from the blood. However, a considerable portion of the administered dose appears to be retained in fat tissue.[29,32] PCP has been detected in body tissues for 3 months after a severe intoxication, although urine assays for PCP tend to be negative within the first 24 hours.[29,30,32] Persistence of PCP in tissues over a long period of time, even with drug-negative urine tests, may be associated with recurrence of the initial psychotic symptoms. It is often necessary to maintain the patient on haloperidol or a comparable drug at a daily dose of 2 to 5 mg for 2 to 4 months after the initial episode. I have observed several patients whose initial psychosis cleared in a matter of a few days, the antipsychotic agent was discontinued, and the PCP-induced psychotic state returned two to five days later. In these situations, after reinstituting haloperidol the symptoms again cleared, though the second course of treatment tended to produce a somewhat slower response than the initial treatment.

Consistent with current theories of psychotic illness, it is interesting that PCP increases availability of dopamine centrally, by facilitating its release and inhibiting its reuptake.[24] This compound also blocks reuptake of norepinephrine, which may explain its peripheral sympathomimetic effects and the increased risk of serious hypotensive reactions if chlorpromazine is administered.[24]

Although pleasurable reactions may be experienced by some users, the risk of a serious and persistent toxic psychosis is exceedingly high.[29] Clinical studies have suggested that some individuals are relatively immune to the severe toxic psychotic reaction to PCP while others are exceedingly vulnerable. This perhaps explains the severe reactions in novice users and the tendency of regular, experienced users not to have severe reactions.[2] It is conceivable that this epidemiologic and pharmacologic information regarding the actions of PCP at neurotransmitter receptor sites may eventually be explained on the basis of the underlying propensity of some persons to develop schizophrenic or other psychotic states, most likely based on genetic factors.[24] PCP has been associated with rhabdomyolysis and myoglobinuria. This skeletal muscle damage appears to be the result of excessive involuntary isometric motor activity during PCP intoxication.[33] There has been one report of a severely deformed baby being born of a mother who used PCP during pregnancy.[34]

AMPHETAMINES

A large group of compounds similar either structurally or pharmacologically to the amphetamines produce a variety of CNS and autonomic effects. These drugs are classified as sympathomimetic agents because they mimic the actions of the sympathetic nervous system, producing vasoconstriction, tachycardia, and elevations of both systolic and diastolic blood pressure. These compounds also produce stimulation of the CNS and may provoke tremor, restlessness, increased motor activity, agitation, insomnia, and anorexia.[35] These drugs were initially marketed as appetite suppressants, though this clinical action is prominent only over the first 2 weeks of treatment, after which the anorexic effect diminishes.[35] These drugs were employed early in their history in the treatment of depression, often by physicians who did not clearly recognize the existence of depression but simply noted that the patient was slowed down. Amphetamines are occasionally useful in the treatment of depression and they may be of value in assessing potential response to antidepressant drugs and in enhancing the antidepressant action of conventional pharmacotherapy. These drugs have fallen into disfavor in the treatment of obesity, but are still used in the treatment of pathologic hypersomnia known as narcolepsy. Various compounds of this group have value in treating attention-deficit disorders and hyperactivity associated with minimal brain dysfunction in children.[35]

The amphetamines produce their effects by stimulating adrenergic receptors directly, and indirectly, through release of dopamine and norepinephrine and by mild inhibition of the enzyme, monoamine oxidase.[3,35] The classic drugs in this group, which have been and continue to be abused, are dextroamphetamine and methamphetamine.[2] Other related compounds possessing abuse potential include phentermine, phenmetrazine, phendimetrazine, and phenylpropanolamine. The latter compound is the only one readily available as a component of various over-the-counter medications. The other agents are Class II controlled substances under the Drug Enforcement Administration.[35]

Several other related compounds also have similar pharmacologic effects including methylphenidate, which is chemically unrelated and possesses

$$\langle\bigcirc\rangle-CH_2-\overset{\overset{\displaystyle H}{|}}{\underset{\underset{\displaystyle CH_3}{|}}{C}}-NH_2$$

DEXTROAMPHETAMINE

somewhat less liability for abuse than dextroamphetamine. The desired effect of the amphetamine-related compounds is an elevation of mood, a sense of increased energy and alertness, and a decreased need for both food and sleep. Patients using amphetamines tend to experience increased anxiety, irritability, and loquaciousness.[2] During amphetamine abuse a paranoid psychosis, which may be indistinguishable from paranoid schizophrenia, can occur. Tolerance to the behavioral effects of amphetamines is known to occur. Thus patients need to take increasingly larger doses to achieve the desired pharmacologic effects.

Once drug use is discontinued the individual will experience a withdrawal syndrome, though it is less dramatic than the withdrawal associated with narcotics or barbiturates. Withdrawal symptoms associated with amphetamine-like drugs include increased appetite and weight gain, decreased energy, and increased need for sleep.[3] Patients may develop a voracious appetite and sleep for several days after amphetamines are discontinued.[2,35] Paranoid symptoms may persist during drug withdrawal but generally do not develop as a result of withdrawal. The patient suddenly discontinuing amphetamine use may develop severe depression and become suicidal. Management of amphetamine withdrawal does not require detoxification but does require appropriate and cautious clinical observation of the patient, recognition of depression, and treatment with an appropriate antidepressant drug if clinically necessary.[3] Since amphetamine withdrawal depression appears to be related to depletion of noradrenergic function, antidepressants acting on this neurotransmitter may be clinically superior to those primarily affecting serotonin. The peripheral sympathetic hyperactivity associated with continuous use of amphetaminelike drugs contraindicates low-potency antipsychotic agents such as chlorpromazine and thioridazine in the treatment of paranoid reactions, and indicates the need for high-potency antipsychotic drugs such as haloperidol, generally in relatively low dose.[10]

COCAINE

The euphoric effect of cocaine is similar to that produced by the amphetamines.[36] One study found that subjects familiar with cocaine could not distinguish between the subjective effects of 8 to 10 mg of this drug and those produced by 10 mg of dextroamphetamine, when both were administered IV.[39] The toxic behavioral syndrome associated with cocaine is similar to that produced by high doses of amphetamine. The euphoriant effect of cocaine lasts only about 30 minutes, while that of methamphetamine may persist for hours.[2] Cocaine produces pupillary dilatation, tachycardia, hyperpyrexia, tremor, and sweating, all of which are associated with the administration of amphetamines as well.[2] Persons taking cocaine may become hyperreactive, paranoid, and impulsive, and may participate in repetitious-compulsive behavior patterns.[2] Paranoid psychotic reactions, similar to those seen with amphetamines, may occur during cocaine use.[2,36] Likewise, a withdrawal syndrome is known to occur following discontinuation of cocaine. This syndrome includes marked fatigue, hyperphagia, and hypersomnia, as well as irritability and depression.[2] Cocaine withdrawal symptoms are very similar to those of amphetamine withdrawal.[36] Detoxification from cocaine is not necessary, but appropriate observation of the patient is necessary to detect the development of depression, which may require psychiatric treatment, including pharmacologic management.[36]

Cocaine inhibits nerve reuptake of norepinephrine, potentiating the actions of this neurotransmitter, similar to the effect of tricyclic antidepressants.[2] There is also evidence that cocaine may bind to serotonergic sites in the brain.[36] Cocaine activates mesolimbic or mesocortical dopaminergic pathways, which appears to explain its euphorigenic effect.[39]

Cocaine may be used by IV injection, nasal snorting, and inhalation of smoked "crack" or free-base cocaine, and through admixture of free-base cocaine with tobacco or marijuana cigarettes.[36] Free-base is prepared by the user by adding a strong alkali, such as ammonia or baking soda, to an aqueous solution of cocaine hydrochloride, producing a relatively pure volatile product. Free-base is then ignited and deeply inhaled from a pipe.[2] "Crack" is another potent form of cocaine commonly used. "Crack" is prepared in the same way as free-base, except that the product is prepared by the dealer, rather than by the user, and sold in small white pebblelike chunks that look like soap and feel like porcelain. Free-based cocaine, the production of which employs highly flammable ether, is less popular now than it was a few years ago. Currently "crack" cocaine which has similarly intense intoxicating effects, has largely replaced "free base" which is dangerous to make.[37]

There are many patterns of cocaine use, ranging from infrequent low-dose usage to periodic binges, which may last for 12 hours or less, but may extend for several days. There are those who use low doses of cocaine on a daily basis, reminiscent of amphetamine abuse. Once a regular pattern of cocaine abuse is established, craving often develops. Craving for cocaine is often intense and compelling and will lead the user to spend large amounts of money for this expensive drug. Those who are compelled to continuously obtain and use cocaine will often, in the process, destroy their business or professional lives, and wreak havoc with their family and social connections.[37,38]

Cocaine use may provoke hallucinations and a psychotic state that may be indistinguishable from hypomania or mania.[36] There is profound stimulation of the sympathetic nervous system and catecholamine release during cocaine use, which may provoke a variety of physiologic symptoms, including tachycardia, hypertension, and hyperpyrexia.[40] Intense stimulation of cardiac rate and force of contraction, as well as generalized vascular constriction, may produce myocardial infarctions, worsen hypertension, and provoke cerebrovascular accidents.[40,41,42] Because of the prominent sympathomimetic effect of cocaine, this drug and the amphetamines are contraindicated in patients being treated with monoamine oxidase inhibitors. I have seen two MAOI-treated patients who developed acute psychotic reactions following the use of cocaine. In neither of these cases was a hypertensive reaction documented; however, there were symptoms suggestive of a mild hypertensive crisis as well. Although cocaine is often snorted or smoked in the form of "crack", it is also commonly taken by intravenous injection and therefore may produce the medical complications seen with other intravenously used substances, including infections and AIDS.[42]

Many patients who abuse cocaine chronically present a past history of depressive episodes and a positive family history for affective illness. Indeed, since cocaine inhibits nerve reuptake of neurotransmitters, resembling the pharmacologic actions of cyclic antidepressants, it is conceivable that it is being used by these patients as self-treatment for their depressive disorder. A study of the antidepressant action of orally administered cocaine revealed some modest mood effect, but no pronounced antidepressant action.[5] It could be argued that the technique of oral administration favored a negative response in that study, and that had the drug been administered through snorting or by another means which would have facilitated its absorption, a more significant antidepressant action might have been seen.

Because of the intense craving for cocaine and the possibility of underlying affective disorders facilitating its continual use, treatment of cocaine dependence is extremely difficult and often ineffective. Intense supportive treatment programs involving the patient and his family are essential for a successful result, though they do not necessarily guarantee a favorable outcome.[38] Several studies have found that the administration of tricyclic antidepressants to patients who have withdrawn from cocaine may produce mood improvement and a greater potential of prolonged abstinence.[38] Desipramine appears to be the most promising drug since it is primarily a noradrenergic antidepressant, and cocaine's primary site of action involves noradrenergic neurotransmission.[36] Imipramine has also produced some favorable results in cocaine abusers.[36]

Most studies of desipramine management of cocaine abuse have found a favorable response more likely to occur in those patients whose cocaine abuse is associated with a diagnosable affective disorder.[38] Although not significantly affecting noradrenergic neurotransmission, fluoxetine has been shown in one open prospective study, at a mean daily dose of 45 mg, in cocaine-dependent methadone maintenance patients, to reduce cocaine use.[44] Eleven of the 16 patients in the latter study were HIV infected, and reduced cocaine use was indicated by patient self reports and by quantitative measurements of cocaine and its metabolite, benzoylecgonine in plasma and urine. That study, which was 9 weeks in duration, did not find significant drug interactions with either cocaine or methadone. One wonders, however, whether the ability of fluoxetine to potentiate a variety of drugs in fact allowed patients to be more comfortable or drug-satisfied at lower doses of concurrently administered cocaine and methadone, although methadone plasma levels were not significantly increased. Lithium has been used clinically and subjected to limited clinical trials in cocaine abuse. Some patients benefit from its use, however, a study in 10 cocaine abusers with bipolar spectrum disorders, failed to find lithium effective in altering cocaine use.[45] Carbamazepine, which has a mood stabilizing effect and in addition, inhibits neuronal kindling, has been shown to reduce cocaine use when administered in daily doses of 200 to 800 mg.[12]

Because of the high recidivism rate among cocaine abusers, it may be too risky to utilize MAOIs for treatment of the underlying affective illness because of the potential serious drug interaction between MAOI antidepressants and cocaine. In a controlled environment, however, if patients can be kept truly abstinent, MAOI antidepressants may produce a favorable therapeutic response, and there have been anecdotal reports supporting this pharmacologic intervention.

Cocaine inhibits reuptake of dopamine, which may be a major mechanism of its euphoriant effect. Chronic administration of cocaine increases postsynaptic dopamine binding sites and decreases brain concentration of dopamine.[47] Depletion of brain dopamine stores may be the chemical basis for cocaine withdrawal symptoms and craving.[47] The dopamine agonists bromocriptine, and pergolide have both been demonstrated to suppress cocaine craving.[12,47] Neuroleptic drugs, which are dopamine antagonists, may provoke cocaine craving in habitual cocaine users.

Reduced cocaine craving has been seen in some studies of the dopaminergic drug, amantadine.[12,46] Bupropion, an antidepressant thought to work through enhanced dopamine neurotransmission, has also been shown to reduce cocaine craving and use in some patients.[12] The noradrenergic/dopaminergic precursor, L-tyrosine, and the serotonin precursor, L-tryptophan, have also occasionally been found to reduce cocaine craving.[36] Although there are suggestions of beneficial effects of a widely divergent group of chemicals, there is inadequate data to strongly recommend any one of them as a standard or reliable treatment, thus more research is essential to gaining some control of the escalating cocaine problem.

MISCELLANEOUS INTOXICANTS

Adverse behavioral effects of over-the-counter drugs have been discussed in chapter 13. Some people will use patent medicines containing anticholinergics or phenylpropanolamine in an attempt to "get high." Some will turn to nonprescription products to get high or modify their feelings or behavior during withdrawal from other drugs including narcotics or sedatives. The pronounced behavioral and toxic effects of these nonprescription products in the management of any patient with a history of drug abuse must be recognized, since the potential for any drug abuser to use multiple substances is exceedingly high.

In addition to conventionally recognized psychoactive substances present in over-the-counter drug products, there are numerous herb-containing teas, cigarettes, and "natural medicines" obtainable in "health food" stores. There are plants and weeds that grow wild throughout the United States that likewise contain potentially psychotoxic substances. Most of these substances, whether harvested from the user's own herb garden, picked in a vacant lot, or purchased at an exorbitant price in a health food store, contain alkaloids with potent anticholinergic action.[48]

The most prevalent clinical manifestation of intoxication with any of these natural products is an anticholinergic delirium. The intoxication should be treated by discontinuation of drug use, administration of a mild short-acting sedative such as lorazepam if necessary, and the possible administration of physostigmine to clarify the diagnosis. In some of these plant-associated intoxications, the use of small doses of high-potency antipsychotic drugs is necessary, though this approach can frequently be avoided once the condition is clarified as an anticholinergic delirium.

A variety of organic solvents may be inhaled and produce a 'high'. Volatile organic solvents, including gasoline, toluene, chloroform, trichloroethylene, and ether, have been used for a number of years, primarily by teenagers, as a means of inducing an intoxicated state.[3] The major advantage of these intoxicants is that they are readily available and inexpensive. The major disadvantage of this form of *high* is that it may have a fatal outcome. Commonly, the organic solvent or solvent-containing glue is placed in a plastic bag from which it is inhaled. The solvents utilized are cardiotoxic and may provoke cardiac arrhythmias and myocardial depression.[3] The danger of these toxic substances is enhanced by hypoxia, which may develop as a result of inhalation from plastic bags.

Tobacco

Tobacco smoking is one of the most ancient and prevalent forms of recreational drug use. Most commonly, tobacco is used in the form of cigarettes. Cigar and pipe smoking are less popular, but for the smoker, more pleasurable forms of tobacco use. The least common technique of tobacco use is in the form of snuff or chewing tobacco. Each of these products delivers nicotine, along with a variety of other organic and inorganic compounds, including polycyclic aromatic hydrocarbons, some of which are documented carcinogens. Chronic use of tobacco is causally linked to a variety of serious diseases, including coronary artery disease and lung cancer. Men who smoke two packs of cigarettes daily, have an overall mortality ratio of 2.0 in comparison to nonsmoking males.

Since ancient times man has continually searched for mood-altering drugs.

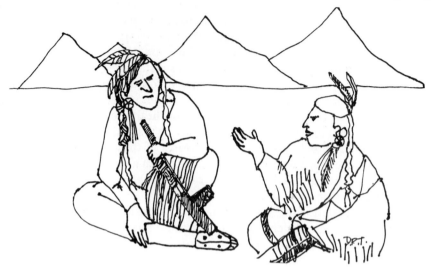

"Please pass the Prozac."

Cigar smoking increases mortality in proportion to the number smoked, but not as sharply as for cigarettes. Those who smoke pipes exclusively show a very slight increase in mortality.[2]

Nicotine is responsible for the majority of the pharmacologic effects of tobacco consumption. Nicotine is readily absorbed and reaches the brain rapidly, where it releases norepinephrine and dopamine.[49] Depending on dose, nicotine may either increase or decrease acetylcholine release.[49] There is evidence that nicotine may also stimulate serotonergic sites in the brain. Nicotine administration to humans exerts an alerting effect, and can facilitate memory and attention, while producing a mild relaxant action. Modest doses of nicotine may decrease irritability and suppress appetite. Most people who discontinue smoking, regardless of the means utilized, experience increased appetite and weight gain, which may be considerable.[49] It is conceivable that the increased appetite associated with discontinuation of nicotine use may relate to changes in serotonergic neurotransmission centrally. Discontinuation of tobacco use is followed by a mild withdrawal syndrome, including a craving for tobacco, increased appetite, irritability, anxiety, restlessness, and difficulty in concentration.[49] Drowsiness, headaches, insomnia, and GI complaints are also common during withdrawal. Nicotine chewing gum containing 2 mg per piece may be a useful adjunct in discontinuing tobacco use. Nicotine gum reduces tobacco craving and diminishes nicotine withdrawal symptoms. The use of nicotine gum may also help to suppress increased appetite, which is one of the more troublesome and persistent sequelae of smoking cessation.[2] Nicotine patch therapy has increasingly supplanted the use of nicotine gum, in that it produces a reliable and stable serum concentration of the drug, and through the use of patches of decreasing potency, allows a convenient means of gradual nicotine detoxification.[50] An analysis of 17 double-blind, placebo controlled nicotine patch studies which included a total of 5098 patients confirmed the efficacy of this treatment modality.[50] In that analysis, it was found that subjects wearing the nicotine containing patch were twice as likely to quit smoking than those wearing a placebo patch, an effect that was seen with either high or low intensity counseling.[50] The public health benefits of cessation of cigarette smoking with respect to cardiovascular and neoplastic disease are well accepted and potentially easier to accomplish through the use of the nicotine patch. An agonizing question, for me, is that over the past two decades as the prevalence of smoking declines, there has been a steady rise in the incidence of Alzheimer's disease. The presence of central nicotinic receptors is well known and one wonders whether there is an association between lesser stimulation of these receptors through smoking and the current epidemic of (AD) Alzheimer's disease. Studies of Alzheimer's patients who had discontinued smoking many years before the onset of their disease noted that patients who eventually developed AD had experienced a lack of desire to smoke and virtual absence of withdrawal symptoms as compared to matched controls who did not develop AD.[51] It was suggested that an alteration of central nicotinic receptors may occur many years before the onset of symptomatic Alzheimer's disease.[51] As discussed in chapter 12, tobacco use induces a number of drug-metabolizing enzymes, and may thus alter plasma levels and therapeutic responses to a variety of drugs.[49]

CAFFEINE

Although not commonly thought of as a drug of abuse, caffeine, in the form of coffee, tea, and carbonated cola beverages, is widely used and often consumed in prodigious amounts. Many patients presenting to the psychiatrist with panic disorder will describe, if properly questioned, use of large amounts of coffee and diet cola, containing caffeine, one of the best documented panicogenic substances. Patients with panic disorder will very often experience a decrease in the frequency or severity of their attacks after eliminating caffeine from their diet. It must be recognized that for the high dose caffeine user, eliminating this drug may produce considerable discomfort and a withdrawal syndrome.[3] Studies of low to moderate dose caffeine users revealed a withdrawal syndrome with 52% complaining of headache, and approximately 10% experiencing symptoms of depression, anxiety, increased fatigue, and decreased vigor.[52] A side issue to heavy caffeine consumption is that the source is often aspartame sweetened diet cola. It has been documented that high dose consumption of aspartame, which is metabolized to phenylalanine, may cause headaches, and rarely with very high doses seizures. Patients, particularly those receiving

MAOIs, should be urged to minimize their use of aspartame. When it is necessary to reduce or eliminate caffeine use, the dosage should be gradually tapered to reduce the likelihood of withdrawal symptoms.

ANABOLIC STEROIDS

The current emphasis on fitness, exercise, and body physique, particularly among young males, has spawned abuse of anabolic and androgenic steroids, drugs previously used only for the management of endocrinopathies in general medicine. Steroids in current use by athletes and body builders are derivatives of the male hormone testosterone. These agents are generally used in large doses, 10 to 100 times their normal replacement dosage, and administered orally or by intramuscular injection and not uncommonly by both routes simultaneously.[53] Anabolic steroids are mostly used by males, but some women also use them ostensibly to enhance muscular growth, although it is not clear that steroid use actually builds muscle mass in either males or females. Steroids are also used to allow more intensive training, increase motivation and endurance, and reduce fatigue and recovery time between workouts.[53]

Anabolic steroid abuse may cause a variety of medical complications including cardiovascular disease, diabetes, liver disease, testicular atrophy, gynecomastia in men, and clitoral enlargement in women.[53] Psychiatric complications include both depression and mania, as well as psychosis, delirium, increased aggressiveness, violence, homicide, and suicide.[53] Both medical and psychiatric complications are likely to be dose dependent, although individual sensitivity to these drugs may yield a dramatic complication in some patients using rather trivial doses. A controlled study of 160 athletes who abused steroids found that 23% had major mood syndromes including hypomania, mania, and major depression. These affective disorders were significantly more likely to be present during steroid use than in the absence of steroids in these subjects.[54]

Steroid abusers may develop tolerance to their effects, increase their dosage, continue to use the drug in spite of adverse effects, and experience a withdrawal syndrome upon discontinuation. These findings support the contention that anabolic steroids can induce addiction.[53] Withdrawal symptoms include depressed mood, fatigue, restlessness, loss of appetite, insomnia, headaches, and decreased libido. Manic symptoms during steroid use may require lithium, alone or along with neuroleptics. Depression occurring during steroid use or withdrawal may necessitate treatment with antidepressant drugs. The physician must be alert to the potential of unpredictable behavior or violence in the abuser of anabolic steroids. A study of anabolic steroid use in ninth grade students found that a significant number of those surveyed also abused other drugs, including cocaine, marijuana, alcohol, tobacco, and injectable drugs.[55] Since many published reports note that steroid abusers, who inject, not uncommonly share needles, thus raising concerns about potential spread of HIV infection in this group of substance abusers.[55]

OPIOIDS

There are a variety of opioids derived from the opium poppy and synthetically manufactured that produce similar pharmacologic effects.[56] In addition, there are several drugs such as propoxyphene and pentazocine, which were initially developed and marketed as nonnarcotic analgesics and subsequently shown to produce addiction of the opiate type.[56] Heroin is the classic opiate with addiction-producing liability. Rapid IV injection of this substance produces a warm flush of the skin and sensations in the lower abdomen that addicts describe as being similar in intensity and quality to sexual orgasm.[2] This rush lasts for about 45 seconds after injection and is followed by a milder pleasurable sensation that may last for two hours or longer. Morphine produces a similar effect, though its intensity is less and its duration longer. Meperidine produces a much less dramatic effect, but of somewhat longer duration, often associated with anticholinergic symptoms.[2] Methadone has a long duration of action, with a half-life approximating 15 hours following the administration of a single dose in nontolerant subjects. With chronic administration the methadone half-life is extended to approximately 22 hours.[2]

Opioids possess analgesic effect and also decrease aggression and sexual drive. Long-term administration of opioids is associated with a decrease in circulating testosterone concentrations in males. Since opioid addicts must continually administer these costly substances, they frequently become engaged in criminal activity to obtain money to support their habit. Fortunately or unfortunately, there is no underground FDA to regulate the quality and purity of illicit drugs sold on the street. Not infrequently, heroin sold illicitly, regardless of price, is impure. Most commonly users of street-obtained narcotics use multiple other drugs, including alcohol, barbiturates, and benzodiazepines, because of the limited pharmacologic action of available narcotic products. Persons unable to obtain opiates will also use propoxyphene and pentazocine, which will satisfy drug hunger and produce their own opioid effect. Pentazocine has both narcotic agonist and antagonist effects, and may, by virtue of the latter action, provoke a narcotic withdrawal syndrome when administered to someone who has been using opiates.[56] Narcotics do not produce hallucinations or toxic psychoses, during use or during withdrawal. Propoxyphene possesses a hallucinogenic effect and hallucinations may also occur with use or also withdrawal of pentazocine.[56,57]

All of these substances produce a true addiction marked by the development of tolerance, wherein the patient must take larger and larger doses to maintain the same pharmacologic effect. Furthermore, the other characteristic of addiction is the development of a withdrawal syndrome, which occurs following abrupt discontinuation of any of these opioids.[2] During withdrawal, most individuals will engage in whatever activity is necessary to obtain a continuing supply of drugs, including polite requests, demands, and manipulations of medical personnel. They may also perform violent acts to obtain the desired drug. The physiologic signs of narcotic withdrawal include lacrimation,

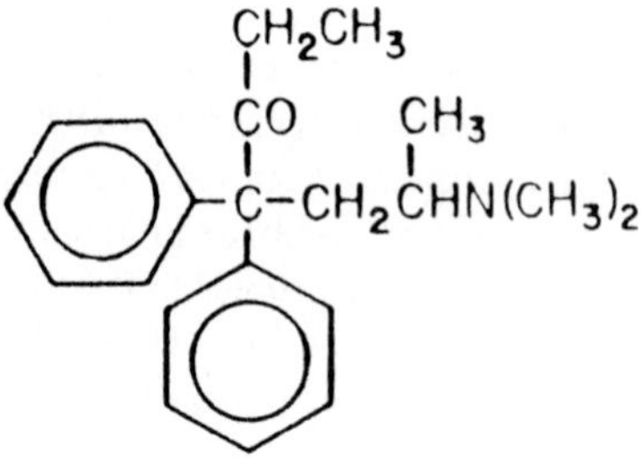

METHADONE

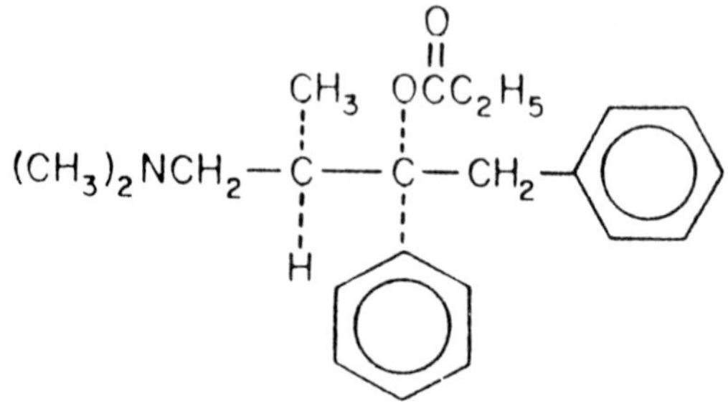

PROPOXYPHENE

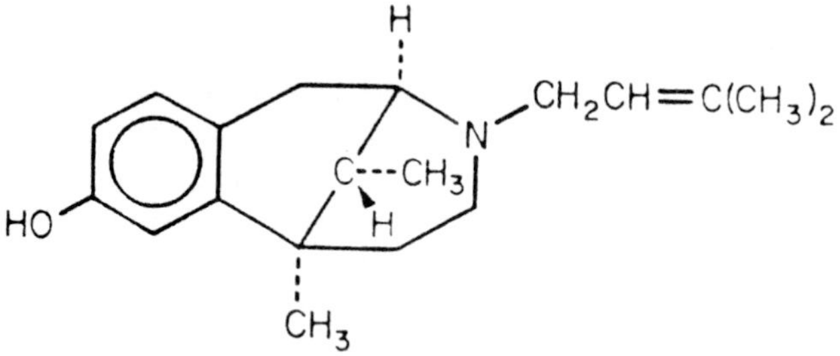

PENTAZOCINE

rhinorrhea, yawning, sweating, and restlessness during the first 12 hours after drug discontinuation. Dilated pupils, anorexia, gooseflesh, irritability, and tremor subsequently develop. Weakness, depression, nausea and vomiting, as well as abdominal pain and diarrhea, also occur during withdrawal. Patients experience an increase in heart rate and blood pressure and may have postural hypotension. Chills, alternating with flushing and associated with excessive sweating, commonly occur with the persistence of gooseflesh. Abdominal cramps and pains in muscles and bones, as well as muscle spasms and kicking movements at times associated with ejaculation in men and orgasm in women, are other signs not infrequently seen as withdrawal progresses. The patient may describe a flulike syndrome with abdominal and GI complaints, as well as anorexia, which may progress to dehydration and weight loss. The classic morphine withdrawal syndrome will gradually disappear in 7 to 14 days if no treatment is administered. The shorter-acting narcotics such as heroin produce a withdrawal syndrome more quickly than does discontinuation of longer-acting narcotics such as methadone. Unlike withdrawal from barbiturates or other sedatives, narcotic withdrawal is not associated with seizures or the potential for a fatal outcome.[2] Most of the above described symptoms of opioid withdrawal are manifestations of noradrenergic hyperactivity, originating in the locus coeruleus, and are reduced by agents such as clonidine which inhibit noradrenergic firing.[58]

The oral administration of an adequate dose of methadone will diminish and terminate the uncomfortable signs and symptoms associated with narcotic withdrawal. Since patients who abuse narcotics often give inaccurate histories regarding the quantity of substance used, and since the purity of street-obtained preparations varies, there is no ideal way to estimate the dose of methadone that must be administered to suppress withdrawal symptoms. When methadone was first used to alleviate narcotic withdrawal symptoms the doses administered generally were excessive. Repeated clinical studies have revealed that 40 mg of methadone daily will generally block withdrawal symptoms associated with narcotic addiction, regardless of the dose of narcotic used.[2,59] The clinician must realize that narcotic users often employ multiple substances and that methadone will not suppress withdrawal symptoms associated with alcohol, barbiturates, or benzodiazepines.

In treating these patients it is important to get the best historical information possible early in the course of evaluation and treatment, so that dependency on other drugs can be simultaneously treated. There is no accurate tolerance test for assessing the level of narcotic dependency comparable to the test utilizing pentobarbital to evaluate sedative addiction. The proper use of methadone in suppressing narcotic withdrawal symptoms is to initially administer 5 mg orally, and observe the patient approximately one hour later for reduction of withdrawal symptoms which will be associated with a decrease in pupillary dilatation. If the desired effect is not observed, an additional 5 to 10 mg may then be administered and the patient re-evaluated one hour later for evidence of decreased narcotic withdrawal symptoms and the appearance of pupillary constriction. The dose of methadone needs to be gradually titrated until withdrawal symptoms are significantly decreased and pupillary size is diminished. However, many of the withdrawal symptoms, including muscle aching and flulike syndrome, will persist for one or more days, even after adequate doses of methadone are administered.[2] The initial signs indicating that the dose is adequate involve changes in pupillary size and a diminution in the autonomic symptoms of withdrawal.

Methadone, in addition to suppressing acute signs of narcotic withdrawal of any of the opioids, is effective for detoxification of patients from narcotics. By federal law methadone can be administered for detoxification only in those inpatient facilities licensed under the DEA for narcotic detoxification. In such facilities methadone can be administered in gradually decreasing doses for a maximum period of 21 days. If it is administered to treat narcotic addiction for a period exceeding 21 days, this is classed under federal laws as methadone maintenance, for which a specific license must be held by the institution.

Methadone cannot be administered on an outpatient basis to addicts except under the auspices of properly licensed methadone maintenance clinics. It should not be administered parenterally to narcotic addicts for detoxification unless a coexisting medical condition prevents the oral administration of the drug. Once the initial response to methadone is assessed during the process of titration, the drug should be administered in two divided doses at approximately 12-hour intervals. Generally, 5 to 20 mg are administered in liquid form twice daily in a blind fashion, wherein the patient does not know the dose that he is receiving. The patient should receive a stable dose of methadone during the first three days of detoxification after which the dose is gradually decreased by 2.5 to 5.0 mg every day or every second day. The process of detoxification may take from 7 to 21 days, depending on the extent of tolerance and the level of previous drug use as judged by the initial response to methadone. Detoxification may be further monitored by periodic determinations of blood pressure in the sitting and standing position 2 or 3 times daily, since the persistence or development of postural hypotension is one relatively objective measurement indicating that detoxification is proceeding too rapidly.

As an alternative approach to methadone detoxification, which may be equally effective, clonidine, a centrally acting alpha-adrenergic agonist, may be administered in a dose of 0.1 to 0.5 mg twice daily.[58] This drug has been repeatedly shown to diminish or abate the signs and symptoms of opiate withdrawal, allowing the patient to be more comfortable following abrupt discontinuation of narcotics.[58,60,61] Alternatively, clonidine may be used along with methadone detoxification to minimize the patient's discomfort. Clonidine is thus far not approved by the FDA for the treatment of narcotic withdrawal, and this use of the drug must therefore be explained to the patient and documented in the record as an unapproved use of an FDA-approved medication. Increasing clinical data support clonidine as being equal or superior to methadone in its efficacy for the treatment of narcotic withdrawal.[60,61]

Although most clinicians think of narcotic addiction in the context of illicit drug use, many patients with trivial or severe medical illnesses receive long-term treatment with narcotics for the purpose of analgesia. Many patients receiving physician-prescribed narcotics become addicted to these drugs. Patients who have become medically addicted to narcotics may need acute treatment of their withdrawal syndrome when the drug is discontinued, and may need methadone detoxification. Clonidine has also been shown to be useful in the detoxification of medically addicted patients.[62] When used for detoxification, the dose must be titrated to the level at which narcotic withdrawal symptoms disappear. The orally administered dose of clonidine can then be gradually reduced until the drug is discontinued without the recurrence of narcotic withdrawal symptoms. Patients addicted to large doses of propoxyphene or pentazocine may need methadone detoxification, following the same course of treatment as those who have been addicted to morphine, meperidine, or other narcotic substances. The one additional caution in patients being detoxified from pentazocine is that hallucinations and other psychotic manifestations may occur during withdrawal from this drug, unlike withdrawal from conventional narcotics. If these symptoms do arise it is best to treat them with relatively low dosages of orally or IM administered haloperidol. These patients generally do not need long-term maintenance with antipsychotic medication, though the use of this medication during detoxification may make the difference between a successful and an unsuccessful course of treatment. Low-potency antipsychotics are to be avoided, because of their pronounced effects on the autonomic nervous system.

It is beyond the scope of this book to discuss the philosophy or clinical value of methadone maintenance. However, repeated documentation in the literature has demonstrated a high correlation between continued methadone maintenance and simultaneous use of alcohol, barbiturates and benzodiazepines. Apparently a relatively small number of patients maintained on methadone over a period of years actually successfully detoxify and remain drug-free.[63] It appears at this time that methadone maintenance is not a desirable approach in the long-term management of narcotic addicts. It is conceivable that the increasing clinical evidence for the efficacy of clonidine in suppressing narcotic withdrawal may eventually lead to the use of this agent in the maintenance of narcotic addicts in an opiate-free state. Furthermore, as our understanding of opiate receptors and the mechanisms of analgesia and addiction become further extended, hopefully more effective and less addicting analgesics will be developed that will eventually reduce the incidence of opiate dependence.[64,65]

Advances in the pharmacologic inhibition of opioid abuse and management of withdrawal have utilized drugs which antagonize opioid receptors or inhibit excess catecholaminergic discharge in the locus coeruleus during withdrawal.[58] Naloxone is an opioid antagonist with a half life of 1 to 4 hours, and will provoke withdrawal symptoms in addicts who are using. This drug also counteracts respiratory depression following an opiate overdose, but its duration of action is often shorter than that of the drug taken in overdose. Naltrexone, which has a duration of action of approximately 24 hours, will also reverse narcotic induced respiratory depression and provoke withdrawal symptoms in patients actively using opioids.[58] Both naloxone and naltrexone will block euphoriant and other pharmacological effects of opioids taken by patients who have been previously given either antagonist.[56] Since naltrexone is devoid of any pleasurable effect, and will block the action of any opioid subsequently taken, it is difficult to get addicts to take the drug consistently and regularly.[56] Several groups have found, however, that patients who remain reliably on naltrexone maintenance will have significantly reduced narcotic consumption.[58] Buprenorphine is a mixed agent with weak opioid agonist effect along with antagonist activity.[58] Clinical studies of sublingual buprenorphine have found this agent to reduce opioid abuse during treatment.[58] One 16 week study utilizing a flexible dosage schedule found buprenorphine to be as effective as orally administered methadone in reducing opioid consumption.[66] Other studies have found buprenorphine more effective than methadone in suppressing illicit opioid abuse.[58] Many opioid abusers also use cocaine but find the latter agent, used alone to produce a somewhat dysphoric effect, and therefore use opioids and cocaine in combination, known as "speedball". Several studies have found that buprenorphine treatment of opioid addicts reduces cocaine use, as documented by measurement of urinary metabolites of cocaine.[58,66] Buprenorphine has also been somewhat effective in reducing cocaine abuse in non-opioid dependent patients. Although the addictive potential of buprenorphine is less than that of opioids, this drug may produce its own dependency problems, the extent of which will not be appreciated until more extensive clinical experience accumulates.

SEDATIVE AND HYPNOTIC DRUGS

There is a large group of substances, widely divergent in their chemical structure, which share the ability to produce generalized depression of the CNS. These agents include approximately a dozen different barbiturates and a similar number of benzodiazepines, as well as other chemically unrelated CNS depressant drugs. The CNS depressant effects of ethyl alcohol do not differ widely from the CNS action produced by this divergent group of sedative-hypnotic agents.

The drugs in this group produce a variety of metabolic and neurotransmitter changes in the CNS. The benzodiazepines act on specific brain receptor sites.[65] Barbiturates and the nonbenzodiazepine sedatives do not bind significantly to these receptor sites. The relative affinity of different benzodiazepines for binding to these receptors varies parallel to their therapeutic potency. Despite the existence of specific benzodiazepine receptors, the chemical compounds classed as sedative-hypnotic agents all produce dose-dependent CNS depression.

Furthermore, there is cross-reactivity between these various sedative compounds.[2] A patient who has developed tolerance to any of the benzodiazepines not only will be tolerant to any other compound in this group, but will also be tolerant to barbiturates and other CNS depressants.[2] Individuals who have become tolerant to the barbiturates will show similar tolerance to benzodiazepines and other CNS depressants. Following abrupt discontinuation of any of these compounds by an individual who has become dependent, the

Table 17-3   Drugs which may produce sedative-type addiction*

Drug	Daily dose (mg)	Duration of administration	Reference no.
Barbiturates			
Pentobarbital	800	6 weeks	67
Secobarbital	800	6 weeks	67
Amobarbital	800	6 weeks	67
Phenobarbital	200	Several years	69
Benzodiazepines			
Alprazolam	1.5-3.0	3-11 months	70, 71
Chlordiazepoxide	300-600	2-6 months	72, 73
Diazepam	15-30	Several years	74, 75
Diazepam	80+	6 weeks	73, 74
Flurazepam	60-90	Several months	76, 77
Lorazepam	8	6 months	78
Lorazepam	12+	6 weeks	78
Oxazepam	30-60	1 year	79
Traizolam	0.5-5.0	2-3 months	73, 80
Miscellaneous			
Chloral hydrate	2000	Several months	76, 77
Ethchlorvynol	2000	Several months	67, 77
Ethinamate	1500	Several months	67, 77
Glutethimide	1000	Several months	67, 77
Meprobamate	1600	Several months	73, 76
Methaqualone	1000	3-6 months	71, 76, 77
Methyprylon	2000	Several months	67, 77

*This list includes commonly used sedatives with addiction potential. Many patients will be able to take these drugs at lesser dosage or in some cases at higher dosage without becoming addicted within the time frame presented in the table. Some persons may become addicted to these agents at much lower doses or following much briefer periods of treatment. The absence of any sedative compound from the table does not imply the absence of addiction-producing liability. It is unlikely, for instance, that any benzodiazepine compound is totally free of the potential to produce addiction if administered in a large enough dosage for a long enough period of time.

administration of any other compound in this group will prevent symptoms of withdrawal. All drugs shown in Table 17-3 are capable of inducing addiction as marked by the occurrence of tolerance, wherein progressively less pharmacologic effect occurs with continued administration of the same dose.

Abrupt discontinuation of any of these compounds is associated with a withdrawal syndrome. The withdrawal syndrome associated with barbiturates, benzodiazepines, and other sedative-hypnotic drugs is identical. Careful clinical observation of patients who have discontinued use of any of these drugs does not allow the clinician to determine which agent has been taken, except that those drugs with longer half-lives tend to produce their withdrawal syndrome later after drug use is discontinued than those substances with short half-lives.[79] A significant proportion of sedative-dependent patients will present a history of having used two or more agents simultaneously. The non–drug-abusing patient being treated by a physician with a single benzodiazepine over a prolonged period of time may gradually develop tolerance and eventually a withdrawal syndrome when the drug is discontinued. Since many benzodiazepines have long half-lives, generally of two to five days, after prolonged periods of administration, the pharmacologic effects of these drugs tend to be cumulative over a period of use. The clinician prescribing benzodiazepines should be aware of both their dependency-producing qualities and their long half-lives and tendency to produce a cumulative effect.[74,79]

The patient receiving continuing treatment with benzodiazepines should be evaluated by the physician, periodically for nystagmus, slurred speech, drowsiness, and ataxia, which are indicative of excessive drug effect, due to the patient escalating his dosage, or to the cumulative action of drugs with lengthy half-lives. Coadministration of SSRIs, particularly fluoxetine, fluvoxamine, or paroxetine with benzodiazepines or barbiturates, are likely to cause increased sedative effect, nystagmus, slurred speech, and ataxia. Reduction in ability to metabolize drugs associated with aging will yield even more prolonged half-lives for these compounds in elderly persons. Some benzodiazepines, particularly diazepam, chlorazepate, flurazepam, and prazepam, can be measured in the blood of patients for as long as seven to 14 days after discontinuation of a prolonged period of usage. More lengthy half-lives are likely to occur in the elderly or patients with impaired drug metabolism.

The classic study of barbiturate addiction, on which much of our knowledge of this type of drug dependency is based, involved the administration of either secobarbital or pentobarbital over a prolonged period of time to a group of former narcotic addicts in a hospital research ward setting.[67] In that study it was found that administration of either of these drugs at a daily dose of 600 to 800 mg for a period of 35 to 57 days was sufficient to produce a clinically significant degree of physical dependence. All of the 18 subjects abruptly withdrawn from barbiturate dosages of 800 to 2200 mg daily had minor abstinence symptoms, while 14 of the 18 had convulsions and 12 had delirium; some subjects had both convulsions and delirium.[67] In that study, the minor abstinence symptoms associated with barbiturates included: postural hypotension, coarse rhythmic intention tremors, hyperreflexia, muscular weakness, aching or twitches, apprehension, insomnia, profuse sweating, and anorexia. These symptoms developed in all patients within the first 24 hours following drug withdrawal, and the symptoms persisted from three to 14 days thereafter. Eighty percent of the patients withdrawn from the short-acting barbiturates developed seizures, initially occurring on the second or third day and persisting over a period of eight days. Sixty percent of the patients developed psychoses or deliria, beginning between the third and eighth day after drug discontinuation and persisting for three to 14 days.[67] The psychotic symptoms usually resembled those associated with delirium tremens, and visual hallucinations were particularly prominent.

In clinical practice seizures and psychotic symptoms often first appear five to seven days following abrupt discontinuation of short-acting barbiturates. The seizures are generally not associated with an aura, and it is important for clinicians to be aware that phenytoin has absolutely no protective value against seizures associated with barbiturate or sedative withdrawal.[81] Patients who become psychotic during sedative withdrawal are frequently disoriented, agitated, and deluded, and have visual and auditory hallucinations. Although fevers were not seen in patients abruptly withdrawn from sedatives in Wikler's study,[67] the author points out that rising core temperature is an ominous sign prognosticating a fatal outcome if not combated vigorously by the administration of barbiturates. It is absolutely essential for clinicians to be aware that exceedingly high temperatures may be seen in the course of sedative withdrawal, with temperatures as high as 108°F reported.[82] If the proper diagnosis is made, the prompt administration of sedating doses of barbiturates may reverse the process and avoid a fatal consequence.

One case report attributes hyperthermia and death to the administration of haloperidol in a patient undergoing withdrawal from methaqualone and barbiturates.[83] Having reviewed both that publication and the patient's clinical record, it appears clear to me that both the fever and the fatal outcome were directly related to sedative withdrawal rather than the administration of haloperidol.

The classic study of barbiturate withdrawal reported by Wikler also noted that meprobamate, all benzodiazepines, glutethimide, ethinamate, ethchlorvynol, and methyprylon are all capable of producing sedative intoxication, as well as the barbiturate-type abstinence syndrome, including both minor and major manifestations.[67] That study provided the initial clinical basis for utilizing pentobarbital as a tolerance test in patients dependent on barbiturates and other sedatives. In evaluating and planning treatment for a sedative-dependent patient it is important to perform a satisfactory pentobarbital test. Data obtained from this test should be used to determine the necessity of detoxification and the dosage level of medication necessary to provide a safe detoxification program.

It must be underscored that pentobarbital should be used for the tolerance test regardless of whether the substance used was a barbiturate, benzodiazepine, or a chemically unrelated CNS depressant drug. Although this technique has generally not been employed with patients addicted to alcohol, it could conceivably be applied in these patients as well.

Pentobarbital Tolerance Test

The proper performance of a pentobarbital test relies on careful clinical observations of the patient before and after the administration of one or more test doses of pentobarbital. The patient should not be drug-intoxicated at the start of the tolerance test. If a patient has been using short-acting barbiturates, the test should be done after waiting six to eight hours after the last dose and being certain that there are no signs of CNS depression such as nystagmus, slurred speech, drowsiness, or ataxia. An individual who has been using longer-acting drugs such as diazepam may need to remain in the hospital under observation for several days, until a satisfactory amount of the intoxicating drug has been metabolized, prior to performing an accurate tolerance test. If the patient has a considerable amount of CNS depressant drug still circulating or present in tissue, the administered dose of pentobarbital will add to the drug already present, and give a false low reading for that patient's level of tolerance. An inaccurately determined tolerance based on this situation could give rise to the decision not to detoxify the patient, or to a program of detoxification that would cease too rapidly, causing the patient to develop withdrawal symptoms during or shortly after detoxification. If the tolerance test is initiated when the patient is relatively drug-free, a reasonably accurate index of the patient's tolerance to sedative drugs, regardless of their chemical type, and satisfactory guidelines for the dosage to be used during detoxification, will be provided.

In a drug-free individual who is not physically dependent on sedative drugs, the administration of 200 mg pentobarbital orally will produce sound sleep within approximately one hour. An individual with a mild degree of tolerance to sedative drugs may become drowsy and have nystagmus, slurred speech, and ataxia following the oral administration of 200 mg pentobarbital, which would indicate that detoxification of this patient is not clinically necessary. Patients who are tolerant to barbiturates or sedatives, when given an initial test dose of 200 mg pentobarbital, frequently show no signs of CNS effect; speech, gait and alertness are unaffected, and there is no nystagmus when the patient is evaluated one hour following the orally administered test dose given in liquid form. In this situation the patient should be given an additional 100 mg of pentobarbital and again evaluated one hour later. If by this time, nystagmus occurs and no other signs of CNS effect are noted, the patient could be said to be tolerant to 300 mg pentobarbital. Assuming that no CNS manifestations of barbiturates are observed at that time, an additional 100 mg pentobarbital is then given in liquid form and the patient is evaluated one hour later. The presence of nystagmus or other CNS signs of barbiturate effect at this time indicates that 400 mg pentobarbital has been required to just exceed this patient's tolerance. If no signs of CNS effect are noted after the cumulative administration of 200 mg, 100 mg, and 100 mg pentobarbital, additional pentobarbital should not be immediately administered, since a significant portion of the initial dose will now have been metabolized, and an accurate estimate of tolerance cannot be obtained. The patient should then remain drug-free for eight hours, at which time the tolerance test can be repeated, starting with an initial dose of 300 mg pentobarbital orally with 100-mg increments given at hourly intervals until CNS signs appear, specifically the presence of nystagmus. In most instances, 200 to 300 mg pentobarbital administered orally will be adequate to produce nystagmus or other signs of CNS effect; that is, it will be adequate to just override the patient's level of tolerance.

Persons who have used exceedingly large doses of benzodiazepines or other sedatives will obviously require a larger amount of barbiturate to exceed their level of tolerance. For optimal clinical practice pentobarbital should be administered in liquid form, by dissolving the somewhat insoluble contents of pentobarbital capsules in warm water, mixing with fruit juice, and administering the suspension orally. An advantage of utilizing liquid forms for the tolerance test, and throughout the course of detoxification, is that the clinician can be certain that the total dose administered has been swallowed. Also, the tolerance test and detoxification can proceed blindly, without the patient knowing, by recognizing the capsules or tablets that he receives, the exact dose of barbiturate administered at any given time.

The tolerance test should be done with the same technique, whether the patient has been using any one of the barbiturates, any of the benzodiazepines, or any other chemically unrelated CNS depressant drug. Once the level of tolerance has been determined, the patient may be stabilized by administering pentobarbital every six hours for a period of three days, and subsequently reducing the daily dose of pentobarbital by 100 mg/day. The dose of pentobarbital required to just exceed the patient's tolerance level is taken as one fourth of the total daily dose; that dose would be administered every six hours during the course of stabilization, with subsequent gradual reduction of the pentobarbital dosage by 100 mg/day. Since the duration of action of pentobarbital is approximately five to six hours, if this drug is chosen it must be administered regularly at six-hourly intervals. Pentobarbital will protect against seizures and other manifestations of withdrawal from any CNS depressant drug. However, pentobarbital itself does not have a specific anticonvulsant effect and may actually lower seizure threshold.[76]

Sedative Detoxification

Although pentobarbital is clearly the drug of choice for performing the tolerance test, it is less than ideal for stabilization and detoxification because of its previously mentioned characteristics. Therefore, once the tolerance test has been done, it is preferred clinical practice to use phenobarbital, a longer-acting barbiturate, during stabilization and detoxification of the sedative-dependent patient. The dose of phenobarbital to be administered can be readily calculated based on 30 mg phenobarbital being equivalent to 100 mg pentobarbital; if 300 mg pentobarbital were required to just exceed a patient's level of tolerance, 90 mg phenobarbital would produce a similar effect and could be administered 4 times daily during stabilization.[59,84]

Subsequently, during detoxification the daily dose of phenobarbital is reduced by 30 mg each day. Since the half-life of phenobarbital approximates 24 hours, it is less critical to administer this compound at six-hourly intervals. Administering the calculated dose 4 times daily with the spacing between dosages approximately equal is satisfactory. Furthermore, one half of the daily dose could be administered in the morning and one half at night, although many patients undergoing detoxification will prefer to receive their medication four times daily. A four times daily schedule, while somewhat more cumbersome, will frequently reduce requests for supplemental medication, which should not be administered during the course of detoxification.

Again, it must be emphasized that phenytoin will not protect against seizures and other symptoms seen during withdrawal from barbiturates, benzodiazepines, and other sedatives.[81] Phenytoin should not be administered during withdrawal unless the patient has a previously existing seizure disorder for which the medication is required. If phenytoin is used during the performance of the tolerance test or during detoxification, the clinician must be aware that therapeutic blood levels of this compound will ordinarily produce prominent lateral gaze nystagmus; therefore, this indicator of barbiturate or sedative effect cannot be utilized in the course of phenytoin administration.

The most critical medication to avoid during sedative withdrawal is chlorpromazine, which produces hypotension and worsens postural hypotension that often occurs during withdrawal.[10,67] Furthermore, the ability of chlorpromazine to lower seizure threshold will significantly increase the risk of seizures occurring during sedative withdrawal and may facilitate the development of status epilepticus, one of the most serious complications of sedative-hypnotic withdrawal.[10,67] If a patient with a coexisting psychotic illness needs an antipsychotic agent during sedative withdrawal, haloperidol is the safest neuroleptic to use, because of its minimal effect on blood pressure and seizure threshold.[10] Neither haloperidol nor any other antipsychotic agent should be used to the exclusion of appropriate barbiturate detoxification for a patient being withdrawn from sedative drugs.

In an emergency, when barbiturates are not available to prevent the recurrence of a withdrawal reaction, diazepam may be administered until an appropriate supply of barbiturates can be obtained. Diazepam, however, because of its time course of action, cannot be used for performing a tolerance test, and it is not good clinical practice to simply take historical information from a patient, place him on a comparable dose of diazepam, and withdraw him. Since minor manifestations of withdrawal from short-acting barbiturates generally occur within the first day and major manifestations may not occur until the fifth to seventh day after discontinuation, it is important to recognize that the disparity between the half-lives of short-acting barbiturates and those of benzodiazepines, particularly the long-acting agents such as diazepam and flurazepam, will modify the time course for the withdrawal syndrome. Minor withdrawal manifestations from the benzodiazepines may not appear until two to four days after discontinuation of the drug, while major manifestations of the withdrawal from these agents may initially occur as late as ten to 15 days after discontinuation. Tolerance testing is not foolproof, particularly if the patient has other sedatives present at the time of the test. It is important to observe patients carefully in a hospitalized setting, not only during the course of detoxification but also for one to two weeks following completion of the detoxification program, so that appropriate emergency management may be instituted in the event of a late-occurring withdrawal syndrome.

In the event that seizures or other manifestations of sudden withdrawal appear during or following detoxification, it is important to administer barbiturates, preferably phenobarbital or amobarbital, IM in a sufficient dose to produce sedation. When the patient awakens, a new tolerance test should be done and an appropriate detoxification regimen reinstituted. I have learned that historical information presented by patients is notoriously inaccurate in dealing with the problem of sedative dependency. One of the first patients I treated for presumed barbiturate addiction gave a history of taking massive amounts of multiple barbiturates; had I followed his recommendation for the necessary dose I would have provided him a fatal overdose, which I learned following an initial tolerance test. This patient died about 6 months later in an auto accident that was apparently suicidally motivated. More commonly, patients will present a history of taking lower doses of sedatives than they actually do take, and often patients will repeatedly deny sedative abuse, with symptoms of sedative withdrawal occurring during treatment for medical, surgical, or psychiatric illness. As discussed in chapter 3, the triazolobenzodiazepines may be particularly difficult with respect to addiction, since patients treated with these drugs may have serious withdrawal symptoms in spite of adequate benzodiazepine or barbiturate treatment during detoxification. As a reminder, commonly prescribed triazolobenzodiazepines include alprazolam, triazolam, and estazolam.

Unsuspected Sedative Dependency

Although clinicians have become increasingly aware of the potential development of sedative addiction in users of "street drugs," it is becoming apparent from the literature and from my clinical experience that patients who do not appear clinically as classic drug abusers may develop severe degrees of sedative dependency during the course of conventional medical treatment with hypnotic drugs or antianxiety agents with CNS depressant effects. We have, unfortunately, at times been lulled into a sense of excessive security regarding the safety of benzodiazepines, and most clinicians assume that patients becoming addicted to these drugs must be taking massive doses. Numerous reports indicate that regular use of relatively small therapeutic doses of benzodiazepines may be associated with withdrawal symptoms.[79,85] Withdrawal psychosis was reported in three patients taking larger-than-ordinary therapeutic doses of diazepam or flurazepam.[74] Another patient using 15 to 30 mg diazepam daily, generally not recognized as an excessive dose of this drug, developed a withdrawal psychosis following abrupt discontinuation of medication.[75] Patients using prescribed dosages of flurazepam, diazepam, or oxazepam over periods of one to ten years have developed prominent withdrawal syndromes with insomnia, panic attacks, agitation, depersonalization, and in some cases, an acute organic brain syndrome.[78] Although chlordiazepoxide was the first benzodiazepine reported to produce a withdrawal syndrome,[72] there are numerous reports of minor abstinence symptoms and occasional reports of major abstinence syndromes including seizures associated with abrupt discontinuation of diazepam,[86] lorazepam, and other benzodiazepines following prolonged use.[78,87] The literature includes multiple reports of tremulousness, irritability, and other minor withdrawal symptoms associated with abrupt discontinuation of diazepam at doses as low as 15 mg/day.[88] It is not surprising that many of these situations are missed clinically, since the minor symptoms of withdrawal are often mistakenly identified by the physician as an indication that the patient had previously responded favorably to the medication and requires continuous maintenance. Withdrawal symptoms have also been associated with the administration of low-dose barbiturates in the course of ordinary medical therapy.[69]

The major therapeutic advantage of short-acting benzodiazepines is their lesser tendency to accumulate and produce progressively increasing sedation with prolonged administration. A disadvantage of the shorter-acting benzodiazepines, however, is the possibility that they may produce a somewhat greater risk of dependency, a more abruptly developing withdrawal syndrome, and greater difficulty of maintaining abstinence in a patient who wishes to discontinue their use. The problem of dependence on short-acting benzodiazepines has increased in recent years with the popularity of relatively high-dose alprazolam regimens in the treatment of panic disorder, agoraphobia, and depression. These regimens commonly employ alprazolam at a daily dose of 2 to 6 mg, and occasionally employ even higher doses. Eight patients receiving alprazolam in doses of 1.5 to 10 mg daily over a period of 8 weeks to 18 months developed withdrawal symptoms following abrupt discontinuation.[77] In two of these cases, diazepam and chlordiazepoxide were unable to suppress withdrawal symptoms, which were subsequently suppressed by readministration of alprazolam. Delirium and seizures occurred with abrupt withdrawal of alprazolam in a 77-year-old man, who had received 1.5 to 5.0 mg daily over the previous 3 months.[70] Withdrawal delirium was reported in a 68-year-old man following discontinuation of alprazolam, which he had received in a dose of 0.5 mg 3 times daily for 11 months.[71] In that case, the delirium was unresponsive to diazepam, but cleared following reinstitution of alprazolam.

Triazolam, the shortest-acting benzodiazepine with a half-life of two to three hours, has also been reported to produce withdrawal symptoms. A 53-year-old man, who had been using 5 mg of triazolam daily for 3 months, experienced psychosis and delirium following withdrawal of the drug.[80] Although the patient had been receiving an extremely high dose of triazolam, withdrawal has also been associated with lower doses of the drug. One patient, a 26-year-old woman, received 0.5 mg of triazolam nightly at bedtime for 3 weeks, followed by 1.25 mg nightly for an additional 2 weeks, at which point she was hospitalized and triazolam was discontinued. Approximately 30 hours after her last dose of triazolam, she experienced a generalized tonic-clonic seizure.[73]

The occurrence of serious withdrawal symptoms with the triazolo-benzodiazepines should alert the clinician to be cautious in their use, particularly when they are employed for prolonged periods of time at high dosage levels. If they are used in this way, very gradual dosage reduction should be undertaken, rather than abrupt discontinuation, because of the risk of significant withdrawal symptoms. Since patients who fail to respond to high-dose alprazolam regimens are likely to be subsequently treated with tricyclic antidepressants, an added note of caution is in order. Withdrawal of benzodiazepines may provoke seizures, while conventional doses of tricyclic antidepressants lower seizure threshold. Thus the combination of initiating tricyclic drug therapy, while discontinuing benzodiazepines, may expose the patient to the risk of a drug-related seizure. The best way to minimize the risk of benzodiazepine dependency is to prescribe the lowest possible dosage, preferably utilizing an intermittent schedule of administration, and to limit the course of benzodiazepine therapy to the shortest possible duration consistent with good patient care. Any patient begun on a benzodiazepine should be alerted to the possibility of developing withdrawal symptoms and told not to discontinue his or her medication abruptly, but to do so on a gradual basis, in accordance with the physician's recommendation.

Although benzodiazepines are the most widely prescribed group of drugs with dependency-producing potential and barbiturates have become less widely prescribed, the latter agents still present considerable risk of addiction and continue to be available both by prescription and from illicit sources. Hypnotics available on the illicit market, including ethchlorvynol, glutethimide, meth-aqualone and methyprylon, continue to be responsible for sedative addiction.[89] Meprobamate, which is prescribed infrequently, also has considerable potential to produce addiction. Unfortunately, this was recognized only several years after the product was initially introduced and prescribed on a very widespread basis.[89] Chloral hydrate is occasionally prescribed as a relatively safe hypnotic agent. However, the regular and persistent use of this substance, particularly with gradually increasing dosage, may produce a syndrome of addiction and the appearance of withdrawal symptoms on discontinuation.[2]

There are a variety of myths and realities associated with methaqualone which have made it a popular illicit drug. Users describe it as possessing less hypnotic action and at the same time a happy, contented high compared with the drowsiness experienced with barbiturates. Although not proved by available data, aphrodisiac qualities and orgasm-promoting effects have been attributed to methaqualone. Methaqualone was initially marketed as nonaddicting. Experience with this drug has shown not only that it produces a high that many people find to be extremely pleasurable, but also that it is capable of producing sedative addiction comparable to that seen with barbiturates.[2] Methaqualone produces tolerance, and following a course of persistent use, a withdrawal syndrome appears on discontinuation.[90] The drug has a very desirable reputation among drug abusers.[91] Fortunately, it has been withdrawn from the United States prescription market. Methaqualone sold on the street is often mislabeled diazepam or, methaqualone smuggled into the United States from other countries. Abuse of any of the nonbarbiturate, nonbenzodiazepine sedatives requires the same cautious and thorough evaluation and treatment that would be employed for the management of barbiturate or benzodiazepine addiction.[92]

REFERENCES

1. Rosner F: *Julius Preuss: Biblical and Talmudic Medicine.* New York, Sanhedrin Press, 1978.
2. Jaffe JH: Drug addiction and drug abuse. In Gilman AG, Rall TW, Nies AS, Taylor P (eds): *Goodman and Gilman's The Pharmacological Basis of Therapeutics,* ed 8. New York, Pergamon Press, 1990, pp 522-573.
3. Winger G, Hofmann FG, Woods JH: *A Handbook on Drug and Alcohol Abuse: Biomedical Aspects,* ed 3. New York, Oxford, 1992.
4. Lewin L: *Phantastica: Narcotic and Stimulating Drugs.* New York, E P Dutton, 1931.
5. Goldstein DB (ed): *Pharmacology of Alcohol.* New York, Oxford University Press, 1983.
6. Himmelhoch JM, Hill S, Steinberg B, et al: Lithium, alcoholism, and psychiatric diagnosis. *J Psychiatr Treatment Eval* 1983;5:83-88.
7. Jacob MS, Sellers EM: Emergency management of alcohol withdrawal. *Drug Ther* 1977;2:28-42.
8. Saitz R, Mayo-Smith MF, Roberts MS, et al: Individualized treatment for alcohol withdrawal: A randomized double-blind controlled trial. *JAMA* 1994;272:519-523.
9. Greenblatt DJ, Shader RI, McLeod SM, et al: Absorption of oral and intramuscular chlordiazepoxide. *Eur J Clin Pharmacol* 1978;13:267-274.
10. Bernstein JG: Drug interactions. In Cassem NH (ed): *Massachusetts General Hospital Handbook of General Hospital Psychiatry,* ed 3. St Louis, Mosby Year Book, 1991, 571-610.
11. Kraus ML, Gottlieb LD, Horwitz RI, et al: Randomized clinical trial of atenolol in patients with alcohol withdrawal. *N Engl J Med* 1985;313:905-909.
12. Gorelick DA: Overview of pharmacologic treatment approaches for alcohol and other drug addiction. *Psychiatr Clin North Am* 1993;16:141-156.
13. Bernstein JG: Medical consequences of marijuana use, in Mello NK (ed): *Advances in Substance Abuse, Behavioral and Biological Research,* Greenwich, Conn, JAI Press, 1980, vol 1, pp 255-387.
14. Thomas H: Psychiatric symptoms in cannabis users. *Br J Psychiatry* 1993;163:141-149.
15. Cohen S: Marijuana, in Frances AJ, Hales RE (ed): *APA Annual Review.* Washington, DC, American Psychiatric Press, 1986, vol 5, pp 200-211.
16. Mendelson JH, Rossi AM, Meyer RE (eds): *The Use of Marijuana: A Psychological and Physiological Inquiry.* New York, Plenum Press, 1974.
17. Babor TF, Mendelson JH, Greenberg I, et al: Marijuana consumption and tolerance to physiological and subjective effects. *Arch Gen Psychiatry* 1975;32:1548-1552.
18. Jones RT, Benowitz NL, Herning RI: Clinical relevance of cannabis tolerance and dependence. *J Clin Pharmacol* 1981; 21:1435-1525.
19. Bernstein JG, Becker D, Babor TF, et al: Physiological assessment: Cardiopulmonary function, in Mendelson JH, Rossi AM, Meyer RE (eds): *The Use of Marijuana: A Psychological and Physiological Inquiry.* New York, Plenum Press, 1974, pp 147-160.
20. Tennent FS, Guerry RL, Henderson RL: Histopathologic and clinical abnormalities of the respiratory system in chronic hashish smokers. *Sub Alcohol Actions Misuse* 1980;1:93-100.

21. Greenberg I, Kuehnle JC, Mendelson JH, et al: Effects of marijuana use on body weight and caloric intake in humans. *Psychopharmacology* 1976:49:79-84.
22. Logan WJ: Neurological aspects of hallucinogenic drugs, in Freidlander WJ (ed): *Advances in Neurology.* New York, Raven Press, 1975, vol 13, pp 47-78.
23. Schwartz RH: Heavy marijuana use and recent memory impairment. *Psychiatric Annals* 1991;21:80-82.
24. Stillman R, Barnett G, Petersen R: Phencyclidine: Epidemiology, pharmacology and pharmacokinetics, in Mello NK (ed): *Advances in Substance Abuse, Behavioral and Biological Research.* Greenwich, Conn, JAI Press, 1980, vol 1, pp 289-303.
25. Gold MS: The epidemiology, attitudes, and pharmacology of LSD use in the 1990s. *Psychiatric Annals* 1994;24:124-126.
26. Miller NS. Gold MS: LSD and Ecstasy: Pharmacology, phenomenology, and treatment. *Psychiatric Innals* 1994;24:131-133.
27. Aghajanian GK: Serotonin and the action of LSD in the brain. *Psychiatric Annals* 1994;24:137-141.
28. McDowell DM, Kleber HD: MDMA: Its history and pharmacology. *Psychiatric Annals* 1994;24:127-130.
29. Grinspoon L, Bakalar JB: Psychedelics and arylcyclohexylamines, in Frances AJ, Hales RE: *APA Annual Review.* Washington, DC, American Psychiatric Press, 1986, vol 5, pp 212-225.
30. Yesavage JA, Freeman AM III: Acute phencyclidine intoxication: Psychopathology and prognosis. *J Clin Psychiatry* 1978;39:664-666.
31. Allen RM, Young SJ: Phencyclidine-induced psychosis. *Am J Psychiatry* 1978;135:1081-1084.
32. Hollister LE: Phencyclidine (PCP) use. *Int Drug Ther Newsletter* 1979; 14:17-20.
33. Cogen FC, Rigg G, Simmons JL, et al: Phencyclidine-associated acute rhabdomyolysis. *Ann Intern Med* 1978;88:210-212.
34. Golden NL, Sokol RJ, Rubin IL: Angel dust: Possible effects on the fetus. *Pediatrics* 1980;65:18-20.
35. Weiner N: Norepinephrine, epinephrine and the sympathomimetic amines, in Gilman AG, Goodman LS, Rall TW, et al (eds): *Goodman and Gilman's The Pharmacological Basis of Therapeutics,* ed 7, New York, Macmillan, 1985, pp 145-180.
36. Kleber HD, Gawin FH: Cocaine, in Frances AJ, Hales RE: *APA Annual Review,* Washington, DC, American Psychiatric Press, 1986, vol 5, pp 160-185.
37. Weddington WW: Cocaine: Diagnosis and treatment. *Psychiatr Clin North Am* 1993;16:87-95.
38. Carroll KM, Rounsaville BJ, Gordon LT, et al: Psychotherapy and pharmacotherapy for ambulatory cocaine abusers. *Arch Gen Psychiatry* 1994;51;177-187.
39. Goeders NE, Smith JE: Cortical dopaminergic involvement in cocaine reinforcement. *Science* 1983;221:773-774.
40. Warner EA: Cocaine abuse. *Ann Intern Med* 1993;119:226-235.
41. Levine SR, Brust JCM, Futrell N, et al: Cerebrovascular complications of the use of the "crack" form of alkaloidal cocaine. *N Engl J Med* 1990;323:699-704.
42. Cherubin CE, Sapira JD: The medical complications of drug addiction and the medical assessment of the intravenous drug user: 25 years later. *Ann Intern Med* 1993;119:1017-1028.
43. Post RM, Kotin J, Goodwin FK: The effects of cocaine on depressed patients. *Am J Psychiatry* 1974;131:511-517.
44. Batki SL, Manfredi LB, Jacob P, et al: Fluoxetine for cocaine dependence in methadone maintenance: quantitative plasma and urine cocaine/benzoylecgonine concentrations. *J Clin Psychopharmacol* 1993;13:243-250.
45. Nunes EV, McGrath PJ, Wager S, et al: Lithium treatment for cocaine abusers with bipolar spectrum disorders. *Am J Psychiatry* 1990;147:655-657.
46. Meyer RE: New pharmacotherapies for cocaine dependence—Revisited. *Arch Gen Psychiatry* 1992;49:900-904.
47. Dackis CA, Gold MS: Bromocriptine as a treatment of cocaine abuse. *Lancet* 1985;1:1151-1152.
48. Siegel RK: Herbal intoxication. *JAMA* 1976;236:473-476.

49. Benowitz NL: Pharmacologic aspects of cigarette smoking and nicotine addiction. *N Engl J Med* 1988;319:1318-1330.

50. Fiore MC, Smith SS, Jorenby DE, et al: The effectiveness of the nicotine patch for smoking cessation: a meta-analysis. *JAMA* 1994;271:1940-1947.

51. Barclay L, Kheyfets S: Tobacco use in Alzheimer's disease. *Prog Clin Res:* Alzheimer's Disease and Related Disorders 1989; 317:189-194.

52. Silverman K, Evans SM, Strain EC, et al: Withdrawal syndrome after the double-blind cessation of caffeine consumption. *New Engl J Med* 1992;327:1109-1114.

53. Brower KJ: Anabolic steroids. *Psychiatr Clin North Am* 1993;16:97-103.

54. Pope HG, Katz DL: Psychiatric and medical effects of anabolic-androgenic steroid use: A controlled study of 160 athletes. *Arch Gen Psychiatry* 1994;51:375-382.

55. DuRant RH, Rickert VI, Ashworth CS, et al: Use of multiple drugs among adolescents who use anabolic steroids. *New Engl J Med* 1993;328:922-926.

56. Jaffe JH, Martin WR: Opioid analgesics and antagonists, in Gilman AG, Rall TW, Nies AS, Taylor P (eds): *Goodman and Gilman's The Pharmacological Basis of Therapeutics*, ed 8, New York, Pergamon, 1990, 485-521.

57. Swanson DW, Weddige RL, Morse RM: Hospitalized pentazocine abusers. *Mayo Clin Proc* 1973;48:85-93.

58. Gold MS: Opiate addiction and the locus coeruleus: The clinical utility of clonidine, naltrexone, methadone, and buprenorphine. *Psychiatr Clin North Am* 1993;16:61-73.

59. Wesson DR, Smith DE: A conceptual approach to detoxification. *J Psychedelic Drugs* 1974;6:161-168.

60. Gold MS, Pottash AC, Sweeney DR, et al: Opiate withdrawal using clonidine. *JAMA* 1980;243:343-346.

61. Charney DS, Sternberg DE, Kleber HD, et al: The clinical use of clonidine in abrupt withdrawal from methadone. *Arch Gen Psychiatry* 1981;38:1273-1277.

62. Charney DS, Kleber HD: Iatrogenic opiate addiction: Successful detoxification with clonidine. *Am J Psychiatry* 1980;137:989-990.

63. Jaffe JH: Opioids, in Frances AJ, Hales RE (eds): *APA Annual Review*. Washington, DC, American Psychiatric Press, 1986, vol 5, pp 137-159.

64. Synder SH: Opiate receptors in the brain. *N Engl J Med* 1977;296:266-271.

65. Synder SH: Opiate and benzodiazepine receptors. *Psychosomatics* 1981;22:986-989.

66. Strain EC, Stitzer ML, Liebson IA, et al: Comparison of buprenorphine and methadone in the treatment of opioid dependence. *Am J Psychiatry* 1994;151:1025-1030.

67. Wikler A: Diagnosis and treatment of drug dependence of the barbiturate type. *Am J Psychiatry* 1968;125:758-765.

68. Juergens SM: Benzodiazepines and addiction. *Psychiatr Clin North Am* 1993;16:75-86.

69. Epstein RS: Withdrawal symptoms from chronic low-dose barbiturates. *Am J Psychiatry* 1980;137:107-108.

70. Levy AB: Delirium and seizures due to abrupt alpraxolam withdrawal: Case report. *J Clin Psychiatry* 1984;45:38-39.

71. Zipursky RB, Baker RW, Zimmer B: Alprazolam withdrawal delirium unresponsive to diazepam: Case report. *J Clin Psychiatry* 1985;46:344-345.

72. Hollister LE, Motzenbecker FP, Degan RO: Withdrawal reaction from chlordiazepoxide. *Psychopharmacologia* 1961;2:63-68.

73. Tien AY, Gujavarty KS: Seizure following withdrawal from triazolam. *Am J Psychiatry* 1985;142:1516-1517.

74. Preskorn SH, Denner LJ: Benzodiazepines and withdrawal psychosis. *JAMA* 1977;237:36-38.

75. Dysken MW, Chan CH: Diazepam withdrawal psychosis. *Am J Psychiatry* 1977;134:573.

76. Rall TW: Hypnotics and sedatives; ethanol, in Gilman AG, Rall TW, Nies AS, Taylor P: *Goodman and Gilman's The Pharmacological Basis of Therapeutics*, ed 8. New York, Pergamon, 1990, 345-382.

77. Browne JL, Hauge KL: A review of alprazolam withdrawal. *Drug Intell Clin Pharm* 1986;20:837-841.
78. Soni SD, Smith ED, Shah A, et al: Lorazepam withdrawal seizures: Role of predisposition and multi-drug therapies. *Int Clin Psychopharmacol* 1986;1:165-169.
79. Busto U, Sellers EM, Naranjo CA, et al: Withdrawal reaction after long-term therapeutic use of benzodiazepines. *N Engl J Med* 1986;315:854-859.
80. Heritch AJ, Capwell R, Roy-Byrne PP: A case of psychosis and delirium following withdrawal from triazolam. *J Clin Psychiatry* 1987;48:168-169.
81. Essig CF, Carter WW: Failure of diphenylhydantoin in preventing barbiturate withdrawal convulsions in the dog. *Neurology* 1962;12:481-484.
82. Fraser HF, Shaver MR, Maxwell ES, et al: Death due to withdrawal of barbiturates. *Ann Intern Med* 1953;38:1319-1325.
83. Greenblatt DJ, Gross PL, Harris J, et al: Fatal hyperthermia following haloperidol therapy of sedative-hypnotic withdrawal. *J Clin Psychiatry* 1978;39:673-675.
84. Smith DE, Wesson DR: Phenobarbital technique for treatment of barbiturate dependence. *Arch Gen Psychiatry* 1971;24:56-60.
85. Haskell D: Withdrawal of diazepam. *JAMA* 1975;233:135.
86. Woody GE, O'Brien CP, Greensteiz R: Misuse and abuse of diazepam: an increasingly common medical problem. *Int J Addict* 1975;10:843-845.
87. Howe JG: Lorazepam withdrawal seizures. *Br Med J* 1980;280:1163-1164.
88. Allgulander C: Dependence on sedative and hypnotic drugs. *Acta Psychiatr Scand* 1978; 270(suppl):1-120.
89. Essig CF: Addiction to nonbarbiturate sedative and tranquilizing drugs. *Clin Pharmacol Ther* 1964;5:334-343.
90. Swatzburg M, Lieb J, Schwartz AH: Methaqualone withdrawal. *Arch Gen Psychiatry* 1973;29: 46-47.
91. Inaba DS, Gay GR, Newmeyer JA, Whitehead C: Methaqualone abuse: "luding out." *JAMA* 1973;224:1505-1509.
92. Wesson DR, Smith DE: *Barbiturates: Their Misuse and Abuse.* New York, Human Sciences Press, 1977.

CHAPTER 18

Creative Psychopharmacology: Medication-Intolerant and Refractory Patients

OVERVIEW

1. Creative psychopharmacology demands a broad base of pharmacologic knowledge, which may allow safe combinations of multiple medications to achieve clinical improvement where simpler regimens have failed.

2. Optimal management often requires use of novel drugs or those approved for non-psychiatric indications to treat mood and behavioral disorders.

3. Patients must be monitored clinically and by laboratory tests as indicated to achieve safe treatment and to alert the clinician to potential adverse effects.

4. A thorough knowledge of potential drug interactions is essential, as is a close and caring physician-patient relationship, with adequate communication.

5. Often, lower than usual doses of medications will improve efficacy and eliminate drug induced side effects.

6. The physician must be alert to variant forms of psychiatric disorders, and frequently utilize medications for symptom-targeted pharmacotherapy.

7. Clear documentation of the course of pharmacotherapy in the patient's record as well as reasons for alternative treatment and evidence that the treatment has been explained to the patient who has given consent.

8. Novel approaches can often improve conditions previously not known to be medication responsive, can achieve benefits in psychiatric illnesses which have not responded to prior use of conventional pharmacotherapy, and can eliminate, minimize, or effectively treat adverse effects of necessary psychotropic drugs.

The incense was composed of balm, onycha, galbanum, and frankincense, seventy minas weight of each; myrrh, cassia, spikenard, and saffron, sixteen minas weight of each; twelve minas of costus; three minas of an aromatic bark; nine minas of cinnamon; nine kabs of karsina lye; three seahs and three kabs of Cyprus wine — if Cyprus wine could not be obtained, strong white wine might be substituted for it — a fourth of a kab of Sodom salt, and a minute quantity of *ma'aleh ashan* (a smoke-producing ingrediant). Rabbi Nathan says: A minute quantity of Jordan Amber was also required. If one added honey to the mixture, he rendered the incense unfit for sacred use; and if he left out one of its required ingredients, he was subject to the penalty of death.

TALMUD (Kerithoth 6a)[1]

Pharmacology is an ancient art, with scientific and sacred origins. Indeed, the incense prepared for Temple sacrifices as described thousands of years ago in the Old Testament left no room for error, since the potential side effects were fatal. Although not used as a medicine, the therapeutic powers of incense were profound through their role in religious ritual and the relationship between man and his creator.

In the life, religion, culture, and healing rituals of Native American Indians, herbal medicines played a central role, and their power for good (beneficial) and evil (adverse effects) were well known.[2] Medicine was a power contained in objects revealed in a dream or vision. These objects became part of a "ceremonial bundle" or "medicine bundle" that could be handed down through generations. Uncontrolled or unchanneled power of the "medicine bundle" was seen as wreaking havoc and causing great injury. Most early cultures saw medicines as having a divine origin and therefore had great respect and indeed reverence for these potentially curative and simultaneously potentially dangerous substances. To properly use medicines in the Twentieth Century, one needs knowledge, reverence, caution, and enthusiasm; the latter being the origin of the creativity often necessary to achieve an optimal therapeutic result.

When pharmacologic therapies began to be employed in psychiatry, in the 1950s, the notion arose that a patient should receive only 1 medication at a time and that if 2 or more were simultaneously prescribed, the patient was receiving "polypharmacy" and therefore by definition, the physician was doing something wrong. Some of the most important innovations in psychopharmacology have come from physicians who, trained initially as internists, were accustomed to use multiple medications simultaneously, as in the management of hypertension, congestive heart failure, and infectious diseases. For a number of years, Drs. Jonathan Cole, Alan Schatzberg, and myself have taught a course in Clinical Psychopharmacology at the annual meetings of the American Psychiatric Association. During the panel discussion of our course in 1992, Dr. Jonathan Cole, in his usual humble but insightful manner, coined the term Creative Psychopharmacology. Thinking in these terms about the rational use of multiple medications simultaneously to treat difficult illnesses places psychiatric pharmacotherapy on a par with treatment in other medical specialties, and should help to allay the guilt of the skilled pharmacotherapist who uses multiple medications simultaneously, based on his knowledge of their pharmacology. I am indebted to Dr. Cole for positing this framework and inspiring me to review with the reader some of my experiences and some of the published case reports employing novel approaches to difficult patient management problems.

When employing innovative therapies, the patient may be treated with lower or, occasionally, higher than usual doses of psychotropic medications, may receive novel combinations of medications, be treated with non-psychotropic drugs for psychiatric indications, or may require treatment with pharmaceutical products marketed outside of the United States but not currently available here. Additionally, some innovative treatments may employ natural substances, including vitamins, as in the case of Vitamin E for tardive dyskinesia, or may involve aromatic essential oils for reduction of anxiety, as supported by aromatherapy approaches which have been researched for many years in Europe and the United Kingdom.

Creative psychopharmacology is not an authorization to practice quackery or to treat patients with alternative remedies without scientific knowledge of rational mechanisms to support the novel therapy.[3] It must be recognized that the initial application of a sedating, temperature lowering, antihistamine, chlorpromazine, in the treatment of schizophrenia was an early example of creative psychopharmacology. It is important to know the pharmacology of any drugs that will be used and to inform the patient that the therapy is innovative and may not work and may produce side-effects, which should be discussed openly. Informed consent from the patient and often family members should be obtained and documented in the medical record.

If safe and effective therapies are available, generally innovative approaches are not appropriate. The patient who is receiving novel pharmacotherapeutic approaches must be seen frequently enough, examined as clinically appropriate, and have clinically indicated laboratory studies done. The physician embarking on new approaches to psychopharmacologic management must have enough medical knowledge to evaluate changes in laboratory and clinical findings and should not adopt an unproven therapy as his or her routine approach to clinical problems. The psychiatrist may in some cases want to engage the patient's internist in evaluation and monitoring before and during the innovative treatment. In mentioning that lower or higher than usual doses of psychotropic drugs may need to be used, I should comment that the innovative approach that I have used most often is to employ lower than usually recommended doses, when a patient has experienced drug intolerance. For example, since the advent of SSRIs, it has been my experience that the usually recommended doses are too high for many patients. I have seen many patients previously intolerant to SSRIs respond to daily doses of fluoxetine of 1.25 to 5 mg, many do very well with 12.5 mg per day of sertraline, and occasional patients respond to clomipramine at a daily dose of 5 mg. I have also seen many people, who were intolerant to the side effects of conventional doses and blood levels of lithium, have a favorable enhancement of the efficacy of antidepressants or achieve adequate protection from hypomania with serum lithium levels of 0.3 to 0.5 mEq/L, and occasional patients have benefitted from lithium levels as low as 0.2 mEq/L. Many patients who have less than optimal responses to antidepressants may experience enhanced therapeutic responses with the addition of 1 to 2 mg daily of a neuroleptic such as trifluoperazine, in spite of the absence of psychotic symptoms. Furthermore, some patients with severe obsessive compulsive disorder will respond better to conventional doses of clomipramine or an SSRI when very low doses of a high potency neuroleptic is added than if the dose of clomipramine or SSRI is dramatically increased. In many cases, when an innovative therapy has been employed, it may be useful in the course of treatment to try to eliminate the added drug or resume a conventional medication regimen, to ascertain whether the innovation is really necessary and the source of increased efficacy. It must be understood, however, that some patients receiving innovative therapies are doing so well as compared to prior management that removing the innovation is too frightening for the patient or physician because of the possibility of reverting to the previous symptomatic state of illness. If neuroleptics are being used innovatively, it is important to be aware of the risk of tardive dyskinesia, even with small doses of neuroleptics, and to discuss this risk with the patient.

Many combined treatment approaches to psychiatric illness have been discussed earlier in this volume, and those which have been more extensively investigated have been reviewed elsewhere.[4] In employing creative approaches to pharmacotherapy, it is important to deviate some from a strict diagnostic categorization, and think in terms of differential effects of monoamine neurotransmitters and their imbalance on behavior.[5] Deficient dopaminergic function may be operative in generating inertia and behavioral retardation, since this transmitter appears to be important in governing goal directed behavior.[5]

Noradrenergic deficiency may be seen as underlying anhedonia, therefore restoring adequate functional levels of this transmitter may result in reawakening the depressed patient's ability to experience pleasure.[5] Serotonin on the other hand may partially function as a regulator of mood, aggression, and anxiety.[5] The current discussion will focus on some psychiatric disturbances, categorized either into broad, not necessarily DSM-IV, diagnostic groups and groups of symptoms, which may cut across diagnostic lines but be amenable to pharmacologic intervention. The discussion will focus on medications which have been successfully employed, not necessarily studied by controlled double-blind techniques. Some of the medications have been FDA approved for non-psychiatric indications, while others approved for psychiatric use in other countries have not been approved by the FDA in the United States. Discussion of these alternative treatment approaches is not meant to endorse them or to urge the physician to employ treatments that he does not understand or feel comfortable prescribing. Yet, when faced with a difficult treatment problem, it behooves the physician to consider all potentially beneficial approaches, to review the medical and scientific literature, and consider a creative psychopharmacologic intervention.

ANXIETY DISORDERS

Benzodiazepines have been useful in a variety of anxiety disorders, yet the risk of dependency is a most important consideration, particularly with high dose alprazolam regimens. Clonazepam is generally effective with a lower risk of dependency, particularly with controlled lower-dose regimens. Buspirone has been recommended for generalized anxiety and for social phobia, however, in my experience and in published studies, its major advantage is lack of dependency risk rather than superior efficacy.[6] Monoamine oxidase inhibitors, the best studied of which is phenelzine, thus far show the greatest efficacy in social phobia.[6] Various SSRIs including fluoxetine, fluvoxamine, and sertraline have been employed and studied in social phobia and panic disorder, with considerable efficacy.[6,7,8] Probably the major problem encountered with SSRIs in anxious patients, whether the diagnosis is generalized anxiety, panic disorder, or social phobia, is their use in excessive dosage, which may actually provoke or worsen anxiety. Many patients whom I have seen in consultation because of an unfavorable response to SSRIs, have, with temporary discontinuation and downward dosage adjustment, had satisfactory control of social phobia or panic disorder. In these situations, it may be optimal to initiate fluoxetine at 2.5 to 5 mg daily or sertraline at 12.5 to 25 mg daily often along with low doses (0.25 mg twice daily) of clonazepam and to titrate the SSRI dosage up slowly, in small increments approximately every 2 weeks. Clonazepam may need to be continued, occasionally at higher doses, but often can be discontinued when a response to the SSRI is established.

Although anecdotal reports have suggested potential efficacy of calcium channel blockers, such as verapamil and nifedipine, in anxiety disorders, including panic, there is inadequate data to recommend this treatment.[9] The lack of dependency risk with these drugs would encourage their trial when the physician wishes to avoid benzodiazepines and the patient is intolerant to SSRIs or MAOIs.

Preliminary studies suggest that fluoxetine, and potentially other SSRIs, may be useful in some patients with posttraumatic stress disorder.[10] In my experience, low doses of SSRIs are definitely worth trying in PTSD, and among other potential advantages lack addictive risk which is an important characteristic of medical therapies for this disorder. Another non-addictive drug which has been effective in reducing hyperarousal and hyperreactivity symptoms in PTSD is valproate, which was both effective and well tolerated in an open study in 16 Vietnam veterans.[11] Valproate was also shown to be effective in controlling panic disorder symptoms in a 6 week open trial in 12 patients.[12] Valproate has the advantage of lacking hypotensive effects of the MAOIs and in some panic patients may be better tolerated than SSRIs. Carbamazepine and valproate have both been found somewhat effective in generalized anxiety disorder, with the latter often better tolerated.[13] Valproate may be useful in managing anxiety associated with drug withdrawal, when it is often preferable to avoid dependency producing drugs such as benzodiazepines.[13] A novel approach to reducing anxiety employing odoriferous essential oils, applied in dilute form to the skin, or by allowing the patient to smell the oils in conjunction with relaxation therapy, has shown some efficacy and will be discussed at the end of this chapter.[14]

Obsessive Compulsive Disorder

Although clomipramine and the SSRIs are generally considered the most effective and best studied pharmacotherapies in OCD, many patients either fail to respond to these drugs in ordinary dosage or are intolerant to them, with impaired sexual function being most prominent among adverse effects. Some patients will respond better when higher doses are employed or when fluoxetine or another SSRI is combined with clomipramine, but in these situations, serum concentrations of the latter agent must be closely monitored to avoid seizures and other complications of excessive clomipramine serum concentrations. Often lower doses of clomipramine or SSRI can be employed with greater efficacy if a neuroleptic such as trifluoperazine, haloperidol, or risperidone in low dosage is added to the antiobsessional medication. Efficacy for this combination regimen has been best documented if there is an associated tic disorder, although some benefit of adding a neuroleptic is apparent even in the absence of tics and also has been documented in OCD variants such as trichotillomania.[15,16] Although lithium and thyroid hormones have both been shown to increase efficacy of antidepressant medications, these drugs do not appear to enhance antiobsessional activity.[17] Fenfluramine, which releases serotonin, inhibits its reuptake and has direct serotonin receptor agonist activity, has been shown to improve control of obsessive compulsive symptoms when used in conjunction with clomipramine or SSRIs.[18] Unfortunately some OCD patients do not tolerate clomipramine or SSRIs. In these patients monoamine oxidase inhibitors often produce beneficial results, although they require dietary precautions and may produce postural hypotension. Limited clinical experience indicates that in some patients carbamazepine or valproate may reduce OCD symptoms, while the benzodiazepine, clonazepam, often demonstrates significant anti-OCD effects.[19] I have seen considerable benefit of clonazepam in OCD and in patients with Tourette's Syndrome who have been intolerant to other pharmacotherapies. Individual case reports have also supported a therapeutic trial of calcium channel blockers, such as nifedipine in tic disorders, when other medications cannot be employed. When OCD is associated with tics or psychotic features, optimal therapeutic response often requires coadministration of neuroleptics with antiobsessional drugs.[20] Many variants of OCD exist, including partial symptom OCD spectrum disorders. Serotonin reuptake inhibitors have been shown in an open study to be highly beneficial in the treatment of moral or religious scrupulosity, which fits into the OCD spectrum.[21] Clomipramine has been found useful in the management of both trichotillomania and onychophagia, other OCD spectrum disorders.[22,23] Body dysmorphic disorder, also an OCD variant, is responsive to SSRIs. Perhaps other variants, including hoarding, sexual compulsions, and compulsive shopping, may also prove to be SSRI responsive.[24,25]

Very severe OCD is a major diagnostic and therapeutic challenge, requiring much creativity to achieve success. These patients who wash their hands 20 or 30 times a day, spend hours in showers, and are plagued by continuous repetitive thoughts, or sounds of music that won't quit, most often require more than a simple regimen of SSRIs. Some in fact respond better to clomipramine, which increases availability of both serotonin and norepinephrine. Since many of these patients are intolerant to the anticholinergic effects of clomipramine, I have often found venlafaxine, which is both serotonergic and noradrenergic, to be more effective than ordinary SSRIs, although in these patients, larger doses of 225 to 375 mg are most often required. Since anti-obsessional drugs are slow to act and require gradual dosage titration, coadministration of a neuroleptic is often helpful in achieving a more complete and rapid response. I have often found risperidone at 1 to 3 mg twice daily to be the ideal neuroleptic in severe OCD, since it has, in these doses, no significant anticholinergic, cardiovascular, or extrapyramidal side effects.

An even greater challenge is the OCD patient who suffers from bipolar disorder, wherein any anti-obsessional drug is likely to provoke mania.[26] In these patients, lithium is often helpful, although infrequently adequate protection against mania, therefore other medications must be used to protect against SSRI induced mania. Carbamazepine, valproate, or a neuroleptic, such as risperidone along with lithium and the anti-obsessional drug, often improve the therapeutic response and protect against drug-induced mania. Although clonazepam can have an anti-obsessional action, my impression is that higher doses of this drug or other benzodiazepines, barbiturates, and perhaps narcotics, including buprenorphine, can worsen obsessional thinking, making pharmacotherapy more difficult.

DEPRESSION

Since clinicians frequently encounter depression, which is unresponsive or only partially responsive to standard pharmacotherapy, creative approaches to treatment have been most extensively explored in its treatment. Suicide is a potential outcome in any patient with severe or persistent depression, therefore concerns about suicidal behavior being provoked by pharmacologic therapies is a source of great concern. In the early days of fluoxetine, there was a disturbing report of intense, violent suicidal preoccupation developing in 6 patients, without "recent" suicidal ideation.[27] In reality, though suicidal ideation had perhaps not been "recent" it was indeed previously present in these patients. There was evidence of motor restlessness or akathisia in patients who experienced suicidal preoccupation while taking fluoxetine, which was offered as an explanation of the suicidal ideation. It appears to me from reviewing published data that when suicidal ideation or violence emerges during fluoxetine therapy, the culprit is most likely an excess effect of coadministered benzodiazepines or other disinhibiting drugs, whose blood level and pharmacological effect will be increased by fluoxetine, which impairs metabolic degradation. Extensive chart reviews at the Massachusetts General Hospital have failed to find excessive suicidal ideation or attempts with fluoxetine when compared to tricyclic or monoamine oxidase inhibitor antidepressants. A meta-analysis of 17 double-blind clinical trials of fluoxetine in 1765 patients with major depression compared with 731 tricyclic treated and 569 placebo treated patients, failed to find an increased risk of suicidal preoccupation or suicidal acts in patients who received fluoxetine.[28]

It is often difficult to diagnose depression, in that many patients will present with few symptoms or with unusual symptoms. It has been reported that "anger attacks" may be symptomatic of depression or of panic disorder in some patients, who when treated with antidepressant or antipanic medications experience a dissolution of anger and other symptoms.[29] Adjunctive use of lithium, thyroid hormones, and neuroleptics as adjuncts to enhance efficacy of cyclic, SSRI, and MAOI antidepressants has been discussed in chapters 5, 6, and 8.[30] Combined use of tricyclic and MAOI antidepressants is discussed in chapters 5 and 6, but it must be restated here that clomipramine and the SSRIs must never be combined with MAOIs, because of the potential of a fatal serotonin syndrome occurring. When a patient experiences excessive tiredness or other side effects, or fails to respond to fluoxetine or another SSRI, the physician should consider the possibility that reducing the dose, allowing adequate time for serum concentration to restabilize, may be the most effective therapy, rather than adding other drugs or increasing SSRI dosage. There may in fact be a therapeutic window for optimal fluoxetine response.[31]

Many drugs with noradrenergic or dopaminergic activity have been used to augment responses to conventional antidepressants. Stimulants, including d-amphetamine, methylphenidate, and pemoline, are among the most underutilized, but potentially beneficial augmenting agents. These drugs are used less frequently than may be indicated probably due to their status as DEA controlled substances, the first two being class II, while pemoline is a class IV substance which eases somewhat the difficulty in its prescribing. Psychostimulants may be useful alone in the short term management of depression, particularly in the elderly, the medically ill, and in patients unable to tolerate conventional antidepressants.[32,33] When added to cyclic or SSRIs, stimulants may both speed and enhance the antidepressant response. A more daring combination is the use of stimulants concurrently with MAOI antidepressants, a combination that most people would avoid due to the fear of a hypertensive reaction. A published report found that stimulants are useful and safe adjuncts to MAOI therapy in healthy patients who are carefully followed.[34] I have not infrequently used methylphenidate or pemoline, generally for short periods of time, to augment MAOI response, and have never encountered any significant elevation of blood pressure or other adverse effect. Most commonly I have employed methylphenidate at 5 mg one to three times daily or pemoline at 18.75 mg once or twice daily, although higher doses can generally be safely used.

Increased dopamine activity is another approach to the treatment of the refractory depressed patient. Indeed, nomifensine, a dopaminergic antidepressant, no longer available in the United States due to hematologic toxicity, produced a dramatic response in many patients who were not improved by other antidepressants. I have seen a favorable response to bupropion, which is also dopaminergic, in many patients, including those who had previously responded to nomifensine, although the latter is often more effective. Lithium augmentation of bupropion may enhance its efficacy, as with lithium used with other antidepressants.[35] Bromocriptine is a dopaminergic drug used in Parkinson's disease, as is pergolide, both of which decrease serum prolactin concentrations and improve depressive symptoms occasionally when used alone and more often when used as adjuncts to conventional antidepressants. These dopaminergic adjuncts have been used safely with a variety of antidepressants, including MAOIs. Pergolide is more potent than bromocriptine and its effect lasts approximately 24 hours as compared to 6 to 8 hours for bromocriptine. In an open study of 20 treatment refractory patients with unipolar major depression, pergolide produced improvement, judged to be clinically significant, in 11 patients, at daily doses of 0.25 to 2 mg, most commonly 0.5 to 1 mg.[36] Side effects encountered with bromocriptine or pergolide most commonly include nausea, vomiting, and dizziness. Hypomania is an uncommon adverse effect which may be alleviated by dosage reduction. If bromocriptine is used, dosage may begin at 1.25 mg twice daily with gradual dosage increase as tolerated, and as dictated by clinical response.

It has been proposed that activation of somatodendritic serotonin (5-HT$_{1A}$)

autoreceptors may occur during antidepressant drug therapy and during treatment with SSRIs. Conceivably activation of 5-HT_{1A} receptors during chronic SSRI treatment may reduce neuronal firing, 5-HT synthesis, and terminal release, which may explain the observation that some patients experience reduced responsiveness to these drugs during long-term treatment.[37] The beta-adrenergic antagonist, pindolol, has high affinity for 5-HT_{1A} receptors and has been studied in an attempt to reduce latency between initiating SSRI therapy and response and to facilitate responsiveness to antidepressants in refractory patients.[37] In that uncontrolled study, 5 of 7 non-refractory patients had a better and more rapid response when pindolol 2.5 mg three times daily was given along with paroxetine 20 mg daily.[37] More impressive was the finding that 6 patients out of a group of eight treatment refractory patients responded favorably to the same dose of pindolol added to either an SSRI or MAOI antidepressant.[37] It would appear that antagonism of 5-HT_{1A} receptors by pindolol may be a useful technique of enhancing antidepressant responsiveness. Side effects and contraindications of pindolol are the same as for other beta adrenergic antagonists, although bad dreams and nightmares are more common with this drug.

Yohimbine has often been used to treat psychotropic drug induced sexual dysfunction. This drug which is a centrally acting alpha$_2$ adrenergic antagonist, has also been used with some success to enhance efficacy of antidepressant drugs in treatment refractory patients, and is a reasonable alternative to adjunctive therapy, which is generally well tolerated.[38] Buspirone, discussed in chapter 3, remains a psychotropic drug in search of an indication. An uncontrolled study found an improved antidepressant response when buspirone was added to either fluoxetine or fluvoxamine in 17 of 25 treatment refractory depressed patients.[39] In my experience addition of buspirone to an SSRI is likely to enhance nausea and may provoke or worsen panic attacks. Selegiline (deprenyl) a selective MAO-B inhibitor is helpful in some depressed patients intolerant or non-responsive to other agents. Its antidepressant efficacy may be improved by coadministration of 250 mg of 1-phenylalanine each morning along with selegiline 5 mg once or twice daily.[40] Short-term administration of adrenal corticosteroids may be helpful in some severely depressed treatment-refractory patients.[41] In a preliminary study, HAM-D scores in 16 patients given either 4 or 8 mg of dexamethasone intravenously dropped by 56%.[41] I have occasionally found beneficial effects of orally administered prednisone in a range of 10 to 40 mg daily for 1 week.

MANIA, RAPID CYCLING, AND CYCLOTHYMIA

Patients with dysphoric mania, mixed affective states, and rapid cycling are more difficult to maintain in the euthymic state than other bipolar patients, and most often are only partially responsive to lithium. Alternative treatments for these conditions are reviewed in chapter 8, however, some additional creative approaches have often been useful and necessary. Although hypothyroidism is a potential complication of lithium therapy, according to some investigators, there appears to be a higher incidence of hypothyroidism, particularly grade I, in rapid cycling patients than can be accounted for by lithium therapy alone.[42] It has been proposed by one study that a central thyroid deficit may predispose to a rapid cycling course.[42] Grade I hypothyroidism is defined as decreased serum T_4 or free T_4 index with some clinical signs of hypothyroidism. There is evidence that thyroid hormones function in the CNS by altering neurotransmitter activity. In a series of 11 patients with grade I hypothyroidism, administration of high doses of 1-thyroxine (0.15 to 0.4 mg/day), produced improvement in depressive symptoms in 10 patients and reduced manic symptoms in 5 of 7 in whom they were present at baseline observation.[43] This approach may therefore be clinically useful in rapid cycling patients, who must be carefully evaluated and monitored prior to and during treatment, which should begin with low 1-thyroxine doses, built up gradually as tolerated and as needed for symptomatic improvement. Although I have occasionally seen a favorable response to 1-thyroxine at doses of 0.2 to 0.3 mg per day, one patient reportedly had his rapid cycling arrested by daily thyroxine doses of only 25 μg (0.025 mg).[44]

A variety of other agents have occasionally been found effective in controlling rapid cycling, including calcium channel blockers,[9] propranolol, clonidine, and cholinergic agents such as physostigmine.[45] It has been reported that rapid cycling patients who require antidepressants may improve with the combination of lithium and tranylcypromine, resulting in decreased cycling.[46] I have frequently found this antidepressant less likely to perpetuate rapid cycling than SSRIs or tricyclics. Bupropion has been reported to have a mood stabilizing effect in some bipolar patients, particularly when used in conjunction with lithium. A series of 6 rapid cycling bipolar II patients were reported to experience stabilization and control of rapid cycling when treated with bupropion and lithium.[47] I have seen one patient whose rapid cycling was controlled on bupropion in combination with lithium, but who became manic after discontinuation of bupropion, which he decided to do because he thought he was going to become hypomanic. Valproate, which has demonstrated mood stabilizing activity in bipolar disorder as discussed in chapter 8, has also shown beneficial effects, when administered in lower than usual antimanic doses to patients with milder affective disorders. In a group of 33 patients treated with valproate at a dose of 125 to 500 mg daily (mean serum concentration of 32.5 mcg/ml) 79% sustained partial or complete mood stabilization, including 15 patients who were cyclothymic and 11 who were bipolar II.[48]

Unfortunately, bipolar patients are very prone to discontinuing their medications; since I treat many physicians, I have learned that knowledge does not confer immunity to this error of judgment. One of the lingering questions has been whether interruption of maintenance pharmacotherapy in bipolar disorder contributes to the worsening of this condition or transition to a rapid cycling disorder. A series of 4 bipolar patients whose mood had stabilized over a 6 to 15 year period of lithium maintenance experienced relapses following lithium discontinuation.[49] In these patients it was found that following reinstitution of lithium therapy, it was no longer effective as it had previously been.[49] I have seen several patients with histories of prolonged mood stabilization on lithium as the sole agent, who following a period of self-imposed lithium abstinence, required adjunctive medications along with lithium to maintain euthymia.

PSYCHOSIS

Until rather recently, blockade of dopamine D_2 receptors was seen as the sine qua non of antipsychotic efficacy. Two of the newer neuroleptic drugs are relatively weaker D_2 antagonists with prominent serotonin 5-HT_2 receptor antagonist activity as discussed in chapter 4. These agents, clozapine and risperidone, produce considerably less extrapyramidal side effects than conventional neuroleptics and may ultimately prove safer with respect to tardive dyskinesia. The most striking feature of these drugs is their ability to reduce negative schizophrenic symptoms, which do not respond well to other antipsychotic agents. Schizophrenic patients who are refractory to or intolerant of standard neuroleptics may improve significantly and experience fewer side effects with these newer agents. Clonidine, a noradrenergic antagonist which does not cause D_2 receptor blockade, was shown in preliminary studies some years ago to be effective in controlling psychotic symptoms in some schizophrenic patients and to reduce symptoms of tardive dyskinesia, its major side effects being sedation and hypotension.[50] Unfortunately there have been no large scale controlled studies to provide further documentation of this potentially interesting effect. Interest in calcium channel blockers has waxed and waned in the management of mania, though there is efficacy in some patients. The literature is even more spartan with respect to these drugs in schizophrenia. An open label study in 10 patients with chronic schizophrenia found that nifedipine 30 or 60 mg daily produced some modest improvement with reduction in BPRS scores as well as improvement in tardive dyskinesia, with associated diminution in AIMS scores.[51] Certainly larger numbers of patients would need to be studied at a broader dosage range to clarify whether or not this effect is real and of clinical value. Since many neuroleptics have calcium channel blocking activity, it is conceivable that drugs such as nifedipine may be useful in psychosis, without producing D_2 receptor blockade and associated movement disorders. I have occasionally found that carbamazepine, coadministered with neuroleptics, will improve behavioral control in agitated non-manic psychotic patients, in spite of the fact that carbamazepine may decrease neuroleptic plasma concentrations (whatever they mean clinically) as discussed in chapter 12. Valproate, often useful in mania, has also been used with some success in schizophrenia. Baclofen, a gabaminergic drug, may also enhance efficacy of neuroleptics in schizophrenia, although further studies are certainly necessary.

PERSONALITY DISORDERS

In the not too distant past, suggestions of pharmacotherapy for personality disorders would have been countered with laughter and jeering. Analysts take note! In this, the decade of the brain, personality does indeed have neurobiological underpinnings, thus neurotransmitter alterations are likely to be expressed in variations of personality. The conceptual model proposed by vanPraag wherein alterations in certain transmitters may be linked to altered drives and behaviors, is clearly applicable to the human personality as well as to psychiatric illness.[5] It requires little stretch of the imagination to see shyness as indicative of relatively low central noradrenergic or dopaminergic activity while gregariousness may represent heightened expressions of these transmitters, and perhaps a mild form of hypomania. Patients with dependent personality disorder may be more likely to have symptoms of panic and agoraphobia,[52] while those with avoidant personality disorder may have associated social phobia or panic disorder.[52] Just as SSRIs or MAOIs may be beneficial in patients with panic disorder, agoraphobia, and social phobia, these drugs may alter some of the associated personality characteristics.

Personality disorders have symptoms which may be analogous to those of psychiatric illnesses and potentially, therefore, responsive to drugs that modify a particular neurotransmitter system. For instance, although different in intensity of expression, symptoms of obsessive compulsive personality disorder resemble those of obsessive compulsive disorder and if they interfere with an individual's ability to function, or impair his interaction with others, may justify pharmacologic therapy employing anti-obsessional drugs.

Depersonalization is not uncommonly associated with panic disorder and obsessive compulsive disorder; depersonalization disorder also occurs independently of these axis I disorders, and in either case is likely to be responsive to serotonin selective reuptake inhibitors and clomipramine.[53] Sertraline has been shown to be an effective treatment for impulsive aggressive behavior in personality disordered patients.[54] Consistent with this pharmacologic effect is the finding of abnormal central serotonergic function in personality disordered patients and its association with an increased risk of impulsive aggression in their first-degree biological relatives.[55] m-CPP (m-chlorophenylpiperazine), a partial 5-HT agonist, provokes a "high" in male alcoholics similar to that experienced with alcohol.[56] Patients with borderline personality disorder, when given m-CPP, also may experience a "high" or "spacy" feeling associated with feelings of depersonalization or derealization as well as decreased anger and fear.[56] These findings suggest that treatment of a variety of personality disorders with SSRIs may reduce dysphoria, and perhaps improve social and interpersonal personality dimensions. Fluoxetine in daily doses of 20 to 80 mg has been shown to significantly reduce symptoms in 10 of 16 hypochondriacal patients.[57] Conceptual similarities between hypochondriasis and OCD as well as body dysmorphic disorder are underscored by finding a favorable treatment response to serotonergic anti-obsessional drugs in the former condition. Hypochondriasis and depersonalization/derealization have been well recognized as troublesome conditions, showing minimal change with psychotherapy. Self-defeating personality disorder, which may not be a distinct entity, based on a recently published study, nevertheless causes the individual much failure and disappointment and demonstrates very limited responsiveness to psychotherapy.[58] Based on considerable evidence of favorable responses to SSRIs in other personality disorders, a trial of SSRI therapy would seem to be a logical approach when one encounters a patient showing behaviors consistent with self-defeating personality, furthermore added likelihood of benefit may be expected in these patients who are often depressed and prone to making poor judgments and decisions.

Among personality disorders, the condition subjected to the most extensive trials of pharmacotherapy has been borderline personality disorder, perhaps because these patients are often so skilled at frustrating the psychotherapist. Various regimens have been found to be helpful in the past, most notably lithium in conjunction with low doses of high potency neuroleptics, and occasionally either or both of these agents given with tricyclic antidepressants. In a comparative study of haloperidol with phenelzine in borderline personality disorder, rather discouraging results were found for both.[59] In that study, the only benefit of haloperidol in doses up to 6 mg daily was in the treatment of irritability, while phenelzine produced only modest improvements in irritability and depressive symptoms.[59] In any case, the potential for impulsivity in these patients would generally make MAOI therapy appear too risky for long-term maintenance. Furthermore, this would be a good group of patients in whom to avoid excessive doses or durations of neuroleptics, because of the risk of tardive dyskinesia. Based on the symptom pattern of borderline personality disorder, my preferred approach is judicious use of SSRIs, preferably sertraline or venlafaxine, to minimize the risk of drug interactions, along with carbamazepine, or alternatively lithium.

OBESITY

Obesity is a major public health problem affecting about 30% of Americans in whom it is associated with increased risk of cardiovascular disease.[60] This problem often comes to the attention of the psychiatrist because of its impact on the patient's self image, and because many psychotropic drugs increase appetite, carbohydrate craving and body weight, particularly tricyclic antidepressants, neuroleptics, and lithium.[61] Since smoking cessation, which is being urged as a means to avoid tobacco related illnesses, is associated with increased appetite and weight gain, we are likely to see an increase in the obesity epidemic.

Clearly dietary restriction, particularly the avoidance of high fat content foods, is the most effective treatment for obesity. Increased exercise, with enhancement of muscle mass, facilitates weight loss since muscular tissue burns more calories than does fat tissue. Although it would be reassuring to announce a pharmacologic intervention that truly facilitates weight loss and helps to maintain the reduced weight, no such good news is likely to be forthcoming in the near future.

The most promising drugs which may suppress appetite and facilitate weight loss are fenfluramine, a serotonergic compound, and phentermine and phenylpropanolamine, both of which are sympathomimetics, the latter being available without prescription. Fenfluramine, which has a rather specific ability to decrease carbohydrate craving, has been demonstrated to be effective in counteracting weight gain associated with psychotropic drugs.[61,62] D-Fenfluramine has been shown to suppress weight gain, overeating, and dysphoric mood associated with smoking cessation.[63] In a 34 week randomized double-blind placebo-controlled study of 112 obese individuals, utilizing behavior modification, calorie restriction, and exercise, those subjects treated with either phentermine or fenfluramine lost more weight than those receiving placebo.[64] Both of these drugs are Class IV controlled substances with significantly less risk of dependency than the formerly employed amphetamines. In the United States, only DL-fenfluramine is currently available, while in Europe, D-fenfluramine, which has fewer side effects, is available by prescription. Phenylpropanolamine, which is a non-prescription drug in the U.S., is a sympathomimetic amine with minimal stimulant and euphorigenic effects, which may have a mild thermogenic effect in addition to an ability to diminish appetite.[65] Although chromium picolinate is not an anorexic, it has recently been extensively used to to facilitate weight loss along with calorie restricted diets and exercise; this compound is available over-the-counter and worth using as a potential adjunct to a weight loss diet program.

Among psychotropic drugs the SSRIs generally decrease carbohydrate craving and may facilitate weight loss when used in relatively high doses. In addition, for many people, obesity is associated with obsessional eating patterns, therefore, evidence of OCD or OCPD should be sought in evaluating any obese patient, since in many of those individuals, use of an SSRI in conjunction with calorie restriction may facilitate weight loss and maintenance of desired weight. Bupropion, a dopaminergic antidepressant, will often have an appetite suppressant effect and may thereby facilitate weight loss when used in conjunction with an appropriate reduced calorie diet.

CHRONIC FATIGUE SYNDROME

Chronic Fatigue Syndrome (CFS) is a real and symptomatic disorder which is poorly understood, not infrequently viewed negatively by physicians, and often comes to the attention of psychiatrists, because the patient is functionally impaired and is seeking relief.[66,67] CFS is often preceded by mild flu-like symptoms, and at the outset is associated with low grade fever, sore throat, tender lymphadenopathy, and extreme fatigue.[66] During the chronic course of this illness, myalgias, headaches, gastrointestinal symptoms, cognitive dysfunction, persistent tiredness and fatigue, and depression, anxiety, and irritability are common manifestations. The clinician evaluating CFS patients is tempted to conceptualize this disorder as a depressive illness, following a viral flu-like syndrome. Many CFS patients become preoccupied with their symptoms and illness and show features of obsessional thinking, with compulsive behaviors focused on managing their CFS and daily lives.

I have been impressed by a number of CFS patients whom I have seen as suffering from obsessive compulsive disorder with associated depression. Indeed these two diagnoses commonly coexist in non-CFS patients. There is as yet no safe and reliable treatment for the broad medical manifestations of CFS, although symptomatic management often involves non-steroidal inflammatory drugs, and amantadine has occasionally been found useful.[66] An appropriate approach to the psychiatric symptoms is the use of non-anticholinergic, stimulating antidepressant drugs. Medications with anticholinergic activity are likely to worsen the cognitive disturbance, sedating drugs may increase tiredness and fatigue, and hypotensive agents may add to dizziness which may already be present. Because of the obsessional characteristics often seen in these patients, use of SSRIs such as sertraline or venlafaxine may be beneficial in relatively low doses. If tolerated and not contraindicated by other factors, the energizing MAOI, tranylcypromine, may be extremely beneficial, and I have seen favorable responses to this drug in CFS. Because of the chronic nature of this condition, amphetamines and methylphenidate are generally not desirable because of potential dependency. Some favorable responses have been seen with pemoline, which has a low addictive risk.[66] It would be interesting to explore the efficacy of the dopaminergic antidepressant, bupropion, and possibly other dopaminergic drugs such as bromocriptine and pergolide in patients with CFS.

SEXUAL FUNCTION AND DYSFUNCTION

Psychiatrists are frequently consulted by patients requesting help with problems of low sexual desire, erectile, ejaculatory, and orgasmic dysfunction. Magical aphrodesiacs have been sought for centuries, and when found they often are neither magical or aphrodesiac. The brain is clearly the central command post, both through emotions and through neurochemistry, and indeed the gate keeper of the regions below. Emotions governing sexual attraction, arousal, and satiation are neurochemically driven, and are most likely under control of potent pheromones, sexual attractant hormones, which may or may not flow through the air. Neurochemical studies in animals and limited clinical studies correlate central noradrenergic and dopaminergic activity with sexual arousal and orgasmic function.[68] Central cholinergic activity as well as ACTH and oxytocin are also prosexual in their effects.[68] As most clinicians are aware, increased central serotonergic activity correlates with decreased sexual drive, reduced arousal, and impaired orgasmic function.[69]

Impaired libido and sexual function have long been known to occur with tricyclic and monoamine oxidase inhibitor antidepressants as well as a variety of anti-hypertensive drugs.[69] Although the advent of serotonin selective reuptake inhibitors has been a giant step forward in the management of depression, panic disorder, and obsessive compulsive disorder, they have produced a giant step backward for the genitals of many patients. Although I would consider sexual dysfunction with older antidepressants to be about sixth in importance in the list of side effects, my clinical experience indicates that for SSRIs they would be the most prevalent or second most prevalent patient complaint. A survey of 160 patients, whose depressions were successfully treated with fluoxetine, found 34% complaining of sexual side effects, including 10% with reduced libido, 13% complaining of decreased sexual response, and 11% reporting impairment in both areas.[70] My experience with low to moderate doses of SSRIs is similar to these findings, although I would estimate that among patients whom I have treated, the reduction in erectile and ejaculatory function is closer to 25% and the reduction in orgasmic function in women approximates 20%.

None of the SSRIs is free of sexual side effects, although venlafaxine appears somewhat less problematic in this area. In approximately three out of four patients with SSRI impairment of sexual function, dosage reduction will yield adequate function. In the absence of any contraindications, yohimbine in a dose of 5.4 mg (one tablet) three times a day will most often provide further improvement, if not always complete return to normalcy, particularly in men, often with somewhat less efficacy in women. Several small groups of patients with fluoxetine, or other SSRI induced sexual dysfunction, have been treated successfully with yohimbine, with improvement in libido as well as erectile and orgasmic function.[70] I have also successfully treated this problem by prescribing 25 to 50 mg of trazodone once or twice daily while continuing the SSRI. Many patients in my experience have had to discontinue SSRI therapy to reestablish adequate sexual function. I have occasionally seen SSRI related dysfunction not recur when the patient's regimen is subsequently (after an adequate wash-out period) changed to tranylcypromine. There have been a number of reports in the literature demonstrating the relative lack of sexual side effects with bupropion, which has been used either in conjunction with SSRIs or as a replacement for them.[71] Neuroleptic drugs, including the newer agents, clozapine and risperidone, can also impair libido, erection, and orgasm.[69] Neuroleptics also have potent neuroendocrine effects, they generally increase serum prolactin and may cause amenorrhea, breast engorgement, and lactation, which may be amenable to cautious administration of bromocriptine or pergolide, although these drugs may provoke psychotic symptoms.[69] Although lithium decreases hypersexuality associated with mania and hypomania, it is generally free of significant sexual side effects during maintenance therapy.

Fluoxetine and other SSRIs have been used successfuly to reduce sexual obsessions and compulsions and have also been useful in the treatment of paraphilias, including, pedophilia, exhibitionism, voyeurism, and frotteurism.[69,72]

Male patients with low sexual desire, impairment of erection or ejaculation, in the absence of medication treatment, should have serum testosterone levels measured. Although low testosterone is a relatively uncommon cause of sexual dysfunction, it is potentially treatable by administration of depo-injections of testosterone or application of testosterone patches (Testoderm) to the scrotum. More recently, it has been found that some men with erectile impairment and reduced serum testosterone levels may have decreased secretion of gonadotropin hormone-releasing hormone (GnRH) from the hypothalamus. In these patients, administration of the fertility drug clomiphene alters feedback control, and increases gonadotropin stimulation of testosterone production and release, resulting in increased circulating levels of testosterone and improved erectile function.[73]

Selegiline (deprenyl) used in the treatment of Parkinson's disease and occasionally for depression, has also shown sexual stimulating effects in some patients, and at times has been touted as "an anti-aging aphrodisiac". Selegiline has noradrenergic and dopaminergic activity and may in some people increase libido, and perhaps performance. Other dopaminergic agents used in Parkinsonism, including 1-DOPA, used alone or most commonly with carbidopa, as well as amantadines bromocriptine and pergolide, all may increase libido, sexual arousal, and function.[69]

AROMATHERAPY

Over the last decade, a number of investigators have reported impaired odor identification and sensitivity to test odorants in a variety of psychiatric disorders, including major depression, obsessive compulsive disorder, schizophrenia, Alzheimer's, and Parkinson's disease.[74] There have been conflicting findings in some studies, which may relate to whether odor identification or sensitivity are being measured and to the medication status of patients being studied. One interesting report found no alteration of odor threshold of major depression or obsessive compulsive disorder, compared to normal control, but did find increased odor sensitivity in patients with major depressive disorder, after successful pharmacotherapy.[74] Altered response to odorants and changes in olfactory sensitivity in various psychiatric illnesses suggest that there may eventually be a practical therapeutic application of odorants. Just as there are a wide variety of neurotransmitter receptors in the brain, there are a multitude of odor receptors, waiting to be tapped, explored and stimulated, perhaps with pleasant and even medically beneficial results.

Various plant derived odorants and essential oils have been used for centuries to create pleasant sensations or to effect therapeutic goals, although the term *aromatherapy* is scarcely more than a half century old, and is only becoming known in the United States in the last decade. Indeed aromatherapy, as a medical and scientific discipline, has been practiced in Europe and the United Kingdom since the 1930s and in many circles abroad is accepted as a useful means of altering mood and feelings.[75] In the United States, the most widely accepted use of aromas is in perfumes, which as can be seen from advertisements in any magazine, alter mood, create relaxation, stimulation, or sexual attraction. One psycho-commercial application of aromas which is becoming increasingly used is the instillation of various odorants into circulating air in factories, to calm and enhance work productivity of employees as well as to scent the air of stores and shopping centers, to create a relaxed and presumably acquisitional mind set.[76] Odorants have even been employed in some MRI facilities to calm patients.

The scientific underpinnings of responsiveness to odorants and essential oils have more recently been explored with newer technologies including studies of evoked potentials and brain electrical activity mapping (BEAM) which reveal neurophysiological changes associated with the pharmacologic actions of these potent substances.[76] Although it is impossible here to catalogue the pharmacologic properties of the multitude of plant-derived essential oils, the putative mood and behavioral indications are shown in parentheses, following the name of each oil: Clary Sage (anxiety, depression), Lavender (irritability, insomnia), Rose (anxiety, depression), Rosemary (mental fatigue, obsessions), Ylang Ylang (impotence, frigidity). Often a variety of oils is used in combination to achieve certain emotional or mood effects, as in studies employing aromatherapy in conjunction with relaxation techniques in the management of anxiety.[14]

Various approaches have been used for the administration of essential oils, which are only infrequently recommended for oral administration. One common means of administration is as additives to massage oils, and to water in tub baths or whirlpools. Essential oils are also administered by diffusion into room air by means of an electrical aspirator pump, or by having the patient inhale deeply over a bottle of a specific or mixture of oils. Although much clinical research is indicated in this area, patients who are "pharmacologically challenged", i.e. intolerant to medications, may achieve some anxiety reduction by administration of selected oils in conjunction with relaxation therapy techniques. I have seen some anxious and even a few depressed patients achieve a modicum of benefit from these novel approaches.

NON-FDA APPROVED DRUGS

The role of the physician is to diagnose and treat illnesses, but most importantly to relieve human suffering, using any reasonably safe and potentially effective remedy. The world extends beyond the United States, and competent scientists and clinicians are scattered throughout the world, therefore it is reasonable to assume that novel, effective and potentially safe remedies may exist beyond our shores.[77] Having followed pharmacologic developments during the last half of this century, I am well aware of the many pharmaceutical products developed, marketed, and prescribed elsewhere, which became available in the United States years after their general application elsewhere. For example, lithium was widely used in the United Kingdom since the late 1950s, and was approved by the U.S. FDA in 1970. Clomipramine was in use throughout the civilized world for more than a decade before United States physicians were permitted to prescribe it. Moclobemide, a RIMA, which is potentially safer than conventional MAOIs, has been available throughout the world for several years, and it is uncertain when and if it will be available here.[77] Zopiclone, an apparently safe and highly effective hypnotic, even for geriatric patients, is available throughout the world,[77] except in the United States, where we remain relatively unique in having permission to prescribe triazolam, a drug judged dangerous enough to have been removed from the prescription market in most other countries.

Unfortunately many drugs from other countries face such approval and marketing hurdles in the United States that their patent life and potential costs make it unfeasible for the manufacturers to seek FDA acceptance. Two French drugs are cases in point. One, minaprine, is a unique "activating" antidepressant with serotonergic and dopaminergic activities in addition to cholinergic agonist, rather than antagonist effects.[78] Minaprine often improves libido and sexual function, rather than impairing them as is the case with serotonergic antidepressants which lack dopaminergic and cholinergic activities. Clinical studies indicate that as an antidepressant, minaprine is superior to placebo and comparable to imipramine.[79] The other interesting French drug is adrafinil, which stimulates central alpha$_1$ noradrenergic post-synaptic receptors producing an activating, energizing effect clinically.[80] This drug is used to treat cognitive and memory impairment, and improve alertness in the elderly and in patients with presumed Alzheimer's.[80] Judging by available data, this drug may be no less effective than tacrine, approved in the United States for similar problems, yet the unapproved drug lacks hepatotoxicity.[80] When I discussed potential future availability of these drugs in the United States with the European manufacturers, I was told that, lacking significant patent duration, the hurdles of satisfying FDA requirements, precluded their seeking approval for marketing here.

When faced with a difficult to treat patient, in whom a non-FDA approved drug may be helpful, the imaginative and committed physician may have the option of referring that individual to a recognized specialist in a neighboring country or abroad who can evaluate the patient and if indicated, prescribe the U.S. unavailable medication. The patient may then be evaluated periodically by the consultant in conjunction with monitoring by the local physician. It is legal for an individual patient to receive by mail a non-FDA approved foreign drug which is not a DEA controlled substance, for his or her own use, under appropriate medical supervision.

WHAT WE NEED

Pharmaceutical development and eventual marketing approval is a slow process. Most often when one manufacturer develops a particular type of drug, others follow with chemically or pharmacologically related drugs. Witness the vast array of benzodiazepines, most of which represent commercial rather than therapeutic advances. Likewise, there is a growing family of SSRIs, some of which do in fact have clinical advantages over others. We have virtually no good centrally acting dopaminergic, noradrenergic or cholinergic drugs, which if available may prove to be clinically useful in some forms of anergic depression, impaired libido and sexual function, and cognitive decline of aging as well as in Alzheimer's disease. Such drugs could also be beneficial in improving drive and motivation, and perhaps controlling binging and overeating in obesity and eating disorders. We as yet have no effective and safe thermogenic drugs which could facilitate weight loss and maintenance of lower body weight in obesity. The substance abuse epidemic is crying for help in suppressing drug craving, and antagonizing intoxication induced by drugs of abuse. Beyond the need for drugs with different pharmacologic characteristics and therapeutic potentials, we need physicians to become better educated to the safe and effective use of currently available psychotropic drugs as well as future additions to our therapeutic armamentarium.

REFERENCES

1. Epstein I (ed): *The Hebrew-English Edition of the Babylonian TALMUD: Tractate Kerithoth*, London, Soncino Press, 1989, 6a.
2. Vogel VJ: *American Indian Medicine*. Norman, OK, Univ of Oklahoma Press, 1970.
3. Eisenberg DM, Kessler RC, Foster C, et al: Unconventional medicine in the United States: prevalence, costs, and patterns of use. *N Engl J Med* 1993;328:246-252.
4. Nelson JC: Combined treatment strategies in psychiatry. *J Clin Psychiatry* 1993;54(9, suppl):42-49.
5. van Praag HM, Asnis GM, Kahn RS, et al: Monoamines and abnormal behavior: A multi-aminergic perspective. *Brit J Psychiatry* 1990;157:723-734.
6. Marshall RD, Schneier FR, Fallon BA, et al: Medication therapy for social phobia. *J Clin Psychiatry* 1994;55:(6,suppl):33-37.
7. Louie AK, Lewis TB, Lannon RA: Use of low-dose fluoxetine in major depression and panic disorder. *J Clin Psychiatry* 1993;54:435-438.
8. Hoehn-Saric R, McLeod DR, Hipsley PA: Effect of fluvoxamine on panic disorder. *J Clin Psychopharmacol* 1993;13:321-326.
9. Hoschl C: Do calcium antagonists have a place in the treatment of mood disorders? *Drugs* 1991;42:721-729.
10. Nagy LM, Morgan CA, Southwick SM, et al: Open prospective trial of fluoxetine for posttraumatic stress disorder. *J Clin Psychopharmacol* 1993;13:107-113.
11. Fesler FA: Valproate in combat-related posttraumatic stress disorder. *J Clin Psychiatry* 1991;52:361-364.
12. Woodman CL, Noyes R: Panic disorder: treatment with valproate. *J Clin Psychiatry* 1994;55:134-136.
13. Roy-Byrne PP, Ward NG, Donnelly PJ: Valproate in anxiety and withdrawal syndromes. *J Clin Psychiatry* 1989;50(3, suppl):44-48.
14. King JR: Anxiety reduction using fragrances. In Van Toller S, Dodd GH (eds): *Perfumery: The Psychology and Biology of Fragrance*. London, Chapman and Hall, 1988, 147-165.

15. McDougle CJ, Goodman WK, Leckman JF, et al: Haloperidol addition in fluvoxamine-refractory obsessive-compulsive disorder. *Arch Gen Psychiatry* 1994;51:302-308.
16. Stein DJ, Hollander E: Low-dose augmentation of serotonin reuptake blockers in the treatment of trichotillomania. *J Clin Psychiatry* 1992;53:123-126.
17. Pigott TA, Pato MT, L'Heureux F, et al: A controlled comparison of adjuvant lithium carbonate or thyroid hormone in clomipramine-treated patients with obsessive-compulsive disorder. *J Clin Psychopharmacol* 1991;11:242-248.
18. Hollander E, DeCaria CM, Schneier FR, et al: Fenfluramine augmentation of serotonin reuptake blockade antiobsessional treatment. *J Clin Psychiatry* 1990;51:119-123.
19. Hewlett WA, Vinogradov S, Agras WS: Clonazepam treatment of obsessions and compulsions. *J Clin Psychiatry* 1990;51:158-161.
20. McDougle CJ, Goodman WK, Price LH: Dopamine antagonists in tic-related and psychotic spectrum obsessive compulsive disorder. *J Clin Psychiatry* 1994;55 (3,suppl):24-31.
21. Fallon BA, Liebowitz MR, Hollander E, et al: The pharmacotherapy of moral or religious scrupulosity. *J Clin Psychiatry* 1990;51:517-521.
22. Pollard CA, Ibe IO, Krojanker DN, et al: Clomipramine treatment of trichotillomania: A followup report on four cases. *J Clin Psychiatry* 1991;52:128-130.
23. Leonard HL, Lenane MC, Swedo SE, et al: A double-blind comparison of clomipramine and desipramine treatment of severe onychophagia (nail biting). *Arch Gen Psychiatry* 1991;48:821-827.
24. Hollander E (ed): *Obsessive-Compulsive Related Disorders.* Washington, DC, American Psychiatric Press, 1993.
25. McElroy SL, Keck PE, Pope HG, et al: Compulsive buying: A report of 20 cases. *J Clin Psychiatry* 1994;55:242-248.
26. Keck PE, Lipinski JF, White K: An inverse relationship between mania and obsessive-compulsive disorder: A case report. *J Clin Psychopharmacol* 1986;6:123-124.
27. Teicher MH, Glod C, Cole JO: Emergence of intense suicidal preoccupation during fluoxetine treatment. *Am J Psychiatry* 1990;147:207-210.
28. Beasley CM, Dornseif BE, Bosomworth JC, et al: Fluoxetine and suicide: A meta-analysis of controlled trials of treatment for depression. *Brit Med J* 1991;303:685-692.
29. Fava M, Anderson K, Rosenbaum JF: "Anger Attacks": Possible variants of panic and major depressive disorders. *Am J Psychiatry* 1990;147:867-870.
30. Joffe RT, Singer W, Levitt AJ, et al: A placebo-controlled comparison of lithium and triiodothyronine augmentation of tricyclic antidepressants in unipolar refractory depression. *Arch Gen Psychiatry* 1993;50:387-393.
31. Cain JW: Poor response to fluoxetine: underlying depression, serotonergic overstimulation, or a "therapeutic window"? *J Clin Psychiatry* 1992;53:272-277.
32. Chiarello RJ, Cole JO: The use of psychostimulants in general psychiatry: A reconsideration. *Arch Gen Psychiatry* 1987;44:286-295.
33. Breitbart W, Mermelstein H: Pemoline: An alternative psychostimulant for the management of depressive disorders in cancer patients. *Psychosomatics* 1992;33:352-356.
34. Fawcett J, Kravitz HM, Zajecka JM, et al: CNS stimulant potentiation of monoamine oxidase inhibitors in treatment-refractory depression. *J Clin Psychopharmacol* 1991;11:127-132.
35. Apter JT, Woolfolk RL: Lithium augmentation of bupropion in refractory depression. *Annals Clin Psychiatry* 1990;2:7-10.
36. Bouckoms A, Mangini L: Pergolide: An antidepressant adjuvant for mood disorders? *Psychopharmacol Bull* 1993;29:207-211.
37. Artigas F, Perez V, Alvarez E: Pindolol induces a rapid improvement of depressed patients treated with serotonin reuptake inhibitors. *Arch Gen Psychiatry* 1994;51:248-251.
38. Pollack MH, Hammerness P: Adjunctive yohimbine for treatment in refractory depression. *Biol Psychiatry* 1993;33:220-221.
39. Joffe RT, Schuller DR: An open study of buspirone augmentation of serotonin reuptake inhibitors in refractory depression. *J Clin Psychiatry* 1993;54:269-271.

40. Birkmayer W, Riederer P, Linauer W, et al: L-Deprenyl plus L-phenylalanine in the treatment of depression. *J Neural Transmission* 1984;59:81-87.

41. Arana GW, Forbes RA: Dexamethasone for the treatment of depression: A preliminary report. *J Clin Psychiatry* 1991;52:304-306.

42. Bauer MS, Whybrow PC, Winokur A: Rapid cycling bipolar affective disorder: I. Association with grade I hypothyroidism. *Arch Gen Psychiatry* 1990;47:427-432.

43. Bauer MS, Whybrow PC: Rapid cycling bipolar affective disorder: II. Treatment of refractory rapid cycling with high-dose levothyroxine: A preliminary study. *Arch Gen Psychiatry* 1990;47:435-440.

44. Bernstein L: Abrupt cessation of rapid-cycling bipolar disorder with the addition of low-dose L-tetraiodothyronine to lithium. (letter) *J Clin Psychopharmacol* 1992;12:443-444.

45. Sachs GS: Adjuncts and alternatives to lithium therapy for bipolar affective disorder. *J Clin Psychiatry* 1989;50(12,suppl):31-39.

46. Wehr TA, Sack DA, Rosenthal NE, et al: Rapid cycling affective disorder: contributing factors and treatment responses in 51 patients. *Am J Psychiatry* 1988;145:179-184.

47. Haykal RF, Akiskal HS: Bupropion as a promising approach to rapid cycling bipolar II patients. *J Clin Psychiatry* 1990;51:450-455.

48. Jacobsen FM: Low-dose valproate: A new treatment for cyclothymia, mild rapid cycling disorders, and premenstrual syndrome. *J Clin Psychiatry* 1993;54:229-234.

49. Post RM, Leverich GS, Altshuler L, et al: Lithium-discontinuation-induced refractoriness: preliminary observations. *Am J Psychiatry* 1992;149:1727-1729.

50. Freedman R, Kirch D, Bell J, et al: Clonidine treatment of schizophrenia: Double-blind comparison to placebo and neuroleptic drugs. *Acta Psychiatr Scand* 1982;65:35-45.

51. Stedman TJ, Whiteford HA, Eyles D, et al: Effects of nifedipine on psychosis and tardive dyskinesia in schizophrenic patients. *J Clin Psychopharmacol* 1991;11:43-47.

52. Gitlin MJ: Pharmacotherapy of personality disorders: Conceptual framework and clinical strategies. *J Clin Psychopharmacol* 1993;13:343-353.

53. Hollander E, Liebowitz MR, DeCaria C, et al: Treatment of depersonalization with serotonin reuptake blockers. *J Clin Psychopharmacol* 1990;10:200-203.

54. Kavoussi RJ, Liu J, Coccaro EF: An open trial of sertraline in personality disordered patients with impulsive aggression. *J Clin Psychiatry* 1994;55:137-141.

55. Coccaro EF, Silverman JM, Klar HM, et al: Familial correlates of reduced central serotonergic system function in patients with personality disorders. *Arch Gen Psychiatry* 1994;51:318-324.

56. Hollander E, Stein DJ, DeCaria CM, et al: Serotonergic sensitivity in borderline personality disorder: preliminary findings. *Am J Psychiatry* 1994;151:277-280.

57. Fallon BA, Liebowitz MR, Salman E, et al: Fluoxetine for hypochondriacal patients without major depression. *J Clin Psychopharmacol* 1993;13:438-441.

58. Skodol AE, Oldham JM, Gallaher PE, et al: Validity of self-defeating personality disorder. *Am J Psychiatry* 1994;151:560-567.

59. Cornelius JR, Soloff PH, Perel JM, et al: Continuation pharmacotherapy of borderline personality disorder with haloperidol and phenelzine. *Am J Psychiatry* 1993;150:1843-1848.

60. NIH Technology Assessment Conference Panel: Methods for voluntary weight loss and control. *Ann Intern Med* 1992;116:942-949.

61. Bernstein JG: Psychotropic drug induced weight gain: Mechanisms and management. *Clin Neuropharmacol* 1988;11 (suppl 1):S194-S206.

62. Goodall E, Oxtoby C, Richards R, et al: A clinical trial of the efficacy and acceptability of D-fenfluramine in the treatment of neuroleptic induced obesity. *Brit J Psychiatry* 1988;153:208-213.

63. Spring B, Wurtman J, Gleason R, et al: Weight gain and withdrawal symptoms after smoking cessation: A preventative intervention using d-fenfluramine. *Health Psychol* 1991;10:216-223.

64. Weintraub M, Sundaresan PR, Madan M, et al: Long-term weight control study I (weeks 0 to 34): The enhancement of behavior modification, caloric restriction, and exercise by fenfluramine plus phentermine versus placebo. *Clin Pharmacol Ther* 1992;51:586-594.

65. Morgan JP, Funderburk FR, Blackburn GL, et al: Subjective profile of phenylpropanolamine: Absence of stimulant or euphorigenic effects at recommended dose levels. *J Clin Psychopharmacol* 1989;9:33-38.

66. Krupp LB, Mendelson WB, Friedman R: An overview of chronic fatigue syndrome. *J Clin Psychiatry* 1991;52:403-410.

67. Ware NC, Kleinman A: Depression in neurasthenia and chronic fatigue syndrome. *Psychiatric Annals* 1992;22:202-208.

68. Rosen RC, Ashton AK: Prosexual Drugs: Empirical status of the "new aphrodisiacs". *Arch Sex Behav* 1993;22:521-543.

69. Riley AJ, Peet M, Wilson C (eds): *Sexual Pharmacology* Oxford, Clarendon Press, 1993.

70. Jacobsen FM: Fluoxetine-induced sexual dysfunction and an open trial of yohimbine. *J Clin Psychiatry* 1992;53:119-122.

71. Segraves RT: Overview of sexual dysfunction complicating the treatment of depression. *J Clin Psychiatry*, Monograph Series, 1992;10 (2):4-10.

72. Perilstein RD, Lipper S, Friedman LJ: Three cases of paraphilias responsive to fluoxetine treatment. *J Clin Psychiatry* 1991;52:169-170.

73. Guay AT, Bansal S, Hodge MB: Possible hypothalamic impotence: Male counterpart to hypothalamic amenorrhea? *Urology* 1991;38:317-322.

74. Gross-Isseroff R, Luca-Haimovici K, Sassoc Y, et al: Olfactory sensitivity in major depressive disorder and obsessive compulsive disorder. *Biol Psychiatry* 1994;35:798-802.

75. Tisserand R: *Aromatherapy: To heal and tend the body.* Santa Fe, NM, Lotus Press, 1988.

76. Van Toller S, Dodd GH (eds): *Perfumery: the psychology and biology of fragrance.* London, Chapman and Hall, 1988.

77. Hollister LE: New psychotherapeutic drugs. *J Clin Psychopharmacol* 1994;14:50-63.

78. Kan JP, Mouget-Goniot C, Worms P, et al: Neurochemical profile of minaprine, a new antidepressant drug. In Woodruff GN (ed): *Dopaminergic Systems and Their Regulation,* London, Macmillan, 1986:11-20.

79. Amsterdam JD, Dunner DL, Fabre LF, et al: Double-blind, placebo-controlled, fixed dose trial of minaprine in patients with major depression. *Pharmacopsychiatry* 1989;22:137-143.

80. Laboratoire L. Lafon: *Olmifon (adrafinil): Dossier d'information medicale et pharmaceutique.* Maisons-Alfort, France, Laboratoire L.Lafon, 1994.

APPENDIX A _____

DIETARY AND MEDICATION RESTRICTIONS FOR
MONOAMINE OXIDASE INHIBITORS

Phenelzine (Nardil) and tranylcypromine (Parnate) are monoamine oxidase inhibitors (MAOIs) used for depression. Their side effects may include low blood pressure, dizziness, rapid heart beat, sweating and drowsiness. Certain foods and medications if taken with MAOI drugs can cause increased blood pressure with intense (often pounding) headache, sweating, flushing, rapid pulse, dizziness, faintness, chest pain, neck stiffness, and convulsions. If these symptoms occur, contact your physician and go immediately to a hospital emergency room. Medications in group 1: clomipramine and SSRIs, and group 2: meperidine, can cause a fatal reaction with MAOIs, including selective MAOIs such as selegiline (Eldepryl) and moclobemide (Manerix, Aurorex). Medications in group 1 must be stopped several weeks before starting MAOIs, and group 1 medications must not be started for at least 2 weeks after stopping MAOIs.

While taking MAOIs, the following drugs must be avoided:

1. Clomipramine (Anafranil) and SSRIs including: fluoxetine (Prozac), fluvoxamine (Luvox), paroxetine (Paxil), sertraline (Zoloft), and venlafaxine (Effexor).
2. Meperidine
3. Cocaine
4. Amphetamines, stimulants, appetite suppressants
5. Phenylephrine, phenylpropanolamine, pseudoephedrine (Sudafed), oxymetazoline, ephedrine, isoproterenol, and other decongestants contained in cold medicines, cough syrups, nose drops, and asthma remedies.
6. Local (dental) anesthetics containing epinephrine.

Contact the physician who prescribed your MAOI before taking *any other* medication, with the MAOI.

The following foods *must not be consumed* while receiving MAOI treatment:

1. Cheeses, except American processed, cream cheese, and cottage cheese
2. Broad (fava) bean pods (green beans may be eaten)
3. Chianti and vermouth wines, tap (Draft) beer
4. Sausages, pepperoni, salami, bologna, liver, Spam, and canned ham
5. Pickled herring, sardines, anchovies
6. Any nonfresh or fermented meat, fish, or protein food product
7. Yeast extracts (eg, Marmite, brewer's yeast tablets) or meat extracts
8. Sauerkraut, banana peel

The following food products can be consumed in *limited quantity and with caution* since they may provoke blood pressure elevation if used in excess:

1. Red or white wine—not more than 4 oz per day; ale or beer (NOT TAP)—not more than 8 oz per day.
2. Foods cooked in wine (avoid Chianti and vermouth)
3. Distilled spirits (exaggerated depressant effect, without blood pressure elevation)—not more than 1½ oz per day
4. Avocado (fresh)—not more than one per day
5. Raspberries—not more than 1½ oz per day
6. Soybean paste (tofu)—not more than 4 oz per day
7. Soy sauce—as flavoring for cooked foods
8. Yogurt—8 oz fresh, refrigerated, or frozen; sour cream—fresh, up to 4 oz
9. Cottage cheese and cream cheese, fresh—up to 4 oz each
10. Processed American cheese, fresh—up to 4 oz per day
11. Chocolate candy—up to 4 oz per day
12. Aspartame-containing foods and beverages—not more than three servings per day; monosodium glutamate (in prepared foods, snack foods, Chinese food)—minimize use

There is no evidence that the following foods need be avoided by MAOI-treated patients:

1. Baked goods made with yeast
2. Chocolate-flavored beverages, pastries, ice cream
3. Cola beverages, coffee, tea (caffeine may increase anxiety)
4. Fresh fruits and vegetables, including mushrooms
5. Raisins and canned figs
6. Salad dressing, steak sauces, condiments, meat tenderizers
7. Fresh meats, poultry, and fish products, including canned salmon and tuna.

©1995 by Mosby–Year Book Inc, St. Louis, MO
Bernstein JG: *Handbook of Drug Therapy in Psychiatry, Third Edition*

Generic name index of common drugs used in psychiatry

alprazolam (Xanax)
amitriptyline (Elavil, Endep)
amobarbital (Amytal)
amoxapine (Asendin)
atenolol (Tenormin)
baclofen (Lioresal)
benztropine (Cogentin)
bromocriptine (Parlodel)
bupropion (Wellbutrin)
buspirone (Buspar)
carbamazepine (Tegretol)
chloral hydrate (Noctec)
chlordiazepoxide (Librium)
chlormezanone (Trancopal)
chlorpromazine (Thorazine)
clomipramine (Anafranil)
clonazepam (Klonopin)
clonidine (Catapres)
clorazepate (Tranxene)
clozapine (Clozaril)
dantrolene (Dantrium)
desipramine (Norpramin)
diazepam (Valium)
diltiazem (Cardizem)
diphenhydramine (Benadryl)
divalproex sodium (Depakote)
doxepin (Adapin, Sinequan)
estazolam (ProSom)
fenfluramine (Pondimin)
fluoxetine (Prozac)
fluphenazine (Permitil, Prolixin)
flurazepam (Dalmane)
fluvoxamine (Luvox)
glutethimide (Doriden)
haloperidol (Haldol)
hydroxyzine (Atarax, Vistaril)

imipramine (Tofranil)
lithium carbonate (Eskalith,
    Eskalith CR, Lithane, Lithobid,
    Lithonate, Lithotabs)
lithium citrate syrup
lorazepam (Ativan)
loxapine (Loxitane)
maprotiline (Ludiomil)
meprobamate (Equanil, Miltown)
mesoridazine (Serentil)
metoprolol (Lopressor)
molindone (Moban)
nadolol (Corgard)
nefazodone (Serzone)
nifedipine (Procardia)
nortriptyline (Aventyl, Pamelor)
oxazepam (Serax)
paroxetine (Paxil)
pergolide (Permax)
perphenazine (Trilafon)
phenelzine (Nardil)
phenobarbital (Luminal)
pindolol (Visken)
piperacetazine (Quide)
prochlorperazine (Compazine)
promethazine (Phenergan)
propranolol (Inderal)
protriptyline (Vivactil)
quazepam (Doral)
reserpine (Serpasil)
risperidone (Risperdal)
secobarbital (Seconal)
selegiline (Eldepryl)
sertraline (Zoloft)
temazepam (Restoril)
thiothixene (Navane)

tranylcypromine (Parnate)
trazodone (Desyrel)
triazolam (Halcion)
trifluoperazine (Stelazine)
triflupromazine (Vesprin)
trihexyphenidyl (Artane)

trimipramine (Surmontil)
valproic acid (Depakene)
venlafaxine (Effexor)
verapamil (Calan, Isoptin)
zolpidem (Ambien)

Glossary of trade names of psychotropic drugs and related compounds

Adapin (doxepin)
Ambien (Zolpidem)
Amitid (amitriptyline)
Amytal (amobarbital)
Anafranil (clomipramine)
Artane (trihexyphenidyl)
Asendin (amoxapine)
Atarax (hydroxyzine)
Ativan (lorazepam)
Aventyl (nortriptyline)
Benadryl (diphenhydramine)
Buspar (buspirone)
Calan (verapamil)
Cardizem (diltiazem)
Catapres (clonidine)
Cibalith-S (lithium citrate syrup)
Clozaril (clozapine)
Cogentin (benztropine)
Compazine (prochlorperazine)
Corgard (nadolol)
Dalmane (flurazepam)
Dantrium (dantrolene)
Depakene (valproic acid)
Depakote (divalproex sodium)
Desyrel (trazodone)
Doral (quazepam)
Doriden (glutethimide)
Effexor (venlafaxine)
Elavil (amitriptyline)
Eldepryl (selegiline)
Endep (amitriptyline)
Equanil (meprobamate)

Eskalith (lithium carbonate)
Eskalith CR (controlled release)
Etrafon (amitriptyline combined
    with perphenazine)
Halcion (triazolam)
Haldol (haloperidol)
Inderal (propranolol)
Isoptin (verapamil)
Klonopin (clonazepam)
Libritabs (chlordiazepoxide)
Librium (chlordiazepoxide)
Limbritol (amitriptyline combined
    with chlordiazepoxide)
Lioresal (baclofen)
Lithane (lithium carbonate)
Lithobid (slow release lithium)
Lithotabs (lithium carbonate)
Lopressor (metoprolol)
Loxitane (loxapine)
Ludiomil (maprotiline)
Luminal (phenobarbital)
Luvox (fluvoxamine)
Miltown (meprobamate)
Moban (molindone)
Nardil (phenelzine)
Navane (thiothixene)
Noctec (chloral hydrate)
Norpramin (desipramine)
Pamelor (nortriptyline)
Parlodel (bromocriptine)
Parnate (tranylcypromine)
Paxil (paroxetine)

Permax (pergolide)
Permitil (fluphenazine)
Pertofrane (desipramine)
Phenergan (promethazine)
Pondimin (fenfluramine)
Procardia (nifedipine)
Prolixin (fluphenazine)
ProSom (estazolam)
Prozac (fluoxetine)
Quide (piperacetazine)
Restoril (temazepam)
Risperdal (risperidone)
Seconal (secobarbital)
Serax (oxazepam)
Serentil (mesoridazine)
Serpasil (reserpine)
Sinequan (doxepin)
Stelazine (trifluoperazine)
Surmontil (trimipramine)
Tegretol (carbamazepine)
Tenormin (atenolol)
Thorazine (chlorpromazine)
Tofranil (imipramine)
Trancopal (chlormezanone)
Tranxene (clorazepate)
Triavil (perphenazine combined
  with amitriptyline)
Trilafon (perphenazine)
Valium (diazepam)
Vesprin (triflupromazine)
Visken (pindolol)
Vistaril (hydroxyzine)
Vivactil (protriptyline)
Wellbutrin (bupropion)
Xanax (alprazolam)
Zoloft (sertraline)

Antianxiety Agents and Sedatives

Benzodiazepines
Ativan (lorazepam)
Dalmane (flurazepam)
Doral (quazepam)
Halcion (triazolam)
Libritabs (chlordiazepoxide)

Librium (chlordiazepoxide)
Limbitrol (chlordiazepoxide com-
  bined with amitriptyline)
ProSom (estazolam)
Restoril (temazepam)
Serax (oxazepam)
Tranxene (clorazepate)
Valium (diazepam)
Xanax (alprazolam)

Barbiturates
Amytal (amobarbital)
Luminal (phenobarbital)
Nembutal (pentobarbital)
Seconal (secobarbital)

Other

Ambien (Zolpidem)
Atarax (hydroxyzine)
Buspar (buspirone)
Doriden (glutethimide)
Equanil (meprobamate)
Miltown (meprobamate)
Noctec (chloral hydrate)
Phenergan (promethazine)
Trancopal (chlormezanone)
Vistaril (hydroxyzine)

Antipsychotic Agents

Clozaril (clozapine)
Compazine (prochlorperazine)
Etrafon (perphenazine combined
  with amitriptyline)
Haldol (haloperidol)
Loxitane (loxapine)
Moban (molindone)
Navane (thiothixene)
Permitil (fluphenazine)
Prolixin (fluphenazine)
Quide (piperacetazine)
Risperdal (risperidone)
Serentil (mesoridazine)
Serpasil (reserpine)

Stelazine (trifluoperazine)
Thorazine (chlorpromazine)
Triavil (perphenazine combined
   with amitriptyline)
Trilafon (perphenazine)
Vesprin (triflupromazine)

Antidepressants

Adapin (doxepin)
Anafranil (clomipramine)
Asendin (amoxapine)
Aventyl (nortriptyline)
Desyrel (trazodone)
Elavil (amitriptyline)
Eldepryl (selegiline)
Endep (amitriptyline)
Etrafon (amitriptyline combined
   with perphenazine)
Limbitrol (amitriptyline combined
   with chlordiazepoxide)
Ludiomil (maprotiline)
Luvox (fluvoxamine)
Nardil (phenelzine)
Norpramin (desipramine)
Pamelor (nortriptyline)
Parnate (tranylcypromine)
Paxil (paroxetine)
Pertofrane (desipramine)
Prozac (fluoxetine)
Sinequan (doxepin)
Surmontil (trimipramine)
Tofranil (imipramine)
Triavil (amitriptyline combined
   with perphenazine)
Vivactil (protriptyline)
Wellbutrin (bupropion)
Zoloft (sertraline)

Lithium Preparations

Cibalith-S (lithium citrate syrup)
Eskalith (lithium carbonate)

Eskalith CR-450 (slow-release
   lithium carbonate tablets)
Lithane (lithium carbonate)
Lithobid (slow-release lithium car-
   bonate tablets)
Lithotabs (lithium carbonate)

Nonpsychotropic Drugs Used in Psychiatry

Calan (verapamil)
Catapres (clonidine)
Depakene (valproic acid)
Depakote (divalproex sodium)
Eldepryl (selegiline)
Inderal (propranolol)
Klonopin (clonazepam)
Lioresal (baclofen)
Lopressor (metoprolol)
Parlodel (bromocriptine)
Permax (pergolide)
Pondimin (fenfluramine)
Tegretol (carbamazepine)
Tenormin (atenolol)
Yocon (Yohimbine)

No Longer Marketed in the U.S. — Trade Name (Generic, Class)

Centrax (prazepam, benzodiazepine)
Eutonyl (pargyline, MAOI)
Marplan (isocarboxyzid, MAOI)
Noludar (methyprylon, hypnotic)
Paxipam (halazepam,
   benzodiazepine)
Placidyl (ethchlorvynol, hypnotic)
Quaalude (methaqualone, hypnotic)
Taractan (chlorprothixene, neuro-
   leptic)
L-Tryptophan (serotonin precursor,
   amino acid)

Index

Trade names of psychotropic drugs and related compounds are presented in Appendix B,
p. 548.